System and Circuit Design for Biologically-Inspired Intelligent Learning

Turgay Temel
Bahcesehir University, Istanbul, Turkey

Medical Information Science REFERENCE

MEDICAL INFORMATION SCIENCE REFERENCE
Hershey · New York

Director of Editorial Content:	Kristin Klinger
Director of Book Publications:	Julia Mosemann
Acquisitions Editor:	Lindsay Johnston
Development Editor:	David DeRicco
Typesetter:	Michael Brehm
Production Editor:	Jamie Snavely
Cover Design:	Lisa Tosheff

Published in the United States of America by
Medical Information Science Reference (an imprint of IGI Global)
701 E. Chocolate Avenue
Hershey PA 17033
Tel: 717-533-8845
Fax: 717-533-8661
E-mail: cust@igi-global.com
Web site: http://www.igi-global.com

Library of Congress Cataloging-in-Publication Data

System and circuit design for biologically-inspired learning / Turgay Temel, editor.
p. cm.
Includes bibliographical references and index.
Summary: "The objective of the book is to introduce and bring together well-known circuit design aspects, as well as to cover up-to-date outcomes of theoretical studies in decision-making, biologically-inspired, and artificial intelligent learning techniques"--Provided by publisher.
ISBN 978-1-60960-018-1 (hardcover) -- ISBN 978-1-60960-020-4 (ebook) 1. Neural networks (Computer science) 2. Biologically-inspired computing. 3. Logic circuits. I. Temel, Turgay, 1970-
QA76.87.S97 2010
006.3'2--dc22
2010017198

British Cataloguing in Publication Data
A Cataloguing in Publication record for this book is available from the British Library.

List of Reviewers

Mustafa Aktan, *University of Texas at Dallas, USA*
Osman Aliefendioglu, *Halic University, Turkey*
Yuksel Bal, *Halic University, Turkey*
Jörg Bornschein, *Johann Wolfgang Goethe University, Germany*
Belen Calvo, *Universidad de Zaragoza, Spain*
Damien Coyle, *University of Ulster, UK*
Lokman Erzen, *Fatih University, Turkey*
Olcay Kursun, *Istanbul University, Turkey*
Ziqian Liu, *State University of New York Maritime College, USA*
Nicolas Medrano, *Universidad de Zaragoza, Spain*
Giovanna Morgavi, *IEIIT-National Research Council, Italy*
Girijesh Prasad, *University of Ulster, UK*
Halil Ridvan Oz, *Fatih University, Turkey*
Benjamin I. Rapoport, *Massachusetts Institute of Technology and Harvard Medical School, USA*
Paulo H. da F. Silva, *Federal Institute of Education, Science and Technology of Paraiba, Brazil*
Abdulkadir Subasi, *Sutcu Imam University, Turkey*
Turgay Temel, *Bahcesehir University, Istanbul, Turkey*
Frank Van De Velde, *Leiden Institute for Brain and Cognition, Netherlands*

Table of Contents

Detailed Table of Contents

This chapter reviews research into human and animal forms of learning. It concentrates on two forms of learning in particular. The first is conditioning. The study of conditioning constitutes the first example of experimental research on learning. At first, it seemed to corroborate the view that learning consists of establishing associations. This form of learning was proposed by the early empiricists. The notion of associative learning influenced the emergence of behaviorism, which used conditioning to account for all forms of human and animal behavior. More recent research, however, has shown that conditioning is a more complex form of learning, related to propositional learning. This makes conditioning important for the study of the mechanisms of other, more complex, forms of propositional learning, as found in language and reasoning. The second form of learning reviewed here is visual learning. The study of this form of learning is important for understanding visual processing. And it is important for investigating the neural mechanisms of learning, given the availability of animal models of visual processing.

A general overview of biologically-inspired learning in the paradigm of artificial neural systems is described. In order to have the reader become familiar with fundamentals underlying this paradigm, a substantial and concise hierarchical background from neurophysiology to neuro-computational models is provided with as much clarity as possible. As an application of a well-known artificial neural network algorithm called feed-forward multi-layer perceptron with back-propagation training algorithm is utilized in implementation of an artificial olfactory system also called electronic nose. For improved classification performance, an algorithm as a preprocessing called linear-discriminant analysis is adapted to chosen neural architecture. The main purpose of the preprocessing stage is to lend better scattered input patterns for classes in the feature space compared to that without preprocessing. The performance improvement is also investigated in terms convergence rate, i.e. the number of iteration, given a number of layers, and recalling or generalization capability of the classifier.

This chapter presents an approach of how optimality-oriented stabilization is achieved for recurrent neural networks, which includes both the input-to-state stabilization for deterministic recurrent neural networks and the noise-to-state stabilization for stochastic recurrent neural networks. Owing to the difficulty in solving the Hamilton-Jacobi equation for nonlinear systems, optimal regulation seems to be an unachievable goal in control design for recurrent neural networks. However, a methodology proposed in this chapter solves the problem and obtains optimal stabilization by using the knowledge of Lyapunov technique, inverse optimality, and differential game theory. Numerical examples demonstrate the effectiveness of the proposed design.

This chapter presents a theoretical design of how a global robust control is achieved in a class of noisy recurrent neural networks which is a promising method for modeling the behavior of biological motor-sensor systems. The approach is developed by using differential minimax game, inverse optimality, Lyapunov technique, and the Hamilton-Jacobi-Isaacs equation. In order to implement the theory of differential games into neural networks, we consider the vector of external inputs as a player and the vector of internal noises (or disturbances or modeling errors) as an opposing player. The proposed design achieves global inverse optimality with respect to some meaningful cost functional, global disturbance attenuation, as well as global asymptotic stability provided no disturbance. Finally, numerical examples are used to demonstrate the effectiveness of the proposed design.

The human brain has an amazing ability to recognize hundreds of thousands of different tastes. The question is can we build artificial systems that can achieve this level of complexity? Such systems would be useful in biosecurity, the chemical and food industry, security, in home automation, etc. The purpose of this chapter is to explore how spiking neurons could be employed for building biologically plausible and efficient taste recognition systems. It presents an approach based on a novel spiking neural network model, the evolving spiking neural network with population coding (ESNN-PC), which is characterized by: (i) adaptive learning, (ii) knowledge discovery and (iii) accurate classification. ESNN-PC is used on a benchmark taste problem where the effectiveness of the information encoding, the quality of extracted rules and the model's adaptive properties are explored. Finally, applications of ESNN-PC in recognition of the increasing interest in robotics and pervasive computing are suggested.

This chapter describes a number of modifications to the learning algorithm and architecture of the self-organizing fuzzy neural network (SOFNN) to improve its computational efficiency and learning ability. To improve the SOFNN's computational efficiency, a new method of checking the network structure after it has been modified is proposed. Instead of testing the entire structure every time it has

Algorithmically and energetically efficient computational architectures that operate in real time are essential for clinically useful neural prosthetic devices. Such architectures decode raw neural data to obtain direct motor control signals for external devices. They can also perform data compression and vastly reduce the bandwidth and consequently power expended in wireless transmission of raw data from implantable brain–machine interfaces. We describe a biomimetic algorithm and micropower analog circuit architecture for decoding neural cell ensemble signals. The decoding algorithm implements a continuous-time artificial neural network, using a bank of adaptive linear filters with kernels that emulate synaptic dynamics. The filters transform neural signal inputs into control-parameter outputs, and can be tuned automatically in an on-line learning process. We demonstrate that the algorithm is suitable for decoding both local field potentials and mean spike rates. We also provide experimental validation of our system, decoding discrete reaching decisions from neuronal activity in the macaque parietal cortex, and decoding continuous head direction trajectories from cell ensemble activity in the rat thalamus. We further describe a method of mapping the algorithm to a highly parallel circuit architecture capable of continuous learning and real-time operation. Circuit simulations of a subthreshold analog CMOS instantiation of the architecture reveal that its performance is comparable to the predicted performance of our decoding algorithm for a system decoding three control parameters from 100 neural input channels at microwatt levels of power consumption. While the algorithm and decoding architecture are suitable for analog or digital implementation, we indicate how a micropower analog system trades some algorithmic programmability for reductions in power and area consumption that could facilitate implantation of a neural decoder within the brain. We also indicate how our system can compress neural data more than 100,000-fold, greatly reducing the power needed for wireless telemetry of neural data.

An FPGA-based coprocessor has been implemented which simulates the dynamics of a large recurrent neural network composed of binary neurons. The design has been used for unsupervised learning of receptive fields. Since the number of neurons to be simulated (>104) exceeds the available FPGA logic capacity for direct implementation, a set of streaming processors has been designed. Given the state- and activity vectors of the neurons at time t and a sparse connectivity matrix, these streaming processors calculate the state- and activity vectors for time t + 1. The operation implemented by the streaming processors can be understood as a generalized form of a sparse matrix vector product (SpMxV). The largest dataset, the sparse connectivity matrix, is stored and processed in a compressed format to better utilize the available memory bandwidth.

This work is concerned with the development of a novel diversity-controlled (DC) genetic algorithm (GA) for the design and rapid optimization of frequency-response masking (FRM) digital filters incorporating bilinear lossless discrete-integrator (LDI) IIR interpolation sub-filters. The selection of FRM approach is inspired by the fact it lends itself to the design of practical sharp-transition band digital filters in terms of gradual-transition band FIR interpolation sub-filters. The proposed DCGA optimization is carried out over the canonical-signed-digit (CSD) multiplier coefficient space, resulting in FRM digital filters which are capable of direct implementation in digital hardware. A novel CSD look-up table (LUT) scheme is developed so that in every stage of DCGA optimization, the IIR interpolation sub-filters constituent in the intermediate and final FRM digital filters are guaranteed to be automatically BIBO stable. The proposed DCGA optimization permits simultaneous optimization of the magnitude-frequency as well of the group-delay frequency response of the desired FRM digital filters. An example is given to illustrate the application of the resulting DCGA optimization to the design of a lowpass FRM digital filter incorporating a fifth-order bilinear-LDI interpolation subfilter.

This chapter describes some/new artificial neural network (ANN) neuromodeling techniques and natural optimization algorithms for electromagnetic modeling and optimization of nonlinear devices and circuits. The neuromodeling techniques presented are based on single hidden layer feedforward neural network configurations, which are trained by the resilient back-propagation algorithm to solve the modeling learning tasks associated with device or circuit under analysis. Modular configurations of these feedforward networks and optimal neural networks are also presented considering new activation functions for artificial neurons. In addition, some natural optimization algorithms are described, such as continuous genetic algorithm (GA), a proposed improved-GA and particle swarm optimization (PSO). These natural optimization algorithms are blended with multilayer perceptrons (MLP) artificial neural network models for fast and accurate resolution of optimization problems. Some examples of applications are presented and include nonlinear RF/microwave devices and circuits, such as transistors, filters and antennas.

Preface

Most living biological organisms have developed particular capabilities such that they find viable and successful solutions to challenges and their needs. The development of those capabilities has been known in the form of experiences repeated long enough to reproduce, i.e. *trial and error*. They simply replicate experimental outcomes in the form of codes into genes and pass the associated information to the next generation. The process of learning the most successfully fitting outcome and replicating it can be investigated within the scope of various scientific fields. Moreover, such a process occurs in the scopes ranging from nano, e.g. bacteria, viruses and other cell-based structures to macro, e.g. social structure, (Brabazon, & O'Neill, 2006).

The learning capability and relevant process that biological organisms with a certain degree of intelligence have has inspired humans to devise new methodologies, techniques and systems (Samsonovich, & Muller, 2008), which are attributed to by the phrase *biologically-inspired* systems. Some other terms which have been used commonly in place as substitutions are, *bionics* (Kodogiannis, Lygouras, Tarcynzki, & Chowdrey, 2008; Vincent, 2001) and *biomimetics*, (Cohen, 2006). Although it would be almost impossible to count otherwise examples which would be observed, a comprehensive list of biological mechanisms and inspired system design examples with relevant application and literature details are provided in (Cohen, 2006):

- A very common example of biological inspiration can be given from flying creatures which benefit from their excellent aerodynamics. The body shape of these creatures allows them to fly with superior maneuvering capability. The aircraft systems have been benefiting from these biological systems.
- A well-known and yet to develop further scientific example is of bats, which do not see well and are almost blind. As known, bats can fly in darkness without colliding into any obstacle with the help of their amazing hearing system. Their ear shape differs for differing species. The shape of the bat pinnae causes adaptable directivity patterns which interact with the ear itself. They can direct their ears all directions for localizing the sound sources and recognizing their prey in mixed environments. With their developed skills in navigating and hunting capabilities, they have been a major inspiration of biologically-inspired systems, particularlyrobots, which emulate landmark recognition with navigation and classification of echo sources
- Rats exploit their own whiskers to avoid collision and find food. Whiskers are highly sensitive to touching of environmental objects. Hence, emulating whiskers in rodents can be an inspiration to develop as sensory mechanisms to be used with collision-avoidance robotic systems.
- Elephants can feel and recognize the acoustic wave emitted by another elephant when it rocks its

feet on the ground at long distances, even several kilometers. The hyper-low frequency sound emitted by a whale and transmitted over long distances in the ocean can be recognized by other whales. The mechanism which governs the low-frequency sound wave transmission along the earth and its surface, which has been inspired by these animals, has been used in accelerometers for detection of earthquakes. They have also been used by the sonar systems in submarines.

- Spiders produce silky fiber web which is even tougher than those materials used in bullet-proof vests and stronger than the steel. The fiber web is so sticky that it functions as trap for catching preys. Nano-technology is promising possibilities for making enduring, continuous fibers with use of an electrospinning technique. Velcro which was inspired by seeds that stick to an animal's fur has allowed development in various fields' textile and electric-wires strapping.
- Besides animals, plants also suggest a model for biological inspiration. For example the sunflower directs itself to follow the sun throughout the day for maximum sunlight exposure, which has been an inspiration in developing a cheap solar energy production mechanism with optimality.

Despite a great volume of research and studies in academia and other disciplines with highly successful adaptation into daily life and available technologies, the capability of the biological creatures still excedes the artificially human-made systems that they inspired in terms of adaptivity, sensitivity, and spectral characteristics, (Kodogiannis, Lygouras, Tarcynzki, & Chowdrey, 2008). However, scientific approaches which resort on biologically-developed mechanisms, have made it possible to comprehend the phenomena of interest in biological inspiration and associated principles to devise novel systems and improve their capability, particularly in electronics, or to be more precise, silicon microstructures.

The response of a biological organism to a particular stimulus is mainly determined by the cells which make up associated subsystem to process it. Therefore, it is of prime importance to understand the mechanism and structural functionality demonstrated by the cell structure of associated biological subsystem so it would be possible to realize associated self-assembly silicon circuits, (Saeedi, Kim, & Parviz, 2008). Recently, a considerable effort has exploited micro-/nano- electromechanical systems (MEMS/NEMS) toward realization of cell-based structures, (Tahir, & Aubert, 2010).

It should be stated that in the context of biological inspiration, main design objective generally aims at emulating capabilities of the biological origin in decision making developed on natural feedback for each individual experience. While available design approaches aim at attaining much more diversity in applicable biological fields, those disciplines which prevail intelligence and adaptivity are gaining favor. The biological systems, particularly human, with the capabilities of perception, learning and reasoning with development of reasoning and mind relay vast opportunities for achieving such overwhelming and natural albeit complex structures. How human brain as the main processing unit in the nervous system achieves grasping discernible features of external stimuli was postulated long ago, (Nielsen, 2006). It has been well-publicized that such a system is composed of highly complex information processing units operating in immense parallelism with capability of adapting itself with experience. With this capability of brain, human is able to discriminate a familiar person and associated features in crowd; recognize a blurred image as the original; read writings unseen before etc. Amazing capabilities of nervous system and the brain have been a major inspiration to develop intelligently operating architectures, such as circuits and systems, (Derakshani, & Schuckers, 2002).

Concerning cell-based design, it has been known that major issue for building silicon architectures is to a *neural* model which transforms the external stimuli into coded quantity, transmitted from *sensory* neurons to nervous system, mainly the brain, and then to the motor system which actuates the motor commands as a response. Codified patterns between these systems are in the form of *spiking* impulses, which can be considered as digital words, (Dayan, & Abbot, 2001). However, slow transmission of biological spikes which carry information to be processed by brain makes it possible to exploit the faster conventional electronics to emulate the connectivity of biological networks. It is known that almost 80% of brain energy is consumed for the transmission of impulses along nerve fibers. In low-power artificial implementation of biological counterparts, it is advantageous to adopt analogue design methodologies rather than digital approach, (Dugger, 2003). Analog design readily facilitates major arithmetic operations such as addition, subtraction, exponentiation and integration. Having realization with a pre-specified *threshold* has allowed to build *sparse-coded* decision making based on so-called *integrate-and-fire* (IF) neurons. Design approach with IF-neuron model established the discipline called *neuromorphic engineering,* (Mead, 1989; Eliasmith, & Anderson, 2003). In most neuromorphic circuit designs, active elements, i.e. the transistors, operate in sub threshold region where they simulate the cell membranes of real neurons while voltage- and time-dependent current flows of real ion channels are emulated with external circuitries.

Another major objective of the circuit design with biological inspiration is to introduce *implantable* replacements for those who have lost in sensing, such as silicon retina for the blind, (Boahen, 2005), and cochlea for the deaf, (Sit, & Sarpeshkar, 2008). From an implementation point of view, most artificial systems differ in terms of the design aspects of the sensing stage and relevant interface which transform the stimuli into electrical spike patterns. Mostly, the source identification and associated activity units are implemented as embedded software to fulfill an *artificial neural network* (ANN) algorithm, (Zhang, Sitte, & Rueckert, 2005). Despite considerable studies on other sensory systems, (Cho, et al, 2005; Rulcker, Stenberg, Winquist, & Lundstrom, 2000), outcomes are not mature enough to yield system design with microcircuit realization. Two well-known sensory systems, i.e. vision and hearing, are the two which have been progressed for biologically-inspired microcircuit implementation:

Some well-known major circuit realizations of retina for emulating biological vision system are proposed in (Zaghloul, & Boahen, 2006; Santos, Gotarredona, & Barranco, 2007). They resort on the visual sensory system model where a group of *photoreceptors* reflect electrical patterns which represent light intensity difference in the sector of the visual field. The patterns are then conveyed to over a million of ganglion cells as coded spikes depending on the *relative change* in light intensity. In a silicon version, the current between different locations of the silicon chip is controlled by the voltage produced by photoreceptors and the ion channels of optical ganglion cell neurons are excited or inhibited and controlled by active feedback components, e.g. transistors. A digitally programmed interface is usually employed for converting the analog signal so obtained into digital form and then processing it conveniently as well as providing necessary events addressing and controlling signals, (Stocker, 2006).

Since the prominent study in (Lyon, & Mead, 1988) which reveals analog realization of cochlea, there have been a large number of attempts to replicate auditory system depending on the developed models, (Kuszta, 1998; Hamilton, 2008). Generally, it is accepted that the overall cochlea response can be modeled as a filter bank operation which allocates the incoming sound filtered by the outer ear into a number of channels, e.g. gamma tone filter bank model, (Patterson, 1994). Each channel exhibits spectral response mainly determined by spatial features across the cochlea. The output of the first stage is delivered to spike generation. The source of the sound is identified with use of the coded spike ensembles.

Biologically-inspired design is mainly concerned with thorough understanding of the behavioral and functional association of the system of interest. In the belief that compact organization and arrangement of the circuit and system design will be a major factor in attaining the pursued benefits of biological systems, the book is intended to contain fundamental topics as well as up-to-date studies for even fresh readers to make a smooth transition to system design from principles. Bearing this in mind, the chapters and their scope are organized in a hierarchical manner from abstract fields such as psychology to more concrete topics including circuit design as follows:

Chapter 1 is concerned with evolution of skill and preference development processes in time. It focuses on the impact of literature and experience on learning with competence and relevance to development of models in learning. It has been extended to adaptive learning.

Chapter 2 discusses the correlative interactions between learning components. The author presents detailed neuro-informative background concerning how dynamics in learning is achieved with cognition. Symbolic and expressive embodiment with cognitive information processing toward learning is discussed. Formation of knowledge with underlying reasoning consisting in overall dynamics of neural architecture is shown to be the main factor for grounded generalization. Temporal and local connections form an integrated mechanism with grounding which leads symbols to be exploited as embedding representations globally processed dynamically. The chapter investigates productivity in learning resulting from interactions with environment and experience.

Chapter 3 attempts to reveal prominent associative models in learning namely conditional and visual learning as well as propositional model. These learning models are also investigated with relationship to understanding and reasoning with neural architectures for association, which is the major source for learning paradigms.

Chapter 4 introduces a thorough overview of artificial neural systems and learning. Relevant biophysiological aspects are explained in a hierarchy, i.e. functional transition from neural cells to brain. The main objective of the chapter is to get the reader familiar with the principles of artificial mechanism inspired biologically which pursues learning for decision making given an appropriately arranged input. Major learning algorithms which can be come up with biological organisms are specified in terms of generalization capability so that they can be embedded into a system design. The chapter also presents an application of a well-known learning algorithm to emulate biological olfaction.

Chapter 5 describes a new method toward optimality-oriented stability for deterministic and stochastic neural networks. The approach proposed in the chapter attains a solution of Hamilton-Jacobi equation for nonlinear systems, which is involved in recurrent neural networks by using Lyapunov technique, inverse optimality and differential game theory. The chapter also exemplifies the proposed method.

Chapter 6 focuses on noisy modeling recurrent neural networks for global robustness. The algorithm is developed with use of Hamilton-Jacobi-Isaac equation as well as Lyapunov technique, differential minimax theory and the inverse optimality similar to the previous chapter where each input vector is considered a player against the noise-built player vector. The algorithm is shown to achieve global robustness given some predefined cost functions.

Chapter 7 is mainly concerned with building an evolving adaptive neural network which grants biologically-plausible coded spike populations to represent taste recognition system. Taste is a relatively neglected sensation with respect to vision and hearing. For this reason, it is expected that the study has importance to those who desire to study in this research field.

Chapter 8 presents some scenarios to augment the learning performance and computational efficiency performance of well-known self-organizing fuzzy neural network (SOFNN). Modified network architecture is partly traced while progress of training through the use of a record which keeps the firing strength of the neurons involved in training stage. A new improved-performance SOFNN is also proposed with new feedback connections at a particular layer. Owing to feedback connections which can be added/ removed, it is shown that new recurrent network is able to learn temporal behavior of the input.

Chapter 9 deals with approximate reasoning and inference based on fuzzy logic and their circuit realization. The fuzzy logic has been a principle expert system tool and exploited in various disciplines such as control and machine learning. Based on the axiomatic norms and rules, fuzzy logic yields considerably simple expressions which can be straightforwardly realized in circuits. It should be noted that the norms being used in fuzzy logic provide a mechanism valid for most classification algorithms, fuzzy logic design is an elegant solution to most biologically-inspired system and circuit design. The chapter finalizes its argument by introducing a fuzzy classifier circuit based on concurrent use of complementary norm circuits recently brought into literature.

Chapter 10 proposes an ANN-based biomimetic algorithm for decoding neural cell ensemble signals. It also proposes a computationally efficient, low-power CMOS analog circuit which can be used in real-time neuromorphic signal processing. The decoding algorithm implements a continuous-time ANN utilizing adaptive linear filter bank represented by kernels to simulate synaptic dynamics such as local field potentials and spike rates where the filters transform neural signal inputs into control-parameter outputs. As the realization of the algorithm, the proposed circuit is able to learn with active elements operating in sub threshold region. The experimental results verify that the proposed architecture operates as predicted for the applications considered.

Chapter 11 presents a digital FPGA-based coprocessor implementation of a recurrent neural network to emulate unsupervised learning with a large number of neurons involved. The architecture is able to operate process-and-store based to simulate a connectivity sparse matrix to represent association given an input database, which employs and is conditioned on state- and activity vectors.

Chapter 12 is concerned with implementation and performance issues of programmable analogue ANNs for sensor conditioning in embedded systems. The chapter also investigates the effect of weight selection on performance for a given task such as training by using perturbation algorithm and associated tuning.

Chapter 13 illustrates a digital implementation of ANN architecture with dedicated units operating in fixed-point mathematics. For a fast operation, the overall architecture brings in simplicity and use of mere combinational circuitry. The proposed hardware indicates relevant software which provides the sequence of hardware computation, inputs, weights and biases.

Chapter 14 exploits diversity-controlled (DC) GA for rapid development and optimization of frequency-response masking (FRM) digital filters which incorporates BIBO-stable bilinear lossless discrete-integrator (LDI) IIR filter. Use of DCGA facilitates simultaneous optimization of the magnitude-frequency as well of the group-delay frequency response of the desired FRM digital filters.

Chapter 15 applies ANN paradigm to obtain the electromagnetic model of nonlinear devices and circuits while it optimizes them by using genetic algorithm (GA) with particle swarm optimization (PSO). The ANN being used is of single hidden layer multilayer perception (MLP) trained with back propagation algorithm. The chapter also covers applications of the proposed scheme.

We hope that the book will be a useful resource to those who wish to be familiar with intelligent systems and their implementation.

Turgay Temel
Bahcesehir University, Istanbul, Turkey

REFERENCES

Boahen, K. (2005). Neuromorphic Microchips- Compact Electronics Based on Neural Wiring Could Yield Implantable Silicon Retinas to restore Vision, as well as Robotic Eyes and other Smart Sensors. *Scientific America Perspectives, 292*(5), 56-63.

Brabazon, A., & O'Neill, M. (2006). *Biologically-inspired Algorithms for Financial Modeling*, Berlin, Germany: Springer.

Cho, S. M., et al. (2005). Monolithic Electronic Nose System Fabricated by Post CMOS Micromachining. *Proceedings of IEEE on Sensors,* 420-423.

Cohen, Y. B. (2006). Introduction to Biomimetics: The Wealth of Inventions in Nature as an Inspiration for Human Innovation. In Y. B. Cohen (Ed.). *Biomimetics: Biologically-inspired Technologies*, (pp. 1-40), Boca Raton, FL: Taylor & Francis.

Dayan, P., & Abbot, L.F. (2001). *Theoretical Neuroscience: Computational and Mathematical Modeling of Neural Systems.* Cambridge, MA: MIT Press.

Dugger, J. (2003). *Adaptive Analog VLSI Signal Processing and Neural Networks*. PhD Dissertation.

Eliasmith, C., & Anderson, C. H. (2003). *Neural Engineering: Computation, Representation, and Dynamics in Neurobiological Systems*. Cambridge, MA: MIT Press.

Derakshani, R., & Schuckers, S. A. C. (2002). Biologically Inspired Evolutionary Temporal Neural Circuits. In *Proceedings of IEEE International Joint Conference on Neural Networks, (IJCNN)*, 1357-1361.

Hamilton, T. J. (2008). *Analogue VLSI Implementations of Two Dimensional, Nonlinear, Active Cochlea Models*, PhD Thesis.

Kodogiannis, V. S., Lygouras, J. N., Tarcynzki, A., & Chowdrey, H. S. (2008). Artificial Odor Discrimination System Using Electronic Nose and Neural Networks for the Identification of Urinary Tract Infection. *IEEE Trans. Information Technology in Biomedicine, 12*(6), 707-713.

Kuszta, B. (1998). Silicon Cochlea. In *Proceedings of IEEE WESCON*, 282-285.

Lyon, R. F. & Mead, C. (1988). *An Analog Electronic Cochlea. IEEE Transactions on Acoustics, Speech, and Signal Processing*, *36*, 1119-1134.

Mead, C. (1989). *Analog VLSI and Neural Systems*. Reading, MA: Addison-Wesley.

Nielsen, R. H. (2006). Mechanization of Cognition. In Y. B. Cohen (Ed.). *Biomimetics: Biologically-inspired Technologies*, (pp. 58-125), Boca Raton, FL: Taylor & Francis.

Patterson, R. D. (1994). The Sound of a Sinusoid: Spectral Models. *Journal of American Society of Acoustics, 96*(3), 1409-1418.

Saeedi, E., Kim, S., & Parviz, B. A. (2008). Self-assembled Crystalline Semiconductor Optoelectronics on Glass and Plastic. *Journal of Micromechanics and Microengineering*, *18*, 1-7.

Samsonovich, A. V., & S. T. Muller. (2008). Toward a Growing Computational Replica of the Human Mind. *Proceedings of AAAI Symposium on Biologically-inspired Cognitive Architectures*, 1-4.

Santos, J. C., Gotarredona, T. S.-, & Barranco, B. L. (2007). A Spatial Contrast Retina with on-chip Clibration for Neuromorphic Spike-based AER Vision Systems. *IEEETransactions on Circuits Syst. I, Regular Papers*, 54(7), 1444–1458.

Sit, J. J. & Sarpeshkar, R. (2008). A Cochlear-Implant Processor for Encoding Music and Lowering Stimulation Power. *IEEE Pervasive Computing*, 7(1), 40-48.

Stocker, A. A. (2006). *Analog VLSI Circuits for the Perception of Visual Motion.* New York: John-Wiley & Sons.

Tahir, F. A., & Aubert, H. (2010). Equivalent Electrical Circuit for Designing MEMS-controlled Reflect Array Phase Shifters. In *Proceedings of Progress in Electromagnetics Research*, (PIER), 100, 1-12.

Vincent, J.F.V. (2001). Stealing Ideas From Nature. (2001). In S. Pellegrino (Ed.), *Deployable Structures*. (pp. 51-58), Berlin, Germany: Springer-Verlag.

Zhang, L., Sitte, J., & Rueckert, U. (2005). Local Cluster Neural Network Chip for Control. In *Proceedings of the International Conference on Adaptive and Natural Computing Algorithms,* 116-119.

Zaghloul, K. A., & Boahen, K. (2006). A Silicon Retina that Reproduces Signals in the Optic Nerve, *Journal of Neural Engineering*, *3*(4), 123-135.

Chapter 1
Biologically-Inspired Learning and Intelligent System Modeling

Giovanna Morgavi
IEIIT-National Research Council, Italy

ABSTRACT

Artifacts having to perform in the real world should be able to cope with uncertain situations and react quickly to changes in the environment. Living systems, starting from a pre-structured set of functions, develop competence to better adapt to the environment all life long, from childhood to maturity. This phenomenon is called growing up. A developmental intelligence for growing up robots must be able to generate autonomously representations for unknown knowledge and skills. Models of development can play an important role in specifying the minimal preferences, faculties, and processes needed for this skill to emerge. A perspective on the analysis of some adaptive learning processes originating from literature and experiments in natural world result in some suggestion intelligent system architecture modeling.

INTRODUCTION

Biological organisms have evolved to perform and survive in a world characterized by rapid changes, high uncertainty, indefinite richness, and limited availability of information. Industrial systems, in contrast, operate in highly controlled environments with no or very little uncertainty. Artifacts having to perform in the real world should be able to cope with uncertain situations and react quickly to changes in the environment.

DOI: 10.4018/978-1-60960-018-1.ch001

Over the last decade, a number of researchers have suggested a developmental perspective on artificial intelligence and robotics. The ultimate shared goal among them seems to be the idea of bootstrapping high-level cognition through a process in which the agent interacts with a real physical environment over extended periods of time (Kuniyoshi, Y. and Berthouze, L.. 1998; Metta, G. et al. 1999; Asada, M. et al., 2000). Although many challenges remain, concepts from biologically inspired (bio-inspired) artifacts can enable researchers to engineer machines for the real world that possess at least some of the desirable properties of biological organisms, such as adaptivity, robustness, versatility, and agility. Natural systems provide an exceptional source of inspiration. Given the vastness of the information available, the question arises as to what insights from biology could and should be exploited for designing robots. Simply copying a biological system is either not feasible (even a single neuron is too complicated to be synthesized artificially in every detail) or is of little interest (animals have to satisfy multiple constraints that do not apply to robots, such as keeping their metabolism running and getting rid of parasites), or the technological solution is superior to the one available in nature (for example, the biological equivalent of the wheel has yet to be discovered). Rather, to work out some principles of biological systems that can be in some way used as inspiration in robot designing is very important. Epigenetic systems, whether natural or artificial, share a prolonged developmental process through which varied and complex cognitive and perceptual structures emerge as a result of the interaction of an embodied system with a physical and social environment. The usage of robots to instantiate and investigate models, originating from developmental psychology, and the necessity to design robotic systems with a better autonomy, adaptability and sociability by means of the application of the insights gained from the ontogenetic development studies are suggested. Interdisciplinary theory and empirical evidence are used to inform epigenetic robotic models, and these models can be used as theoretical tools to make experimental predictions in developmental psychology and other disciplines studying cognitive development in living systems. From one hand, biologists and psychologists can provide the detailed empirical findings and theoretical generalisations that can guide the implementations of robotic systems capable of cognitive development. On the other hand, these implementations can help in clarifying, testing, and even developing psychological theories, which, due to the complexity of the interaction processes involved, often cannot be exhaustively tested (Bertouze, L. and Prince, C.G. 2003). Biologically motivated intelligent computing has in recent years been successfully applied to solving complex problems. Biological organisms have evolved to perform and survive in a world characterized by rapid changes, high uncertainty, indefinite richness, and limited availability of information. Industrial systems, in contrast, operate in highly controlled environments with no or very little uncertainty. Artifacts having to perform in the real world should be able to cope with uncertain situations and react quickly to changes in the environment. New approaches where intelligence is not given to the system from outside, but is acquired by the system through learning, have proven much more successful.

BACKGROUND

One of the fundamental methodological assumptions is, that cognition is embodied, which means that it arises from bodily interactions with the world and that it is continuously meshed with them (Lakoff, G. and Johnson M. 1980; Johnson, M. et al. 1998; Varela F.J. et al., 1991, Lungarella M. et al.2001). In other words, thinking emerges from real life experiences, from sensory-motor coordinated interactions, and from exploration of the surrounding environment. Robotic models are fundamentally preferable to standard computer models for capturing distributed cognition and/or social interaction. Computer models, indeed, make many more presumptions about how information about the world is reduced, encoded, and represented. The environmental context of learning (physical setting, spatial arrangement of people and objects, etc.) is centrally important. Modelling the 'real' environment would be prohibitively difficult, and any simulation of it requires so many assumptions that its results could be questionable. Robotic models, on the contrary, circumvent this problem by using a realistically complex physical environment. The complexity of living being is much higher then the complexity of actual artefacts but, even if one could “raise” a robot in environments that are deliberately reduced in various ways, to determine what ecological conditions are salient for the emergence of adaptive skills such as social interaction and knowledge representation and only few experiments can be done, the increase of this perspective is very important to understand the mechanisms involved in adaptation and in intelligent behaviour. The exploratory behavior seems to “shape” the information flow in various sensory channels. Human infants, for instance, exhibit a wide range of exploration strategies: mouthing, banging, fingering, scratching, squeezing, waving, and listening (Kellman, P.J. and Arterberry, M.E. 1998). Through its own action, living beings are able to generate stable sensory patterns in different sensory channels, which can be exploited to form cross-modal associations. In humans these associations seem to be a basic prerequisite for concept formation (Thelen S. and Smith, L. 1994), which is of fundamental importance for what might be called high-level cognition.

With time, a brain-like natural or an artificial embodied system, under the control of its intrinsic developmental program (coded in the genes or artificially designed) can develop mental capabilities through autonomous real-time interactions with different environments (including its own internal environment and components) by using its own sensors and effectors. Such computational studies are necessary to understand the mechanisms of thinking.

Our human genetic program has evolved to use our body well. Analogously, the developmental programs for robots should be body-specific, or specific to robot “species”, like traditional programs. An artifact permits to focus on the traits that allow adaptation to emerge. The precision of knowledge required, in order to identify these mechanisms on robots, will improve our chances of answering some of the major open questions in cognitive science: how does the human brain develop a sense of the world around it? Advances in creating robots capable of autonomous mental development are likely to improve the quality of human life.

The dynamic systems approach (Thelen S. and Smith, L.1994; Elman J. L. 1995) attributes the emergence of complex cognitive skills (e.g., finding objects, imitation, word learning) to basic processes of attention and pattern learning in subsymbolic distributed networks (Deák, G.O. et al. 2000; Diedrich F.J. et al, 2002). Robotic models of development can play an important role in specifying the minimal preferences, faculties, and processes needed for these skills to emerge. These models could provide access to internal states as a behaviour develops. Psychological experiments can provide rich and subtle accounts of infant behaviour as it changes with age, but it is more difficult to track and describe internal changes. Robotic models permit us to correlate the model’s changing behaviours in real time and space with all changes in internal representations and processes shown.

A developmental intelligence for developmental robots must be able to generate autonomously representations for unknown knowledge and skills. Through an analysis of some classical psychological and biological experiments, both cognitive and comparative, let try to achieve suggestions and indications for developmental robot architecture. This research has been grounded above all on those experiments, with animals or with very young children, which have the aim of identify and ratify animal’s and children’s perception of the environment, their orientation in it, their knowledge of events and of the environment’s characteristics.

Learning as Adaptation

Like humans and animals, the robots must learn in real time while performing “on the fly.” A cognitive developmental process is also an open-ended cumulative process: a robot cannot learn complex skills successfully without first learning necessary simpler skills. The Darwinian gradualist concept of evolution considers development as the cumulative result of a large number of very small changes that occur over a long period of time. This gradual continuous process is driven by the blind process of natural selection. Successful biological adaptation was fuelled by a process of random variation and mutation. Highly homogeneous species have limited chances of survival if the environment changes beyond certain bounds. Vested or acquired features keep the system from mutation. This equilibrium lasts until the system is no longer able to assimilate demands for change into its existing structure. A great deal of current research work in robotics and autonomous systems is still focused on getting an agent to learn to do some task such as recognizing an object or going to a specific place. The learning process may be supervised, unsupervised or a process of occasional reinforcement, but the whole aim in such work is to get the robot to achieve a task that was predefined by the researcher. The Artificial Neural Network (ANN) models are defined within this paradigm. ANNs are budded from the observation and the simulation of some characteristics of the neuron network running in Nature. These computational models allow the optimization of learning of specific functions in specific environments (Smith S.S., et al. (Eds.), 1995):

- Supervised ANN models take care of the influence and the conditioning of the environment on learning
- Unsupervised ANN take care of the internal classification criteria.

Some ANN are able to generate explicit rules, but none of them can mime the 'cognitive jump' of using something that has been learned as a starting point for reaching a new level of learning. Ability that is pretty common in human being.

The Piaget theory on development of cognitive functions, says that the behaviour that is accomplished both in an action or in a thought can be considered as an adaptation step of the organism in the environment.

Also little evolved animals, answer to the environmental stimulations and rather they integrate the information coming from different senses to build a representation of the world in which they live.

Learning can be defined "*both as an adaptive modification of the behaviour and as an improvement of the "machine" of sensory and neural apparatuses which function is the behaviour*" (Lorenz, K.1977).

The integration of information coming from different senses allows the organism to perform an adaptive behaviour in the environment where it lives. Adaptation becomes a learning process when the experience is memorized by the organism and it results reusable in other occasions; vice versa if a mechanism of temporary elaboration (i.e. mechanical mechanism) is used, the information is acquired, processed, but then it is "forgotten."

Adaptation can be considered as a form of intelligent behaviour, when adaptation foresees a learning process. Some simple organisms (i.e. prokaryotes), react exclusively to external stimuli genetically determined as dangerous for the maintenance of the organism: through "behaviours of escape", they react estranging themselves from dangerous stimulus. They are sensitive to the "favourable" environment situations they can draw nourishment and they behave remaining in these favourable environment situations.

K. Lorenz wrote: "Information about external reality that reaches our nervous system by way of our sense organs never or only exceptionally, reaches the level of our subjective experience in its original form as separate sense date absorbed by individual receptors ...(information travels from receptor to the mind through the process of evaluation or interpretation in some way)" (Lorenz, K. 1977).

R.L. Gregory wrote: "We will describe perception as a continually changing hypothesis of the world, which is tested by sensory data and stored by generalizations based on past experience... "(Gregory, L.R. 1974)

That means that our individual experience is very important for our next cognition. This mechanism of our pre-understanding of the world is also the ground for differentiation between relevant and irrelevant information processes. Learning can be seen as a way living beings use to attempt to identify key aspects of a fluctuating environment: to detect its regularities and ignore the distracting "noise" which is not important for them.

We can give some definitions of learning:

- the process through which experience modifies pre-existing behaviour and understanding
- relatively persistent change in behaviour as a result of experience
- an individual's adaptation to environmental events

One of the most remarkable aspects of the living system learning process is its capability to increase its own internal complexity. Cohen and Cashon (Cohen, L.B. and Cashon, C.H. 2003) postulate that infants organize stimuli into categories based on criteria such as frequency, invariance and co-occurrence. Moreover, infants then build higher-level representations by applying these criteria to lower-level representations.

Perception and Interaction with the Environment

Li P. (Li P. et al. 2003) tested how children learn some spatial concepts and their reference words such as "left, right, north and south". Some studies show that most children do not understand or use these spatial words, like left, right, north, and south, reliably until they are seven years old. In addition, words like left and right, which are relative to the body, may be learned in very different ways than words like north and south, which are relative to the environment. To explore these differences, the researchers attempted to teach four-year-old children some of these spatial words by using feedback and clear examples of the words' usage. Using different terms (left and right or north and south) the teaching has been varied with different groups of subjects. Within each of these groups, half of the children were taught the words as they pertained to their bodies (e.g., "Can you flap your north/right arm?") and the other half were taught using objects at their sides ("The surprise is in the box on the north/right side. Can you find it?") Children showed a strong tendency to interpret the words relative to the environment, yielding a correct first hunch for north and south, but an incorrect first hunch for left and right. Children trained in the Left-Right condition were often unable to overcome their incorrect first guess, and this group (on average) did not learn the words during the training session. By contrast, children in the North-South condition were very successful with the training, mastering these terms rapidly and robustly. Learning was especially dramatic for the children who were taught north and south using objects at their sides. To see how thoroughly children had understood the terms north and south, a follow-up study has been conducted. Children were quickly taught north and south using objects and then asked to generalise these terms to new puzzles. In the first puzzle, a stuffed animal was placed at the child's side with two objects on each side of the animal. In this situation, all of the toys would be on one side (e.g. the north) of the child, but it was possible to ask for the toy to the north or south of the stuffed animal. Children found this game trivially easy (over 80% correct answers). In the second puzzle, children were taken out of the training room into the hallway and they were asked to point to the north and south from various points in the hallway. Children were incredibly successful at this game as well (again over 80%

correct). These results make a very surprising point: children learning spatial reference terms find it much easier to learn words that are defined relative to the environment (north and south) than words that are defined relative to themselves (left and right)."

From psychology, to neurobiology and to computer vision, especially animate vision, there are evidences on the salience of sensory-motor coordination in self developing artefacts and living beings. But what are the reasons behind it? Why is it so ubiquitous?

- *Perceptual nature* purpose: sensory-motor coordination implies that both sensory and motor processes play an integral part in perception. From this it follows that in ontogenetic development the two abilities should co-evolve otherwise there could be no coordination. For robots this means that sensory and motor abilities should "match" in complexity, they should obey the principle of ecological balance. The same principle can again be observed in infants. It has been found that very often infants must have certain motor capabilities before the corresponding perceptual abilities can emerge
- *Physical control over objects*. Needless to say, having control over objects like food items or building materials has many advantages for survival and has therefore a strong functional character. This type of sensory-motor coordination has been found to be important in infants' discovery of an object's 3-D structure. Infants generate the visual information necessary to detect the 3-D structure of an object by rotating the object held in the hand. It has been found that inspections of objects held in the hand are also conducted at a close distance. This means that the objects are unlikely to be occluded by other objects; hence, there is less ambiguity regarding their full contours than if the same objects are viewed from a long distance.

Moreover, the relatively constant distance from which hand-held objects are viewed makes real size relationships readily apparent. In sum, the visual information related to an object's 3-D structure is especially clear and accessible when the object is viewed while held and manoeuvred in the hand: the infant has physical control over the object.

- The third purpose is more of an information-theoretic nature: sensory-motor coordination *induces correlations*, reducing, thus, the high dimensional sensory-motor space to a low-dimensional sub-space. These correlations are largely due to the agent's self-motion. They are essential enablers of categorisation and learning and provide a natural focus-of-attention mechanism.
- Sensory-motor coordination allows the *integration of several sensory modalities*, visual or auditory. This can be achieved by forming associations according to space-temporal correlations that exist between various sensory modalities. Sensory-motor coordination has an exploratory function: new relationships can be discovered.

And finally the most obvious purpose of sensory-motor coordination is learning to master sensory-motor coordination itself. The hand-eye coordination, for example, is essential in reaching and grasping behaviour. This can be learned from the correlation of sensory signals produced by self-motion.

In robotics's field some o these principle have been applied. Metta's graduate work (Metta, J. et al 1999), i.e., revolved around "Babybot", a humanoid robot consisting of a 5-DOF stereoscopic head and a 6-DOF torque-controlled arm. The robot follows a developmental progression tied extensively to results in developmental psychology and cognitive science. Babybot learns to look at and reach out to real objects. However, Babybot is rewired to learn precisely this task and the component faculties, which lead up to it. Without enough sensory stimulation, Babybot may fail to learn this task, but no amount of training will ever make it learn to do anything else. The qualitative structure of what Babybot can and cannot do is predetermined by the connections of the very specific models, which are coded into it.

Lungarella and Metta in (Lungarella, M. and Metta,G. 2003) studied the role of changes in the acquisition of primary motor abilities: learning to *pendulate* (to swing like a pendulum) or bounce. In the first case the study was conducted with a small-sized humanoid robot that learned to *pendulate*. They performed a comparative analysis between the outright use of all degrees of freedom (left and right hip and knee), and the progressive involvement of all degrees of freedom by using a developmental mechanism of initial freezing and freeing. They observed that a freezing of the peripheral degree of freedom (knee) led to increase of the range of neural control parameters associated with a stable oscillatory behaviour.

Billard's DRAMA (Dynamical Recurrent Associative Memory Architecture) (Billard, A. et al. 1998) bills itself as a complete bottom-up learning system. It tries to develop a single control architecture that enables a robot to learn and act independently of a specific task, environment or robot used for the implementation. The core of the system is a recurrent ANN that learns relations between sensor states and motor activity. These relations can include time delays. DRAMA was implemented on mobile robots, both in simulation and the real world. Two types of experiments were performed. In the first, a hard-wired "teacher" robot would trundle about a world populated with coloured boxes (and, in simulation, sloped hills). As it encountered different landmarks, it would emit a pre-programmed radio signal describing the landmark. A "learner" robot would follow the teacher, and learn the radio names for landmarks (as it experienced them via its own sensors).

In the second set of experiments, the learner would follow the teacher through a constrained twisting corridor and learn the time-series of sensory and motor perceptions as it navigated the maze. Inspecting the connections learned by the DRAMA network and verifying that the expected associations were made and that the knowledge was "in there" evaluated the results of experiments. It is not clear, however, how that knowledge could later be put to use by the robot. (Once the trained learning robot is let loose itself in the environment, would it emit the right radio signals at the right landmarks?) The sensor and motor encoding are still overly simple, however although DRAMA can learn the time delays between sensor and motor bit-flips, it has no mechanism for abstraction. DRAMA cannot condense patterns of activation into new bits of state. The structure of the network is fixed from start to end.

Categorization

Animals can discriminate between food and non-food, can recognise their nest, and can differentiate between co-specifics and individuals of other species. This competence is called *classification* or *categorization*. Some aspects of this capacity can be innate or pre-defined such as the taste of particular foods or the recognition of co-specifics. Others, like the shape of the food items and their location, might vary greatly, depending on the kind of environment and sensors that are used.

What do we mean by categorisation? In most textbooks categorisation is defined in terms of mappings of sensory stimulation onto internal representations (e.g. category nodes). Many psychological models of categorisation, for example, consist of an input layer that codes the object features and an output layer that represents the categories. The goal is to learn an association or a mapping between activations in the input layer and the corresponding activations in the category layer.

In (Vallortigara, G. et al, 2000) are explained some experiments with few-days-old chicks that have to find some food hidden under the sand in the middle of a flat arena are described. The chicks had as only reference point the walls of the box containing the flat arena and the shape of the box varied from trial to trial. All the chicks, although no food was hidden in the middle of the arena, looked for food exactly in the centre of the arena, notwithstanding the shape of the walls. It looks as if chicks could "calculate" the position of the eventual food in a specific position respect the wall and is able to make inferences on exact equidistance of the centre from the all the walls, independently from the absolute value of that distance. Chicks seem to learn something very similar to the concept of centre. Some hints for the re-projection are suggested by this experiment. The first one concerns the organisation of the knowledge of the environment. If very "primitive" beings are able organise their space perception and in some way build a sort of "concept", a sort of "prediction" of a precise point in the space that we call *centre of the arena*, a similar behaviour could be expected by a robot. The question is if the concept of *centre* is present before the experience and if the capacity of calculating the distance from the wall is innate.

Brown et al. (Brown, M. et al. 1996) demonstrated that rats could locate hidden goals using the spatial pattern of the goal. In the set of experiments described in the article, the authors examined the possibility that two spatial patterns –a square and a line- can simultaneously control spatial choice. After a training period, the experiments reveal that rats were able, also without using the olfactory perceptions, to predict correctly the disposition of a baited goal, either on a line or on a square disposition, and behave consequently to reach the goal. This experiment was based on olfactory perception, ability that is not re-projectable nor designable in a robot, but also on memory and on map making concepts. From the experiment emerges that, for rats, geometrical cues could be an easy and predictable tool to enlarge the environment's knowledge.

Sovrano et al. (Sovrano, V.A. et al. 2002) made a similar experiment to demonstrate the ability of simple-minded fish to use purely geometric information to get the task of escaping. In a rectangular isolation cell inside a tank, a fish could escape and rejoin its companions by pushing an opaque door put in one of the corners of the rectangular cell. Even in condition of new information hints, the fish continued in pursuing its disambiguation of patterns recognised as valid to pursue the task of escaping already experienced.

Hauser (Hauser, M.D. 1994) in an experiment with monkeys who were cracking nuts with a stone proposed them some coloured stones and they did not care this feature as salient for their task. They seem to be more sensitive to the functionally relative features, ignoring differences that have no impact on the task.

Similarly a robot for collecting garbage has to be able to distinguish between garbage and non-garbage, the garbage truck from other trucks, other garbage robots from human agents; it has to be able to recognise the charging station, etc. While a garbage robot might have a predefined way of identifying the charging station or of recognising the garbage it should collect once it is nearby, the location of the charging station, or the visual appearance of the garbage might vary from city to city.

How are robots endowed with the capacity to categorise? One way is to predefine the categories by either incorporating special sensors (e.g. for colour or conductivity), another by predefining configurations in sensory space that correspond to various categories. While the former is easily achievable, although we do not gain a lot of insights on the nature of intelligence, the latter turns out to be very difficult. Especially if we take into account that the robots move around the environment and that one and the same object leads to a large variety of proximal stimulation of the sensors. Although in simulated environments predefining activation patterns might still be possible, it will no longer work in a general sense in more complex ones. In mobile robots, there is a large variation in proximal sensory stimulation originating from the same object. For that reason the categorisation behaviour is hard to achieve, and there have been limited successes in the past in solving this problem. There are some papers, in literature, suggesting that concepts are firmly grounded in sensory-motor coordination, rather than being information-processing constructs (e.g. (Kelso, J.A: 1982); (Lakoff, G. and Johnson, M.1980)).

But *what type of categories can be considered interesting by an artefact?*

If we look at the behaviour of the robot, it makes sense to attribute to the robot the following concepts: "graspable objects", "pushable objects", and "uninteresting objects". We can ask how these categories are represented internally.

Embodied models of categorisation are not passively exposed to sensory data, but through movements and interactions with the environment, are able to generate "good" sensory data.

Growing Up Learning

Piaget (Piaget, J. 1952) proposed a mechanism by which infants integrate experience into progressively higher-level representations, which he called "constructivism." According to constructivism, infants progress from simple to sophisticated models of the world by use of a "change mechanism" that allows the infant to build higher-level representations from lower-level ones. This is a powerful model of grounded knowledge acquisition (Drescher, G.L. 1991; Cohen, P.R. et al.1997), but constructivism, though, has long been criticized for its vagueness regarding the precise nature of the change mechanism. The lack of detail in this area has hampered the production of more powerful models of cognitive development, and has led someone to suggest that the primitives of the infant's world model (such as solidity and causality) are innate (Spelke, E.S. et al., 1992). However, recent studies of infant cognitive development (Cohen, P.R.; 1970 Cohen, P.R. and Amsel, G. 1998; Cohen P.R. et al., 1998) have provided strong evidence that these primitives are indeed acquired and, in doing so, they have shed light on the details of the change mechanism itself.

Given a task, there are different ways in which an organism might behave, i.e., the organism readily may produce the behaviour needed to attain its goal (the organism knows what to do), and the episode comes to an end. This can be done as an innate reaction or a learned one. If prior learning is not sufficient for success, past experience can get in the way; something new and different must be done to achieve the goal.

In nature, the stage theories of development reflect a discontinuous qualitative change from one stage to another (Ross, P. et al. 2003; Kellman, P. and Arterberry, M.E. 1998). Each person develops through a successive, mostly invariant sequence of stages. Each stage is characterised by being more complex than the preceding one and having in its structure subsumed all the cognitive, relational and organised structures of the previous stages (Thelen, E. and Linda S. 1994).

While at the levels of physiological nature the regulations are essentially conservative, the specificity of the behaviours is the extension to a continuous overcoming in the double direction: toward an extension of the environment and toward a growth of the powers of the organism. In the cognitive field there is therefore a direct activity on the environment, able to extend its limits on increasing degree, receiving the information, organizing and integrating their contents, and anticipating their transformations to the goals to reach the best adaptation.

In humans the stage sequence is, in some way, always affordable and flexible: a person in a later stage is able to afford to a schemata belonging to an earlier stage.

The transition between stages, denoting the growing up process, is possible through the assimilation and accommodation dynamic: the assimilation represents the system's bias to stability. The system maintains itself stable until environment, events and different circumstances will allow it. The sequence of stages derives from the integration of several subprocesses. Each subprocess is unsynchronized with development in other subprocesses (Guastello J. 1995.). This process called 'growing up' involves among others, the processing of perception, the knowledge organization, the emotions, the value system, the motivations and drives, the experiences and the social interactions (Weisberg, R. W. 1995). Through the developmental perspective, artefacts can grow up and can acquire new adaptive abilities. A developmental intelligence for growing up robots must be able to generate automatically representations for unknown knowledge and skills. The next logical step along the road towards truly autonomous robots that can dive in unpredictable environments is to investigate how one might design robots that are capable of evolve through experience.

We can find out different levels of learning and growing up, all of them are in some ways complexity increasing:

- Concept building is an enlargement of the knowledge internal map. The object of knowledge, once defined and processed as a set (i.e. a set of perceptions felt at angle "a" is stored and called "angle a"), can be compared with older knowledge belonging to different contests (i.e. are there other elements that are "similar"?). From the knowledge level, i.e. processing and analysis, this growing up can introduce new level of comprehension of the objects in relationship to other known objects and this can produce meaning. How do we build our ideas of what the environment look like? How do we build concepts?
- Abstraction. The new object (i.e. from angle "a" and angle "b" to "angle"), representation can be more abstract and it strikes roots in the experience connected to a preceding familiar object. Abstraction leads to a growing up in knowledge, in mapping of the environment, in progression to language acquisition and production.
- Insight. Insight is the highest level of growing up. In (Köhler W. 1969) a chimpanzee was confronted with a problem that required a creative solution by Köhler: a bunch of bananas was placed outside the cage beyond the reach of the chimp, and long sticks were inside the cage. The chimp used a stick as a sort of rake to pull the bananas closer to the cage so the chimp can eat them. The chimpanzee's solutions may reflect a mental trial and error process - the animal formed a mental representation of the problem, manipulated components of the representation, and then solved the problem. The solution appeared to be sudden because the researchers did not have access to the chimpanzee's mental process. The solution was available thereafter because a mental representation persists over time, and the solution is transferable because the representation is abstract enough to cover more than the original situation. Thorndike (Thorndike, E.L. 1911) referred growing up as "trial and error accidental success". Maltzman (Maltzman, I. 1955) said that growing up is nothing more than switching to a new combination of responses associated with a problem situation or a new combination of habit strengths within a habit family hierarchy.

A mechanism common to these growing up aspects is that the system shifts to a new level that can "slave" the level(s) below, or it can show a kind of co-evolution towards greater complexity. A living artefact grows up when its capabilities (abilities/knowledge) shift to a further level of complexity (i.e. the complexity rank of its internal capabilities performs a step forward).

In individual learning, 'growing up' would involve the processing of perception, the knowledge organization, the emotions, the value system, the motivations and drives, the experiences and the social interactions and can be called also 'creative thinking'.

In (Weisberg, R.W. 1995) Weisberg and Ward empathize the importance of prior knowledge in creative endeavours – Weisberg from the stand point of knowledge retrieval and Ward in terms of antecedent cognitive structures that underlie concept generation and exploration. Incubation, spreading activation, contextual fluctuation have been attributed to normal cognitive mechanisms. Everybody agree saying that growing up is a fundamental step for adaptation to new environment, for diving with new environment and new experiences, for leading to use what has been learned to reach new goals.

Growing up is not a simple and unified process, but rather a complex product of multiple cognitive structures that, although often undetected in the product of creative thinking, combine to set the stage for a new level of knowledge.

Finke et. al. (Finke R.A. et al. 1992) have indicated that the foundation of growing up in cognition is the reflexive activity that promotes the creative analysis and may be revealed through the use of analogues, metaphors, mental transformations or a variety of cognitive strategies. By continuing, modifying and regenerating these strategies the individual would identify the emergent structure of a conclusion or solution. Once that conclusion was determined, a different set of mental representations can be generated through different types of mental processes, to explore or critique the applicability of former conclusions.

Growing up is an emergent mechanism (Ross, P. et al. 2000.). This means that it cannot be reduced to its parts. In other words, it exists at one level of structure but cannot be fully explained in terms of structure at a lower level. Many artefacts consist of a mobile artefact in a static environment where the artifact must learn some functions (Nolfi, P. and Parisi, D. 1997). These "goal states" are defined spatially by unique coordinates so that it is easy to assess how well the individual is doing by comparing the known optimal solution to the actual solution. As tasks require increasingly complex behavior, this type of metric becomes difficult to define. A critical problem in trying to evolve complex behaviours is that the strategies that emerge are often temporary elaborations. These strategies yield reasonable performance in terms of maximizing a fitness measure, but do not exhibit the kind of intelligent responsiveness to the environment that is required to ultimately accomplish the objective. Seeming competence in the task is often only a sideeffect of the "mechanical" strategy; the artefact does not learn the general task, but instead learns a relatively primitive environmentspecific behavior. For example, an artefact being evolved to find an object or a place may exhibit a simple strategy of moving back and forth or in a circle through the environment, because this behaviour is easy to evolve and guarantees better fitness than moving very little. Once in this pathological region, it is unlikely that a good solution will be found since the nonmechanical, general behaviour required to accomplish the task can be very different from the mechanical behaviour.

Complex behaviours are difficult to evolve primarily because usually a reactive response to the current state is not enough; such behaviours require memory, that is, an ability to predict future states based on information about previous states. Looking for model evolving complex general behaviour incrementally, instead of evaluating the learning process of one complex task, the learning process on a relatively easy tasks (i.e. "feel some changes in perceptions that are interesting) should be evaluated before then increasingly harder tasks (name object, concept building, find object, etc), in an effort to build towards the goal behaviour.

The dynamic systems approach (Ward, T.B., et al. 2004.) attributes the emergence of complex cognitive skills (e.g., finding objects, imitation, symbol grounding) to basic processes of attention and pattern learning in sub-symbolic distributed networks. Robotic models of development can play an important role in specifying the minimal preferences, faculties, and processes needed for a skill to emerge. A better understanding of the growing up mechanism can be very useful for the knowledge of what really is intelligent behavior.

There are many skills that a robot might acquire that are uninteresting or unproductive for observers or even unrecognizable, such as the ability to percept, to classify objects, places and situations that are not intelligible for human beings. We feel that higher-level skills should be skills that are manifested on appreciably longer time-scales than lower-level ones. The ability to recognize a certain location, for example, involves internal and external activity over a longer time scale than the ability to avoid collisions.

From the knowledge level, i.e. processing and analysis of input data coming from sensors, growing up introduces a new level of comprehension of objects in relationship to other known objects. In the language research field, abstraction is an example of growing up (Weisberg, R.W. 1995). A better understanding of this mechanism could be very useful for the knowledge of what really happen in a growing up process.

But how does this process happen in nature, what kinds of procedures do people activate to turn up the abstraction? What mechanisms are trigged off? In (Morgavi G. and Marconi, L. 2008) an experiment on the modalities through which pre-school children (4-5 years old) turn up a growing up process is presented. Children have been asked for the research of meaning of metaphors hidden in common idiomatic sentences in their native language. This operation requires an abstraction process, even if the cognitive development of children of this age do not include the ability of abstraction, but they are able to explain the process they are thinking. When the children realized that in the proposed sentences there were some contradictions in comparison with the script of their concrete knowledge, at first, they tried to apply different strategies to reach an acceptable internal configuration. Children reach the abstraction through the combination/integration of such different subprocesses. The collective answers have been recorded, analyzed and classified, resulting in a set of mechanisms that can be used for suggestions for new architecture for growing up robots.

If they were not successful, the children propose alternate strategies by returning to the generation phase of identifying new structures until he/she hits upon an emergent structure that appears to satisfy the task at hand.

As in human being an efficient developmental architecture shows a hierarchy of basic parallel path to process different aspects of knowledge, to let the 'growing up' phase to emerge, an artificial architecture should be able to parallel process a combination of different paths in an internal representation. Children try to make logical connection among the scripts elicited by the sentence, stating cause-effect relationship between their memories and words in the sentence. Some time they failed in tautologies. The motivational system should maintains a connection between actual state and previous and next step

Children try to build a context, a localization to find out a logical sense to the new sentence. They try to integrate the unknown situations within their reality or they try to build a coherent fantastic reality. They build stories that give meaning to phrases. Drawings are also examples of this subprocess. They built many cause-effect relationship between stories and words. The artifact should have some kind of motivational system to maintains a connection between actual state and previous and next step. In literature only few work begin to evaluate the importance of generating motivational states to simulate future needs, and to made possible anticipatory planning (Gulz, A. 1991, Kursun, O. and Favorov, O. 2004, Favorov, O. and Ryder D. 2004).

Children scanned memory by using images, sound and emotions as index. Their memories were elicited from similar characteristics (i.e. colors, shapes, dimension, position) or from similar labels. Words with similar sounds were associated to the same meaning. Information in memory should be stored in such a way that the sensorial perspective should be respected. The structure memories work should follow a fuzzy logics. This probably will shorten the retrieve algorithms. Children keep explanations as close as possible to their sensorial perceptions. The sensorial modality most used was the visual sensors, followed by the auditory one. It seems that children have the habit to store in their mind most single information under images.

Sometime children choose a word similar to the ones in the sentence to build a interpretation script. The similarity can be based on parasynonimy, on assonance or on functional similarity.

These results give some suggestion for the storage organization for information in memories.

Ambiguity in the structure of the problem stimulus, tends to expand creative interpretations or possibilities, and further lends itself to creative exploration. Implicit meaningfulness is the implied meaning in a structure that the individual perceives.

Novelty, is certainly a key factor in exploration and discovery. Although common structures can be interpreted in novel ways, it is often helpful in creative cognition if the structure of the problem stimulus was novel rather than common.

Emergence is the extent to which unpredicted features or unexpected relations can occur. Two existing forms can be synthesized to create a new form. Emergence as the discovery in the novel structure of unexpected characteristic or Emergence as inclusion (none of these pieces seem to fit together...how are they similar?) or exclusion (only one part of the puzzle doesn't fit it. how is it different?). Incongruity is the contrast between dissimilar properties in the 'old' structure. This experiment on Growing up in cognition addresses the different types of cognitive functions that rely upon many highly differentiated mental processes that constitute the act of creative thinking.

Only a part of the input was processed. The attention was a function of many variables. Their previous experiences, their mood, their values, their emotions, their motivation system, their drive, their goal were fundamental triggers for the choice of the words to be processed. This filter shows a very complex behaviour and is connected to motivation, affective relationships, value systems, emotions, experiences, knowledge system etc.

But the most important result in this experiment was the importance of the emotional based drive. The emotional and social world seems to be driving each level and to be involved in each information processing step. As confirmed in (Balkenius, J. Moren, A 1988),whether called emotional control or merely an equivalent version of reinforcement learning with critic (evaluative control), these methods should be increasingly being utilized by control engineers, robotic designers and decision support systems developers and yielding excellent results.

The emotion world seems to be driving each level and it seems to be involved in each information processing box Some papers on controllers based on emotional learning have shown very good robustness and uncertainty handling properties (Ogden, C. K. e Richards, I. A. 1960).

Although, for a long time, emotion was considered as a negative factor hindering the rational decision making process, the important role of emotions in human cognitive activities is progressively being documented by other psychologists (Piaget J. 1952; Greene, J. et al. 2001).

Motivation, drive, value system and emotions are very difficult to separate: they are strongly related with very strong feedback each other. The motivation is related to some well known variables which include epistemic needs (needs of structure, for desired outcome), values, goals, and mood.

Motivational system maintains a connection between actual state and next step Another suggestion that come out from the experiment is that human being do not act according to the objective situation, but on the basis of their "own perception of the situation". Since this has a major impact on the resulting behavior, a minimal cognitive apparatus performing characterization and/or classification using the robot's values should be provided. There is no need to produce a complete world view by designing a complex ontology, only the most important decision criteria should be provided.

One of the basic questions we always have to ask ourselves is what to define or design into the agent, and what the agent ought to acquire by itself. One extreme position is that everything - sensors, morphology, control - has to be evolved. The other extreme is that everything can be designed into the system. Intelligent behaviour can be explained at various levels. We find the most powerful explanations. In the experiments described in this chapter, we focus on learning and development, starting with a given genetic set-up, letting the agent interact with the environment, trying to understand how its behaviour develops over time.

Once the morphology, the sensors, the motor system, the learning mechanisms have been defined, we have to consider the value system. There is an implicit and an explicit aspect to the value system. The explicit one actually consists of mechanisms, typically neuronal ones, which are connected to the sensory-motor apparatus. An example would be that if a particular behaviour can be executed, a reinforcement signal is automatically generated. For example, grasping is associated with intrinsic pleasure: the act of grasping is itself rewarding. It is therefore a good idea for the learning mechanism to reinforce the sensory-motor sequence before the successful event.

The implicit aspect of the value system is the observer attributes to the behaviour of an agent. In a sense, anything on the robot constitutes value. For example, we, as observers, say that it is good for an agent not to hit obstacles. Thus, avoiding obstacles is of value. It is also of value to be near objects, because being near bears the potential for physical control over the objects, say, for eating or building a nest. Moreover, it is of value to the agent if it can grasp objects.

It is a general-purpose reinforcement scheme, and any interactions with the environment leading to success (i.e. value signals being generated) can be learned in principle. The reinforcement learning algorithm itself is part of the implicit value system. The algorithm is based on the assumption that it is good for the agent to maximise value over time.

In this perspective, the reflexes have a number of functions. First, they provide a certain amount of coarse adaptivity to a particular environment. Second, they tend to lead to sensory-motor coordination that can be exploited by the agent. And third, they increase the probability of successful interactions with objects.

In order to guarantee survival, physical integrity, and task performance of any artefact, a value system has to be predefined by the designer. It includes basic reflexes, basic reinforces, and reinforcement learning schemes. The basic reinforces can be defined by analogy to biological systems. If the robot has been successful at grasping an object, this is considered intrinsically rewarding and a signal is generated by the value system. The same holds for pushing large objects and avoiding very large ones. The value signal thus generated influences the learning process. Picking up objects and pushing objects are what the artefact is supposed to do. They are therefore associated with intrinsic value. Avoiding very large objects also has value, because the agent is prevented from engaging in useless behaviours, i.e. behaviours that are not associated with value.

In the pure value-based case, the "representation" is given by the association strengths between the nodes in the input layer and the networks for the various processes. This connectivity matrix is the reason that for certain activation patterns of the sensory-motor space, certain process networks receive significant activation. In this sense, the categories of the agent are fully grounded. "Representation" is put in quotes because it is the observer that makes this correspondence between internal state and the outside world, not the agent itself.

Darwin V (Breazeal, C. L. 2000) was designed to provide a concrete example for how the computational weights of neural circuits are determined by the behavioural and environmental interactions of an autonomous device. Through real-world interactions with physical objects, Darwin V developed a capability for position-invariant object recognition, allowing a transition from simple behaviours to more complex ones.

CONCLUSION

If we observe an infant picking apples from a table, while leaving the newspapers, we say that his behaviour is based on a category that we might want to call "apple". Note that this is an attribution made to the infant by an observer. Moreover, it is an attribute of the infant as a whole, not of one part of the infant, as its brain. We do not have to postulate any kind of representation in order to describe its behaviour. Thus, if an agent consistently displays one kind of behaviour when it encounters one type of object but not when it encounters other objects, it is reasonable to talk about categories for the agent. If an infant initially picks different kinds of things off the table and over time only chooses apples, we say that it has learned the category that we call "apples". Again, learning is attributed by the observer to the agent as a whole. We observe a change in his behaviour over time: the agent begins to consistently show certain behaviours in reaction to objects that he did not exhibit before. We are not talking about internal representations whatsoever. How this change comes about, is an entirely different story. It is then of interest to correlate behaviour and internal mechanism in order to further our understanding of how this behaviour comes about. Hopefully this will also shed light on the question of what we might want to call a representation.

Piaget (Piaget, J. 1952) proposed a mechanism by which infants integrate experience into progressively higher-level representations, which he called "constructivism." According to constructivism, infants progress from simple to sophisticated models of the world by use of a "change mechanism" that allows the infant to build higher-level representations from lower-level ones.

Cohen (Cohen, P.R.1970) postulates that infants organise stimuli into categories based on criteria such as frequency, invariance and co-occurrence. Moreover, infants then build higher-level representations by applying these criteria to lower-level representations.

Given a task, there are different ways in which an organism might behave. I.e., the organism readily may produce the behaviour needed to attain its goal (based on its value system), and the episode comes to an end. This can be done as an innate reaction or a learned one. If prior learning is not sufficient for success, past experience can get in the way; something new and different must be done to achieve the goal. The growing up is a shift of capabilities (abilities/knowledge) to a further level of complexity.

Experiments on robots are motivated because:

- Structures and processes requested are very concrete and so it is clear how the theoretical assumptions have been transformed in procedures.
- We can use real-world situations, i.e. physical objects, human interactions, etc. to get realistic presuppositions and realistic sources of input. This is particularly important when studying social learning, which relies heavily on the intervention of the mediator, grounded in reality

- We can extract data about internal states of the learning process, which is not possible with human beings. Internal states of children going through a developmental or learning process cannot be observed at all.
- We can easily examine alternative hypotheses. For example, we can compare the level of abstraction that can be achieved through a specific mechanism with same data as a social learning process.
- But there are also important limits to this methodology:
- We do not expect at all that robotic experiments could model in any realistic way animal or children nor the environments in which they typically operate
- It is an extraordinary challenge to build and maintain physical robots of a required complexity.

Some experiments can be done to answer some specific questions like: Can an evolving artefact make growing up? Can it build super-ordered categories? Can a robot learn information about its own dimensions (i.e. if a gate is large enough to go across)? If not what kind of mechanism should be implemented or hard wired? If we implement a Cartesian/metric map is the Robot able to learn left/ right concepts? Or if it builds a topological map self referred is it able to learn concepts like North and South? And back to psychology, what are the steps and the child's mechanisms involved in the adapting end in learning? How are they connected to the value and the emotional system?

REFERENCES

Asada, M., Mac Dorman, K. F., Ishiguro, H., & Kuniyoshi, Y. (2000). Cognitive developmental robotics as a new paradigm for the design of humanoid robots. In *Proc. Of the 1st IEEE-RAS Int. Conf. on Humanoid Robotics*, Cambridge, MA: MIT Press.

Balkenius, J., & Moren, A. (1988). Computational Model Of Emotional Conditioning In The Brain. In *Proceeding of the workshop on Grounding Emotions in Adaptive* Systems, Zurich.

Baron-Cohen, S. (1995). The eye direction detector (EDD) and the shared attention mechanism (SAM): Two cases for evolutionary psychology. In Moore, C., & Dunham, P. (Eds.), *Joint attention: Its origins and role in development* (pp. 41–59). Hillsdale, NJ: Erlbaum.

Bateson (1980) *Mind and Nature - A Necessary Unity*. New York: Bantam Books.

Berthouze, H., Kozima, D., Bullock, G., & Stojanov, C. (Eds.). (2003) *Balkenius*. In *Proceedings of the Third International Workshop on Epigenetic Robotics: Modeling Cognitive Development in Robotic Systems*. Lund, Sweden: Lund University Cognitive Studies Volume 101.

Berthouze, L., & Prince, C. G. (2003) Introduction *The Third International Workshop on Epigenetic Robotics.*

Billard, A., Dautenhahn, K., & Hayes, G. (1998). *Experiments on human robot communication with robots: an imitative learning and communicating doll robot*. (Technical Report CPM-98-38), Centre for Policy Modelling

Bloom, P. (2000). *How children learn the meanings of words*. Cambridge, MA: MIT Press.

Breazeal, C. (2000, May). *Social Machines: Expressive Social Exchange Between Humans and Robots*. (PhD Thesis), Cambridge, MA: Massachusetts Institute of Technology.

Brown, M., Di Gello, E., Milewsky, M., Wilson, M., & Kozak, M. (2000). Spatial pattern learning in rats: conditional control by two patterns. *Animal Learning & Behavior*, *28*(3), 278–287.

Caton, R. (1875). The electric currents of the brain. *British Medical Journal*, *2*, 278.

Cohen, L. B., & Amsel, G. (1998). Precursors to infants' perception of causality. *Infant Behavior and Development, 21*(4), 713–732. doi:10.1016/S0163-6383(98)90040-6

Cohen, L. B., Amsel, G., Redford, M. A., & Casasola, M. (1998). The development of infant causal perception. Chapter. In Slator, A. (Ed.), *Perceptual Development: Visual, auditory and speechperception in infancy*. London: UCL Press and Taylor and Francis.

Cohen, L. B., & Cashon, C. H. (2003). Infant object segregation implies information integration In R. Lerner, A. Easterbrooks, and J. Mistry (Eds.), *Comprehensive handbook of psychology. Volume 6, Developmental Psychology*. II. Infancy. (pp 65-89) New York: Wiley and Sons.

Cohen, L. B., & Younger, B. A. (1984). Infant perception of angular relations. *Infant Behavior and Development, 7*, 37–47.doi:10.1016/S0163-6383(84)80021-1

Cohen, P. R., Atkin, M., Oates, T., & Beal, C. R. (1997). Neo: Learning conceptual knowledge by sensorimotor interaction with an environment. In *Proceedings of the First International Conference on Autonomous Agents*. 170-177.

Cohen (1970). *Il linguaggio del bambino*, La nuova Italia Editrice, Bologna.

Deák, G. O., Flom, R., & Pick, A. D. (2000). Perceptual and motivational factor affecting joint visual attention in 12- and 18-month-olds. *Developmental Psychology, 36*, 511–523.

Diedrich, F. J., Roberts, B., Diller, D. E., MacMillan, J., & Deutsch, S. (2002). Hybrid Team Training Testbed for AWACS Aircraft Controllers. In *Proceedings of the Human Factors and Ergonomics Society 46th Annual Meeting*, Baltimore, MD.

Drescher, G. L. (1991). *Made-Up Minds: A Constructivist Approach to Artificial Intelligence*. Cambridge, MA: MIT Press.

Elman, J. L. (1995). Language as a dynamical system. In *R. F. Port and T. Van Gelder. Mind as motion. Explorations in the dynamics of cognition* (pp. 195–226). Cambridge, MA: Bradford Book/MIT Press.

Favorov, O., & Ryder, D. (2004). SINBAD: a neocortical mechanism for discovering environmental variables and regularities hidden in sensory input. *Biological Cybernetics, 90*, 191–202. doi:10.1007/s00422-004-0464-8

Finke, R. A., & Ward, T. B. Smith S. M (1992). *Creative cognition: theory, research and application*. Cambridge MA: MIT Press.

Greene, J., Sommerville, R. B., Nystorm, L. E., Darley, J. M., & Cohen, J. D. (2001). An FMRI Investigation of Emotional Engagement in Moral Judgment. *Science, 293*, 2105–2108. doi:10.1126/science.1062872

Gregory, R. L. (1974). A look at biological and machine perception. In Meltzer, B., & Michie, D. (Eds.), *Machine intelligence 7*. Edinburgh, UK: Edinburgh University Press.

Guastello, J. (1995). *Chaos catastrophe and human affairs*. Upper Saddle River, NJ: Lawrence Erlbaum Ass.

Gulz, A. (1991). *The planning of action as a cognitive and biological phenomenon*. Lund University Cognitive Studies 2.

Hauser, M. D. (1994). How monkeys feel about how they see the world. *Language & Communication, 14*, 31–36. doi:10.1016/0271-5309(94)90018-3

Jean, P. (1952). *The Origins of Intelligence in Children*. New York: Norton.

Johnson, S., Slaughter, V., & Carey, S. (1998). Whose gaze will infants follow? The elicitation of gaze-following in 12-month-olds. *Developmental Science, 1*, 233–238. doi:10.1111/1467-7687.00036

Kellman, P. J., & Arterberry, M. E. (1998). *The Cradle of Knowledge*. Cambridge, MA: MIT Press. A Bradford Book.

Kohler, W. (1969). *The task of Gestalt psychology*. Princeton, NJ: Princeton University Press.

Kuniyoshi, Y., & Berthouze, L. (1998). Neural learning of embodied interaction dynamics. *Neural Networks*, *11*, 1259–1276. doi:10.1016/S0893-6080(98)00085-9

Kursun, O., & Favorov, O. (2004). SINBAD automation scientific discovery: From factor analysis to theory synthesis. *Natural Computing*, *3*(2), 207–233. doi:10.1023/B:NACO.0000027756.50327.26

Lakoff, G., & Johnson, M. (1980). *Metaphors We Live By*. Chicago, IL: The University of Chicago Press.

Li, P., Abarbanell, L., & Shusterman, A. (2003). *Spatial Reference, Laboratory of Development at the Cambridge*. MA: Harvard.

Lorenz, K. (1977). *Behind the mirror*. London: Methuen and co Ltd. Oxford University Press

Lungarella, M., & Metta, G. (2003). Beyond Gazing, Pointing, and Reaching: A Survey of Developmental Robotics. In *Proceedings of the 3rd International Workshop on Epigenetic Robotics*. (pp.81-89). Boston

Lungarella, M., Pfeifer, R., & Iida, F. (2007). Self-Organization, Embodiment, and Biologically Inspired Robotics. *Science*, *318*, 1088–1093. doi:10.1126/science.1145803

Maltzman, I. (1955). Thinking: From a behaviorist point of view. *Psychological Review*, *62*, 275–286. doi:10.1037/h0041818

Metta, G., Sandini, G., & Konczak, J. (1999). A developmental approach to visually-guided reaching in artificial systems. *Neural Networks*, *12*, 1413–1427. doi:10.1016/S0893-6080(99)00070-2

Mitri, S., Floreano, D., Magnenat, S., & Keller, L. (2007). Evolutionary Conditions for the Emergence of Communication in Robots. *Current Biology*, *17*(6), 514–519. doi:10.1016/j.cub.2007.01.058

Morgavi, G., & Marconi, L. (2008). Growing Up of Autonomous Agents: an Emergent Phenomenon. In *AIP Proceedings* 1051 (pp.187-194). Dubois Ed.

Morgavi G., Morando M., Biorci G., & Caviglia D. (2005, June). Growing up: emerging complexity in living being. *Cybernetics and Systems: an International Journal.* Boca Raton, FL: Taylor and Francis ed.

Nolfi, S., & Parisi, D. (1997). Neural networks in an artificial life perspective., In W.Gerstner, A.Germond, M.Hasler, and J.D.Nicoud (Eds.) *Artificial Neural Networks (ICANN97).* In *Proceedings of the 7th International Conference on Artificial Neural Networks*. Berlin, Germany: Springer Verlag, pp. 733-738

Ogden, C. K., & Richards, I. A. (1960). *The Meaning of Meaning. A Study of the Influence of Language upon Thought and of the Science of Symbolism.* London: Routledge.

Pierce, D., & Kuipers, B. (1997). Map learning with uninterpreted sensors and effectors. *Artificial Intelligence Journal*, *92*, 169–229. doi:10.1016/S0004-3702(96)00051-3

Ross, P., Hart, E., Lawson, A., Webb, A., Prem, E., Peolz, P., & Morgavi, G. (2003). *Requirements for getting a robot to grow up*. Lectures Notes in Artificial Intelligence.

Rothenberg, A. (1990). Creativity health and alcoholism. *Creativity Research Journal, 3*, 179–202. doi:10.1080/10400419009534352

Rumelhart, D. E., Hinton, G. E., & Williams, R. J. (1986). Learning Representations by Backpropagating Errors. *Nature, 32*, 533–536. doi:10.1038/323533a0

Scassellati, B. M. (2002). Theory of mind for a humanoid robot. *Autonomous Robots, 12*(1), 13–24. doi:10.1023/A:1013298507114

Scott, K. J. A. (1982). Concepts and issues in human motor behavior. In Scott Kelso, J. A. (Ed.), *Human Motor Behavior: An Introduction*. Hillsdale, NJ: Lawrence Erlbaum Associates.

Severinson-Eklund, K., Green, A., & Hüttenrauch, H. (2003). Social and collaborative aspects of interaction with a service robot. *Robotics and Autonomous Systems, 42*, 223–234. doi:10.1016/S0921-8890(02)00377-9

Sinclair-de-Zwart, H. (1973). Language acquisition and cognitive development. In Moore, T. (Ed.), *Cognitive development and the acquisition of language*. New York: Academic Press.

Smith, S. S., Ward, T. B., & Finke, R. A. (Eds.). (1995). *The creative cognition approach* (pp. 27–52). Cambridge, MA: MIT Press.

Sovrano, V. A., Bisazza, A., & Vallortigara, G. (2002). Modularity and spatial reorientation in a simple mind: encoding of geometric and nongeometric properties of a spatial environment by fish. *Cognition, 85*, B51–B59. doi:10.1016/S0010-0277(02)00110-5

Spaepen, L. (2003). *Goal oriented reaching*. Cambridge, MA: Harvard University Press.

Spelke, E. S., Breinlinger, K., Macomber, J., & Jacobson, K. (1992). Origins of knowledge. *Psychological Review, 99*(4), 605–632. doi:10.1037/0033-295X.99.4.605

Steels, L. (1999). Discovering the Competitors. *Journal of Adaptive Systems, 4*(2).

Thelen, E., & Smith, L. (1994). *A Dynamical Systems Approach to the Development of Cognition and Action*. Cambridge, MA: MIT Press.

Thorndike, E. L. (1911). *Animal intelligence. New York: Macmillan. Watson, J. B. (1958). Behaviorism*. Chicago: University of Chicago Press.

Vallortigara G, Regolin L., Tommasi L., Zucca P., (2000). *Altro che cervello di gallina*, Le Scienze n.387

Varela, F. J., Thompson, E., & Rosch, E. (1991). *The Embodied Mind: Cognitive Science and Human Experience*. Cambridge, MA: MIT Press.

Ward, T. B., Patterson, M. J., & Sifonis, C. M. (2004). The role of specificity and abstraction in creative idea generation. *Creativity Research Journal, 16*, 1–9. doi:10.1207/s15326934crj1601_1

Weisberg, R. W. (1995). Prolegomena to theories of insight in problem solving: Definition of terms and a taxonomy of problems. In Sternberg, R. J., & Davidson, J. E. (Eds.), *The nature of insight* (pp. 157–196). Cambridge, MA: MIT Press.

Wertheimer, M. (1959). *Productive thinking*. New York: Harper and Row.

Chapter 2
Representation of Neuro-Information and Knowledge

Frank van der Velde
Leiden University, The Netherlands

ABSTRACT

Human cognition integrates grounding, productivity and dynamics. This chapter discusses how combinatorial structures can be created by forming temporal interconnections between grounded representations of concepts (words). Specific architectures are required so as to allow these temporal connections to be formed. A crucial aspect of these architectures is that they do not copy and transport symbols. Instead, the representations they use remain "in situ", such that each representation of a concept used in a combinatorial structure is always the same grounded representation of that concept. These architectures therefore combine productivity of cognition with grounding of representations. Because they consist of neural structures, they are also inherently dynamic, which ensures the ability to interact dynamically with the environment. Grounded representations as constituents in combinatorial structures provide both local and global information. As constituents, they can affect specific (local) combinatorial structures, but without losing their embedding in the global information structure of which they are a part. The constraints that grounding, dynamics and productivity impose on each other have consequences for processing, learning and development. These consequences will be discussed and illustrated.

INTRODUCTION

There is clearly a close relation between our ability to learn and the way information (knowledge) is stored in the brain. On the one hand, our learning capacity determines what knowledge is stored and how it is stored. But, on the other hand, the way the brain represents knowledge also determines what we can learn and how we learn.

Representation of knowledge in the brain is affected by (at least) three important features that underlie human cognition. These features are the productivity of human cognition, our ability to interact dynamically with the environment, and

DOI: 10.4018/978-1-60960-018-1.ch002

the fact that our conceptual representations are grounded in perception, action, associations and semantic relations. Because these features influence the way information is represented, they would also influence the interaction between learning and representation.

One can assume that each of these features (productivity, dynamics and grounding, for short) evolved as a response to specific constraints imposed on cognition. Productivity of cognition refers to the ability to combine learned knowledge to form and process combinatorial structures, as found in language, reasoning, planning or navigating in (visual) environments. With productivity, we can process and produce much more information that we can learn in a lifetime. For example, we can understand (or produce) more sentences than we could ever learn. In this way, a community of people can share each others knowledge, and humans can pass their knowledge on to later generations (e.g., in a written or verbal form). So, with productivity we can accumulate knowledge over time (evidence of that can be found in any library). Our ability to interact dynamically with the environment ensures that we can process information about events in the real world as they unfold. This is an essential feature of cognition because the dynamics of events in the outside world are mostly beyond our control. Grounding entails that our conceptual knowledge is determined by the way we interact with our environment and other people. It also ensures, as I will argue, that our conceptual knowledge is activated in a direct way by the information we receive and process, and that conceptual knowledge can steer our actions in a direct way as well.

Although productivity, dynamics and grounding are each important features of cognition, it is in particular their combination that is important. Indeed, it may be their combination that sets human cognition apart from cognition as found in animals or artificial systems. Dynamical interaction is quite clearly an important feature of animal cognition, and grounding can be achieved with associative neural networks, as found in animal brains as well. Productivity, on the other hand, is clearly found in artificial forms of information processing, as in digital computers. However, productivity to the extent of human cognition is not found in animals, and dynamics and in particular grounding are missing in artificial forms of cognition.

The purpose of this chapter is to illustrate that when productivity, dynamics and grounding are combined, they impose constraints on each other that require specific systems (architectures) for their combined implementation. Because these architectures are different from the symbolic architectures of classical cognitivism, I will briefly discuss symbolic architectures first. This also serves to illustrate that the lack of grounding in artificial cognition is related to the symbolic way information is represented and processed in these systems,

BACKGROUND

The classical theory of cognition, or classical cognitivism for short, arose in the 1960s. It emphasized the importance of productivity for human cognition, and the demands it imposes on cognitive architectures (e.g., Anderson, 1983; Newell, 1990). Classical cognitive architectures achieve productivity because they use symbol manipulation to process or create compositional (or combinatorial) structures.

Symbol manipulation depends on the ability to make copies of symbols and to transport them to other locations. Newell (1990) argued that symbols are needed for cognition because only a limited amount of information can be stored physically at a given location. The symbol token is then needed to obtain more information when that is required for a given process. In Newell's words:

The symbol token is the device in the medium that determines where to go outside the local region

to obtain more structure. The process has two phases: first, the opening of access to the distal structure that is needed; and second, the retrieval (transport) of that structure from its distal location to the local site, so it can actually affect the processing. (...) Thus, when processing "The cat is on the mat" (which is itself a physical structure of some sort) the local computation at some point encounters "cat"; it must go from "cat" to a body of (encoded) knowledge associated with "cat" and bring back something that represents that a cat is being referred to, that the word "cat" is a noun (and perhaps other possibilities), and so on. (Newell, 1990, p. 74)

The symbol token is thus needed to obtain more information when that is required for a given process. Symbols can be used to access and retrieve information because they can be copied and transported. For the same reason, symbols can be used to create combinatorial structures. For example, we could use symbols to create the sentence *The cat is on the mat* in the following way (ignoring *the*). A specific symbol, say *101*, represents *cat* (we can use a string like *101* as a single symbol). Another symbol represents *mat* (e.g., *010*) and yet another (e.g., *110*) represents the phrase *is on*. It's arbitrary which symbol represents which word. The symbol *101* could just as well represent *mat* or *is on*, instead of *cat*. But once a choice is made, we need to use the same symbol throughout.

So, with symbols it is easy to make constituents like words. Because symbols can be copied and transported, they can be used to create complex combinatorial structures based on these constituents. What is required is a suitable computational architecture to implement these processes. That's why classical cognitivism saw the Turing machine or the Von Neumann computer as the basic model for this architecture. Of course, actual symbol architectures would be more complex and refined as these model architectures, but they shared the same feature that knowledge is represented using symbols that can be copied and transported (even over the internet in present times), and can be used to create or process complex symbol strings. For example, the symbolic combinatorial structure of *cat is on mat* could be represented with *101-110-010* (using - for a blank symbol).

When information is represented using symbols, representing complex combinatorial (e.g., sentence-like) forms of information is easy. This is why symbolic architectures excel in storing, processing and transporting huge amounts of information, ranging from tax returns to computer games. The capacity of symbolic architectures to store (represent) and process these forms of information far exceeds that of humans. But interpreting information in a way that could produce meaningful answers or purposive actions is far more difficult with these architectures. In part, this is due to the ungrounded nature of symbols.

When a symbol token is copied and transported from one location to another, all its relations and associations at the first location are lost. For example, the perceptual information related to the concept *cat* is lost when the symbol token for *cat* is copied and transported to a new location outside the location where perceptual information is processed. At the new location, the perceptual information related to cats is not directly available. Indeed, as noted by Newell in the quote above, a significant role of a symbol is to escape the limited information that can be stored at one site. So, when a symbol is used to transport information to other locations, at least some of the information at the original site is not transported.

The ungrounded nature of symbol tokens has consequences for processing. Because different kinds of information related to a concept are stored and processed at different locations, they can be related to each other only by an active decision to gain access to other locations, to retrieve the information needed. This raises the question of who (or what) in the architecture makes these decisions, and on the basis of what information. Furthermore, given that it takes time to search and retrieve information, there are limits on the amount of information that can be retrieved and the frequency with which information can be renewed.

So, when a symbol needs to be interpreted, not all of its semantic information is directly available, and the process to obtain that information is very time consuming. And this process needs to be initiated by some cognitive agent. Furthermore, implicit information related to concepts (e.g., patterns of motor behavior) cannot be transported to other sites in the architecture.

The ungrounded nature of symbol tokens has consequences for learning as well. Because different kinds of information concerning a concept are stored at different locations, the changes that occur at one location have no effect on the information stored at another location, unless again an active process is initiated to transfer the new information to the other locations. Furthermore, new information that is learned in an implicit manner cannot be transferred in this way.

The nature of information representation in symbolic architectures also differs from the way information is represented in the brain. As I will argue in the next section, information is stored in the brain in the form of network structures that are always grounded, and that cannot be copied and transported as symbols.

GROUNDED NATURE OF REPRESENTATION

In human cognition, conceptual representations are grounded in experiences (perception, action, emotion) and (conceptual) relations (e.g., Harnad, 1991; Barsalou, 1999). In the brain, the grounded representation of a concept consists of a network structure distributed over the cortex (and other brain areas).

Figure 1 (left) illustrates the grounded structure of the concept *cat*. It interconnects all aspects related to cats. For example, it includes all perceptual information about cats. It also includes action processes related to cats (e.g., the embodied experience of stroking a cat, or the ability to pronounce the word *cat*), emotional content associated with cats, and all other information related to or associated with cats, such as the (negative) association between cats and dogs and the semantic information that a cat is a pet or has paws.

As figure 1 aims to illustrate, the grounded structure of the concept *cat* consists of a network structure that develops over time in a continuous fashion (that is, it can and will be adjusted continuously). For example, the network labeled "perception" indicates that networks located in the visual cortex learn to identify cats or learn to categorize them as animals. In the process of learning to identify or categorize cats they will modify their connection structure, by growing new connections or synapses or by changing the synaptic efficacies. Other networks will be located in the auditory cortex, or in the motor cortex or in parts of the brain related to emotions. For these networks as well, learning about cats results in a modified network structure. Precisely because these networks remain located in their respective parts of the cortex, learning can be a gradual and continuous process. Moreover, even though these networks are located in different brain areas, connections can develop over time between them because their positions relative to each other remain stable as well.

The grounded network structure for *cat* illustrates why grounded concepts are different from symbols. When *cat* is represented by a symbol like *101*, it is clear how copies of the representation of *cat* can be used to represent different sentences like *cat is on the mat* or *cat chases dog*. But when the conceptual representation of *cat* is embodied in a network structure as illustrated in figure 1, it is difficult to see what should be copied to represent *cat* in sentences like these.

For example, the grey oval in figure 1, labeled *cat*, plays an important role in the grounded representation of the concept *cat*. It represents a central neural population that interconnects

Figure 1. Left: illustration of the grounded structure of the concept "cat". The circles and ovals represent populations of neurons. The central population labeled "cat" can be used to bind the grounded representation to combinatorial structures. Right: without the overall connection structure, the central population no longer forms a representation of the concept "cat"

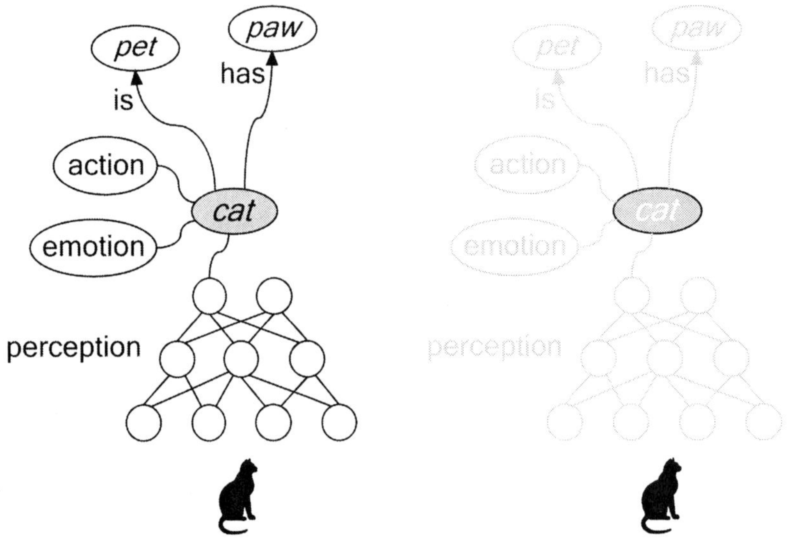

the neural structures that represent and process information related to cats. However, it would be wrong to see this central neural population itself as a neural representation of *cat* that could be copied and transported like the symbol *101*. As Figure 1 (right) illustrates, the representational value of the central neural population labeled *cat* derives entirely from the network structure of which it is a part. When the connections between this central neural population and the other networks and neural populations in the structure of *cat* are disrupted, or when the other networks and populations are removed, the central neural population no longer constitutes a representation of the concept *cat*. For example, because it is no longer activated by the perceptual networks that identify cats. So, when the internal network structure of the central neural population (or its pattern of activation) is copied and transported, the copy of the central neural population is separated from the network structure that represents *cat*. In this way, it has lost its grounding in perception, emotion, action, associations and relations.

Grounded Representations and Productivity

Because grounded representations cannot be copied and transported, the question arises as to how they can be used to represent combinatorial structures, which form the basis of the productivity of (human) cognition.

At face value, there seems to be a tension between the grounded nature of human cognition and its productivity. The grounded nature of cognition depends on structures as illustrated in figure 1. At a given moment, they consist of a fixed network structure distributed over one or more brain areas (depending on the nature of the concept). Over time, they can be modified by learning or development, but during any specific instance of information processing they remain stable and fixed. Indeed, it is precisely because they are stable and fixed that they can be modified and can develop over time. When the core of the structure is (relatively) fixed and stable, it forms an anchor to which new information (e.g., new relations) can be connected in a gradual way.

However, productivity requires that new combinatorial structures can be created and processed on the fly. For, example, humans can understand and (potentially) produce in the order of 10^{20} sentences or more (Miller, 1967). This numbers exceeds the lifetime of the universe in seconds, so it precludes that these sentences are somehow encoded in the brain by learning or genetic coding. Thus, most of the sentences humans can understand are novel combinatorial structures (based on familiar words), never heard or seen before. Symbolic architectures have no problem with creating new combinatorial structures, because they can make copies of symbols (e.g., representing words) on the fly and paste them in new combinatorial structures. Indeed, this ability was a main motivation for the claim that human cognition depends on symbolic architectures (e.g., Fodor & Pylyshyn, 1988).

Yet, the process of copying symbols results in ungrounded (word) representations. On the other hand, grounded structures seem to preclude the ability to create new combinatorial structures on the fly. Somehow, though, the combination of grounding and productivity is instantiated in the human brain, given that they are fundamental characteristics of human cognition.

Figure 2 illustrates that grounded representations of the words *cat*, *is*, *on*, and *mat* can be used to create a combinatorial (compositional) structure of the sentence *The cat is on the mat* (ignoring *the*). The structure is created by forming temporal interconnections between the grounded representations of *cat*, *is*, *on*, and *mat* in a "neural blackboard architecture" for sentence structure (van der Velde and de Kamps, 2006a). The neural blackboard consists of neural populations that represent syntactical type information such as sentence (S_1), noun phrase (here, N_1 and N_2), verb phrase (V_1) and prepositional phrase (P_1). In the process of creating a sentence structure, the populations representing specific syntactical type information (or syntax populations, for short) are temporarily connected (bound) to word structures of the same syntactical type. For example, *cat* and *mat* are bound to the noun phrase populations N_1 and N_2, respectively. In turn, the syntax populations are temporarily bound to each other, in accordance with the sentence structure. So, *cat* is bound to N_1, which is bound to S_1 as the subject of the sentence, and *is* is bound to V_1, which is bound to S_1 as the main verb of the sentence. Furthermore, *on* is bound to P_1, which is bound to V_1 and N_2, to represent the prepositional phrase *is on mat*.

All bindings in this architecture are of a temporal nature, represented by the double line connections in Figure 2. Binding is a dynamic process that activates specific connections in the architecture. The syntax populations play a crucial role in this process, because they allow these connections to be formed. For example, each word structure corresponding to a noun has connections to each noun phrase population in the architecture. However, these connections are not just associative connections. Instead, they consist of neural circuits that control the flow of activation through the connection. In figure 2, these circuits are represented by the small circles in between the syntax populations. For example, the circle labeled "n" represents the circuit that binds N_1 to S_1 as its subject.

To make a connection active, its control circuit has to be activated. This is an essential feature of the architecture, because it provides control of activation, which is not possible in a purely associative connection structure. In this way, relations instead of just associations can be represented. Figure 1 also illustrates an example of relations. They consist of the conditional connections between the word structure of *cat* and the word structures of *pet* and *paw*. For example, the connection between *cat* and *pet* is conditional because it consists of a circuit that can be activated by a query of the form *cat is*. The *is* part of this query activates the circuit connection between *cat* and *pet*, so that *pet* is activated as the answer to the query. Thus, in

Figure 2. Illustration of the combinatorial structure "The cat is on the mat" (ignoring "the"), with grounded representations for the words. The circles in the neural blackboard represent populations and circuits of neurons. The double line connections represent conditional connections. The bottom of the figure shows a symbolic representation of the sentence "The cat is on the mat" (N, n = noun; P, p = preposition; S = sentence; V, v = verb.)

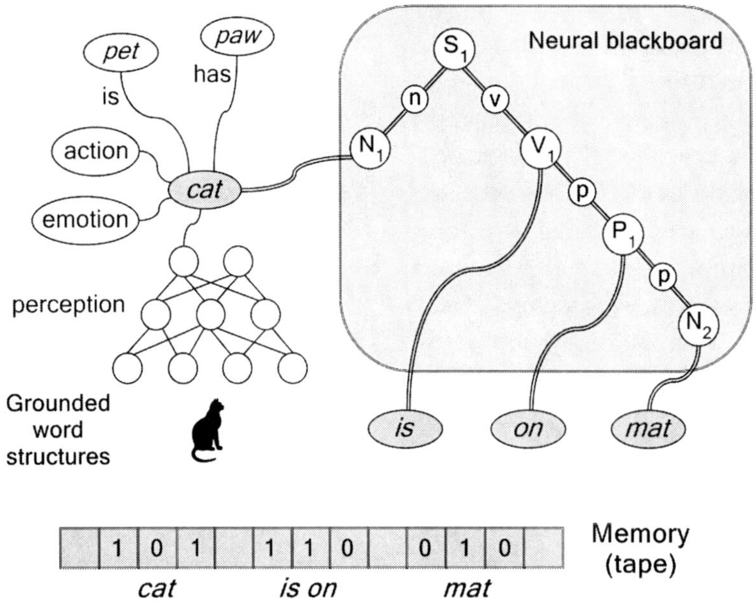

conditional connections the flow of activation can be controlled. For example, the *is* and *has* labels in Figure 1 indicate that information of the kind *cat is* or *cat has* controls the flow of activation between the word structures.

In Figure 2, the connections in the neural blackboard and between the word structures and the blackboard are also conditional connections, in which flow of activation and binding are controlled by circuits that parse the syntactic structure of the sentence. These circuits, for example, detect (simply stated) that *cat* is a noun and that it is the subject of the sentence *cat is on mat*. However, the specific details of the control and parsing processes that allow these temporal connections to be formed are not the main focus of this chapter. Details can be found in van der Velde and de Kamps (2006a). Here, I will focus on the general features that are required by any architecture that combines grounded representations in a productive way.

First, the representations of *cat*, *is*, *on*, and *mat* remain grounded in the whole binding process, and the structure of the sentence is compositional. As I noted, the syntax populations play a crucial role in this process, not just because they represent aspects of syntactic information but also because they allow temporal connections to be formed between grounded word representations. For example, the productivity of language requires that we can form a relation between an arbitrary verb and an arbitrary noun as its subject. But we can hardly assume that all words structures for nouns are connected with all word structures for verbs, certainly not for noun verb combinations that are novel. But we can assume that there are connections between words structures for nouns and a limited set of noun phrase populations, and that there are connections between words structures for verbs and a limited set of verb phrase populations. And we can assume that there are connections between noun phrase and verb phrase populations. So, using the indirect link provided by syntax populations we can create new (temporal) connections between arbitrary noun and verbs, and temporal connections between words of other syntactic types as well, as between *on* and *mat* in Figure 2.

Second, the use of conditional and temporal connections is crucial. Conditional connections can be used to encode relational information. By controlling the flow of activation the architecture can answer specific queries such as *where is the cat* or *who is on the mat*. Without such control of activation, only associations between word (concept) structures could be formed. Because the connections are temporal (that is, their activation is temporal), arbitrary and novel combinations can be formed in the architecture. And, the activations in the architecture could guide the forming of more permanent combinatorial structures (see van der Velde & de Kamps, 2006a).

Third, the syntax populations eliminate the need for copying representations to form sentences. Grounded concepts cannot be copied, yet some sentences seem to require copies of words. For example, in the sentence *The cat is on the cat*, the noun *cat* has the role of subject, but also the role of a noun in a prepositional phrase. A symbolic architecture can solve this problem easily. Figure 2 shows a symbolic representation of the sentence *cat is on mat*, with symbols stored in a memory (tape). All that is required to form *cat is on cat* is to replace the symbol for *mat* with a copy of the symbol for *cat*, as illustrated in Figure 3.

Figure 3 illustrates how this problem can be solved in an architecture of grounded cognition. Instead of making a copy, the grounded representation of *cat* is connected twice to the sentence structure of *The cat is on the cat* in the neural blackboard for sentence structures. This can be achieved because the grounded structure for *cat* is now bound to two noun phrase populations, N_1 and N_2. Because N_1 is bound to S_1, *cat* is the subject of the sentence. But *cat* is also the noun in the prepositional phrase because N_2 is bound to P_1. Both representations of *cat* in the sentence remain grounded in this way.

The fact that the two copies of *cat* in the symbolic representation of *cat is on cat* are not grounded results from the fact that one cannot copy all information related to cats and insert that in the slots for *cat* in the sentence structure of *The cat is on the cat*. For example, one cannot copy all neural structures or activations in the grounded representation of *cat* in figure 1, even if it were possible to copy its central neural population (the oval labeled *cat*). Instead, in the symbolic representation in figure 3, the symbol for *cat* is used as a kind of pointer that can be used to retrieve information about cats when needed. This is indeed the way Newell described the use of symbols in his quote given earlier.

But in that case we could perhaps use symbols as pointers to "reground" the symbolic representations of *cat* in the sentence *The cat is on the cat*. So, when we need perceptual information about cats to see if the statement expressed by sentence is correct, we could use the symbol for *cat* to retrieve that information. Again, this is indeed the way symbols are used in the symbolic architecture as described by Newell. But this procedure is faced with the difficulties outlined earlier: it requires an active decision to obtain that information, which raises the question who or what makes that decision. It also raises the question of when (e.g., how often) these decisions are made, given that it takes time to execute the process and retrieve information. And it raises the question about learning. For example, do we update our knowledge about cats on the basis of the information expressed in a sentence like *The cat is on the cat*? Or do we restrict updating to "important" information only? And who or what decides what is important in this respect, and on what basis?

Figure 3. Illustration of the combinatorial structure "The cat is on the cat" (ignoring "the"), with grounded representations for the words. The circles in the neural blackboard represent populations and circuits of neurons. The double line connections represent conditional connections. The bottom of the figure shows a symbolic representation of the sentence "The cat is on the cat" (N, n = noun; P, p = preposition; S = sentence; V, v = verb.)

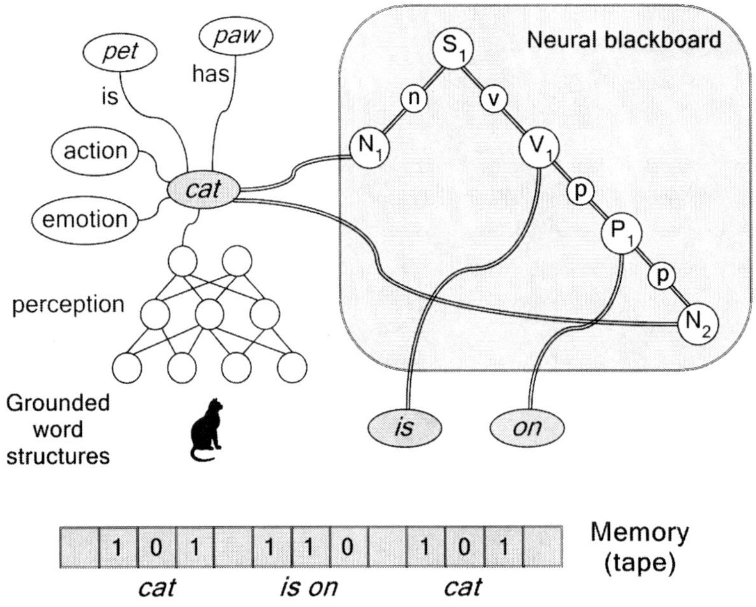

Visibility of Grounded Representations

In one aspect, symbols and grounded representations are alike. Both are explicit forms of representation, in the sense that they remain accessible or "visible" in combinatorial structures. For example, the symbol *101* for *cat* is a (recognizable) constituent in the symbol structure for *The cat is on the mat*, and the grounded representation for *cat* is a (recognizable) constituent in the grounded structure for that sentence as well (Figure 2).

Some connectionist models eliminate the use of explicit constituent representations in processing combinatorial structures. The aim of this "eliminative connectionism" was to show that networks can process complex combinatorial structures without relying on explicit constituent representations like words. In this way, networks would constitute a genuine alternative to symbolic architectures of cognition, instead of just implementing these architectures in networks.

Two examples of are illustrated in Figure 4. The first (Figure 4A) is the recurrent network used by Elman (1991) in a word prediction task. This type of network can process sequential information. In the word prediction task, the network learns to predict the kind of word that can follow in a given sentence context. For instance, with the sentence *cat is on mat*, it learns to predict that a noun will follow after *on*. The network uses two kinds of representations for words. In the input layer and the output layer, each word is represented by a designated node. So, the sentence *cat is on mat* is presented to the network by activating the input node for each word in the sentence in a sequential manner. The network responds by activating one or more of its output nodes. For example, after the (sequential) presentation of *cat is on*, the net-

Figure 4. (A) A recurrent neural network for sentence representation. The network has input and output representations of words, given by nodes in the input and output layer. Representations for the words in a sentence structure are formed by the connection weights in the network. (B) The reduced vector representation of "cat is" (diagonal vector), based on the vector representation for "cat" (horizontal vector) and "is" (vertical vector)

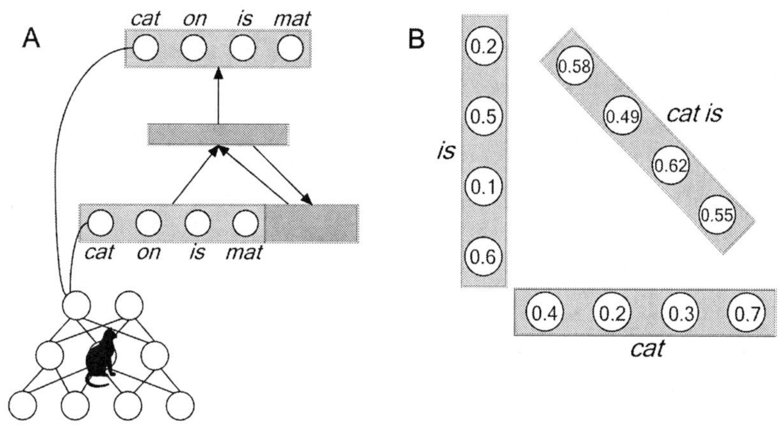

work has to activate the node for *mat* (or nodes for other nouns).

The individual words are represented explicitly in the input and output layers (Marcus, 2001). They are also grounded. Figure 4A illustrates how the nodes that represent *cat* can be grounded in visual perception. But words are not represented as visible constituents in sentence structures. To see this, consider how a sequence like *cat is on mat* is processed by the network. Each word in the sentence activates its node in the input layer. But the middle (hidden) layer of the network also activates a part of the input layer. The network then learns to activate the output node of the word that could be the next word in the sentence, based on the overall activation of the input layer. For example, when the word *on* is presented as input, it is combined with the activation in the network's hidden layer produced by the previous input (*cat is*). In this way, the input reflects that *on* is part of the sequence *cat is on*. For this input, the network has learned to activate a node like *mat* as output.

So, the network activates the output *mat* when it has processed the sequence *cat is on*. But it has not used or formed a constituent representation of *cat is on*, using visible representations of the words *cat*, *is* and *on*. In general, there are no constituent representations for any of the sentences the network has learned. Instead, the network has formed sentence representations in its connection weights when it learned to perform this task. These weights, in particular those of the connections between the hidden layer and the output layer, form a "state space" representation of the sentences the network has learned. When the network processes a sentence like *cat is on mat*, it moves along a trajectory in this state space. In this way, the network has eliminated the use of (visible) constituent representations when it processes complex structures like sentences.

But as a result, the representations of the words in a sentence are ungrounded, because they are "invisible" from the outside. For example, the representation of *cat* in the state space of the network is not activated when a cat is seen. Conversely, the state space representation of *cat* cannot influence processing in the visual system either, to look for a cat in the environment. Nor can it influence the pronunciation of *cat*, when a sentence like *cat is on mat* needs to be pronounced.

Of course, the word *cat* can be pronounced by activating the output node for *cat*, using the state space representation of the sentence *cat is on mat* or *cat is on cat*. But at the level of the output nodes, the representation of the sentence structure has disappeared. Thus, either we have a representation of *cat* in a sentence structure, or we have a representation of *cat* used for pronunciation, but we never have a combined representation of both. So, when the word *cat* is pronounced, information about its sentence context, e.g., the difference between *cat is on mat* versus *cat is on cat* is lost.

Figure 4B illustrates loss of grounding in the reduced vector representation of combinatorial structures (e.g., Plate, 2003). In this kind of model, constituents like words are represented as vectors, like the four dimensional vectors for *cat* and *is* in figure 4B. A combinatorial structure such as *cat is* is represented by a reduced vector representation, derived from the vectors for the constituents *cat* and *is*. The reduced vector representation results from an intricate mathematical operation know as circular convolution. The details of this operation are not important here, except the fact that it takes the constituent vectors as input and produces a representation of a combinatorial structure that has the same magnitude (dimension) as the vectors of the constituents. So, the vector for *cat is* is also a four dimensional vector, as illustrated in figure 4B. This vector reduction for combinatorial structures eliminates the problem of the increasing dimensions of tensors for hierarchical combinatorial structures (Plate, 2003). Continuing in the same manner, a reduced vector representation can be made of the sentence *cat is on mat*.

It is clear from figure 4B that the vector for *cat* (or *is*) is not accessible (visible) in the reduced vector for *cat is* (or that of *The cat is on the mat*). This is a direct consequence of using reduced vector representations for combinatorial structures. Because the vector of the combinatorial structure has the same dimension as the constituent vectors, it has to be different from each of these. The vector for *cat* itself can be grounded, and it can be retrieved from the reduced vector representation of the sentence *The cat is on the mat*. But when the vector is retrieved, the structure of the sentence is lost (e.g., there is no way to tell the difference between *cat is on mat*, *cat is on cat*, or *mat is on cat* is that case).

Because the representation of a constituent (e.g. *cat*) is not accessible in combinatorial structures provided by eliminative connectionist models such as recurrent networks or reduced vector coding, the representation of *cat* is not grounded in these combinatorial structures. In this aspect, eliminative connectionism is on a par with symbol manipulation. Both produce ungrounded combinatorial structures.

This shows that grounded combinatorial structures provide an alternative to both symbol manipulation and eliminative connectionism. It resembles the latter in that its individual constituent representations are grounded. It resembles symbol manipulation in that constituent representations remain visible in combinatorial structures. In this way, constituent representations remain grounded in combinatorial structures. As a result, they can influence the process by which these combinatorial structures are formed and they can be influenced by these combinatorial structures as well.

So, because the representation of *cat* remains visible in the structure of a sentence like *The cat is on the mat*, the connection structure of *cat* can be activated when *cat* is part of a sentence. In this way, the word structure for *cat* can influence the binding process that produces the sentence structure, or it can generate a motor program to pronounce *cat* in the pronunciation of *The cat is on the mat*. Furthermore, new information given by the sentence, e.g., a relation between *cat* and *mat* (e.g., cats are on mats and not vice versa), can be integrated with the word structures for *cat* and *mat*.

Figure 4 illustrates that accessibility (visibility) is a necessary requirement for a representation to be grounded. But it is not sufficient. The symbol tokens in Figures 2 and 3 are accessible (visible), but they are not grounded. Instead, a representation is grounded when it is accessible (visible) and remains "in situ", that is, when its information structure always remains intact, as illustrated in figure 1.

Visibility of Grounded Representations in Combinatorial Structures

Because grounded representations are visible (accessible), they can influence the combinatorial structures of which they are a part. Figure 5 illustrates this with the sentences *Time flies like an arrow* and *Time the race*.

The usual interpretation of *Time flies like an arrow* is in terms of a metaphor, that states that time changes very fast. In this interpretation, *time* is a noun and *flies* is a verb. But there are (at least) four other interpretations of this sentence (Pinker, 1994). In some of these, *time* is a verb and *flies* is a noun. For example, the sentence could mean that one should measure the speed of flies in the way as one measures the speed of an arrow. Ambiguities of this kind are common in language and cognition in general, but humans often do not notice them (Baars & Franklin, 2003; Baars, 2006). This is also the case for the sentence above. Whereas humans usually end up with one interpretation, a computer program of sentence analysis (based on symbol manipulation) gave all five interpretations (Pinker, 1994).

Figure 5 illustrates how ambiguity resolution could occur in a neural architecture of grounded cognition. In the architecture, dynamical interactions can occur between encoded sentences (van der Velde & de Kamps, 2006a). Similar interactions can also influence the binding process, that is, the process by which a sentence structure is formed. Figure 5A shows the competing sentence structures of *time flies*. The word *time* activates two word structures, one for *time* as a noun ($time_N$) and one for *time* as a verb ($time_V$). In the same way, *flies* activates $flies_N$ and $flies_V$.

Initially each of the word structures binds to corresponding syntax populations, such as N_1 and V_1. These syntax populations form competing sentence structures. In Figure 5A, the grey nodes and ovals indicate the sentence structure for $time_N$ $flies_V$, with $time_N$ as the subject of the sentence and $flies_V$ as the main verb. The white nodes and ovals (and S_1) form the sentence structure for $time_V$ $flies_N$. Here, $flies_N$ is the theme (t) of the verb $time_N$, which results in a different binding structure (van der Velde & de Kamps, 2006a).

But there is a dynamic competition between the sentence structures and between word structures. In particular, the word structures for $time_N$ and for $time_V$, and those for $flies_N$ and $flies_V$, inhibit each other. This competition implements the constraint that a word can have only one interpretation at the same time in a sentence structure. Between the sentence structures there is a competition (inhibition) between the circuits that activate conditional connections of the same kind (in Figure 5A those for the verb connections), and an inhibition between similar syntax populations (e.g., between the noun phrases N_1 and N_2 and between the verb phrases V_1 and V_2).

The dynamic interaction in the architecture is resolved when there is a clear advantage for one of the competing structures (van der Velde & de Kamps, 2006a). In figure 5A, an advantage for one of the sentence structures can arise from the fact that the interpretation of *time* as a noun is more frequent than the interpretation of *time* as a verb. In that case, the activation of $time_N$ will be stronger than that of $time_V$, so that the first inhibits the second. Then, $flies_V$ inhibits $flies_N$, because $flies_V$ is activated by $time_N$ through the sentence structure, whereas N_2 is inhibited by N_1 (this inhibition becomes stronger with increasing activation of $time_N$). In this way, the grey structure in figure 5A remains as the active structure to which the rest of the sentence, *like an arrow*, binds.

Figure 5. Competing neural blackboard structures for "time flies" (A) and "time the race" (B). The ovals and circles represent populations as in figures2 and 3. Grey circles and ovals are active. (N, n = noun; S = sentence; t = theme; V, v = verb.)

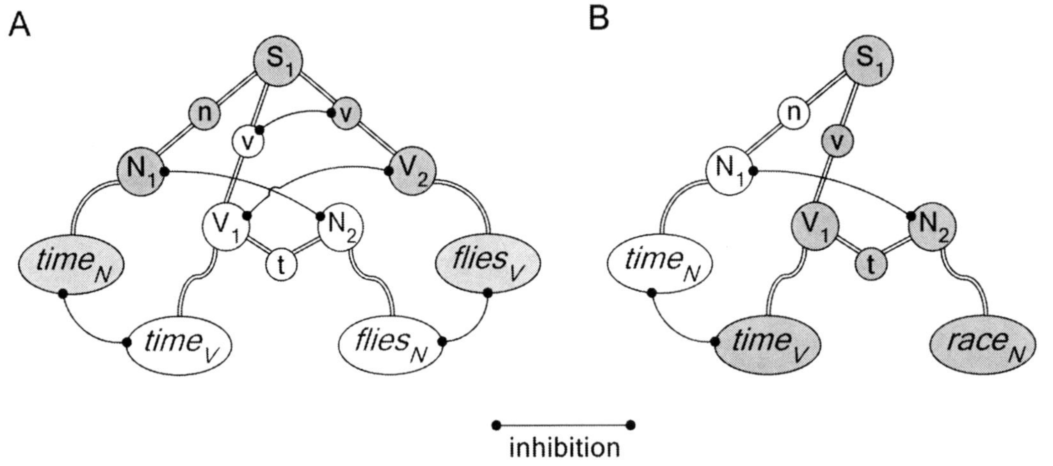

Figure 5b shows how *time*$_V$ will inhibit *time*$_N$ in the sentence structure *time the race*. The noun phrase *the race* matches *time*$_V$ as its theme (verb object). Through the active theme conditional connection, *race*$_N$ enhances the activation of *time*$_V$, which affects the inhibition of *time*$_N$ by *time*$_V$. Furthermore, N_1 is inhibited by N_2. The resulting activation pattern favors the interpretation of the sequence *time (the) race* as a verb and its object over the interpretation of this sequence as two nouns.

The outcome of a dynamic competition as illustrated in Figure 5 depends on the competition between the word structures and the sentence structure to which they are bound. This interaction process illustrates the importance of the accessibility (visibility) of grounded representations in combinatorial (e.g., sentence) structures. When word representations are encoded in combinatorial structures, as in Figure 4, such a competition is not possible. The node or vector for *cat*, for example, cannot influence the structures for *cat is on mat* in these models, because it is detached from the representation of *cat* in this sentence.

The competition in Figure 5 also illustrates why grounded representations are important, and why they have to remain grounded in combinatorial structures. The competition that solves the ambiguity of *time flies*, for example, results from the interaction between the structures of *time*$_N$ and *time*$_V$. The assumption is that *time*$_N$ wins this competition because it is used more frequently than *time*$_V$ in natural language. Due to the grounded nature of representations, the more frequent use of *time*$_N$ will affect the grounded representation of *time*$_N$ directly, because this representation is always used to represent *time*$_N$. Furthermore, the difference between *time*$_N$ and *time*$_V$ is found only in sentence contexts, thus in combinatorial structures. So, when grounded representations remain grounded in combinatorial structures, the more frequently used type of combinatorial structure can influence the grounded structures involved directly.

Putative Origin of Grounded Representations in Combinatorial Structures

Because the grounded representations are visible in combinatory structures, they can influence these structures by a dynamic process, as illustrated in

Figure 5. The converse is also true. A dynamical process within a combinatorial structure activates the grounded constituent representations directly (e.g., see van der Velde & de Kamps, 2006a). For example, when the structure of the sentence *cat is on mat* is activated, the sentence can be pronounced because the word structures are activated as well. Learning to speak consists of a prolonged training process in which (simply stated) word representations activate the muscles in the face and throat. Again, the grounded nature of word representations is crucial here, because in this way a word representation can gradually develop (or be linked to) a motor program that is needed to pronounce the word.

Motor programs could in fact be a basis for the development of grounded representations. After all, muscles are by nature "grounded". That is, we have just one set of muscles that we use for making specific movements. For example, consider moving the fingers of one hand in playing music (e.g., keyboard). To play the index finger, its muscles have to be activated. To play the same finger again, the same muscles have to be activated. In this way, the set of muscles that produces a particular movement is grounded: it is always the same set that is used. Hence, a complex movement pattern in which alternate fingers have to be moved in a specific way can be seen as a combinatorial structure based on grounded representations.

For example, consider a combinatorial finger pattern in which the fingers 1 (thumb), 2 (index finger) and 3 (middle finger) have to be played in a specific sequence like 2-1-3-2. The pattern seems to consist of a sequence of copies of specific fingers, and in symbolic architectures it would be represented as such. But in the execution of the pattern there are no copies. The index finger is moved by the same set of muscles, whether it is played as the first or as the fourth finger in the sequence. The motor program that executes this sequence has to activate this set of muscles at these positions in the sequence. This resembles the pronunciation of, for example, *cat is on cat*, where the grounded structure for *cat* has to be activated at the first and fourth position in the sentence.

Because muscles are grounded by nature, a complex motor program could be seen as a combinatorial structure based on (visible) grounded representations, consisting of the neural populations that activate (sets of) muscles. Over time, these populations would learn to control their muscles in a more precise way, which again shows the benefit of having grounded representations. Complex motor programs could then develop on the basis of these representations, based on blackboard architectures that allows combinatorial motion patterns to be formed.

So, the existence of combinatorial structures based on grounded representations in cognition could have a precursor in the existence of combinatorial motor programs. Or course, human evolution is not based on the need to play complicated musical instruments. But the fact that we can do so illustrates that we have developed the ability to execute and memorize complex motor programs, which would consist of combinatorial structures based on grounded representations. In the course of evolution, some of the grounded motor representations could have evolved into more conceptual representations, for example, by combining perceptual input with motor output. And some of the blackboard architectures for combinatorial motion patterns could have evolved into blackboard architectures for other forms of cognitive processing, using these grounded conceptual structures as constituents.

Blackboard Architectures for Cognitive Processing

The combination of productivity and grounding requires certain architectures in which the grounded representations can be combined temporarily into combinatorial structures. The neural blackboard for sentence structure illustrated in Figures 2 and 3 is an illustration of such an architecture.

The question arises as to how may of these architectures would be needed. Any type of approach that aims to account for human cognition has to assume that some kind of machinery exists for a given cognitive process. This is true for symbol manipulation, eliminative connectionism and theories of grounded cognition. In the case of symbol manipulation, for example, we have to assume that a kind of machinery exists that can execute the required forms of symbol manipulation. Indeed, this assumption is the basis for classical cognitivism. In the words of Fodor and Pylyshyn:

Classical models of the mind were derived from the structure of Turing and Von Neumann machines. They are not, of course, committed to the details of these machines as exemplified in Turing's original formulation or in typical commercial computers; only to the basic idea that the kind of computing that is relevant to understanding cognition involves operations on symbols. ... the idea that the brain is such a machine is the foundational hypothesis of Classical cognitive science. (Fodor and Pylyshyn, 1988, p4, p30)

If the mind/brain is some kind of machine as described by Fodor and Pylyshyn then it would have, say, registers to store the copies of symbols needed to form combinatorial structures. It would also have the programs needed to manipulate symbols. Such programs, combined with the machinery to store and manipulate symbols, constitute the basis for specific cognitive processes as found in human cognition.

The grounded representations as illustrated in Figure 1 cannot be copied, so registers and the like would not be of any use (even assuming that they can be implemented in neural tissue). Yet, specific cognitive processes do require that specific operations on representations can be executed. Some kind of machinery is needed as the basis for these processes. The suggestion made here is that specific cognitive processes, certainly processes requiring combinatorial structures, each depend on some kind of neural blackboard.

The neural blackboard illustrated in Figures 2 and 3 provides the ability to form sentence structures. But words, for example, also have a phonological structure, and these structures are productive (combinatorial) as well. So, words would also be a part of a phonological neural blackboard (see van der Velde & de Kamps, 2006b). Words (concepts) can be used in reasoning processes based on sentence structures, which would require a specific blackboard architecture as well (see van der Velde & de Kamps, 2006a). But words could also be a part of non-sentence like sequences, which could be used for other specific forms of reasoning (Hadley, 2008). Because the sentence blackboard is not suitable for these sequences, a specific sequence blackboard is required as well.

Figure 6 illustrates the notion of specific neural blackboards for specific cognitive processes. It shows that the grounded word structure for *cat* will be embedded in neural blackboards for sentence structure, phonological structure, sequences and reasoning processes, and potential other blackboards as well. One might argue that this is overly complex. But complexity is needed to account for human cognition. Such complexity is hidden in symbol manipulation as well. For example, when a specific symbol manipulation process is executed on a computer, a lot of its complexity is hidden in the underlying machinery provided by the computer. As a model of cognition, this machinery has to be assumed as a part of the model as well.

Furthermore, the situation illustrated in Figure 6 is a direct consequence of the grounded nature of representations. Because these representations always remain "in situ", they have to be connected to architectures like blackboards to form combinatorial structures and to execute processes on the basis of these structures. Figure 6 suggest that specific blackboards will arise for specific kinds of processes, instead of some gen-

Figure 6. A grounded conceptual representation is embedded in several specialized neural blackboard architectures, needed for specific cognitive processing based on specific combinatorial structures

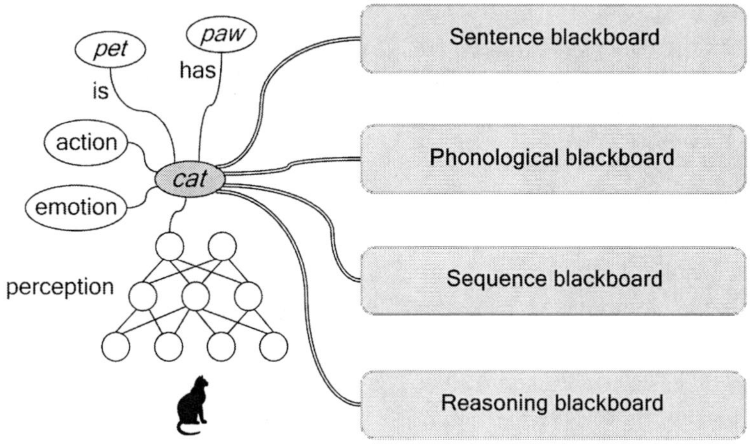

eral kind of blackboard that could serve for all purposes. Figure 6 also illustrates the crucial role played by grounded representations. Because they are grounded, they are a part of each specific blackboard architecture. In this way, they form the link between these architectures. When processes occur in one blackboard, the grounded representation can also induce processes in the other blackboards, which could in turn influence the process in the first blackboard. In this way, an interaction occurs between local information embodied in specific blackboards and global information embodied in grounded representations. The resolution of ambiguity in Figure 5 is an illustration of this interaction.

FUTURE RESEARCH DIRECTIONS

If cognition arises from the interaction between grounded representations and blackboard architectures, it raises the question of how these systems develop and how learning occurs in these systems.

The nature of grounded cognition suggests that these overall questions can be reduced to more special ones. First, learning and development occurs with grounded representations themselves. The visibility of grounded representations plays a crucial role in this respect. For example, over time associations between representations can develop due to their grounded nature, as illustrated in Figure 1. In a similar vein, relations between grounded representations can be developed or learned over time, when these representations interact frequently in specific blackboards (van der Velde & de Kamps, 2006a). Because the grounded (word) representations and their associations and relations develop/learn independently from the architectures needed for specific cognitive processes, the overall system scales well under enlargement, and newly learned words and concepts can integrate easily in the architecture.

The blackboards themselves are a major topic for further investigation, in particular the way in which these architectures can develop and how they provide a basis for learning. We can distinguish here between the issue of learning control in a blackboard architecture and the development of the architecture itself. Figures 2 and 3 illustrate that a sentence like *cat is on mat* is bound to a (temporal) sentence structure in a sentence blackboard. This process presupposes the existence of the blackboard and the grounded representations. The process also requires a control of the binding process.

We investigated learning control of binding by training a feedforward network (FFN) to control the binding of a set of sentence structures (van der Velde & de Kamps, 2008). Figure 7 illustrates how an FFN can learn to control the binding of the sentence *cat is on mat*. The input layer of the network receives information about the word types of the words in the sentence. So, *cat* and *mat* activate the *noun* node in the input layer, *is* activates the *verb* node and *on* activates the *preposition* node in the input layer. The network also receives feedback from the developing sentence structure as input. Here, it receives information that *on* is bound as a preposition phrase. This information can be used by the network to learn that the next noun is the noun of the preposition phrase.

The output layer of the network produces the binding signals that control the binding process. So, with *cat is on mat*, *cat* activates the *noun* node. The network has learned (based on training with a set of training sentences) that the first noun is the subject of the sentence. It thus activates the output node *subject*. This initiates the binding of N_1 with S_1 as its subject (for details of this binding process, see van der Velde & de Kamps, 2006a). In a similar way, it has learned to bind the verb (*is*) as the main verb of the sentence, that is, after the presentation of *is*, the output node *main verb* is activated, which initiates this binding. For *on*, the FFN activates the output node for *preposition*. This initiates the binding of the preposition phrase P_1 to V_1. The activation of P_1 also generates input to the FFN. The network has learned to combine this activation with the next activation of the input node *noun* (by *mat*) to bind that noun as the noun of the preposition phrase. That is, to generate the binding signal that results in the binding of P_1 and N_2.

In our study (van der Velde & de Kamps, 2008) we trained FFNs on basic input-output relations to control the binding process in the architecture, as illustrated in Figure 7. The networks then dealt successfully with more complex and recombined sentence types, such as sentences with relative clauses. The reason that learning basic input-output relations with an FFN suffices even for complex sentence structures is due to the fact that a substantial part of what a sentence structure can be is embodied in the architecture itself, that is, in the neural blackboard of sentence structure.

This raises the issue of how the structure of the architecture itself emerges. This could be the result of a different kind of process that might be referred to as "development" instead of just learning. The FFN used in figure 7 shows what could be the difference between learning and development. The FFN learns by an adaptation of its weights, but its structure does not change. Perhaps one could introduce a structure change by allowing new connections to be formed in the FFN. But even then, the structure change is not on a par with that is needed to develop the structure of the blackboard architecture. The latter requires the development of different kinds of syntax populations and the neural circuits by which these populations can be bound (van der Velde & de Kamps, 2006a).

The success of learning control of binding with an FFN thus perhaps suggest that language learning (and cognition learning in general) is the result of a dual process, consisting of an adaptation of control in combination with a structural development of a binding architecture for grounded representations. This dual process proceeds alongside with the learning process that occurs with grounded representations, as outlined above. The dual process might motivate the search for two different kinds of learning (development) mechanisms in the design of systems and circuits. One for the structural development of the architectures needed, such as the language architecture illustrated in figure 7, and one for control, based on feedback from these architectures, as the FFN illustrated in figure 7. The first mechanism could perhaps be better referred to as development than (just) learning, because it is primarily related to structural

Figure 7. Learning control of binding in the sentence architecture, using a feedforward network. The sentence structure is the one illustrated in figure 2. The input nodes of the feedforward network receive activation from the words and the combinatorial structure in the neural blackboard. The output nodes of the feedforward network activate the circuits in the neural blackboard that produce specific bindings between syntax populations

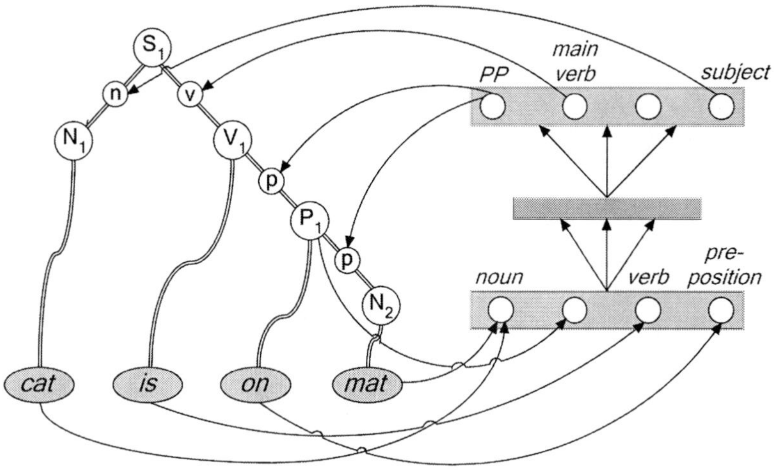

changes that might occur only at an initial stage. The latter could be referred to as learning, based on continuously updated information.

CONCLUSION

The importance of the combination of productivity, dynamics and grounding is that they impose constraints on each other. In turn, these constraints can reveal fundamental aspects of human cognition. For example, combinatorial structures can be created with grounded representations, but not all structures are equally feasible. For example, not all sentence structures are equally feasible in the language architecture illustrated in Figure 2 (van der Velde & deKamps, 2006a). And, as illustrated in figure 5, the combinatorial structures formed are influenced by dynamics, which provides additional constraints on the ability to create combinatorial structures. The examples given in Figure 5 show that these constraints prevent the excessive production of sentence interpretations, as found in systems with unlimited productivity based on symbol manipulation. But, on occasion, it can also result in misrepresentations, as found in human cognition.

Fodor, who has supported the computational view of cognition from its beginning, has more recently argued that a computational (symbol manipulation) account of cognition is incomplete (Fodor, 2000). In his view, computational processes based on symbol manipulation do not capture the global flexibility of cognition, which is perhaps the most important feature of human cognition (Fodor, 2000). The reason for that is that computational processes are always local (as indeed illustrated in the quote from Newell, given earlier). Connectionism, in his view, cannot fill this gap, because it lacks the productivity of human cognition.

However, grounded cognition, as presented here, is both local and global, and it is productive. Specific processes, such as the creation of sentence structures, are local. But the representations involved are grounded, and grounded representations are global. As figure 6 illustrates, this combination provides a basis for the productivity and global flexibility of cognition.

REFERENCES

Anderson, J. R. (1983). *The architecture of cognition*. Cambridge, MA: Harvard University Press.

Baars, B. J. (2006). Conscious cognition and blackboard architectures. *The Behavioral and Brain Sciences*, *22*, 70–71.

Baars, B. J., & Franklin, S. (2003). How conscious experience and working memory interact. *Trends in Cognitive Sciences*, *7*, 166–172. doi:10.1016/S1364-6613(03)00056-1

Barsalou, L. W. (1999). Perceptual symbol systems. *The Behavioral and Brain Sciences*, *22*, 577–660.

Elman, J. L. (1991). Distributed representations, simple recurrent networks, and grammatical structure. *Machine Learning*, *7*, 195–225. doi:10.1007/BF00114844

Fodor, J. A. (2000). *The mind doesn't work that way*. Cambridge, MA: MIT Press.

Fodor, J. A., & Pylyshyn, Z. W. (1988). Connectionism and cognitive architecture: A critical analysis. In Pinker, S., & Mehler, J. (Eds.), *Connections and symbols* (pp. 3–71). Cambridge, MA: MIT Press.

Hadley, R. F. (2008). The problem of rapid variable creation. *Neural Computation*, *20*, 1–23.

Harnad, S. (1991). The symbol grounding problem. In Forrest, S. (Ed.), *Emergent computation: Self-organizing, collective, and cooperative phenomena in natural and artificial computing networks*. Cambridge, MA: MIT Press.

Marcus, G. F. (2001). *The algebraic mind*. Cambridge, MA: MIT Press.

Miller, G. A. (1967). *The psychology of communication*. London: Penguin.

Newell, A. (1990). *Unified Theories of Cognition*. Cambridge, MA: Harvard University Press.

Pinker, S. (1994). *The Language Instinct*. London: Penguin.

Plate, T. A. (2003). *Holographic Reduced Representation*. Stanford, CA: CSLI Publications.

van der Velde, F., & de Kamps, M. (2006a). Neural blackboard architectures of combinatorial structures in cognition. *The Behavioral and Brain Sciences*, *22*, 37–70.

van der Velde, F., & de Kamps, M. (2006b). From neural dynamics to true combinatorial structures. *The Behavioral and Brain Sciences*, *22*, 88–108.

van der Velde, F., & de Kamps, M. (2008). The role of recurrent networks in neural architectures of grounded cognition: learning of control. In L. D. Raedt, B. Hammer, P. Hitzler, W. Maass (Eds.) *Recurrent Neural Networks- Models, Capacities, and Applications. Dagstuhl Seminar Proceedings 08041* (pp. 237-288). http://drops.dagstuhl.de/opus/ volltexte/2008/1421.

ADDITIONAL READING

Amit, D. (1995). The Hebbian paradigm reintegrated: Local reverberations as internal representations. *The Behavioral and Brain Sciences*, *18*, 617–657. doi:10.1017/S0140525X00040164

Barsalou, L. W., Simmons, W. K., Barbey, A. K., & Wilson, C. D. (2003). Grounding conceptual knowledge in modality-specific systems. *Trends in Cognitive Sciences*, *7*, 84–91. doi:10.1016/S1364-6613(02)00029-3

Batista, A. P., Buneo, C. A., Snyder, L. H., & Andersen, R. A. (1999). Reach plans in eye-centered coordinates. *Science*, *285*, 257–260. doi:10.1126/science.285.5425.257

Bechtel, W., & Abrahamsen, A. (2002). *Connectionism and the mind.* Malden, MA: Blackwell.

Biedenstock, E., & Gemand, S. (1995). Compositionality in neural systems. In Arbib, M. A., Adelman, G., & Arbib, P. H. (Eds.), *The handbook of brain theory and neural networks* (pp. 223–226). Cambridge, MA: MIT Press.

Bierwisch, M. (1999). Words in the brain are not just labeled concepts. *The Behavioral and Brain Sciences*, *22*, 280–282. doi:10.1017/S0140525X99221826

Bloom, P. (2000). *How children learn the meanings of words*. Cambridge, MA: MIT Press.

Calvin, W. H. (1995). Cortical columns, modules, and Hebbian cell assemblies. In Arbib, M. A., Adelman, G., & Arbib, P. H. (Eds.), *The handbook of brain theory and neural networks* (pp. 269–272). Cambridge, MA: MIT Press.

Calvin, W. H., & Bickerton, D. (2000). *Lingua ex Machina: Reconciling Darwin and Chomsky with the Human Brain*. Cambridge, MA: MIT Press.

Caplan, D. (1992). *Language: Structure, processing and disorders*. Cambridge, MA: MIT Press.

Chelazzi, L., Miller, E. K., Duncan, J., & Desimone, R. (1993). A neural basis for visual search in inferior temporal cortex. *Nature*, *363*, 345–347. doi:10.1038/363345a0

Chomsky, N. (2000). *New horizons in the study of language and mind*. Cambridge University Press.

Churchland, P. M. (1995). *The engine of reason, the seat of the soul*. Cambridge, MA: MIT Press.

Dennett, D. C. (1991). *Consciousness explained*. London: Allen Lane.

Duncan, J. (2001). An adaptive coding model of neural function in prefrontal cortex. *Nature Reviews. Neuroscience*, *2*, 820–829. doi:10.1038/35097575

Durstewitz, D., Seamans, J. K., & Sejnowski, T. J. (2000). Neurocomputational models of working memory. *Nature Neuroscience, 3* (sup), 1184-1191.

Felleman, D. J., & van Essen, D. C. (1991). Distributed hierarchical processing in the primate cerebral cortex. *Cerebral Cortex*, *1*, 1–47. doi:10.1093/cercor/1.1.1-a

Fodor, J. A., & McLaughlin, B. P. (1990). Connectionism and the problem of systematicity - Why Smolensky's solution doesn't work. *Cognition*, *35*, 183–204. doi:10.1016/0010-0277(90)90014-B

Fuster, J. M. (1995). *Memory in the cerebral cortex*. Cambridge, MA: MIT Press.

Gibson, E. (1998). Linguistic complexity: Locality of syntactic dependencies. *Cognition*, *68*, 1–76. doi:10.1016/S0010-0277(98)00034-1

Gonchar, Y., & Burkhalter, A. (1999). Connectivity of GABAergic calretinin-immunoreactive neurons in rat primary visual cortex. *Cerebral Cortex*, *9*, 683–696. doi:10.1093/cercor/9.7.683

Hebb, D. O. (1949). *The organisation of behaviour*. New York: Wiley.

Hubel, D. (1995). *Eye, brain, and vision*. New York: Scientific American Library.

Jackendoff, R. (2002). *Foundations of language*. Oxford: Oxford University Press. doi:10.1093/acprof:oso/9780198270126.001.0001

Livingstone, M. S., & Hubel, D. H. (1988). Segregation of form, colour, movement and depth: Anatomy, physiology, and perception. *Science*, *240*, 740–749. doi:10.1126/science.3283936

O'Reilly, R. C., & Rudy, J. W. (2001). Conjunctive representations in learning and memory: Principles of cortical and hippocampal function. *Psychological Review*, *108*, 311–345. doi:10.1037/0033-295X.108.2.311

Oram, M. W., & Perrett, D. I. (1994). Modeling visual recognition from neurobiological constraints. *Neural Networks*, *7*, 945–972. doi:10.1016/S0893-6080(05)80153-4

Palmer-Brown, D., Tepper, J. A., & Powell, H. M. (2002). Connectionist natural language parsing. *Trends in Cognitive Sciences*, *6*, 437–442. doi:10.1016/S1364-6613(02)01980-0

Pinker, S. (1998). *How the mind works*. London: Penguin.

Rao, S. C., Rainer, G., & Miller, E. K. (1997). Integration of what and where in the primate prefrontal cortex. *Science*, *276*, 821–824. doi:10.1126/science.276.5313.821

Sag, I. A., & Wasow, T. (1999). *Syntactic theory*. Stanford, CA: CSLI Publications.

van der Velde, F. (1995). Symbol manipulation with neural networks: Production of a context-free language using a modifiable working memory. *Connection Science*, *7*, 247–280. doi:10.1080/09540099550039246

van der Velde, F. (1997). On the use of computation in modelling behavior. *Network (Bristol, England)*, *8*, 1–32. doi:10.1088/0954-898X/8/1/002

van der Velde, F., & de Kamps, M. (2001). From knowing what to knowing where: Modeling object-based attention with feedback disinhibition of activation. *Journal of Cognitive Neuroscience*, *13*, 479–491. doi:10.1162/08989290152001907

Van Gelder, T. (1990). Compositionality: A connectionist variation on a classical theme. *Cognitive Science*, *14*, 355–384. doi:10.1016/0364-0213(90)90017-Q

Wasow, T. (1989). Grammatical theory. In Posner, M. I. (Ed.), *Foundations of Cognitive Science* (pp. 161–205). Cambridge, MA: MIT Press.

Chapter 3
Learning:
A Psychological Perspective

Frank van der Velde
Leiden University, The Netherlands

ABSTRACT

This chapter reviews research into human and animal forms of learning. It concentrates on two forms of learning in particular. The first is conditioning. The study of conditioning constitutes the first example of experimental research on learning. At first, it seemed to corroborate the view that learning consists of establishing associations. This form of learning was proposed by the early empiricists. The notion of associative learning influenced the emergence of behaviorism, which used conditioning to account for all forms of human and animal behavior. More recent research, however, has shown that conditioning is a more complex form of learning, related to propositional learning. This makes conditioning important for the study of the mechanisms of other, more complex, forms of propositional learning, as found in language and reasoning. The second form of learning reviewed here is visual learning. The study of this form of learning is important for understanding visual processing. And it is important for investigating the neural mechanisms of learning, given the availability of animal models of visual processing.

INTRODUCTION

The ability to learn is one of the most important features of intelligence. Without it, it is hard to negotiate a complex environment and to deal with ever changing circumstances. Speculations as to how humans learn can be dated back to ancient (Greek) philosophy. From the early days on, the issue of learning is related to the nature-nurture debate. That is, are we born with certain forms of knowledge or abilities, or are all forms of knowledge acquired through experience?

Roughly two opposing positions can be discerned in this debate. The first one is that of rationalism, defended by Plato and, later on, by Descartes. According to this view, the core of human knowledge is inborn. By reasoning, we can expand our knowledge. Experience can be useful

DOI: 10.4018/978-1-60960-018-1.ch003

to focus the mind on certain issues, but it is not the primary source of our knowledge. The opposing view is that of (epistemological) empiricism, as defended by Locke in his *Essay concerning Human Understanding*, first published in 1690. According to empiricism, the mind is a blank slate at birth. No ideas are inborn, Instead, the mind gradually acquires ideas though experience.

Learning is of primary importance for empiricism. Locke described how we acquire ideas through our sense (simple ideas) and how these ideas combine into more complex ideas through experience. So, first we would have ideas like round (shape), green (color), smooth (texture), and sweet (taste), derived from our senses. Later on we combine these simple ideas into the complex idea of 'apple', based on our recurrent experience with apples. Complex ideas derive from simple ideas by the process of association.

The 17th century empiricists aimed to discover the laws that determine how ideas become associated through experience (learning). They argued that we tend to associate ideas because they are in opposition to each other, like white and black or round and square (law of contrast). Or, we associate ideas because they resemble each other (law of similarity). But the most important law of association suggested by the empiricists is the law of contiguity. We associate ideas when they (frequently) co-occur together in time and place. In this way, we learn for example that the combination of round (shape), green (color), smooth (texture), and sweet (taste) constitutes the idea of an apple, because these simple ideas co-occur in time and place whenever we encounter (certain types of) apples.

Later generations of empiricists also formulated laws of association that would account for the strength of an association. So associations between ideas are stronger when our experience of their combination is more frequent, when our experience is more recent, or when our experience is more intense (e.g., more emotional). However, the study of the process of association (learning) was still based on a theoretical analysis. It became an experimental science when Pavlov discovered the process of conditioning, by which perceptions of different events can become associated (or so it seems). The discovery of conditioning forms the beginning of the scientific research into learning, at first dominated by behaviorism.

BEHAVIORISM

In his classical conditioning experiment, Pavlov (1927) showed how an initially neutral stimulus such as the sound of the bell can become the trigger of a response like salivation, that is normally triggered by a food stimulus. The food stimulus is referred to as the unconditioned stimulus (UCS). The salivation response triggered by the food in referred to as the unconditioned response (UCR). Normally, a stimulus like the sound of a bell would not trigger the response of salivation. In the learning stage of the experiment, the bell sound is combined with the food stimulus. That is, the bell sound precedes the presentation of the food. After some time, the bell sound alone triggers the response of salivation. In the terminology of conditioning, the bell sound has become the conditioned stimulus (CS) and the response of salivation has become the conditioned response (CR) when it is triggered by the CS.

At face value, conditioning resembles the process of association proposed by the early empiricists. The CS becomes associated with the UCS (or with the UCR) because the CS and UCS are presented together for some time. This resembles the law of contiguity, one of the association laws proposed by the empiricists. Or course, Pavlov conducted his experiments with animals (dogs) and not humans. But in the mean time, Darwin had proposed his theory of evolution, so animal learning could be seen as a precursor of human learning, because the latter evolved from the first.

Behaviorism combined evolution theory and conditioning into an account of human behavior.

Barring a few inborn reflexes, such as the salivation reflex triggered by food, human behavior develops on the basis of learned associations between stimuli and responses. The learning process is that of conditioning. At first, behaviorists like Watson studied a form of condition known as classical conditioning. This is the form of conditioning pioneered by Pavlov. It begins with an UCS that triggers an UCR. The UCS is then combined with a stimulus (the CS) that, by itself, does not trigger the UCR. Due to the combination of the CS with the UCS, the CS becomes associated with the UCR, which now becomes the CR. That is, the CS on its own can produce the CR.

Watson and Rayner (1920) applied this process to human learning. A classical example is that of little Albert, an 11-month infant. Initially Albert showed no fear of rats, playing with a white rat in a hospital room. Albert was afraid, however, of load noises. The fear for load noises is one of those inborn reflexes, like the salivation reflex. Watson and Rayner used a load noise as the UCS and combined it with a white rat as the CS. So, when little Albert played with the rat, he heard a loud noise that startled him. After a while, the white rat alone was sufficient to trigger the fear response, which thus became the CR. In fact, he showed the fear response for furry white objects such as a rabbit or a white beard. This shows that learning by conditioning can generalize to objects that resemble the CR, a phenomenon known as generalization.

Due to classical conditioning, a response of the organism can be triggered by a stimulus that did not produce that response before. But the response itself is not a novel one. That is, the organism already produces the response as a reaction to an UCS. Thus, using classical conditioning, familiar behavior can be modified. So, little Albert showed no fear in response to a white rat, but after conditioning he did. Conversely, classical conditioning can be used to reduce or eliminate a fear response that occurs, for example, in phobia. In this process, the fear response to a feared stimulus is gradually extinguished by combining the feared stimulus with stimuli that do not result in fear, or in fact trigger comfort.

To redirect behavior, that is, to induce a different response pattern, another form of conditioning is needed. This form, known as operant conditioning, was introduced by Skinner. With operant conditioning, certain forms of behavior, that can occur by chance, are rewarded or punished. The effect is that the behavior is reinforced or reduced (or even extinguished). The difference with classical conditioning is that no specific stimulus response pattern (UCS → UCR) is needed as a basis for conditioning. Instead, in the case of reinforcement, the experimenter waits until a desired form of behavior occurs. If it does, it is rewarded. The result is that the behavior is repeated more often. In this way, an animal can learn a complex pattern of behavior, such as finding its way in a complex maze. Initially, the first correct steps are rewarded. Later on, only more complex moves are rewarded, bringing the animal closer to the goal. Finally, only the complete desired behavior is rewarded, until it is a regular part of the animal's behavior.

ASSOCIATIVE MECHANISMS OF LEARNING

Behaviorism assumed that, with classical and operant conditioning, the basis forms of learning were available to account for human behavior. Watson and Skinner used conditioning to study observable behavior. But Hull aimed to derive a full account of the mechanisms that produce human behavior, based on forms of conditioning. To understand the work of Hull in relation to that of Watson and Skinner, it is necessary to distinguish two forms of behaviorism.

Before behaviorism, introspection was the preferred method of experimental psychology (Pavlov was a physiologist). In an introspection experiment, a stimulus is presented and the task of the subjects is to report what they perceived. In this way, the response obtained in the experiment is the subjects' account of their observations. The negative aspects of this method are obvious. The experimenter has no way of knowing whether the subjects' account is accurate or even meaningful. Furthermore, asking subjects to monitor the process of perceiving a stimulus could easily affect that process itself, which would destroy the purpose of the experiment.

Behaviorism introduced an experimental method in which the experimenter controls both the presentation of the stimulus and the registration of the response. Basically, a stimulus is presented, and the experimenter observes the behavior of the subject in response to the stimulus. The subject's account of their observations is eliminated in this method. In fact, it's viewed as unscientific, because it cannot be checked by an outside observer.

The focus on observable behavior is prominent in the version of behaviorism advocated by Watson and Skinner, which is the version of behaviorism one usually finds in psychology textbooks. Although they were interested in the stimulus-response (S-R) associations underlying behavior and the learning process that established these S-R associations, the process of S-R association was assumed to occur in a "black box". When a specific S was presented to the black box, the associated R emerged from it. But the mechanism in the black box that produced this S-R association was ignored because it could not be observed.

It is important to realize that this form of "radical" behaviorism consists of a combination of two independent views. The first one is the notion that behavior results from S-R associations. The second one is the notion that science is about what is directly observable. This is a view about science itself (not about behavior or cognition), known as positivism. The positivist view on science, endorsed by people like Mach, eschews any use of theoretical entities or constructs like atoms or molecules in physics or black box mechanisms in psychology. These theoretical constructs are rejected because they cannot be observed directly.

The fact that radical behaviorism is indeed a combination of a view about the nature of behavior and a view about the nature of science can be seen in the work of Hull. As a behaviorist, he studied behavior in terms of S-R relations that resulted from learning (conditioning). But in contrast to radical behaviorism, Hull had a clear interest in the mechanisms that produced behavior. In his book on the history of experimental psychology, Boring described Hull's interests, based on his personal acquaintance with him:

He was also concerned with the question of the robot: can machines be built which will duplicate the capacities of the conscious human organism? Hull thought that they could, and that kind of interest grew with his behavioristic kind of thinking. (Boring, 1950, p.652)

From his papers it is clear that Hull wanted to give a truly mechanical account of behavior. But as a behaviorist, he believed that this mechanical account should be given in terms of S-R associations that resulted from learning (in the form of conditioning).

To illustrate what such a theory would look like, I have reproduced some of the S-R mechanisms presented by Hull. Figure 1 (left) illustrates how an organism can internalize a sequence of S-R associations (based on Hull, 1930). First, there is a sequence of stimuli (the S_i's) in the outside world (W). Each stimulus results in a response (the R_i's) of the organism (O), but the responses are initially unrelated. Over time, however, each response produces feedback (the s_i's) and the feedback of a given response becomes associated with the next response in the sequence. In the end, this results in an internalized sequence of responses that can be triggered by a single stimulus in the outside world. So:

... the organismic reactions (R's) which at the outset were joined only by virtue of the energies operating in the outer world sequence of S's, are

Figure 1. Examples of S-R relations presented by Hull. Left: Due to learning, a sequence of stimuli (S_i) in the world (W) produces a sequence of associated responses (R_i) and feedback (s_i) in the organism (O), which can be triggered by a single stimulus. Right: Part of an action sequence determined by S-R relations, feedback (r-s, s-r) and internal drives (S_D)

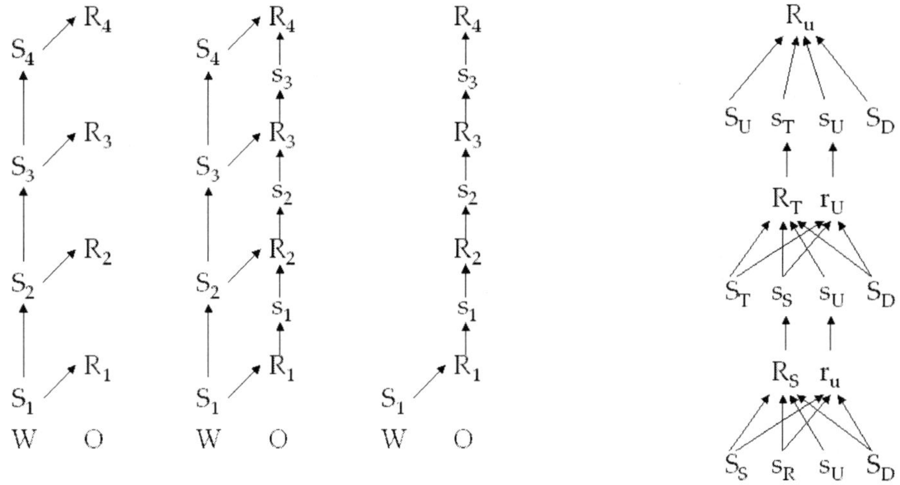

now possessed of a genuine dynamic relationship lying within the organism itself. (Hull, 1930, p. 513)

Figure 1 (right) illustrates a part of an action sequence that results from learned S-R associations, internal drives and feedback within the organism (based on Hull, 1935). Hull used action sequences like these to show how forms of problem solving could produce complex behavior (as that of a rat trying to find the shortest route in a maze). A number of action sequences are available for an organism. The conjunction of external stimuli (e.g., S_S, S_T, S_U), internal drives (S_S) and activated forms of feedback (the r-s or s-r associations) determines the selection of a specific action sequence. The mechanistic nature of these S-R models is clear from Hull's description of their purpose:

So far as the writer is able to see, there is no a priori impossibility of constructing a mechanism which will display genuine thinking ability. Indeed, it is expected with some confidence that such a mechanism will ultimately be constructed. (Hull, 1935, p. 220)

In this behavioristic view, cognitive processing results from long and complex chains of S-R associations, triggered by external stimuli and internal drives. The S-R associations are learned by conditioning. Over time, some of them "internalize" by means of feedback and internal stimulus-response (r-s or s-r) associations, forming complex S-R chains. Behavior at any moment results from a specific conjunction of external stimuli, feedback and internal drives.

Cognitive models of this kind seem to be very complex, and at the same time very fragile and limited. As formulated by Amsel and Rashotte:

While the papers [of Hull] are brilliant in many respects, for the modern reader they raise once again the nagging question of whether an analytical S-R account of complex behaviors is viable. ... The sheer number of individual associative bonds and the problem of quantifying their individual and combined momentary status to predict behavior is mind-boggling. (Amsel & Rashotte, 1984, p. 52-53)

Around 1960, doubts of this kind resulted in the emergence of "classical" cognitive psychology. Moreover, the associative learning principles involved were in doubt as well.

COGNITIVE MECHANISMS OF LEARNING

Conditioning seems to be a form of associative learning. In the view of behaviorism, the CS becomes associated with the UCR, which then becomes the CR. The form of association seems to be that of contiguity, as suggested by the early empiricists. In modern brain terminology, it fits well with Hebbian learning. Hebb (1949) proposed that when neurons are active simultaneously, they become interconnected ('neurons that fire together, wire together'). Because the CS is followed almost directly by the UCS, neurons encoding for the CS might still be (partially) active when the UCR is initiated by the UCS, so these neurons might wire together. After a while, the CS alone would suffice to initiate the UCR (making it the CR).

But doubts about this learning scheme arose even before the emergence of cognitive psychology. In the 1930s, Tolman conducted a series of experiments that showed that rats learn in a different manner as proposed by behaviorism. He used a maze as illustrated in Figure 2 (Tolman, 1948). The rat can take one of three routes (R1, R2 or R3) to go from the start (S) to the goal. After reaching the goal, the route taken is rewarded by food. So, in terms of behaviorism, the behavior of the rat is shaped by operant conditioning, based on reinforcement. Behavior shows that rats take the shorter route more frequently. So, the reward for R1 is stronger than the reward for R2, which in turn is stronger than the reward for R3. This determines the (descending) strength of association between S → R1, S → R2, and S → R3.

Figure 2. Maze use by Tolman to show that rats acquire a spatial map. R1, R2 and R3 are different routes from start (S) to the goal (food). The rats are first trained without any blocks. Then, Block A or Block B is applied. The purpose is to see which alternative route is taken

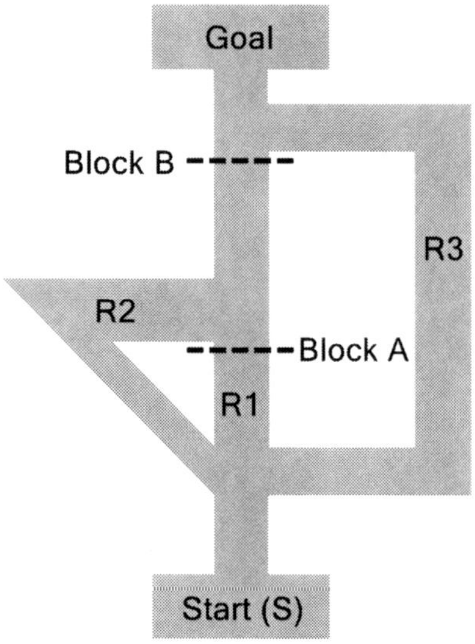

Based on that difference, one can predict what happens when a route is blocked. When block A is applied, rats should eventually take R2, because the association S → R1 is reduced (by extinction), so that the association S → R2 is now the strongest. When block B is applied, rats would first take R2 after extinction of S → R1. Only after extinction of S → R2 would they take R3. However, the rats took the shortest route in both occasions. So, with block A they took R2 straight away, and with block B they immediately took R3, without first taking R2. According to Tolman, this showed that the rats had learned a spatial (cognitive) map of the maze. Based on that map, they could take the shortest route for each block.

Furthermore, learning a spatial map did not depend on a reward. In one experiment, Tolman trained three groups of rats in a complex maze for a number of days. The first group had one trial in the maze each day, without any food reward at the goal of the maze. This group showed little improvement over time in reaching the goal. The second group also had one trail each day, but they received a food reward when they reached the goal. Their behavior improved considerably on a day by day basis. The third group was treated as the first for 10 days. After the 10th day, however, they were treated as the second group, receiving a food reward as they reached the goal. These rats improved dramatically in one day. On day 11, their behavior was as bad as that of group 1. But from day 12 onwards, their behavior was just as good as that of group 2, if not better. Tolman argued that the rats in group 3 (and group 1) had in fact learned the spatial map of the maze, in the same manner as the rats in group 2. But they did not show the explicit behavior of going to the goal, because there was no food there. So, learning can occur even if it is not explicit in the behavior. Tolman referred to this kind of learning as latent learning. The food reward had no effect on the learning process itself, as behaviorism assumed. Instead, it made the effect of learning become explicit in the behavior.

Cognitive View of Classical Conditioning

Tolman's experiments are directed against associative learning in the form of operant conditioning. According to behaviorism, including Hull, an organism would learn a route by a gradual process of conditioning, as illustrated in figure 1. Instead, rats and other animals (and humans) acquire a spatial map, which directs their movements, also when something changes in their environment.

Doubts have also raised about associative learning in the form of classical conditioning. In the version of behaviorism, classical conditioning results in an association between the CS and the CR. But, in fact, Pavlov (1927) had a different theory. In his view, the association produced by classical conditioning was that between the CS and the UCS. In turn, the UCS (activated by the CS) would produce the response. This view is more in line with the early empiricists, who also viewed learning as associations between ideas. In modern terms, these associations would arise between the representations of the CS and the USC. This is already a more cognitive version of association than the association between the CS and response advocated by behaviorism.

Experiments by Rescorla (1973) showed that the cognitive version is more likely. He conditioned rats using a load sound as the UCS. The sound produces a fear response (as in the case of little Albert), which is thus the UCR. The CS was a signal light. After conditioning, the rats showed the fear response (freezing) with the light stimulus only. Rescorla then habituated the fear response to the loud sound in half of the conditioned rats. Habituation results when, after a prolonged series of presenting load sounds, the rats no longer respond to the sound. Rescorla then tested the rats on the light stimulus (CS). If classical conditioning results from the association between the CS and the UCR (CR), then these rats would show the fear response with the light signal. But if classical conditioning results in an association between the CS and the UCS, then the light signal would not produce the fear response, because the UCS itself no longer produces this response. Rescorla's results supported the latter version of classical conditioning. After habituation, the fear response to the light signal (CS) was greatly reduced.

A number of experiments, with different animals, favors the version of classical conditioning in which the CS becomes associated with the UCS instead of the (U)CR (Anderson, 2000).

Classical Conditioning as Learned Expectancy

The CS → UCS association is more cognitive than the CS → UCR association, because it suggest an association between mental representations of the CS and UCS. But it can still be seen as an association as intended by the early empiricists. And it still fits the Hebbian learning scheme, in fact even better than the CS → UCR association. Because the CS and USC activate mental (neural) representations in sequence, these representations could be simultaneously active for a while, allowing Hebbian learning to occur.

However, a number of experiments have shown that this view is too simple. First, the timing of the sequence is very important. For classical conditioning to be effective, the CS has to (slightly) precede the UCS. Classical conditioning commonly does not occur when the CS and the USC are presented simultaneously, or when the UCS (slightly) precedes the CS. In terms of association or Hebbian learning, the order of presentation should make no difference. In fact, the strongest Hebbian learning should be expected when the CS and USC simultaneously activate their representations.

Furthermore, a stimulus can precede the UCS as a CS, but not result in conditioning. Conditioning also requires that the UCS is not presented without the CS. That is, if the UCS occurs both with and without the (preceding) CS, no conditioning occurs (Rescorla & Wagner, 1972). In terms of association or Hebbian learning, the absence of the CS on certain trials should have no effect on the association between the CS and the UCS. For this association to occur, the CS should always be followed by the UCS whenever the CS is presented. The presentation of the UCS without the CS should not have an effect. But it does.

Finally, a stimulus will not become a CS for a UCS when there is already a good CS for that UCS. This is a phenomenon known as blocking. Kamin (1969) showed that a second stimulus combined with a CS does not become a CS itself. In a more schematic presentation, blocking is found in the following procedure. First, a stimulus A (e.g., a sound) is trained to be the CS for an USC (e.g., a shock), which produces an UCR (+). After training, A alone results in the response related to the shock, that is A+ is learned. After that, A is combined with another stimulus B (e.g., a light) and the combination AB is trained until AB+ occurs (thus, AB has become a CS). What happens when A and B are presented alone? When A is presented, A+ occurs, as before. But when B is presented, noting happens, that is, B- occurs: B is not followed by the (U)CR. Apparently, the presentation of A in the combination AB has prevented B to become a CS. This is not what one would expect with association or Hebbian learning. The representation of B is simultaneously active with that of the USC, but does not become associated with it.

In retrospect, many of the differences between conditioning and association or Hebbian learning can be seen in Pavlov's original experiment. There were a lot of stimuli available that did not result in the salivation response. For example, the room in which the experiment occurred or the light in the room etc. For conditioning to occur, the CS has to have some kind of predictive value. After conditioning, the presentation of the CS should increase the expectancy that the UCS, and with it the UCR, will occur. This explains that when the UCS is simultaneous with the CS or even precedes the CS no conditioning occurs. The CS has no predictive value for the UCS in these cases. It also explains the blocking effect. When A already predicts the USC, B has no additional predictive value for the UCS when it is presented together with A. Therefore, the conditioning B+ does not occur.

Cognitive Effects on Conditioning

Associative learning in the form of Hebbian learning is not sufficient to account for the fact that the CS has to have a predictive value to obtain the CS → UCR pairing. Other forms of representation, perhaps of a more propositional nature (Mitchell, De Houwer & Lovibond, 2009), would be required instead. A number of experiments have shown that other cognitive factors influence conditioning, which makes conditioning an even more cognitive form of learning.

Attention, for example, has a clear effect on conditioning. Dawson (1970) and Dawson &

Biferno (1973) used an auditory perception masking task that required participants to answer several questions at the and of each trial concerning the pitch of a series of six tones. One tone (A) was paired with a shock (A+). Another tone (B) was never paired with shock (B-). Due to the masking task, subjects paid less attention to the tones. In particular, they were not aware of the difference between the tones in terms of their relation to the shock (one preceding the shock, the other not). The results showed that the tones failed to be distinguished as predictors of the shock. That is, they showed no difference in conditioning between A and B.

In a similar vein, De Houwer and Beckers (2003) studied the effect of attention (work load) on blocking. Normally, A+ prevents the learning of B+ when B is learned in the combination AB+. De Houwer and Beckers used a secondary task in the learning and test stage of AB+. They found that blocking in human contingency learning was less pronounced when the secondary task was demanding compared to an easy task. Thus, the increased demands of the secondary task also increased the B+ outcome. It seems that, due to the second task, subject were prevented from reasoning that B is redundant when it is presented in the context of A.

The fact that reasoning plays a role in conditioning was investigated by Shanks and Darby (1998). They presented A+, B+, AB-, C-, D-, CD+ trials together with I+, J+, M-, and N- trials. Thus, in an A+ or B+ trial, the A or the B stimulus is followed by an UCR, whereas in an AB- trial, the combination of the stimuli A and B is not followed by an UCR. Relations of that kind between stimuli and UCR apply to the other combinations as well. After learning, the subjects judged that the UCR was more likely to occur after the combination MN than after the combination IJ, even though these combinations were not used during learning. Apparently, subjects learned from the A+, B+, AB-, C-, D-, CD+ trials that the result of combinations of two stimuli (AB-, CD+) is the reverse of the result of the individual stimuli involved (A+, B+, C-, D-). On the basis of this observation, subjects reasoned that the same applied to the MN and IJ combinations.

An even more striking effect of cognition on conditioning results from the effect of verbal instructions on conditioning. Lovibond (2003) trained the combination AB+ (i.e., AB followed by an UCS that produces a shock as UCR) and then trained A- (A without the UCS that produces the UCR). The A- training increased the B+ response. That is, the (U)CR resulted from presenting B alone (even though B+ was not trained). This is a phenomenon known as release from overshadowing, which could result from reasoning. For example, the subject knows that the combination AB produces a shock and that A alone does not. So, the shock must be produced by B. However, Lovibond (2003) also found release from overshadowing when the AB+ and A- trials were described verbally, or when the AB+ trials were presented, but the A- trials were described verbally. So, verbally acquired knowledge and perceptual experience have the same effect on conditioning.

Based on this and other experimental evidence, Mitchell, De Houwer & Lovibond (2009) argued that associative learning, as found in conditioning, depends on high-level cognitive processes and result in propositional knowledge. Viewed in this way, learning as found in conditioning is not separated from other cognitive processes such as attention, memory and reasoning. Instead learning is the consequence of the combined operation of these processes. Conditioning is thus an inferential process. The CS becomes a predictor of the UCS, which allows the organism to avoid or seek the UCS, depending on the nature of the response produced by the UCS. The fact that conditional learning requires attention and cognitive resources such as memory, and that it is influenced by verbal instructions and reasoning processes supports this view.

VISUAL LEARNING

Conditioning has been studied extensively in psychology, but the neural mechanisms involved are not well known. Hebbian learning has been related to neural processes like long-term potentiation, by which the strength of neuronal synapses can be modified for a longer period of time. But, as we have seen, conditioning is not just Hebbian learning. Instead, it consists of a form of expectation, and it is influenced by cognitive factors like attention and language. Indeed, it could be a form of propositional learning, in which the organism learns that if the CS occurs, the CR is likely to follow. Unfortunately, the brain mechanisms of propositional learning as virtually unknown.

However, a topic for which the neural mechanisms are being investigated extensively is visual learning. This is, of course, related to the fact that much is known about the structure of the visual cortex, due to the availability of suitable animal models (e.g., Felleman & van Essen, 1991).

Visual learning can be studied in relation to its development. When the visual cortex develops, an organism will learn tasks like object recognition when the suitable visual environment is available. Interestingly, however, experience-based plasticity is also found in the adult visual system. In recent years many psychophysical studies have shown learning-dependent changes in adults related to the discrimination and recognition of visual stimuli. The stimuli for which learning is found vary from simple features, such as line orientations (Fahle, 2004), to complex visual objects (Fine & Jacobs, 2002).

Why would learning of visual information occur with adults? Of course, conditioning occurs with adults, and other forms of learning as well. But in the case of language, for example, learning a native language is usually restricted to childhood. The well known plasticity-stability dilemma may be a crucial factor in this respect. To learn, the brain needs to be plastic, allowing changes in connectivity and connection strength to occur. However, stability demands that previously learned knowledge is guarded against loss. Too much plasticity might result in loss of previously learned knowledge, but too much stability might result in inflexibility.

In the case of language, what is learned in childhood is the structure of the native language. This structure does not very much in a lifetime, so it is safe to guard the learned structure for loss by reducing plasticity. Furthermore, language itself provides a different way to learn about the word. Sentences provide information that can be stored as knowledge. This kind of learning, using language as an instrument, remains in adulthood.

But the visual environment could change, so the visual cortex has to be plastic enough to match these changes. At the same time, these changes will depend on the statistical regularities in the environment, which for the most part do not change rapidly, giving the system time to adjust. In this way, learning to respond selectively to an object (e.g., in discrimination of recognition) might consist of learning which simpler features are combined in the world in a statistically regular way. These elementary features, activating neurons at the lower level areas of the visual cortex, might be combined in higher level areas of the cortex, where neurons would learn to respond to specific combinations of these features. This kind of learning could be repeated at several levels of the hierarchy of the visual system, resulting in selectivity for progressively more complex preferred stimulus configurations.

A number of studies have investigated the way in which the visual cortex learns to identify visual information. The areas that support identification of visual information and object recognition are primarily localized in the so-called ventral visual stream (e.g., Felleman & van Essen, 1991). Figure 3 illustrates that the ventral stream consists of an hierarchy of cortical areas that begins in the primary visual cortex (area V1), and then runs through the areas V2 and V4 to the posterior inferior temporal cortex (PIT) and the anterior inferior temporal

Figure 3. Illustration of the main areas in the ventral stream of the visual cortex. V1 = visual area 1 (primary visual cortex), V2 = visual area 2, V4 = visual area 4, PIT = posterior inferior temporal cortex, AIT = anterior inferior temporal cortex, LOC = lateral occipital complex

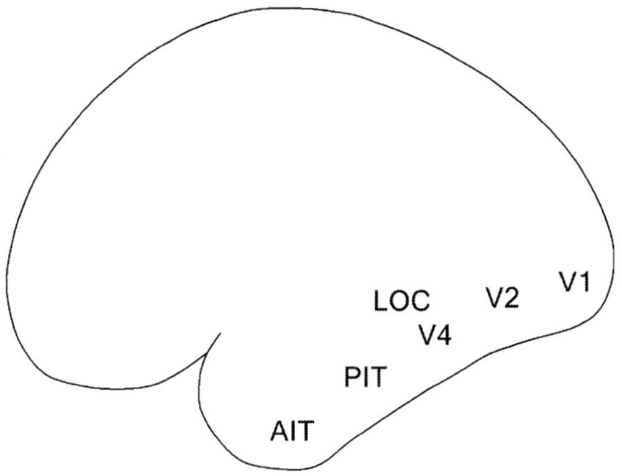

cortex (AIT). The highest stages of this stream (i.e., the anterior inferior temporal cortex in the monkey, and the lateral occipital complex (LOC) in the human) support object recognition directly, to the extent that object identity can be extracted from the patterns of neuronal activity in these areas (e.g., Quiroga et al., 2005; Grill-Spector). Learning effects have been demonstrated in each of these areas, ranging from V1 to inferior-temporal cortex or IT (PIT and AIT combined).

Given the nature of representation in V1 (oriented lines), learning in this area has been studied by training subjects specific line orientations. Furmanski, Schluppeck and Engel (2004) showed that behavioral performance in the discrimination of oblique orientation patterns improved through training, and fMRI responses in V1 increased for these orientations as well. This demonstrates a link between experience dependent behavioral improvement and neural plasticity in the primary visual cortex. Perceptual learning in the areas V1, V2 and V4 (the lower areas of the visual cortex) was investigated in monkey studies as well. Results showed that learning effects occur in each of these areas, in particular in area V4. Neurons in this area showed increased orientation selectivity and better population discrimination performance after training. (Ghose, Yang & Maunsell, 2002).

Due to the nature of representation in the areas from V1 to IT, object learning can be expected to occur in area IT. Research has shown that neurons in monkey IT cortex show enhanced selectivity after training for novel objects (Logethitis, Pauls, & Poggio, 1995; Kobatake, Wang & Tanaka, 1998). Furthermore, learning can influence the categorization of objects by modulating the selectivity of neurons in the inferior temporal cortex (and frontal cortex) for features that determine the specific classes to which novel objects belong (Rosenthal, Fusi & Hochstein, 2001; Sigala & Logothetis, 2002; Freedman et al., 2003).

For example, Freedman et al. (2005) found improved neural selectivity in IT related to enhanced performance in object learning in the context of a categorization task. These learning effects were specific to the trained object features. Moreover, they we also observed for objects to which the monkeys were passively exposed (next to the objects with which the monkeys were explicitly trained). This suggests that learning can occur with supervised training and with passive experience. In both cases, neural plasticity mechanisms can result in the modification (e.g., sharpening) of the underlying neural responses.

Complex shapes of objects could be seen as consisting of combinations of more elementary shapes (e.g., the shape of a bicycle includes that of circles as given by the wheels). So, learning complex shapes could begin by learning associations between shapes. Messinger et al. (2005) showed that some neurons in the inferotemporal cortex represent arbitrary associations between pairs of stimuli. These memorized associations represented in the inferior temporal cortex could be a precursor for the representation of complex shapes, perhaps represented in other brain areas, such as the prefrontal cortex.

A difference in representation between the ventral stream areas and the prefrontal cortex was observed by Rainer and Miller (2000) and Rayner, Lee and Logothetis (2004). They showed that when monkeys learn to discriminate noisy images of natural scenes, neurons in the lower areas of the ventral stream enhance the selective processing of the crucial features for the detection of object targets. Instead, the effect of learning for neurons in the prefrontal cortex appears to result in a facilitation of efficient object processing independent of noise. So, perhaps behavioural performance in discriminating degraded images after training is mediated by different neural plasticity mechanisms in lower visual areas (V4) and the prefrontal cortex (Rainer & Miller, 2000). Whereas stimulus degradation due to noise resulted in decreased responses of V4 neurons to novel images, learning enhanced their responses to degraded stimuli in that area. In contrast, the number of responding neurons in the prefrontal cortex decreased as images became familiar with training, whereas their object selectivity increased.

A difference in learning between lower and higher cortical areas could be related to the difference between bottom-up and top-down processing. Lower cortical areas are more directly influenced by visual experience, so learning in these areas could be more experience driven (bottom-up). In contrast, learning in higher areas could be more driven by expectancy (top-down). The difference between bottom-up and top-down is important for visual search tasks. In a visual search task, a subject has to find (e.g., locate or identify) a target object in a display. The display could consist of the target with a number of distractors, or of the distractors alone (target absent trials). For example, the target could be a horizontal line and the distractors could be vertical lines. The question is whether the detection of the target, as given by the reaction time, is influenced by the presence of the distractors, in particular by the number of the distractors. If the number of the distractors has no effect, search is efficient. If, instead, the increase in the number of distractors slows down the reaction time for the target, the search is inefficient.

Sigman et al. (2005) investigated learning in a visual search task. Initially, a visual search task could be inefficient, but due to learning it could become efficient, because the target and the distractors become familiar. Sigman et al. found a large-scale reorganization in cortical networks due to learning a visual search task. Learning to detect a target among distractors resulted in increased activations in retinotopic (lower) areas of the ventral stream. In contrast, decreased activations were observed in the higher cortical areas of the ventral stream that are involved in shape analysis and in the frontal and parietal areas that are involved in attentional processing. So, perhaps learning shifts shape representation from higher to the lower visual areas, because the lower areas support efficient search and detection of objects in cluttered scenes independently of attentional control.

These results are consistent with the notion that learning could begin at higher stages of visual analysis and proceed in a top-down manner to earlier stages when finer analysis of the stimulus is necessary (Ahissar & Hochstein, 2004). In the case of visual search, learning could affect object representations by enhancing the processing of feature detectors with increasing complexity in a bottom-up manner and by taking into account the relevant task dimensions and demands in a top-down manner.

In this way, learning in different cortical areas supports functions that are important for different tasks, ranging from the bottom-up detection and integration of target features in visual scenes in the areas of the ventral stream to the top-down selection of familiar objects in the prefrontal cortex. In line with this view, neuroimaging studies (Dolan et al., 1997; Buchel, Coull & Friston, 1999; McIntosh, Rajah & Lobaugh, 1999) suggest that learning might enhance the functional interactions between the areas of the ventral stream that encode bottom-up stimulus experiences and the parieto-frontal circuits that encode expectations and interpretations.

Besides object identification, invariance is very important in visual processing. Objects frequently change due to difference in position, distance or pose. Selective object representations must be tolerant to these changes, also after learning. However, Cox et al. (2005) found that perhaps the most fundamental type of invariance, the ability to identify an object irrespective of its position, can be modified by visual experience. Under normal conditions, the same object is seen at different positions across short time intervals due to rapid eye movements that result from exploring the visual world. To test the idea that this experience might underlie the position tolerance of recognition, undetected changes in object identity were introduced during eye movements. Due to this manipulation, the position tolerance (invariance) of object recognition was disrupted in healthy adult observers. So, when the identity of an object is changed during normal eye movements that bring the object from one retinal position to another over short time intervals, later recognition of the object across those same retinal positions is disrupted. This shows that position tolerance is plastic even in adults. Apparently, this fundamental property of primate object recognition has to be maintained by natural visual experience throughout the life span.

In conclusion, visual learning occurs in adult life as well. Learning occurs in virtually all visual areas, but the kind of learning seems to be task dependent. The continued plasticity of the brain, and the combination of bottom-up and top-down effects of learning suggest that the brain is moulded by experience and expectation throughout life.

FUTURE RESEARCH DIRECTIONS

Visual learning shows that the brain is plastic throughout life. Of course, brain plasticity is needed to account for the effects of conditioning as well. The question arises what the neural mechanisms are that sustain conditioning. The fact that associations between visual shapes can be learned in the inferotemporal area of the visual cortex suggests that associations could be learned in higher brain areas as well. But, as noted above, conditioning is already more complex than pure associative learning. It seems to depend on an expectancy that the CS produces the CR, resulting from a kind of propositional learning (learning the proposition "If CS than CR").

Propositional learning is at the heart of other cognitive abilities as well, such as language and reasoning. The mechanisms by which these abilities can be learned are an important topic for future research. The relation with conditioning could provide information about how propositional learning could proceed.

In a different chapter in this volume, I argue and illustrate that human cognition results from a combination of (at least) three important factors: dynamics, productivity and grounding. Propositional learning is at the basis of productivity. Grounding and dynamics refer to the nature of the representations involved. Instead of symbolic (or numerical) representations that can be copied and pasted to create combinatorial structures like propositions, grounded representations remain "in situ". That is they cannot be copied and pasted, because that would destroy the grounded nature of these representations.

Yet, combinatorial structures can be created with grounded representations by embedding them in blackboard architectures. In these architectures temporal connections between grounded representations can be created, in agreement with the combinatorial structure needed. Different blackboard architectures are needed to obtain different forms of combinatorial structures. A basic one is an architecture that provides the ability to represent sequential information. Other architectures, such as the ones for language or reasoning allow the creation and manipulation of more elaborate hierarchical structures.

Perhaps conditioning is the kind of learning that occurs in a sequential blackboard, that allows elementary propositions of the form "If A than B" to be created and learned. The fact that conditioning is found in animals is in agreement with this view. Animals lack language and complex forms of reasoning, so the more complex blackboards for these forms of cognition will be missing in animals. But a basic blackboard that allows sequential patterns of representations to be created could exist in animal as well.

Even more so, because grounded cognition is closely related to motor behavior. Motor planning is grounded because muscles cannot be copied and pasted like symbols. Yet, animals are clearly capable of performing and learning complex motion patterns. So, the neural mechanisms to create these patterns are available in animals. These neural mechanisms could form the basis for the development of blackboard architectures for sequential processing of representations, which in turn could form the basis for more complex blackboards for language and reasoning. Thus, studying the mechanisms by which grounded complex sequential (motor) patterns can be learned and executed could be the basis for understanding the learning mechanisms of more complex forms of cognitive processing as well.

CONCLUSION

Learning is at the heart of intelligence. In this chapter, I reviewed research into two important domains of learning, consisting of visual cognition and conditioning.

Learning in visual cognition shows that brain plasticity continues in adult life. The learning effects in visual cognition, such as fact that even position invariance of object recognition can be affected by learning in adulthood, suggest that brain structures are continuously moulded by experience and expectancy.

At first conditioning seemed to consist of a form of associative learning, in line with the learning mechanisms proposed by the early empiricist. To date, conditioning is still one of the most studied learning phenomena in psychology. Over time, this research has shown that conditioning is a highly cognitive form of learning, quite unlike the basic form of associative learning it seemed to be. Conditioning succeeds when it creates an expectancy that the conditioned stimulus will be followed by the conditioned response. This expectancy seems to depend on propositional forms of learning, in the form of learning "If CS, then CR". This view about conditioning is enhanced by the fact that conditioning is influenced by cognitive factors like attention and (in humans) by language.

The fact that conditioning could be a form of propositional learning is interesting, because it entails that the study of the mechanisms of conditioning could provide a basis for the study of the mechanisms of other, more elaborate, forms of propositional learning, as found in language and reasoning.

REFERENCES

Ahissar, M., & Hochstein, S. (2004). The reverse hierarchy theory of visual perceptual learning. *Trends in Cognitive Sciences*, *8*, 457–464. doi:10.1016/j.tics.2004.08.011

Amsel, A., & Rashotte, M. E. (1984). *Mechanisms of adaptive behavior: Clark Hull's theoretical papers, with commentary*. New York: Columbia University Press.

Anderson, J. R. (2000). *Learning and memory* (2nd ed.). New York: Wiley.

Boring, E. G. (1950). *A history of experimental psychology* (2nd ed.). New York: Appleton-Century-Crofts.

Buchel, C., Coull, J. T., & Friston, K. J. (1999). The predictive value of changes in effective connectivity for human learning. *Science*, *283*, 1538–1541. doi:10.1126/science.283.5407.1538

Cox, D. D., Meier, P., Oertelt, N., & DiCarlo, J. J. (2005). 'Breaking' position invariant object recognition. *Nature Neuroscience*, *8*, 1145–1147. doi:10.1038/nn1519

Dawson, M. E. (1970). Cognition and conditioning: Effects of masking the CS-UCS contingency on human GSR classical conditioning. *Journal of Experimental Psychology*, *85*, 389–396. doi:10.1037/h0029715

Dawson, M. E., & Biferno, M. A. (1973). Concurrent measurement of awareness and electrodermal classical conditioning. *Journal of Experimental Psychology*, *101*, 55–62. doi:10.1037/h0035524

De Houwer, J., & Beckers, T. (2003). Secondary task difficulty modulates forward blocking in human contingency learning. *Quarterly Journal of Experimental Psychology*, *56B*, 345–357.

Dolan, R. J., Fink, G. R., Rolls, E., Booth, M., Holmes, A., Frackowiak, R. S., & Friston, K. J. (1997). How the brain learns to see objects and faces in an impoverished context. *Nature*, *389*, 596–599. doi:10.1038/39309

Fahle, M. (2004). Perceptual learning: a case for early selection. *Journal of Vision (Charlottesville, Va.)*, *4*, 879–890. doi:10.1167/4.10.4

Felleman, D. J., & van Essen, D. C. (1991). Distributed hierarchical processing in the primate cerebral cortex. *Cerebral Cortex*, *1*, 1–47. doi:10.1093/cercor/1.1.1-a

Fine, I., & Jacobs, R. A. (2002). Comparing perceptual learning tasks: a review. *Journal of Vision (Charlottesville, Va.)*, *2*, 190–203. doi:10.1167/2.2.5

Freedman, D. J., Riesenhuber, M., Poggio, T., & Miller, E. K. (2003). A comparison of primate prefrontal and inferior temporal cortices during visual categorization. *The Journal of Neuroscience*, *23*, 5235–5246.

Freedman, D. J., Riesenhuber, M., Poggio, T., & Miller, E. K. (2006). Experience dependent sharpening of visual shape selectivity in inferior temporal cortex. *Cerebral Cortex*, *16*, 1631–1644. doi:10.1093/cercor/bhj100

Furmanski, C. S., Schluppeck, D., & Engel, S. A. (2004). Learning strengthens the response of primary visual cortex to simple patterns. *Current Biology*, *14*, 573–578. doi:10.1016/j.cub.2004.03.032

Ghose, G. M., Yang, T., & Maunsell, J. H. (2002). Physiological correlates of perceptual learning in monkey V1 and V2. *Journal of Neurophysiology*, *87*, 1867–1888.

Grill-Spector, K., & Malach, R. (2004). The human visual cortex. *Annual Review of Neuroscience*, *27*, 649–677. doi:10.1146/annurev.neuro.27.070203.144220

Hebb, D. O. (1949). *The organisation of behaviour*. New York: Wiley.

Hull, C. L. (1930). Knowledge and purpose as habit mechanisms. *Psychological Review*, *37*, 511–525. doi:10.1037/h0072212

Hull, C. L. (1935). The mechanism of the assembly of behavior segments in novel combinations suitable for problem solution. [Reprinted in Amsel, A. & Rashotte, M. E., 1984.]. *Psychological Review*, *42*, 219–245. doi:10.1037/h0063473

Kamin, L. J. (1969). Predictability, surprise attention and conditioning. In B. A.Campbell & R. M. Church (Eds.), *Punishment and aversive behavior* (pp. 279-296). NewYork: Appleton-Century – Crofts.

Kobatake, E., Wang, G., & Tanaka, K. (1998). Effects of shape-discrimination training on the selectivity of inferotemporal cells in adult monkeys. *Journal of Neurophysiology*, *87*, 324–330.

Logothetis, N. K., Pauls, J., & Poggio, T. (1995). Shape representation in the inferior temporal cortex of monkeys. *Current Biology*, *5*, 552–563. doi:10.1016/S0960-9822(95)00108-4

Lovibond, P. F. (2003). Causal beliefs and conditioned responses: Retrospective revaluation induced by experience and by instruction. *Journal of Experimental Psychology. Learning, Memory, and Cognition*, *29*, 97–106. doi:10.1037/0278-7393.29.1.97

McIntosh, A. R., Rajah, M. N., & Lobaugh, N. J. (1999). Interactions of prefrontal cortex in relation to awareness in sensory learning. *Science*, *284*, 1531–1533. doi:10.1126/science.284.5419.1531

Messinger, A., Squire, L. R., Zola, S. M., & Albright, T. D. (2005). Neural correlates of knowledge: stable representation of stimulus associations across variations in behavioral performance. *Neuron*, *48*, 359–371. doi:10.1016/j.neuron.2005.08.035

Mitchell, C. J., De Houwer, J., & Lovibond, P. F. (2009). The propositional nature of human associative learning. *The Behavioral and Brain Sciences*, *32*, 183–198. doi:10.1017/S0140525X09000855

Pavlov, I. (1927). *Conditioned Reflexes: (1927)*. New York, NY, US: Oxford University Press.

Quiroga, R. Q., Reddy, L., Kreiman, G., Koch, C., & Fried, I. (2005). Invariant visual representation by single neurons in the human brain. *Nature*, *435*, 1102–1107. doi:10.1038/nature03687

Rainer, G., Lee, H., & Logothetis, N. K. (2004). The effect of learning on the function of monkey extrastriate visual cortex. *PLoS Biology*, *2*, E44. doi:10.1371/journal.pbio.0020044

Rainer, G., & Miller, E. K. (2000). Effects of visual experience on the representation of objects in the prefrontal cortex. *Neuron*, *27*, 179–189. doi:10.1016/S0896-6273(00)00019-2

Rescorla, R. A. (1973). Effect of US habituation following conditioning. *Journal of Comparative and Physiological Psychology*, *82*, 137–143. doi:10.1037/h0033815

Rescorla, R. A., & Wagner, A. R. (1972). A theory of Pavlovian conditioning: Variations in the effectiveness of reinforcement and non-reinforcement. In Black, A. H., & Prokasy, W. F. (Eds.), *Classical Conditioning II*. New York: Appleton-Century-Crofts.

Rosenthal, O., Fusi, S., & Hochstein, S. (2001). Forming classes by stimulus frequency: behavior and theory. *Proceedings of the National Academy of Sciences of the United States of America*, *98*, 4265–4270. doi:10.1073/pnas.071525998

Shanks, D. R., & Darby, R. J. (1998). Feature- and rule-based generalization in human associative learning. *Journal of Experimental Psychology. Animal Behavior Processes*, *24*, 405–415. doi:10.1037/0097-7403.24.4.405

Sigala, N., & Logothetis, N. K. (2002). Visual categorization shapes feature selectivity in the primate temporal cortex. *Nature*, *415*, 318–320. doi:10.1038/415318a

Sigman, M., Pan, H., Yang, Y., Stern, E., Silbersweig, D., & Gilbert, C. D. (2005). Topdown reorganization of activity in the visual pathway after learning a shape identification task. *Neuron*, *46*, 823–835. doi:10.1016/j.neuron.2005.05.014

Tolman, E. C. (1948). Cognitive maps in rats and men. *Psychological Review, 55,* 189-208.
Watson, J. B., & Rayner, R. (1920). Conditioned emotional reactions. *Journal of Experimental Psychology*, *3*, 1–14.

Yang, T., & Maunsell, J. H. (2004). The effect of perceptual learning on neuronal responses in monkey visual area V4. *The Journal of Neuroscience, 24*, 1617–1626. doi:10.1523/JNEUROSCI.4442-03.2004

ADDITIONAL READING

Barlow, H. (1990). Conditions for versatile learning, Helmholtz's unconscious inference, and the task of perception. *Vision Research, 30*, 1561–1571. doi:10.1016/0042-6989(90)90144-A

Brady, M. J., & Kersten, D. (2003). Bootstrapped learning of novel objects. *Journal of Vision (Charlottesville, Va.), 3*, 413–422. doi:10.1167/3.6.2

Dickinson, A. (1980). *Contemporary animal learning theory*. Cambridge: Cambridge, University Press.

Evans, J. St. B. T. (2003). In two minds: Dual process accounts of reasoning. *Trends in Cognitive Sciences, 7*, 454–459. doi:10.1016/j.tics.2003.08.012

Fodor, J. A. (2003). *Hume variations*. Oxford, UK: Clarendon Press.

Gardner, H. (1985). *The mind's new science: A history of the cognitive revolution*. New York, NY, US: Basic Books.

Ghose, G. M., Yang, T., & Maunsell, J. H. (2002). Physiological correlates of perceptual learning in monkey V1 and V2. *Journal of Neurophysiology, 87*, 1867–1888.

Gilbert, C. D., Sigman, M., & Crist, R. E. (2001). The neural basis of perceptual learning. *Neuron, 31*, 681–697. doi:10.1016/S0896-6273(01)00424-X

Holland, P. C. (1990). Event representation in Pavlovian conditioning: Image and action. *Cognition, 37*, 105–131. doi:10.1016/0010-0277(90)90020-K

Hung, C. P., Kreiman, G., Poggio, T., & DiCarlo, J. J. (2005). Fast readout of object identity from macaque inferior temporal cortex. *Science, 310*, 863–866. doi:10.1126/science.1117593

Johnson-Laird, P. N. (1983). *Mental Models*. Cambridge: Cambridge University Press.

Le Doux, J. E. (2000). Emotion circuits in the brain. *Annual Review of Neuroscience, 23*, 155–184. doi:10.1146/annurev.neuro.23.1.155

Li, W., Piech, V., & Gilbert, C. D. (2004). Perceptual learning and top-down influences in primary visual cortex. *Nature Neuroscience, 7*, 651–657. doi:10.1038/nn1255

Pearce, J. M. (1987). A model for stimulus generalization in Pavlovian conditioning. *Psychological Review, 94*, 61–73. doi:10.1037/0033-295X.94.1.61

Sagi, D., & Tanne, D. (1994). Perceptual learning: learning to see. *Current Opinion in Neurobiology, 4*, 195–199. doi:10.1016/0959-4388(94)90072-8

Schacter, D. L. (1987). Implicit memory: History and current status. *Journal of Experimental Psychology. Learning, Memory, and Cognition, 13*, 501–518. doi:10.1037/0278-7393.13.3.501

Seligman, M., & Johnston, J. (1973). A cognitive theory of avoidance learning. In McGuigan, F. J., & Lumsden, D. B. (Eds.), *Contemporary approaches to conditioning and learning* (pp. 69–110). Washington: Winston.

Sigala, N., & Logothetis, N. K. (2002). Visual categorization shapes feature selectivity in the primate temporal cortex. *Nature, 415*, 318–320. doi:10.1038/415318a

Sigman, M., & Gilbert, C. D. (2000). Learning to find a shape. *Nature Neuroscience*, *3*, 264–269. doi:10.1038/72979

Sloman, S. A. (1996). The empirical case for two systems of reasoning. *Psychological Bulletin*, *119*, 3–22. doi:10.1037/0033-2909.119.1.3

Stanovich, K. E. (1999). *Who is rational? Studies of individual differences in reasoning*. Mahwah, NJ: Lawrence Erlbaum Associates, Inc.

Thompson, R. F. (2005). In search of memory traces. *Annual Review of Psychology*, *56*, 1–23. doi:10.1146/annurev.psych.56.091103.070239

Wagner, A. R., & Brandon, S. E. (1989). Evolution of a structured connectionist model of Pavlovian conditioning (AESOP). In Klein, S. B., & Mowrer, R. R. (Eds.), *Contemporary Learning Theories: Pavlovian conditioning and the status of traditional learning theory* (pp. 149–189). Hillsdale, NJ: Lawrence Erlbaum Associates.

Wang, G., Obama, S., Yamashita, W., Sugihara, T., & Tanaka, K. (2005). Prior experience of rotation is not required for recognizing objects seen from different angles. *Nature Neuroscience*, *8*, 1768–1775. doi:10.1038/nn1600

Chapter 4
Biologically-Inspired Learning: An Overview and Application to Odor Recognition

Turgay Temel
Bahcesehir University, Istanbul, Turkey

ABSTRACT

A general overview of biologically-inspired learning in the paradigm of artificial neural systems is described. In order to have the reader become familiar with fundamentals underlying this paradigm, a substantial and concise hierarchical background from neurophysiology to neuro-computational models is provided with as much clarity as possible. As an application of a well-known artificial neural network algorithm called feed-forward multi-layer perceptron with back-propagation training algorithm is utilized in implementation of an artificial olfactory system also called electronic nose. For improved classification performance, an algorithm as a preprocessing called linear-discriminant analysis is adapted to chosen neural architecture. The main purpose of the preprocessing stage is to lend better scattered input patterns for classes in the feature space compared to that without preprocessing. The performance improvement is also investigated in terms convergence rate, i.e. the number of iteration, given a number of layers, and recalling or generalization capability of the classifier.

INTRODUCTION

An ANN is an information processing paradigm that is inspired by the way biological nervous system, mainly human and primates, process sensory information. It is proposed in that environmental information in biological central nervous system (CNS) undergoes three processing stages as shown in Figure 1, (Arbib, 2003; Haykin, 2003; Dayan, & Abbot, 2001).

1. Conversion into *encoded* electrical signals by the sensory systems, e.g. auditory, vision etc, and transmission to central nervous system, mainly the brain, through forward links,
2. Generation of motor commands through both internal and external feedback lines for verification,
3. Supervision of the motor organs given motor commands.

DOI: 10.4018/978-1-60960-018-1.ch004

Figure 1. Block diagram of the nervous system and the information flow through the links

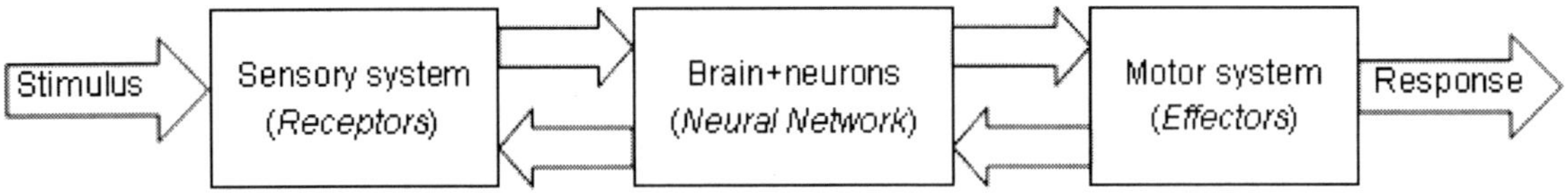

The brain is the main information processor and it is mostly represented as a neural network. It receives and evaluates the coded sensory impulses continuously for appropriately decision-making based on comparison to stored information. The outcome of the processing by the brain is the commands to motor organs, called *effectors*, through forward links. The main function of the effectors is to convert coded electrical impulses coming from the brain into distinct system output responses. During this processing, central nervous system also supervises motor organs by feedback lines. It is seen that the operation which is performed by nervous system exhibits similarity to a closed-loop control system, (Potter, 2007).

It has been known for long that the processing of sensory information is performed by the *associated unit*(s) in the brain in parallel by enormous number nerve cells called *neuron*, (Sherrington, 1933). The the brain is composed of 10^{14} connections (synapses) shared by 10^{11} neurons. Therefore, each neuron carries and process approximately 1200 incoming information. This is the main reason of enormous processing speed by biological systems despite almost 10^{7} times lower speed in signal transmission per connection compared to its silicon counterpart. Such a huge parallel architecture has evolved while developing natural features for respective sensory and motor system patterns. Nevertheless it is still not completely known which selective features are employed and how they are formed even for the best-known sensory perception mechanisms, such as visual and audio, (Guyon, & Elisseeff, 2003).

Contrary to natural processing carried out by nervous system, however, processing with sequential computer systems solely relies upon predefined algorithms and modeled stimuli so as to reproduce a desired pattern flow. Due to sequential nature, the latter conjugates best suitable algorithm, if possible, only if it is available among others. Despite many scientific, and mathematical tasks including numerical problem solving; database management; computer graphics, there are many problems unsolvable by such systems including sensing, perception and most automated recognition of objects, (Porto, & Pazos, 2006).

Inspired by the operational capability of biological information processing, it is desirable to mimic such systems with closest performance to real counterparts. Developing biologically-inspired systems poses a need for modeling the physical and functional understanding of the relationships between input and output quantities. Therefore, at elementary level, it is customary to elucidate and pass through the biology and physics and interrelate both so as to attain the furthest possible scenario for applying it to real-world problems.

Although not much has revealed about activities inside the brain, there has been enough experimental evidence which complies with even presumed models, which can be attributed to artificial neural network (ANN). However, as it will be seen almost all details are hidden within the physiology of individual neurons in terms of incoming and outgoing information flow. In the following sections, we will present a general overview of biological structure and physiological functioning to understand happenings inside the brain and as an introduction to construction of ANN systems.

Figure 2. Physical and some of the functional units of the brain, e.g. Vernicke's area is involved in the understanding of written and spoken language while Broca's area processes speech and language information, Web: Brain of violinsts, http://www.joansviolinlessons.com/a_brain.html

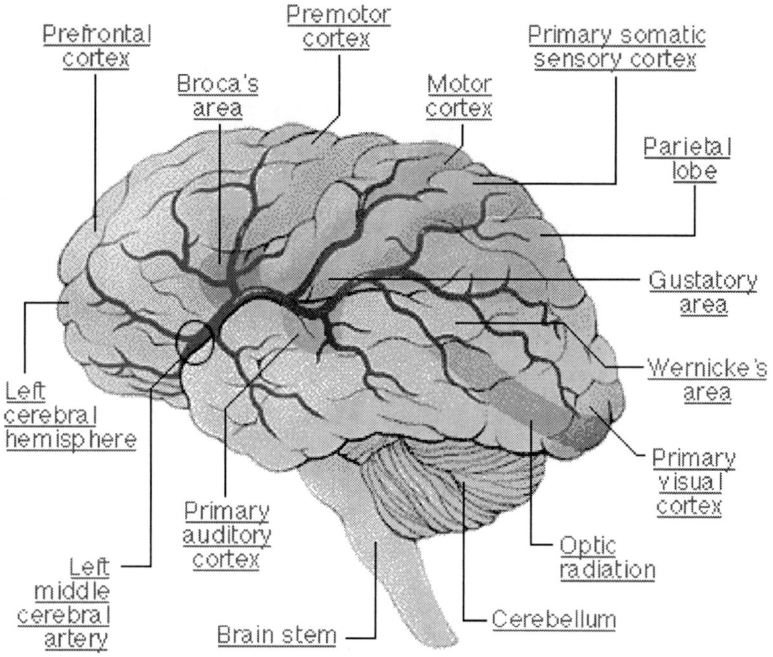

BIOLOGICAL NEURAL NETWORKS

Hierarchical Organization with Elementary Neurophysiology

A large number of researches on the brain reveal that the brain has compartmental structure with each compartment functioning at different level on incoming sensory stimuli patterns, (Kolb, & Whishaw, 2008). This structure is composed of interconnected systems which interact in specific hierarchy with different functionality: For example the *cortex* resides on the highest complexity and deals with cognition and reasoning while the *brainstem* is on the bottom which performs on reflexive stimuli, Figure 2.

Aside from the view of system organization, functional organization of the brain can also be viewed in both hierarchical and topological mapping (Roy, Steinmetz, et al. 2007; Kreiman, 2004). In *behavioral level* which is the uppermost in the brain hierarchy, whole brain represents cognition, thinking, conscious and reasoning. At the second level is the *topographic maps* by which behavioral level stimuli are handled by interconnected and/or overlapped brain compartments, e.g. cortices etc. Beneath the topographic maps is the neuron circuitry each locally processing stimulus. The neuron and its *dendritic subunits* lie beneath the local circuitries. Dendritic subunits are followed by the *neural microstructure* with varying functionalities along with *synapses*. The lowest level is occupied by *synaptic junctions* where nerve cells transmit/receive signals from one to another.

It should be noted that the brain is in fact a network of neurons. Within this network is an aggregation of stimuli-dependent chemical and structural changes in neurons, which is the basis of memory formation. Therefore, a thorough com-

Figure 3. A single neuron and a neural network. Web: Neuroscience for kids, http://faculty.washington.edu/chudler/calpyr.html

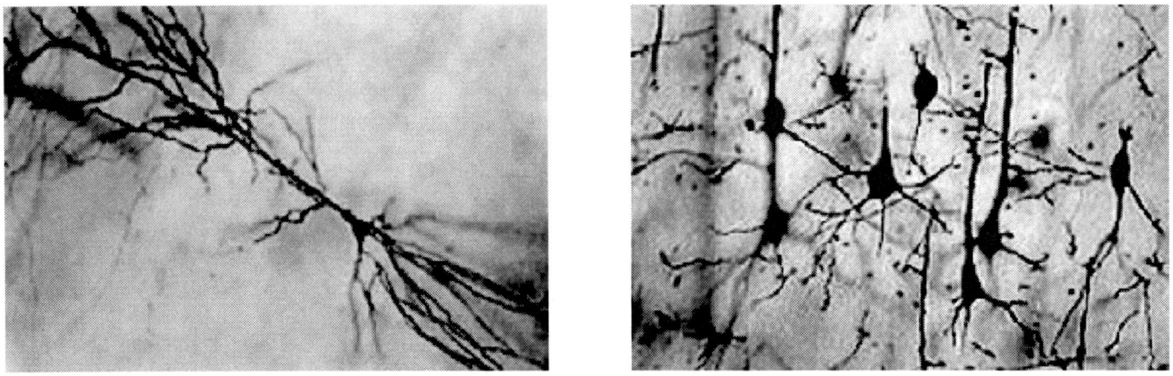

prehension of overall functionality of the nervous system involves familiarity with physiology of the neuron which exhibits diversity in shape and size as shown in Figure 3.

Figure 4 shows a simplified schematic diagram of *generic neuron* with its main components labeled as *cell body* also called *soma, axon, dendrit*es. The intracellular plasma is separated from the external fluid by a *membrane*. The variation in permeability of the membrane to certain ion types, such as Na+, K+ and Cl- is the key for converting sensory stimuli into electrical impulses as will be discussed in more detail later. The electrical branch called the axon is covered with *myelin sheath* layers intercepted at *Ranvier nodes*. The myelin sheath is electrically insulates the axon or the neuron membrane while Ranvier nodes act as channels for ion transfer (Ariniello, McComb, 2002).

The soma is the main processing unit of the neuron with its nucleus which accommodates the genetic material. Besides providing energy to the neuron whole, the soma integrates and modulates the impulses coming from other neurons through the dendrites. The dendrites are the receptors of the neuron for the electrical signals coming from other cells or neurons.

Synapses and Synaptic Junction

Neurons both cooperate and compete with each other in regulating the overall state of the neural system. Chemical signals received by the dendrites from the axon of a neuron that contact them are transformed into electrical signals. Connections to a neuron from other neurons occur at various locations on the cell that are known as synapses. The axon operates like a transmission line which conveys the signal generated by soma to the synaptic end terminal of the cell. The decision about whether to pass an electrical signal to elsewhere or not is determined by the aggregated effect of signals incoming from other synapses.

The brain contains large number of diversities in shape and size of neurons and synaptic junctions between neurons, (Ariniello, McComb, 2002). Figure 5 shows *neurotransmissional interaction* between *presynaptic* and *postsynaptic* neurons at a synapse. At the synapse, the preysnaptic neuron liberates chemical substances called *neurotransmitters* through its axon, which then diffuses across the synaptic cleft. At the other side of the junction the postsynaptic neuron absorbs or receives the diffused neurotransmitters through receptors located within its dendrites. Chemical action of

Figure 4. The principal structures of a typical nerve cell. Web: http://www.web-books.com/eLibrary/Medicine/Physiology/Nervous

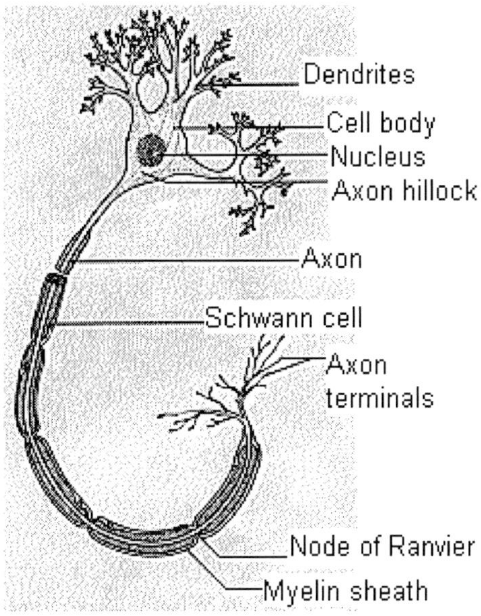

Figure 5. Neurotransmission at a synaptic junction between presynaptic and postsynaptic neurons. Adapted from Web: http://scienceblogs.com/purepedantry/upload/2007/03

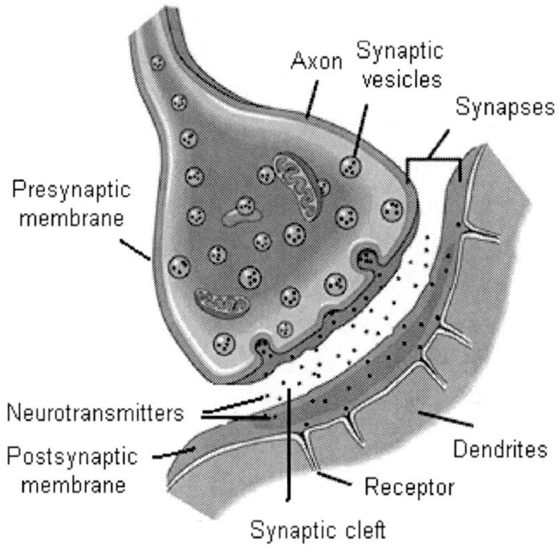

neurotransmitters absorbed by the postsynaptic neuron membrane changes the permeability of the membrane at postsynaptic membrane for particular ions. The synaptic interaction can be of excitatory or inhibitory effect on the receptive neuron. The postsynaptic cell converts the chemical signal back into an action potential which then propagates to other neurons of the neural system.

An important notion with synapses is the *synaptic strength* or *plasticity*: The ability to learn and form memories, things, because of the ability of neurons to change the way in which they communicate with each other. How synaptic plasticity and learning and memory are linked to each other is still not well known. It is believed that synapses that are active and actively changing are kept, the rest are *pruned*. The post-synaptic response to stimulation, i.e. synaptic strength or synaptic weight can be modulated for hundreds of milliseconds, which is called *short-term memory* (STM) or for the long term hours, days or even weeks or *long-term memory* (LTM). Synaptic strength can be varied by altering the amount of post-synaptic depolarization by changing response of receptors to varied time-length they are active, the number of receptors or the amount of L-glutamate liberated into the synaptic cleft, (Riedel, Platt, & Micheau, 2003; Alberini, Milekic, & Tronel, 2006).

Resting and Input Potentials

With no external excitation, the potential of the intracellular fluid of the membrane is about -70 mV relative to that of the extracellular. In this case the cell membrane is said to be polarized with *resting potential* with respect to the extracellular fluid taken as 0 V. Across the membrane, the potential gradient is maintained by special ion channels called *ion pumps*. For example, the concentration of $Na+$ outside the membrane is higher than that of the inside while the inverse holds for $K+$. Under the resting, flow of ions is mainly due to both voltage and concentration gradients across the membrane. Hence any current flow out/into the cell changes the polarity, i.e. making the membrane more negative (or positive), which is termed *hyperpolarization /inhibitory* effect (or *depolarization/excitatory* effect) on the resting potential. For example, an influx of positive ion species into the cell will depolarizes the membrane, which is an excitatory effect. Similarly influx of negative ions causes hyperpolarization, which is an inhibitory effect. However, both effects are local and they spanning a short distance into the cell body, which are aggregated at the *axon hillock*. If the aggregation of an ion flow depolarizes the membrane with greater value than a *threshold*, an internal positive feedback is initiated and an *action potential* is triggered. Action potential is a fluctuation of about 100 mV, across the membrane, Figure 6, (Perelman, & Ginosar, 2008).

The ion flow is not the only reason for action potential to be fired. Due to protein processing inside, the recent firing history of the cell is also another factor for refiring. However, in a few milliseconds just after a cell has fired, which is called the *absolute refractory period*, almost no action potential would be expected. For a time period of tens of milliseconds after firing called the *relative refractory period* it is more difficult to stimulate an action potential, (Furber, & Temple, 2007).

Excitation Propagation

Application of an action potential changes the voltage difference between the intracellular and extracellular surface of the membrane. The influx of positive Na+ ions drives the positive ions down the axon. The charge displacement near the membrane is compensated by outside Na+ ions, and so on, which causes excitation impulse to propagate along the axon.

As the impulse propagates it meets disruption along the membrane whose conductivity varies sharply at the Ranvier nodes. Since the myelin sheath is an insulator with varying thickness at

Figure 6. Action potential variation with time. Adapted from Web: http://content.answers.com/main/content/img/oxford/Oxford_Sports/0199210896.action-potential

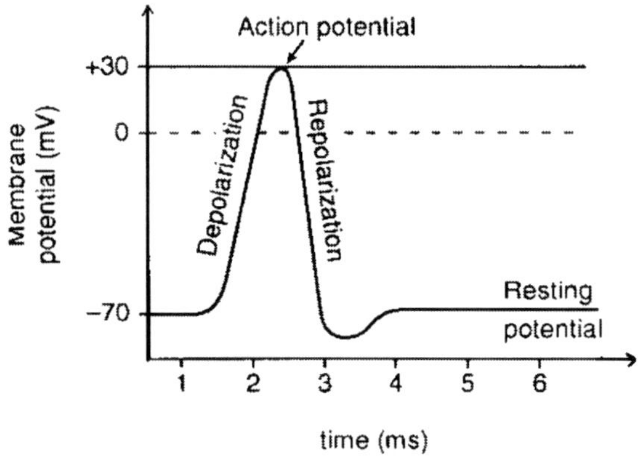

Ranvier nodes, the impulse is not stored and its speed increases from 0.5-2 m/s in unmyelinated section to around 100 m/s in myelinated nerve fiber. This propagation is called *saltatory propagation*. As illustrated in Figure 4 a neuron axon is covered with a *myelin sheath* and the nodes of Ranvier nodes at which the propagation of the action potential is re-excited and restored along the fiber for a short time of about 1 ms, (Perelman, & Ginosar, 2008).

When the propagating impulse arrives at the presynaptic synapse, the permeability change leads K+ ions to influx. These ions bond the vesicles containing the neurotransmitters and the presynaptic membrane for release of neurotransmitters into the synaptic cleft.

The Hodgkin-Huxley model given by (Hodgkin, & Huxley, 1952) quantitatively accounts for the mechanism of neuronal membrane voltage dynamic. The model considers the membrane permeability for each ion type as a non-linear conductance that is driven by the ion-Nerst potential, (Orna, & Stock, 1989). The reader is referred to (Furber, & Temple, 2007) for a detailed treatment on modeling of neural activities.

COMPUTATION WITH ARTIFICIAL NEURAL NETWORKS

In a broad sense, an *artificial neural network* (ANN) (or *neurocomputer*) is a biologically-inspired neural computing paradigm with networks of adaptable nodes. The process of learning with an ANN is simply in the form of storing the experiential knowledge in terms of connection strengths or *weights* between the nodes learned from the task examples. Concerning this definition is the *learning algorithm* which is defined as a procedure used for modifying synaptic strength or so-called weights.

In contrast to a typical computer which requires memory unit(s) for storage and central processing unit(s) for executing instructions sequentially, artificial neural networks are constituted with many simple processing elements that can typically perform on the summation of weighted inputs. In neural networks, information is represented as a result of optimization constructed at an equilibrium state of the network structure. The interconnection-based computation facilitates the accession to partial content of the information as a *content-addressable memory*, (Anderson, 1972).

From the above description it is seen that ANNs are physical cellular systems which receive, store, and employ experiential knowledge about environmental stimuli. Due to algorithmic nature which resorts on optimization rule ANNs have been applied in many fields which involve following properties, (Pandya, & Macy 1995):

1. **Adaptiveness:** Self-adaptability of learning algorithms makes ANNs a favorable tool for processing in a continually changing environment.
2. **Nonlinear processing:** ANNs have the capability to operate in tasks which involve nonlinear relationship with noise-immunity such as classification and prediction
3. **Parallel processing:** Owing to large number of parallel processing units and interconnectivity, ANNs have concurrent and distributed information processing capability.

As its biological counterpart, ANN is defined as architecture of layered and interconnected neuronal units. Each neuron processes the aggregation of weighted inputs through a nonlinear transfer function called *activation function*. The input layer has one neuron for each sensory signal which may represent a *feature* or attribute of the input stimuli as well as a direct measurement Output layer has one neuron for each of the different sample properties that should be predicted such as class of input stimulus. In most applications, as will be shown later, one or more intermediate layers known as *hidden layers* are employed between input and output layers.

ANN is established with *training phase* at which the weights and transfer function characteristics are adapted for desired input-output relationship till they reach equilibrium. Once the structure has been fixed, in *recall phase* network is expected to remember the algorithm or rule for unseen input data which belong to a certain solution space taught at the training phase.

In the following sections, we will present important concepts gained from neurophysiology to the idealized structures that form the basis of most ANN architectures. We in turn will describe well-known ANN models in neural computation and will apply neural learning to realization of an artificial olfactory system.

Neuron as a General Processing Element

By adopting the biological neuron, an artificial neuron as a processing element (PE) can be depicted as shown in Figure 7 where x_j and w_j, $j = 1, 2 \ldots n$ indicate the j-th feature of the n-dimensional input vector or pattern, and the synaptic weight or just weight which process it, respectively, (Pandya, & Macy, 1995). The function $f(.)$ stands for the (nonlinear) processing called the *activation func-*

Figure 7. A general neuron as an information processing unit

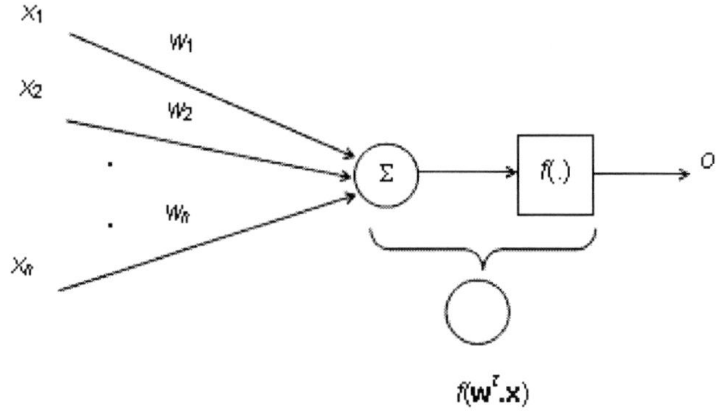

tion performed by the soma or cell body while '*o*' refers to the neuron output. From now on the summation and nonlinear blocks will be packed into a single nonlinear processing function block with empty circle and the nonlinear processing function will be implicit when omitted. Further, if there is any other parameter, e.g. threshold etc. it will be indicated inside the circle, Figure 7.

In case the neuron is the *i*-th component or member of a network *layer*, then it will be appropriate to adopt vector notation **x** and **w** for input and weight, respectively. The output is denoted with o_i. Each neuron operates on a *net-input* value defined as

$$net_i = \sum_j x_j w_{ij} = \mathbf{x}.\mathbf{w}_i^{\,t} = \mathbf{w}_i.\mathbf{x}^t \qquad (1)$$

where the index *j* runs over all connections to the neuron and '*t*' refers to transpose while '.'is the dot-product. It should be noted above notation accounts for the excitation and inhibition effect implicitly in the sign of the weights. Once the net input has been calculated, it is transformed into an *activation value,* or simply *activation,* for the neuron considered through *f*(.). It should be noted that a neural network can be thought of as a *dynamical system* — that is, a system that evolves over time. In ANN terminologies, the network dynamics is expressed as a *learning law*.

In the following (sub)sections, well-known ANN algorithms will be presented along with historical perspective in due order.

McCulloch-Pitts ANN Model

The simplest and first well-known neuro-computational model unit was given by (McCulloch, & Pitts, 1943). McCulloch-Pitts neuron is shown in Figure 8. In the network, inputs x_i and w_i for $i = 1, 2, ..., n$, are the *i*-th input and weight vector component, respectively. The parameter θ is a *threshold value* while o is the output of the neuron defined as

$$o_i = f\left(net_i\right) \qquad (2)$$

The McCulloch-Pitts neuron is characterized by a binary activation function for firing

$$f(u) = \begin{cases} 1 & \text{if } u \geq \theta \\ 0 & \text{otherwise} \end{cases} \qquad (3)$$

It can be shown that by appropriately choosing weight vector and threshold, logic operators AND, OR and NOT can be realized. It is known that these operations constitute a sufficient set for expressing any multivariate combinatorial logic function, Figure 9 (a)-(c). Moreover by inserting

Figure 8. McCulloch-Pitts neuron with threshold element θ

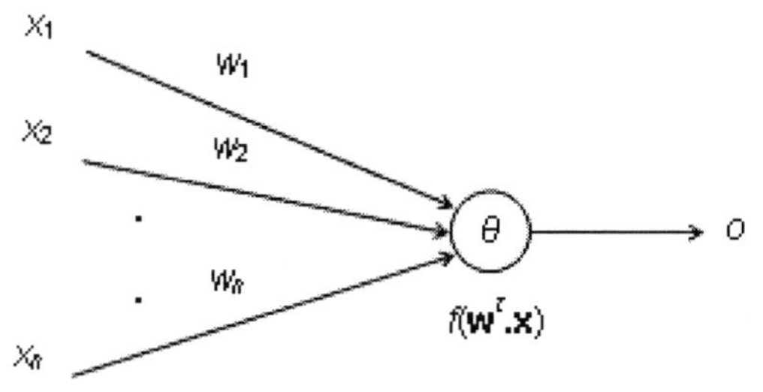

a unit-delay between the output and the input the neuron it is possible to implement storage element for sequential logic functions, Figure 9 (d).

McCulloch-Pitts neuron model consists in following assumptions, (Freeman, & Skapura, 1991):

1. Neurons operate an all-or-none process.
2. A certain number of synapses (> 1) need to be excited within a period of latent addition for a neuron to be excited.
3. The only significant delay within the nervous system is synaptic delay.
4. The activity of any inhibitory synapse absolutely prevents excitation of the neuron at that time.
5. The interconnection of networks does not change with time.

Binary nature of the McCulloch-Pitts neuron was the main inspiration for Wiener to establish the computer-brain analogy known as *cybernetics* (Wiener, 1948). By using idealized switch-delay elements derived from the neuronal models of McCulloch and Pitts, vonNeumann suggested possibilities for building brain-like machines (von Neumann, 1958).

Hebbian Learning

Hebbian learning rule postulated by Hebb in (Hebb, 1949) states that biological neural systems evolve with knowledge resulting from interactions between neuronal units. Learning is the experiential process of incorporating new information by modifying the network in time. Information can be stored in synaptic connections. Synaptic strengths between neurons are updated as learning takes place, which results in continuous connectivity changes in the brain, which was stated by Hebb as

When an axon of cell A is near enough to excite a cell B and repeatedly or persistently takes part in firing it, some growth process or metabolic changes take place in one or both cells such that A's efficiency as one of the cells firing B, is increased.

Hebb also theorized that the synaptic junction area increased during learning. As per Hebb's axiomatic view, more recently it has been acknowledged that learning results from an increase in the rate of neurotransmitter release by the presynaptic neuron with synaptic activation between neurons reinforcing other responses as whole, (Porto, & Pazos, 2006).

Perceptron

The *perceptron* postulated by (Rosenblatt, 1958) is a neuron-like trainable classifier. Rosenblatt utilized the probability theory in modeling and analysis because he believed that the overall structure that biological neural system develops contains a large number of randomly connected networks. For representation of such systems, he developed a theory known as *statistical separability*, (Rosenblatt, 1962).

A simple perceptron consists of the layers called *sensory elements* (S elements), *association units* (A units), and *response units* (R units), respectively, Figure 10.

The connectivity pattern between layers of the perceptron is random. The structure may contain inhibitory feedback connections from the response layer to the association layer as well as lateral connections between R units. The perceptron

Figure 9. Implementation of (a) NOT gate; (b) OR gate; (c) AND gate, and (d) delay or memory element with use of a feedback, one unit of time, z^{-1}. Adapted from Pandya, & Macy, 1995

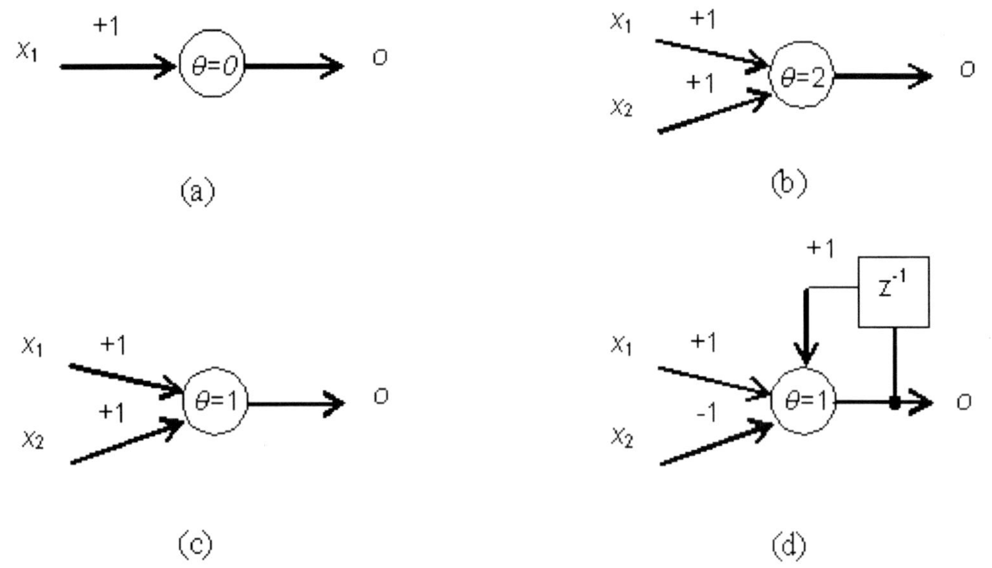

Figure 10. A simple perceptron and its neuron layer units

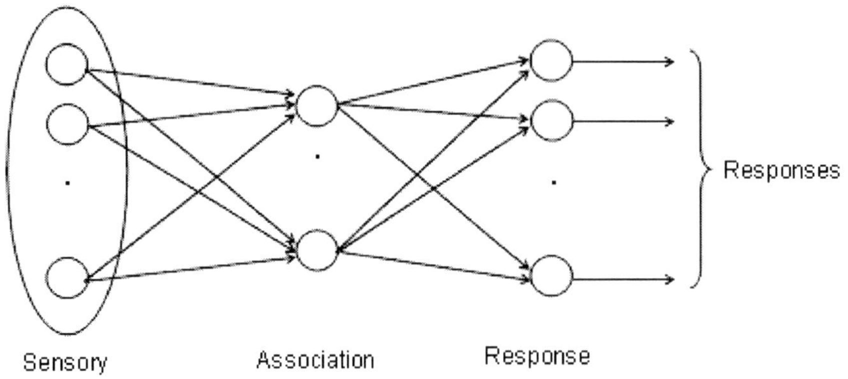

makes use of the assumption that only a single unit given an input pattern wins in the response layer. R units respond in much the same way as do A units. If the sum of their inputs exceeds a threshold, they produce an output value of +1; otherwise, the output is -1.

Training phase of the network involves that the output of A units be either increased or decreased depending on the contribution of individual A units to the active R unit being the correct one or not. If the correct response unit was active, termed the *winner*, outputs of the A units contributing to it were increased, otherwise decreased. The perceptron learning algorithm at training is as follows:

1. Set the weight and thresholds of the neuron to random values and present an input.
2. Calculate the output of the neuron.
3. Alter the weights to reinforce correct decisions and discourage wrong decisions, hence

Figure 11. The ADALINE neural network structure consisting of the adaptive linear combiner, ALC, in the dashed box, and a bipolar output function

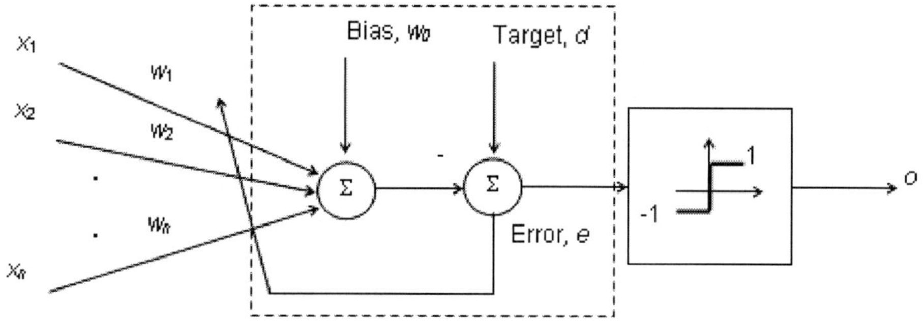

reducing the error. So for the network to learn increase the weights on the active inputs so that the output is active otherwise decrease the weights for the output to be inactive.

4. Now present the next input and go to (2) and proceed until no further weight update is possible.

A perceptron with a single R unit (neuron) can classify two classes. It is possible to classify more than two classes by adding more R units. Rosenblatt (Rosenblatt, 1958; Rosenblatt, 1962) also developed the learning procedure (algorithm) for adjusting the free parameters in the perceptron known as *perceptron convergence algorithm*. The proof of the algorithm has led to conclusion that if the parameters used to train the perceptron are drawn from two linearly separable classes, then the perceptron algorithm converges with a decision surface in data *hyperplane* between the two classes.

In (Minsky, & Pappert, 1969), Minsky and Papert presented a detailed analysis of the perceptron architecture concerning its capabilities and limitations with predicate calculus. Their study demonstrated that the single-layer perceptron fails to differentiate patterns if the samples are not *linearly separable* such as those picked from the hyperplane separated according to XOR operation, (Freeman, & Skapura, 1991).

Adaline and Madaline

As acronym to *ADAptive LINear Element*, (Widrow, & Hoff, 1960), the ADALINE network shown in Figure 11 consists in the learning model known as *Widrow-Hoff learning rule*. The term MADALINE is acronym to *Multiple-ADALINE* (Widrow, 1962). It is an extension of the ADALINE and proposed for those problems, such as XOR, which are not solvable by two-input ADALINE.

The learning algorithm of the ADALINE involves minimization of the mean squared error in the output as previously described neural models do. However, instead of the output mapping via threshold function, the ADALINE uses the net output without mapping. The algorithm also exploited a *bias* term w_0 as a modification in contrast to them. A simple ADALINE algorithm consists of a unit called the *linear combiner* (LC) and the bipolar output function. If the output of the LC is positive, the ADALINE output is +1 otherwise -1.

The LC generates the sum-of-products using the input and weight vectors. If a fictitious term x_0=1 is devised then in vector notation, the output is computed as *inner-product* of input, $\mathbf{x}=[1\ x_1\ \ldots\ x_n]$, and weight $\mathbf{w}=[w_0 w_1\ \ldots\ w_n]$ vectors as

$$y = \mathbf{x}.\mathbf{w}^t = \mathbf{w}.\mathbf{x}^t \quad (4)$$

Since the weights of the linear combiner are determined adaptively in order to allow the network to produce the *correct* (*desired* or *target*) output value given an input, the ADALINE is an adaptive algorithm.

LMS Learning Rule

Suppose we have a set of input vectors, $\{\mathbf{x}_1, \mathbf{x}_2, \ldots, \mathbf{x}_N\}$, each with its own (perhaps) unique, *correct* or *desired* output value, d_k, $k = 1..N$ such as the labels they belong to or mapping to a particular function. The problem is to find a single weight vector that can successfully associate each input vector with its respective desired output value. Finding such a weight vector is referred to as *training* the LC. The weight adjustment procedure which results from minimized error between the linear combination of the input and weight vectors and the desired output is known as the *least mean squared error* (LMS) algorithm.

For the *training set* examples, $\{\mathbf{x}_i, d_i\}_{i=1\ldots N}$, the *best* or optimum weight vector, **w***, for LC which maps the input vectors to a particular function is found by minimizing the difference between the desired output and the actual output for each input vector. If the actual output value is y_k for the k-th input vector, then the corresponding error term is $e_k = d_k - y_k$. The mean squared error value of the error is given by

$$\xi(\mathbf{w}) = \langle e^2 \rangle = \langle \mathbf{e}, \mathbf{e}^t \rangle \frac{1}{N} \sum_{i=1}^{N} e_k^2 \quad (5)$$

where N is the number of input vectors in the training set and '<>' stands for *statistical mean* or average of the dot-product of involved quantities. Assuming that the training set is *stationary*, i.e. first-order statistics do not change or slowly change in time, and samples are statistically independent. Equation (5) can be factorized by defining *correlation matrix* of **x** as $\mathbf{R} = \langle \mathbf{x}^t, \mathbf{x} \rangle$ and the vector as $\mathbf{p} = \langle \mathbf{x}, \mathbf{d}^t \rangle$. Identifying the mean error value as $\xi(\mathbf{w}) = \langle e^2 \rangle$, reduces Equation (5) to

$$\xi(\mathbf{w}) = \langle d^2 \rangle + \mathbf{w}^t\mathbf{R}.\mathbf{w} - 2\mathbf{p}.\mathbf{w}^t \quad (6)$$

The weight vector **w***corresponding to the minimum (or least) mean squared error is found by differentiating ξ with respect to **w** and setting it to zero. Thus,

$$\mathbf{w}^* = \mathbf{R}^{-1}\mathbf{p} \quad (7)$$

At the optimum weight vector the mean squared error is then given by

$$\xi_{\min} = \xi(\mathbf{w}^*) = \langle d^2 \rangle - \mathbf{p}^t.\mathbf{w}^* \quad (8)$$

The Steepest Descent Method

Because in most cases the dimension of **R** is too large for its inverse to be computed, while in small data set estimation may not represent the statistical nature of **R** and **p**, instead of calculating the optimum weight vector analytically, an iterative search is preferred to find the minimum of the error function of the weights. The search algorithm is summarized as follows: Initialize weight vector randomly, and move in a direction with negative slope on the error surface. Update the weight vectors in small amount so that a new minimum error has been reached. As an example consider an arbitrarily formed two-dimensional error surface and its cross-section shown in Figure 12.

In the figure arrows indicate the iterative updates of weights and corresponding track on the error surface while $\mathbf{w}_0$ refers to an initial random guess for the weights. Usually, initially the negative gradient may not point directly at the minimum. Assuming that the weight vector at the k-th training-step or iteration, i.e. when the k-th input

*Figure 12. Steepest descent algorithm in two-dimensional case with all quantities normalized. Initial weight vector **w(0)** is arbitrarily or randomly chosen*

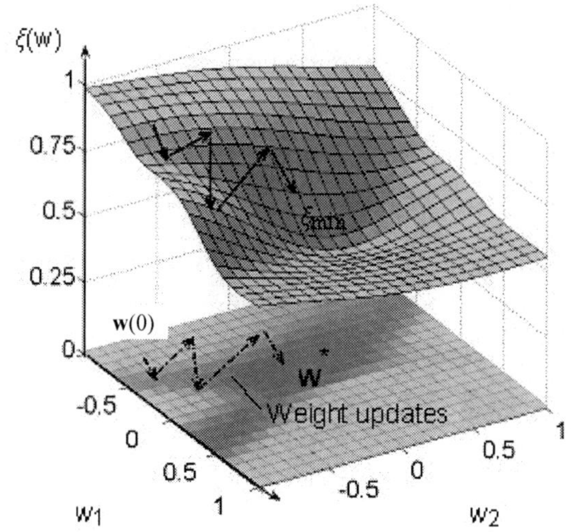

vector $\mathbf{x}(k)$ has been inserted at the network inputs in *sequential-mode*, is $\mathbf{w}(k)$, the weight vector at the next step is assumed to be

$$\mathbf{w}(k+1) = \mathbf{w}(k) + \Delta\mathbf{w} \tag{9}$$

Equation (9) is known as *delta rule*. In delta-rule given above, $\Delta\mathbf{w}(k)$ is the iterative change in $\mathbf{w}$ at the k-th iteration. The problem is to find the direction of the steepest descent at each point on the error surface of $\xi(\mathbf{w})$. It is seen that the negative gradient of $\xi(\mathbf{w})$ is in the direction of *steepest descent*. The magnitude of the change is usually taken proportional to gradient by a suitable constant, μ called *learning rate*, as

$$\mathbf{w}(k+1) = \mathbf{w}(k) - \mu\nabla\xi(\mathbf{w}) \tag{10}$$

The learning rate parameter μ is chosen so that the stability of the algorithm associated with an appropriate speed of convergence toward minimum mean squared error is assured. For analytical determination of $\mathbf{w}^*$, $\mathbf{R}$ and $\mathbf{p}$ still need to be known in advance which is equivalent to knowledge of the error surface shape. To overcome this difficulty, following iterative approximation for the gradient can be adopted:

1. Apply an input vector, $\mathbf{x}(k)$ to ADALINE inputs at the k-th iteration and calculate the error $e(k)$ and its squared value from

$$e^2(k) = [d_k - \mathbf{w}^t(k) \,.\, \mathbf{x}(k)]^2 \tag{11}$$

2. Calculate the approximation to $\nabla\xi\mathbf{w}(k)$ as

$$\nabla e^2(k) = -2e(k)\mathbf{x}(k) \tag{12}$$

3. Update the weight vector by using

$$\mathbf{w}(k+1) = \mathbf{w}(k) + 2\mu . e(k)\mathbf{x}(k) \tag{13}$$

4. Repeat steps (1) through (3) with successive input vectors until the error has been reduced to an acceptable value.

Because of the approximating, the path of the weight vector as it moves down toward the minimum will not be as smooth as that expressed by Equation (13). For guaranteeing a minimum, change in the weight vector must be kept relatively small at each step. Otherwise the weight vector could wander about the surface without finding the minimum.

The value of parameter μ plays a significant role on convergence. If it is chosen too large it is likely that no convergence will occur. Its value can be determined in terms of the input signal statistics. For convergence, it is shown that the value of μ must satisfy the following condition, (Haykin, 2003)

$$\frac{2}{\lambda_{max}} > \mu > 0 \tag{14}$$

Figure 13. Feed-forward multi-layer perceptron architecture

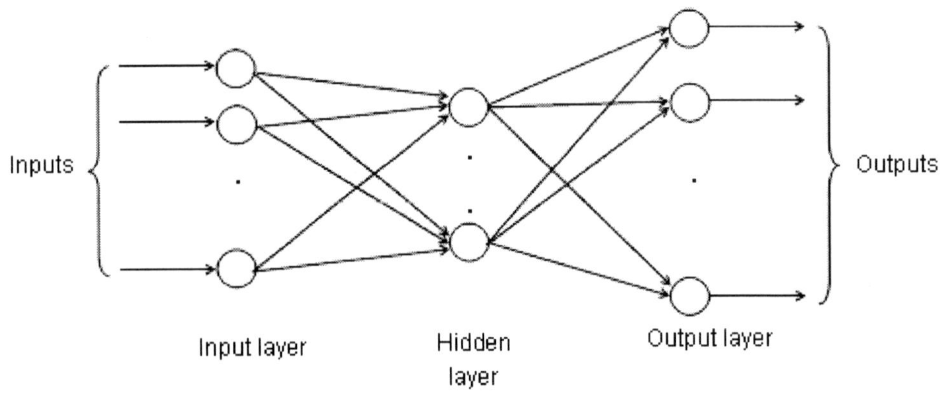

where λ_{max} is the largest eigen-value of **R**. Mostly input statistics is not known explicitly but can be estimated from training examples. The reader is advised to refer to (McDonough, 2004) for elegant derivation of statistical and relevant spectral quantities given an input signal.

FEED-FORWARD MULTI-LAYER PERCEPTRON

The ADALINE which is in fact a generalized version of the single-layer perceptron suffers similar shortcomings in forming a decision surface for linearly separating input-output mappings as in XOR. It is, however, possible to discriminate such mappings by using *multi-layer perceptron*, known since 1960s, (Nilsson, 1965; Werbos, 1974). The multi-layer perceptron was formally devised and termed the *feed-forward multi-layer perceptron* (FFMLP) by (Rummelhart, & McClelland, 1986). FFMLP network trained with error *back-propagation* (BP) is perhaps the most popular neural architecture.

MLP networks with a single-hidden layer and a nonlinear activation function are inherently able to discriminate classes with decision boundaries of arbitrary complexity, (Hartman, Keeler, Kowalski, 1990; Haykin, 2003). Similar to previously discussed models, learning is achieved with weight-update following one of the optimization methods, such as the gradient-descent. The activity in the FFMLP network is propagated forward to output layer via hidden layers where some function, possibly feature extraction, of the net activation is calculated. During training, weights of hidden layers need to be updated accordingly. It is obvious that the LMS rule can be adopted for calculating errors for layers backward from the output. In the BP algorithm, the learning error in response is distributed to the weights of hidden units as *credit* or *blame* terms (*credit assignment*).

Owing to generic learning formalism in the network architecture theoretically it is possible to include as many hidden layers as desired. However, a network with more hidden layers will need longer training time.

A typical FFMLP network with input, output and hidden layers is shown in Figure 13. Generally such a network is referred to by the number of neurons in its each layer such as 6-4-3-2. In this configuration, 6 and 2 represent the number neurons in the input and the output layers, respectively. Remaining numbers 4 and 3 refer to the first and the second hidden layers, respectively.

Features of an input vector to be classified or identified are applied to the input layer neurons and their activations are propagated to subsequent hidden layers and finally to the output layer via weights. There is no dissimilarity between the

Figure 14. (a) Sigmoid and (b) hyperbolic tangent function for various temperature (Q_0) values

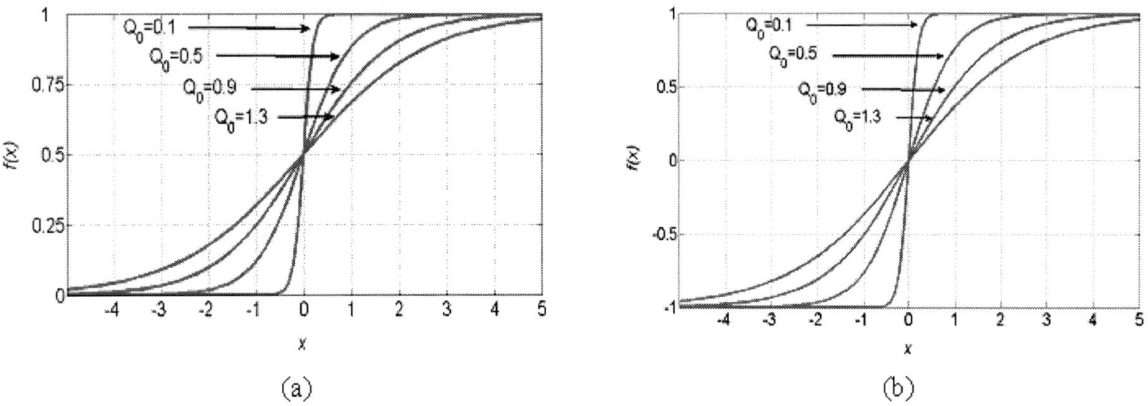

operation carried out by neurons employed in this and the previously described models. Each neuron in a specific layer of interest operates by taking the sum of its weighted inputs and passing the result through a suitable nonlinear activation function. The output of i-th neuron in the l-th layer is given by

$$o_{l,i} = f(net_{l,i}) = f\left(\sum_{j=1}^{m} w_{l,ij} o_{l-1,j} + \theta_{l,j}\right) \quad (15)$$

where $o_{l-1,j}$ is the output of the j-th neuron in the layer preceding the l-th layer and m is the number of neurons in the l-1-th layer. There are several conventionally used choices for the nonlinear activation function f. One of those frequently employed is the sigmoid function given by

$$f(x) = \frac{1}{1 + e^{-x/Q_0}} \quad (16)$$

The term Q_0 in Equation (16) is known as the *temperature* of the neuron. It mainly determines the slope of the function in the non-saturated region. The higher the temperature is the more gently the sigmoid changes while as it becomes smaller the function approaches a step function. Figure 14(a) illustrates the sigmoid function for a variety of temperature values. Note that the function behaves almost linearly in the region surrounding x=0. It has also been suggested that the anti-symmetric sigmoid function shown in Figure 14(b) with property $f(-x)=-f(x)$ offers some better characteristics compared to symmetric sigmoid function.

$$f(x) = \frac{1 - e^{-x/Q_0}}{1 + e^{-x/Q_0}} \quad (17)$$

Training with Back Propagation

The BP algorithm searches for weight vectors that minimize the total error of the network over the set of training examples in forward and backward direction as illustrated in Figure 15 by using credit assignment.

In the forward pass the network is activated given an input example and the error of each neuron in the output layer is computed while in the backward pass the network error is used for updating the weights. This process is more complex than the LMS algorithm formerly adopted for ADALINE because hidden nodes are linked to the error not directly but by means of the nodes of the next layer. Therefore, starting from the output layer, the error is propagated backward

Figure 15. Backpropagation adjusts the weights of the NN in order to minimize the network total mean squared error

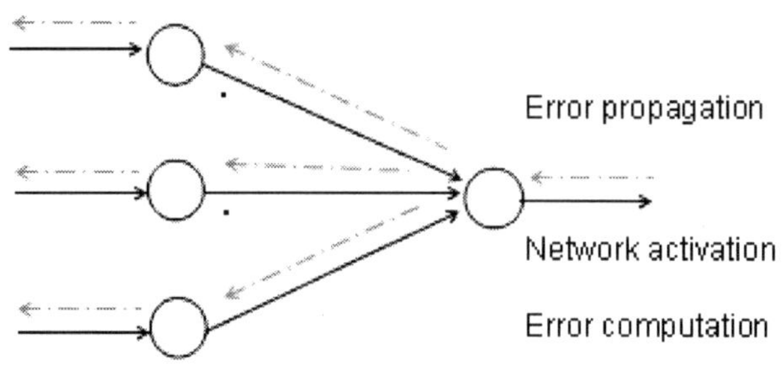

through the network layer-by-layer. This is done by recursively computing the local gradient of each neuron. An appropriate choice for the error measure with the BP training algorithm can be in the mean squared sense despite the fact that some other any differentiable cost error functions can also be considered for this purpose. The mean square error can be computed in terms of network error

$$E(k) = \sum_{\forall j \in \text{ output layer}} e_j^2(k) \tag{18}$$

where $e_j(k)=d_j(k)-y_j(k)$ is the j-th output neuron error, $y_j(k)$ is the computed neuron output and $d_j(k)$ is the desired or target of the j-th neuron at the k-th training sample. The total mean squared error is then given by

$$E_{AV} = \sum_{\forall k} E(k) \tag{19}$$

The weight update rule of BP algorithm is based on the gradient descent method which takes a step in the direction yielding the maximum decrease of the network error E. Consider the flow-graph in Figure 16 which illustrates how errors are back-propagated to the hidden neuron j.

If the link weight w_{ji} from i-th node to j-th node just after the k-th sample applied is $w_{ji}(k+1)= w_{ji}(k)+\Delta w_{ji}(k)$ then

$$\Delta w_{ji} = -\eta \frac{\partial E}{\partial w_{ji}} \tag{20}$$

with time-stamp k dropped. Δw_{ji} is in the opposite direction of E. The input of a neuron j is $net_j = \sum_{i=1...m} w_{ji} y_i$. From the chain rule $\frac{\partial E}{\partial w_{ji}} = \frac{\partial E}{\partial net_j} \frac{\partial net_j}{\partial w_{ji}}$. If a term called *local gradient* of neuron j is introduced as $\delta_j = -\partial E / \partial net_j$. Then from $\partial net_j / \partial w_{ji} = y_i$ it is concluded that

$$\Delta w_{ji} = \eta \delta_j y_i \tag{21}$$

Depending on the j-th node being an output or hidden layer neuron

If j-th output neuron is considered then using the chain rule, since $e_j=d_j-y_j$ and $y_j=f(net_j)$

$$\delta_j = -\frac{\partial E}{\partial net_j} = -\frac{\partial E}{\partial e_j} \frac{\partial e_j}{\partial y_j} \frac{\partial y_j}{\partial net_j} = e_j f'(net_j) \tag{22}$$

Substituting δ_j in $\Delta w_{ji} = \eta \delta_j y_i$ yields

$$\Delta w_{ji} = \eta (d_j - y_j) f'(net_j) y_i \tag{23}$$

If the neuron belongs to a hidden layer

Figure 16. Backward error propagation based on gradient of nonlinear function f(.)

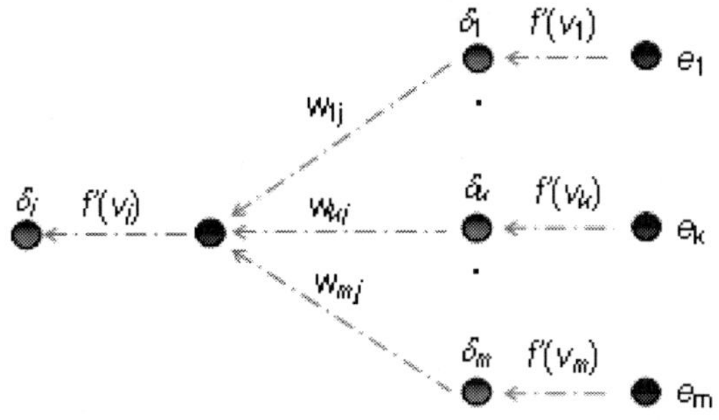

$$\delta_j = -\frac{\partial E}{\partial net_j} = -\frac{\partial E}{\partial y_j}\frac{\partial y_j}{\partial net_j} \tag{24}$$

Observe that

$$-\frac{\partial E}{\partial y_j} = -\sum_{k\in C} e_k \frac{\partial e_k}{\partial y_j} = -\sum_{p\in C} e_p \left[\frac{\partial e_p}{\partial net_p}\right]\frac{\partial net_p}{\partial y_j}$$

where C is the next layer. Since:

$$-e_p \frac{\partial e_p}{\partial net_p} = e_p f'(net_p) = \delta_p \text{ and } \frac{\partial net_p}{\partial y_j} = w_{pj}$$

then $-\dfrac{\partial E}{\partial y_j} = \sum_{p\in C} \delta_p w_{pj}$

For the j-th neuron of a hidden layer considered it can be written

$$\delta_j = f'(net_p)\sum_{p\in C}\delta_p w_{pj} \tag{25}$$

and finally

$$\Delta w_{ji} = \eta y_j f'(net_j)\sum_{p\in C}\delta_p w_{pj} \tag{26}$$

Therefore as a summary of delta rule with generic term $\Delta w_{ji} = \eta\delta_j y_i$ holds with

$$\delta_j = \begin{cases} f'(net_j)(d_j - y_j) & \text{if output layer} \\ \eta . y_i f'(net_j)\sum_{p\in C}\delta_p w_{pj} & \text{if hidden layer} \end{cases} \tag{27}$$

If the activation function chosen is sigmoid then $f'(net_j) = ay_j(1 - y_j)$.

Having defined the performance criterion in terms of mean squared-error, the BP is performed as a gradient descent (or steepest-descent) algorithm, i.e. minimization of total error by adjusting the weights layer-by-layer. Varying number of neurons in each layer also leads to varying dimensional weight vector for each hidden layers. The weights are taken as independent variables in error space. Thus, the shape of the resulting error surface will depend on the error function in combination with the training set.

Generally, the delta-rule algorithm including BP starts with randomly initialized weights of small values and a suitable value for learning rate. If η is small then the algorithm learns the weights very slowly, while if η is large then the large changes of the weights may cause an unstable behavior with oscillations of the weight values. A technique for tackling this problem is the introduction of a term called *momentum constant* $0<\alpha<1$ in the delta rule. The momentum constant takes into account the *previous updates*, which keeps up the *moving average* of the individual weight changes. Momentum term accelerates the descent in steady downhill direction so that it stabilizes the effect in direction that oscillates in time. Resultant weight update expression is called the *generalized delta rule*

$$\Delta w_{ji}(k) = \pm\Delta w_{ji}(k-1) + \eta\delta_j(k)y_i(k) \qquad (28)$$

In the forward phase the actual output values are utilized. In the backward phase a new set of weight values are reached for decreasing total error. Some other heuristics for accelerating the convergence of the BP algorithm through η adaptation is to either assign a value of η for every weight or everyη being allowed to vary from one iteration to the next. The dynamic behavior of the weights during training can be visualized by using *Hinton diagram*, (Pandya, & Macy, 1995).

General Training Issues

The available data set is normally split into three sets as follows: Training set is used to update the weights. Patterns in this set are repeatedly applied in random order. The weight-update equation is applied after a certain number of patterns, which is usually one. Test set is used to test or assess the recalling performance called the *generalization* of the neural network. It is not a part of the neural network development cycle.

One full presentation cycle of all the training examples is known an *epoch*. At training, when the weights do not change over a full epoch, or if the total network error falls below a pre-established threshold, the network is said to have converged. The error does not need to converge steadily since the total network error may exhibit local fluctuations. FFMLP usually has complex error surfaces such as plateaus, long valleys etc., Figure 17, with no single minimum.

The training needs to stop with some criterion to indicate the convergence of the algorithm. In total mean- squared stopping criterion the BP is considered to have converged when the absolute rate of change in the average squared error per epoch is sufficiently small (in the range [0.01, 0.1]). In generalization-based criterion after each epoch the NN is tested for assessing the recalling capability called *generalization* by using a different set of examples called the *validation set*. If the generalization performance is satisfactory, then the BP algorithm stops.

If test samples are not salient, the network will not have good generalization performance (Bishop, 2004). Instead of direct test set, the method of *validation set* can be used to decide when to stop training only by monitoring the error. In this method a *hold-out* validation set is kept aside. The *accuracy* of the network, defined as $N_{correct}/N_{test}$ where $N_{correct}$ is the number of correctly classified examples within N_{test} examples, after each epoch is considered. The weights leading to the best performance among the validation sets are retained and the training is stopped. Detailed description various validation techniques can be found in (Efron, & Tibshirani, 1993).

ANNs generalize the training algorithm to the examples which have not been seen yet, within an error tolerance. The training strategy and arrangement of training set has significant role in generalization of the network. For example restricting training to an excessively low error tolerance leads the network to recall minutiae of the training set and loses its ability to generalize, which is known as *overfitting*. However, a non diverse training set will cause *overtraining* (Bishop, 2004), Figure 18.

Training Strategies: Avoiding Local Minima

Two important issues concerning training are *early convergence* and *slow convergence* (or *non-convergence*). Early or premature convergence is caused mainly when neurons operate in saturation of the activation function resulting in ineffective training due to dependency on derivative. Initialization of weights with large values and choice of inadequate training parameters, i.e. α and η, are

Figure 17. Typical and simple error surface corresponding to single weight for FFMLP

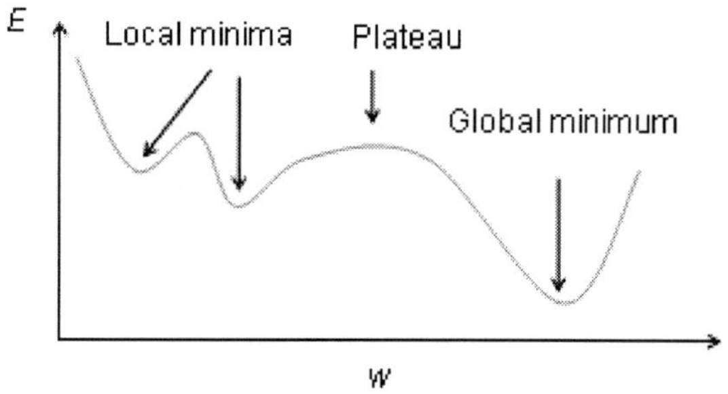

Figure 18. Overtraining and overfitting diagram, Adapted from (Bishop, 2004;Pandya, & Macy, 1995)

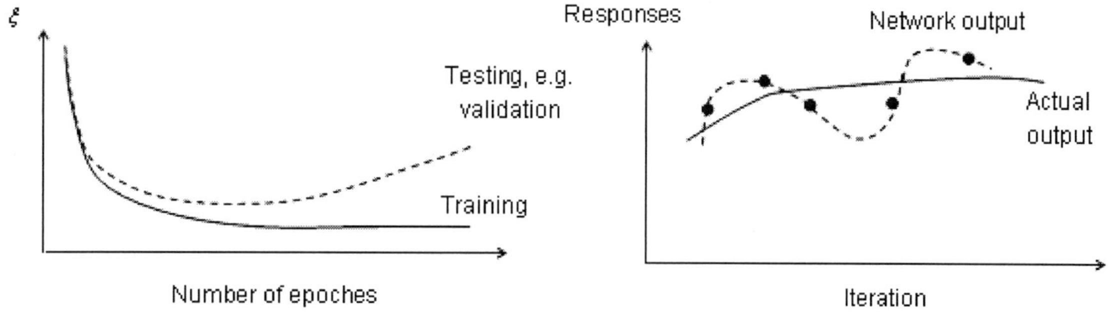

major factors to drive the weights and relevant neurons into saturation. In order to avoid saturation, ALOPEX, (Pandya, & Venugopal, 1991), or similar algorithms which do not depend on the derivative of the activation function can be considered.

An approach to drive the network into converge faster makes use of *data pruning*, (Lee, Oh, Song, & Kim, 1992). In this method, data is divided into learning and idle sets. The latter is the group of redundant or ineffective data applied to the network only a number of epochs, (Tsai, Hong, & Chieng, 1992). The slow convergence may arise in cases of local minima and flat (or shallow) error surface. If the error surface is shallow enough, round-off errors drive the gradient descent algorithm into spurious behavior.

Another approach which is widely adopted for network to converge faster is to adaptively update the learning rate at successive iterations, mainly due to varying convergence for varying dimension across the error surface. The *delta-bar-delta* (Jacobs, 1988) and the *decoupled momentum* (Soucek, 1992) are such two well-known algorithms in this manner although most other schemes are empirical.

During training with BP the objective is to converge to a global minimum rather than local minima. Depending on the error surface a local minimum can be approached falsely as if being global minimum. The major methods to avoid falsely resorting on local minima are *simulated annealing*, *genetic algorithms* and *noise injection*. In simulated annealing, temperature term in the activation function is decreased accordingly during training while in case of using genetic algorithms the solution space is searched for best fitting solution in probabilistic rules. In noise injection, the amount of noise is adjusted (mostly decreased) by a generator as convergence is achieved, (Pandya, & Macy, 1995).

Box 1.

```
1.  Choose a randomized ordering for selecting the examples in the training set in order to avoid poor performance.
2.  k=0, initialize w(k) randomly;
3.  while (stopping criterion not satisfied and k<max_number_of_iterations)
        for each example (x(k),d_k)
            run the network with input x(k) and compute the output y_k
            update the weights in backward order starting from those of the output layer using the (generalized or simple) delta rule
        end-for
    k = k+1;
    end-while;
```

Training Strategies: Variations for Gradient Descent

The behavior of the first and second-order gradients of the error function is affected by frequency of update. There are two types of network training in terms of how frequently the input patterns are applied to the network, namely called *incremental* or *sequential* (on-line, stochastic, or per-pattern) and *batch* modes.

In the first method the weights are updated after each pattern is presented. Following is the incremental mode for backpropagation algorithm, (see Box 1)

In the *batch mode* (off-line or per -epoch) the weights are updated after all the patterns are presented. In the batch-mode the weights are updated only after all examples have been processed using the formula

$$\Delta w_{ji}(k) = \Delta w_{ji}(k-1) + \sum_{\forall x \in \text{ training set}} \Delta w_{ji} \tag{29}$$

The learning process continues on an epoch-by-epoch basis until the stopping condition is satisfied. After each epoch the accumulated changes need to be reset for the next iteration if the network still needs further training.

Sequential mode requires less storage. Random order of presentation and updating per pattern means that search of weight space is stochastic, hence reducing the risk of local minima. It also has the advantage of retaining any redundancy in training set (i.e. same pattern occurs more than once in training set, especially for large training sets). It is simpler to implement. However, batch mode is faster than the sequential mode.

Network Design Issues

In a neural network design, the following issues should be considered:

1. *Data representation* depends on the problem. In general NNs work on continuous (real valued) attributes. Symbolic attributes are encoded into continuous ones. Since attributes of different types having different ranges of values affect the training process, *normalization* may be used. In this case the following scaling can be applied to attributes so each attribute will be between 0 and 1,

$$\overline{x_j} = \frac{x_j - \min_{\forall j}(x_j)}{\max_{\forall j}(x_j) - \min_{\forall j}(x_j)} \tag{30}$$

or a predetermined range for each value of *i*-th attribute.

2. *Network topology* mostly concerns the number of layers and the number of neurons for each layer. It depends on the specification of the task to be fulfilled by the network. Network topology affects the decision surface. For faster training and avoiding a

possible *overfitting* it is desirable to have a network topology with the fewest possible neurons in hidden layer(s).

To attain a network topology with satisfactory training and generalization performance, two types of adaptive algorithms are suggested:

a. Start from a large network and successively remove some neurons and links until the network performance degrades. In the *link-pruning* method (Lee, Oh, Song, & Kim, 1992) the candidate nodes for pruning are identified are identified as those with unchanging output for all training patterns or those with weight vector whose magnitude is relatively much smaller than the others and the output layer.
b. Begin with a small network and introduce new neurons until the performance is satisfactory.

3. *Initialization of the weights*: In general, the initial weights are randomly chosen. Typical values are taken between -1.0 and 1.0 or -0.5 and 0.5. If some inputs are much larger than others, random initialization may bias the network to give much more importance to larger inputs. In such a case, weights can be initialized as follows:

$$w_{ji} = \pm \frac{1}{2N} \sum_{i=1}^{N} \frac{1}{|x_i|} \tag{31}$$

for weights from input to the first layer

$$w_{kj} = \pm \frac{1}{2N} \sum_{i=1}^{N} \frac{1}{f(\sum w_{ji} x_i)}$$

for weights from the previous layer to the next layer.

4. *The size of the training set* must be large. The training set also needs to be diverse enough to optimally represent the problem domain. The size of the training set is mainly determined by the dimension of the input space, network size, e.g. number of neurons, and the desired accuracy.

The required number of training samples grows exponentially with the dimension of the input space, (Kneer, Personnaz, & Dreyfus, 1992), which is termed the *curse of dimensionality*. Feature extraction can be used to reduce the input space dimension while retaining sufficient information. As a rule of thumb the number of training samples is usually at least five to ten times the number of weights. A minimum number of the training examples can be empirically set as

$$N \geq \frac{\text{number of weights}}{1 - a} \tag{32}$$

where a is a desired network accuracy.

Conjugate Gradient Method

A fast search for an optimum weight vector can be achieved by determining a *direction vector* for weight update. Based on Taylor's expansion of the error function it is possible to derive an expression in terms of second-order derivative of the error-function called the *Hessian matrix*. As can be recalled from previous discussions, delta-rule learning with momentum term can be expressed as

$$\mathbf{w}(k+1) = \mathbf{w}(k) + \Delta\mathbf{w}(k) + \alpha\Delta\mathbf{w}(k-1) \tag{33}$$

We demand that the subsequent direction, $\Delta\mathbf{w}(k)$, obey

$$\Delta\mathbf{w}^t(k-1)\mathbf{H}\Delta\mathbf{w}(k) = 0 \tag{34}$$

where $\mathbf{H}$ is the Hessian matrix of the error function defined as second-order derivative with respect to overall weight connections. Above descent direction vector update pairs $\Delta\mathbf{w}(k\text{-}1)$ and $\Delta\mathbf{w}(k)$ in Equation (34) are called *conjugate*. If the Hessian is proportional to the identity matrix, then such directions are orthogonal in weight space.

A global solution for weight vector direction and its size would be to devise an expression which allows the momentum term to be iteration-dependent as

$$\Delta\mathbf{w}(k) = -\nabla\xi(\mathbf{w}(k)) + \beta_k \Delta\mathbf{w}(k-1) \qquad (35)$$

where the term β_k can be computed from the *Fletcher-Reeves' formula* (Fletcher, & Reeves, 1964; Griva, Nash, & Sofer, 2009) as

$$\beta_k = \frac{\nabla\xi(\mathbf{w}(k))^t \nabla\xi(\mathbf{w}(k))}{\nabla\xi(\mathbf{w}(k-1))^t \nabla\xi(\mathbf{w}(k-1))} \qquad (36)$$

An important advantage of the conjugate-gradient method over back-propagation is the elimination of trial-and-error search for determination of learning parameters. It also converges faster than the BP. However, it has the drawback that it is computationally intense and more importantly it requires the batch-mode input since the Hessian matrix is defined over full training set.

SELF-ORGANIZING MAP NEURAL NETWORKS

Biological plausability is shown that the brain is organized into regions that correspond to different sensory stimuli such as linguistically localized units. This localization is exploited to extract associated features from environmental input stimuli in *self-organizing* (*feature*) *map* (SOM) developed by Kohonen, (1982, 1990, 1993). SOM is one of the most commonly used neural network models, which represents regularities within input without supervision, hence so-called unsupervised NN. SOM was mainly inspired from biological systems' ability to learn and extract common attributes found in the retinal cortex, which can be represented as aggregated *competing* cluster centers.

A SOM consists of fully connected input and output layers, the latter also being called the *Kohonen layer*. Figure 19 depicts one and two-dimensional SOM network topologies, respectively. Although higher dimensional networks are possible, they are rare.

The connection weights between input neurons and a particular output neuron i constitutes a vector $\mathbf{w}_i$ in an n-dimensional space. A main characteristic of SOM networks is the *competitive learning* where output layer neurons compete to gain the precedence to response/fire to input patterns as the *winner*. Mostly the winner neuron is the output neuron whose weight vector most resembles the input pattern in the input space so as to reflect typical features shared by the input ensemble. Therefore, SOM is a "*the winner-take-all*" paradigm, where only the winner output neuron determines the class, the label, or the feature to which the input vector belongs.

Another important characteristic of SOM networks is the *lateral-feedback* which represents excitatory or inhibitory interaction between neighboring output neurons. In such a network topology, the lateral feedback is represented as a connection weight between neurons involved. Lateral feedback retains topological organization of output layer neurons. Figure 20 illustrates some of the possible lateral-feedback connections in dotted-lines between output layer neurons for one-dimensional case.

Lateral-feedback weights between neighboring neurons are supposed to monotonically decrease with distance which can be expressed by the so-called *Mexican hat function*, $h(.)$, shown in Figure 21.

Figure 19. Architecture of the Kohonen networks,for one-dimensional, two-dimensional cases. In two-dimensional case the weight connections are depicted for a particular input layer neuron and other input layer neurons are similarly connected to output layer neurons

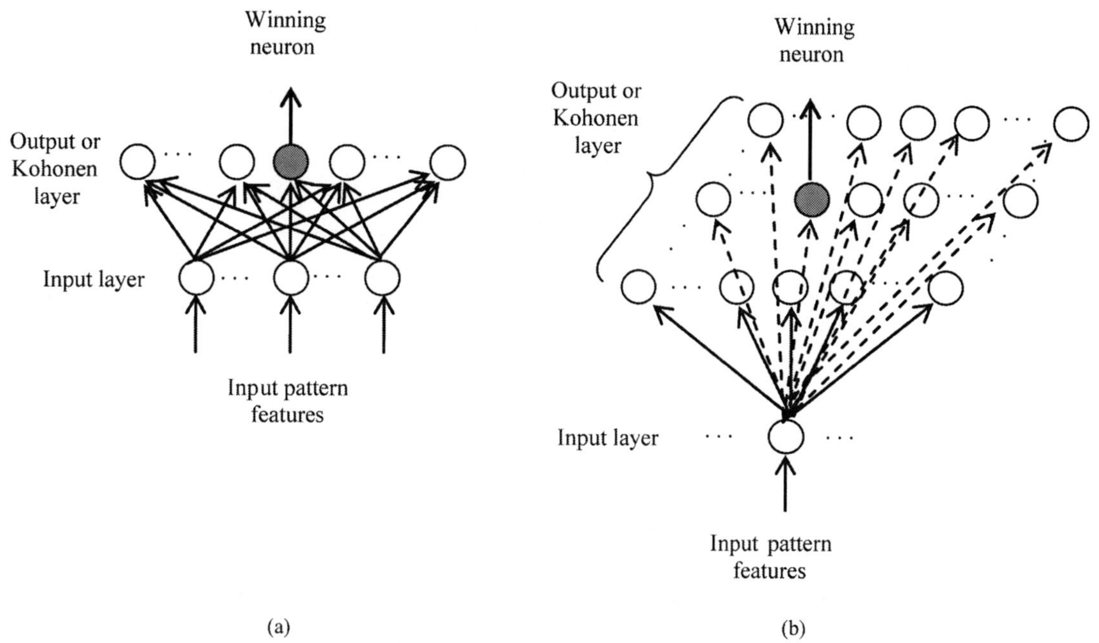

Figure 20. Some of the possible lateral feedback connections (dotted lines) in one-dimensional Kohonen layer

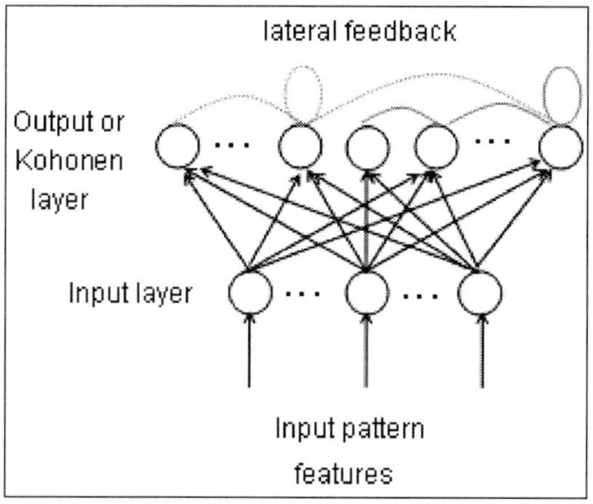

The K-means Algorithm

Consider an n-dimensional input space and a vector, $\mathbf{x}=[x_1, x_2, ..., x_n]^T$ whose *Euclidean norm* or length is defined as $\|\mathbf{x}\| = \left[\sum_{i=1}^{n} x_i^2\right]^{1/2}$ while its distance to a vector $\mathbf{z}$ is given by $d(\mathbf{x},\mathbf{z}) = \|\mathbf{x}\text{-}\mathbf{z}\| = \left[\sum_{i=1}^{n} (x_i - z_i)^2\right]^{1/2}$

K-means is an algorithm which partitions input space based on *a priori* knowledge of the number of partitions (clusters) K. Assuming that the cluster centers are represented by vectors $\mathbf{z}_1, \mathbf{z}_2, \dots \mathbf{z}_K$. A cluster C_j is the set of all points whose distance to cluster center $\mathbf{z}_i$ is smaller than those to other cluster centers. Formally, K-means algorithm is summarized as follows:

Figure 21. Mexican hat function, h(x). Note the regions of positive and negative reinforcement

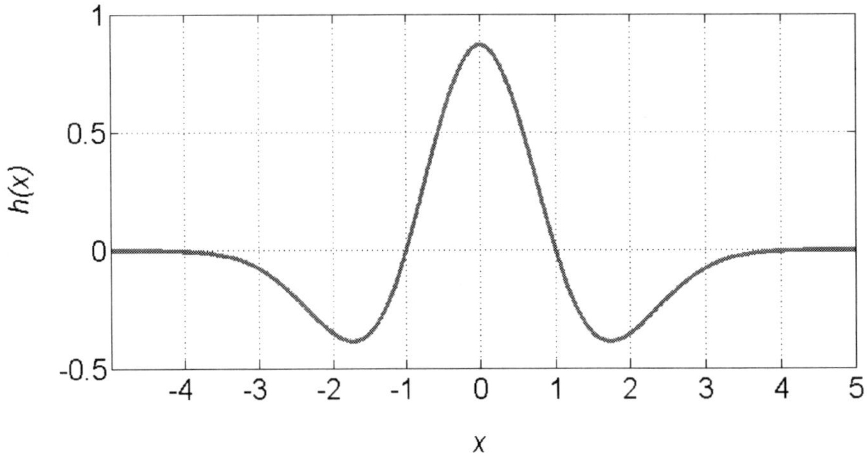

1. Assume $\{\mathbf{z}_1(k), \mathbf{z}_2, \ldots, \mathbf{z}_k(k)\}$ where $\mathbf{z}_i(k)$ represents the value of the i-th cluster center at the k-th iteration, i.e. training sample. If $k=0$ they can be picked up randomly as initialization.
2. Distribute each sample $\mathbf{x}(k)$, based on the minimum distance so $C_i(k)=\{\mathbf{x}(k) | d(\mathbf{x}(k),\mathbf{z}_i) < d(\mathbf{x}(k),\mathbf{z}_j)$ for all $j \neq i\}$
3. Calculate new cluster centers $z_i(k+1) = \frac{1}{N_i} \sum_{\forall x \in C_i} x$
4. If $\mathbf{z}_i(k+1) = \mathbf{z}_i(k)$ for all i then stop, otherwise take $C_i=\{\}$ with $i=1, 2, \ldots K$ with cluster centers formed in (3) and go to (1).

K-means is a simple-to-implement algorithm and it is robust to noise. However, its performance is mainly determined by initialization. It also has the disadvantage of restricting the shape of the clusters to be hyperspherical which makes it sensitive to *outliers*.

Learning Vector Quantization

LVQ allocates categories which are known *apriori* for the inputs to be classified. It simply consists of an *unsupervised* training and regulatory supervised phases, respectively. In the former, the weight or so-called *codebook* vectors are initialized and learned by the SOM. Each output neuron is then assigned a respective class label, Figure 22.

In the supervised stage the codebook vectors are adjusted under the supervision of the codebook vectors and known labels until convergence according to rule

$$w_w(k+1) = w_w(k) \pm \eta[x(k) - w_w(k)] \quad (37)$$

where $\mathbf{w}_w(k)$ is the weight vector connecting input to the winning output neuron at the k-th iteration. The sign of η is taken as '+' if the input sample $\mathbf{x}(k)$ is correctly classified, i.e. *reward* otherwise '-' *punishment*. As FFMLP, the learning rate parameter can be adaptively updated for convergence.

The training algorithm for LVQ may be summarized as follows:

1. Initialize the weight vectors, e.g. randomly, and choose an adequate value for the learning rate.
2. For input vector $\mathbf{x}(k)$ in the training set, find the winning neuron $\mathbf{w}_w$ with $d(\mathbf{x}(k),\mathbf{w}_w) < d(\mathbf{x}(k),\mathbf{w}_i)$ for all i and update it according to Equation (37) while other neurons remain unchanged.

Figure 22. Architecture of the learning vector quantization network

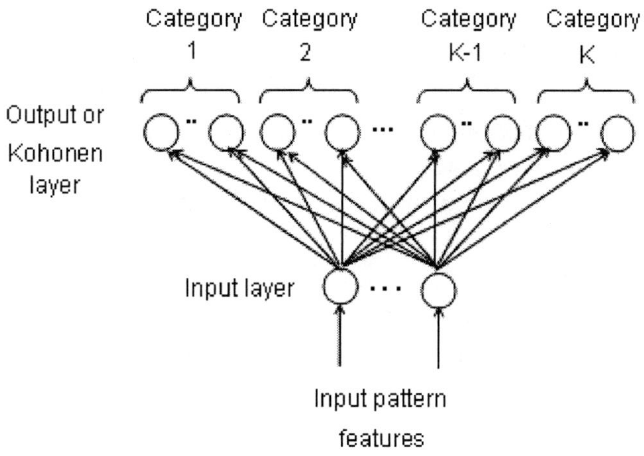

3. Adjust the learning rate, e.g. reduce it as a function of iteration.
4. Terminate if $\mathbf{w}(k+1)= \mathbf{w}(k)$ for all weight vectors otherwise go to (2).

As noticed above, original LVQ algorithm involves update of the winning output neuron only while retaining others intact, which leads degraded topographic mapping around output neurons. Adjustment of other neurons without changing network structure has been considered by several variations of LVQ termed LVQ1, LVQ2 and LVQ3, (Kasabov, 1998)

1. LVQ1 *Algorithm*: Several codebook vectors are assigned to a class, and labeled respectively. Then a correction of the weights with the use of the known labels is performed by applying the algorithm above.
2. *LVQ2 Algorithm*: The nearby output neurons of the winning neuron are adjusted beside the winning neuron. For each input vector incorrectly classified, they are punished while true class neurons are rewarded.
3. *LVQ3 Algorithm*: The same procedure applies as LVQ2 but there is additional weight update, (Kohonen 1995). Based on a window defined for lateral output neurons with codebook vectors C_i and C_j respectively, if the corresponding input neuron can be mapped or fall outside the window, the LVQ2 algorithm is applied. Otherwise, i.e. if the input vectors **w** falls inside the window, then the following algorithm is applied:
    - $\mathbf{w}_i(k+1) = \mathbf{w}_i(k)-\eta[\mathbf{x}-\mathbf{w}_i(k)]$, if **x** falls inside the window and **x** comes from class C_j
    - $\mathbf{w}_j(k+1) = \mathbf{w}_j(k)+\eta[\mathbf{x}-\mathbf{w}_j(k)]$, for $\mathbf{w}_w \in \{C_i, C_j\}$, if **x** falls inside the window and **x** belongs to class C_j
    - $\mathbf{w}_l(k+1) = \mathbf{w}_l(k)+\eta[\mathbf{x}-\mathbf{w}_l(k)]$, for $\mathbf{w}_w \in \{C_i, C_j\}$, if **x** falls inside the window and C_i and C_j represent the same class.

APPLICATION OF ARTIFICIAL NEURAL NETWORKS: LEARNING WITH BIOLOGICALLY-INSPIRED OLFACTORY SYSTEM

An *artificial olfactory system* or *electronic-nose* is a biologically plausible architecture which is usually set up to identify and classify odors, mostly in real-time, (Srivastava, Srivastava, & Shukla, 1997). In most cases the odor classes so overlap that a single ANN operation may fail to classify them reliably, (Wang, Hu, & Zhao, 2007). Usually it is preferred to *pre-process* raw samples to enhance scatter properties of individual classes at least for some features. *Linear discriminant analysis* (LDA) is a widely used method for pre-processing and *feature reduction,* (McLahlan, 1992). It simply dissolves correlation between some features and improves overall class scatter in *feature space*. However, an optimum separation/scatter of classes involves spectral or *eigen-decomposition,* which is not appropriate for real-time operation.

In this study, a modification to a recently proposed pre-processing algorithm proposed by (Temel, & Karlik, 2007) is applied to improve odor classification performance of an FFMLP neural network with BP training algorithm. Experiments with real odor data indicate that the proposed pre-processing algorithm brings in superior performance with adopted classifier, i.e. FFMLP, in identifying odors compared to that which does not use the pre-processing. The scheme is also evaluated in terms of robustness to learning rate variation and the number of iterations for FFMLP to converge in training.

Neurophysiology of Olfactory System

Contrary to significant progress in comprehension of visual and auditory sensory systems, the olfactory system has not been understood as much thoroughly. The reason of this partially hidden and unknown system is somewhat because it is relatively a primal sense with intricate and complicated signal processing involved, (Pardo, & Sberveglieri, 2004). Recently, considerable research in neurobiology has been dedicated to understanding the mechanism underlying how smell information is formed by this sensory system and further processed by the brain. It is now known that the olfactory system is able to distinguish almost very large number of low-concentration chemical compounds with use of about 50 million receptor cells, Figure 23.

Olfaction processing involves the respective odor to reach the olfactory region called *olfactory ephitelium* located in the roof of the two nasal cavities, just below and between the eyes through an air flow. The odorant inhaled through the nose contact is required to have certain properties such as sufficiently high vapor pressure, water solubility, low-concentration etc. to stimulate receptor neurons in ephitelium. The receptor neurons in the ephitelium transduce these molecular features into coded electrical action potential impulses. Considerably evidential works indicate that the diversity of stimuli which can be processed by this sensory system is owing to the fact that each olfactory nerve cell simulates only one particular type of the odor molecular structure. Each odor receptor nerve cell has 8 to 20 cilia that are whip-like extensions of 30-200 microns length. The olfactory cilia are the sites where molecular reception for the smell occurs and sensory transduction starts. Each olfactory receptor nerve cell functions like a switch in responding to a particular chemical which can fit itself, (Leffingwell, 2002). These cells also relay axons to the brain through the olfactory nerve. These axons target *the olfactory bulb* in the brain. The olfactory bulb is responsible for pre-processing the incoming coded information, (Li, & Wang, 2006). It then conveys the processed information to the olfactory cortex and other relevant units of the brain. Main brain regions involved in smell information processing are hippocampus, limbic system and cerebral cortex. They synthesize coded spike trains generated by sensing cells and synthesize various odor features as well as identifying the odor source, (Wachowiak, Cohen, Zochowski, & Falk, 2000).

Pre-Processing for Artificial Olfactory System Design

Most real biological data are multivariate and they have highly involved statistical distribution. Depending on the characterizing features, they

Figure 23. The major processing units of the olfactory system, adapted from (Temel, & Karlik 2007)

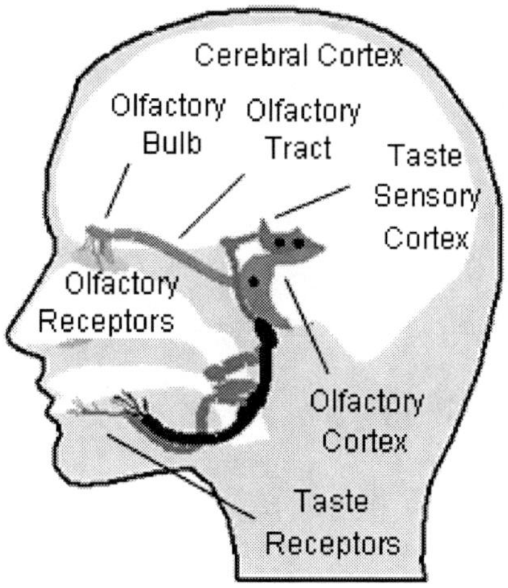

are difficult to discriminate in the sample space, (Osuna, & Nagle, 1999). Moreover, requirement of processing in real-time is a major factor in classification performance of the neural network algorithm to be used. If highly correlated and/or complicated data are to be processed in real-time (on-line) for classification, the network structure may need to be very complicated, i.e. increased number of hidden layers, recurrent design, etc.

Major operations performed by an artificial olfactory system are sensing the odors and identification or recognition of smell pattern ensembles in real-time. Figure 24 illustrates the fundamental block representation of an artificial olfactory system where each varying particular shape in chemical sensor array refers to a respective chemical, (Temel, & Karlik, 2007). The input to the neural network can be taken direct measurement of the sensory array where relevant features are not known or difficult to identify.

Well-known biologically-inspired olfactory system implementation studies are mostly in simulative neural processing nature, (Li, Hopfield, 1989; Caticha, Tejada, Lancet, & Domany, 2002). In order to enhance the training and generalization performance of the neural algorithm employed within an artificial olfactory system the input samples can be pre-processed, Figure 25.

Various pre-processing methods have been developed to be employed in neural information processing systems, (Boukabou, & Bouridane, 2007). They are generally considered for reducing the number of features to avoid *curse of dimensionality* (Bishop, 2004). Despite being in close relevance to feature reduction, the scatter characteristics of raw measurements can be investigated by using discriminant analysis methods without reducing the number of dimensions while preserving the information content. LDA has been extensively applied as a pre-processing algorithm to enhance scatter properties for long, (Liberati, Howe, & Bozdogan, 2009) as a generalization to *Fisher's discriminant analysis*, (Fisher, 1936). The algorithm seeks an optimal linear separation of classes in data space. In order to quantify the LDA algorithm consider a transformation

$$\mathbf{y}=\mathbf{A}\mathbf{x} \tag{38}$$

where $\mathbf{x}$ is the input vector to the pre-processing algorithm. It can be shown that optimum class separation is attained by the following expressions

$$J = \arg\max_{\mathbf{A}} \frac{\left|\mathbf{A}^t \mathbf{S}_b \mathbf{A}\right|}{\left|\mathbf{A}^t \mathbf{S}_t \mathbf{A}\right|} \tag{39}$$

or

$$J = \arg\max_{\mathbf{A}} \frac{tr(\mathbf{A}^t \mathbf{S}_b \mathbf{A})}{tr(\mathbf{A}^t \mathbf{S}_t \mathbf{A})} \tag{40}$$

where $tr(.)$ and $|.|$ are the *trace* and *determinant* of the matrix argument, respectively. Above, $\mathbf{S}_b$, and $\mathbf{S}_t$ refer to the *total between-class,* and the total covariance matrices, respectively. Assuming N data samples represented as row vectors, $\mathbf{x}$, with mean vector $\boldsymbol{\mu}$ coming from c classes they are defined as

Figure 24. Prototype of an electronic nose system where each distinct symbol corresponds to a different odo

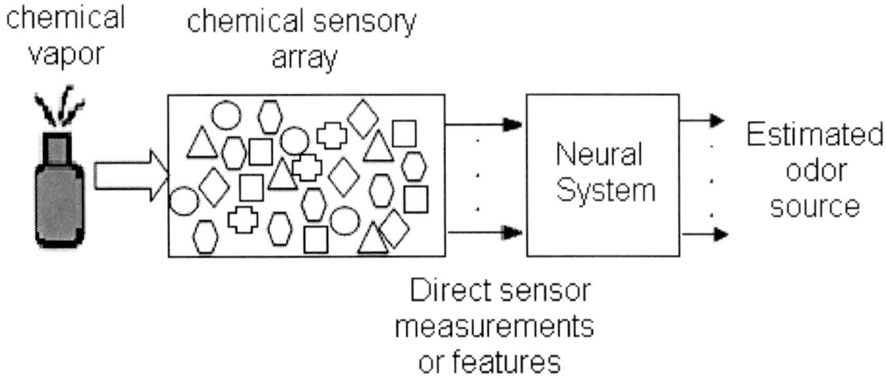

Figure 25. A general neural information system with preprocessing

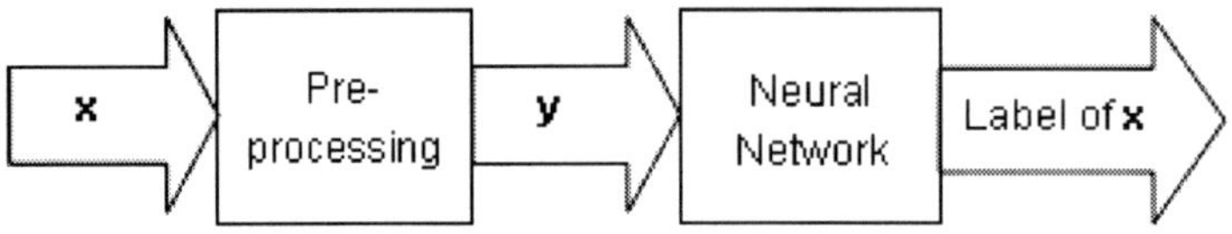

$$\mathbf{S}_b = \sum_{i=1}^{c} N_i(\mu_i - \mu)^t.(\mu_i - \mu)$$

$$\mathbf{S}_t = \sum_{i=1}^{N}(x_i - \mu)^t.(x_i - \mu) = \mathbf{S}_b + \mathbf{S}_w \qquad (41)$$

where $\boldsymbol{\mu}_i$ is the mean vector of the class label i, i.e. C_i, having N_i member patterns. The term $\mathbf{S}_w$ in Equation (41) is the *total within-class scatter* covariance matrix defined as

$$\mathbf{S}_w = \sum_{i=1}^{c}\left(\sum_{x_i \in C_i}(x_i - \mu_i)^t.(x_i - \mu_i)\right) \qquad (42)$$

An analytical solution of Equation (39) or (40) is obtained by exploiting the spectral decomposition, e.g. *principal-component analysis*, (Chen, Shan, & de Haan, 2009), in terms of statistical attributes such as relevant covariance matrices. However, as the dimension of input increases the spectral algorithms with eigen-decomposition methods become unattractive. Particularly biologically-inspired computation which processes large number of instantaneous sensory inputs in real-time may involve an alternative and straightforward, even albeit restrictive, method. Such an alternative approach may be inferred from the mathematical treatment concerning the saliency of feature vectors in a class with respect to overall dataset. Individual class saliency is established by linear transformation expressed in terms of respective class and overall data covariance matrices, (Härdle, & Simar, 2003). A suitable transformation can be of the form

$$y = S_i S_t^{-1} x \qquad (43)$$

as a modified version of the algorithm proposed in (Temel, & Karlik, 2007). In Equation (43) labeled sample **x** belongs to class C_i with covariance matrix $\mathbf{S}_i$, i=1, 2, …, K. It should be noted that the pre-processing needs to be applied at both training and post-training phases while the algo-

Figure 26. Odor classification performance distribution of the FFMLP with (a) raw, and (b) pre-processed patterns

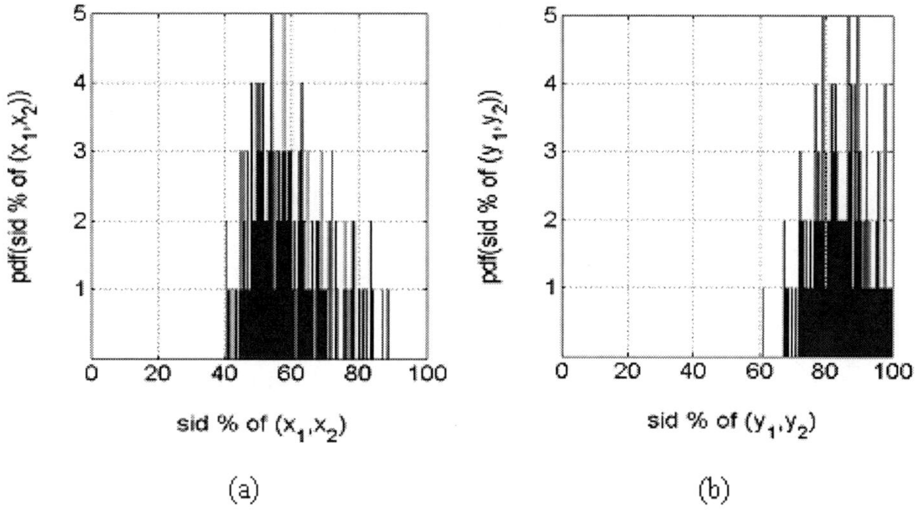

rithm needs matrix multiplication $S_i S_i^{-1}$ to be stored for all the classes given an input sample. These matrices need to be modified as new classes enter the processing.

Experiments and Results

In the experiments 32 samples collected from 20 different odorant perfume s were used. Sampling was performed with two chemical sensors operating in real-time sampling mode. FFMLP weights were updated with the learning rate $\eta(k) = \eta_0 / k$ where η_0 is the initial learning rate and k is the iteration. The collected samples were delivered to BP-trained 2-10-20 FFMLP classifiers with both pre-processing and no-preprocessing simulative blocks to obtain two distinct outputs. Each output neuron of each classifier indicates the computed class labels. The target value for correct classes was taken 0.9 while incorrect classes were identified with output value of 0.1 in order to avoid overfitting and overtraining problems.

In order to evaluate overall odor recognition performance in statistical terms, raw samples were populated by using the boot-strapping, (Gong, 1986), to yield 10 times larger dataset for both FFMLP classifiers. Each classifier was trained and tested with datasets of populated raw and their preprocessed counterparts in 100 distinct experiments. For each experiment conducted, the FFMLP classifiers were cross-validated using 9 labeled training subgroups and one unlabeled testing subgroup for η_0=0.05, 0.1, 0.15, 0.2, while the momentum term was chosen 0.1. For statistical evaluation of performance, each classifier was assessed in respective histogram which indicates the *probability density function* (pdf) of successful identification (sid) of odor samples. Figure 26 reveals that the use of pre-processing brings in superior classification performance for the odorants considered where x_i /y_i refers to raw/preprocessed entry from sensor i=1, 2. A clear improvement in class separation is observed with the preprocessing. The odors were successfully identified at a success score around 85% or higher while the performance score with raw data lies between 40%-80%. Table I presents testing statistics in terms of average (Av.) and standard deviation (std.) of sid and algorithm training convergence performance in the average number of

Table 1. Some statistical values of FFMLP with pre-processing

	η_0=0.05	η_0=0.1	η_0=0.15	η_0=0.2
Av.(it.)	6.2	7.9	7.3	7.1
Av. (sid)	88.5	88.9	83.1	86.7
Std. (sid)	5.3	4.9	6.9	5.1

iterations (Av. it.) for the FFMLP classifier with pre-processing.

An important aspect of the classifier design is its robustness to parametric variations such as learning rate. From Table I it is observed that FFMLP with preprocessing exhibits considerably robust characteristics against adopted range of variations in η_0. This robustness is mainly owing to highly scattered samples given an odor class.

CONCLUSION

In this chapter, fundamental notions of biologically-inspired learning and well-known algorithms are described. The neurobiological mechanism underlying this inspiration is explained as much briefly and concisely as possible for rendering possible problem domain to a diverse solution domain. Starting from major functionalities of neuron, overall nervous system exhibits a profound regularity and hierarchy in responding to environmental or internal stimuli with huge parallelism. Modeling approaches to this hierarchy along with concurrent processing, however, have led to suitable adaptive and effective solutions for most scientific and engineering problems at hand.

The chapter explained delta-rule which reflects the dynamics of synaptic weights at learning phase in artificial neural network units such as basic neuron and perceptron. Least-mean squared-error and steepest-descent methods were also dealt with for analytically expressing the rule in iteratively searching a stable solution. The structure called the adaptive linear element was also introduced. Focus was directed at feed-forward multi-layered perceptron neural network along with the delta-rule. A very elaborate training scheme called back-propagation was visited. Important training and testing issues, such as iterative inspection of global minimum in error function, arrangement of training and testing samples for improved generalization capability, were also discussed. It was explained that the improved performance of a network with back-propagation algorithm stems from reverse credit-assignment to validate forward activation. An important class of neural networks called self-organizing feature maps were exemplified with learning-vector quantization algorithms.

The final section of the chapter was dedicated to an application of artificial neural network paradigm to illustrate design aspects of biologically-inspired system design for artificial olfaction or electronic nose. As a tool for class separation and scatter properties, discriminant analysis was presented. The artificial olfactory system design covered a recently introduced pre-processing scheme for a feed-forward multi-layer perceptron neural network. The neural system with proposed pre-processing scheme was shown to outperform the counterpart without pre-processing.

REFERENCES

Alberini, C. M., Milekic, M. H., & Tronel, S. (2006). Mechanisms of Memory Stabilization and Destabilization. *Cellular and Molecular Life Sciences*, *63*(9), 999–100. doi:10.1007/s00018-006-6025-7

Anderson, J. A. (1972). A Simple Neural Network Generating an Interactive Memory. *Mathematical Biosciences*, *14*, 197–220. doi:10.1016/0025-5564(72)90075-2

Arbib, M. A. (1987). *Brains, Machines, and Mathematics* (2nd ed.). Berlin: Springer-Verlag.

Ariniello, L., & McComb, M. (2002). *Brain Facts: A Primer on the Brain and Nervous System*. Washington: The Society for Neuroscience.

Bishop, C. M. (2004). *Neural Networks for Pattern Recognition* (3rd ed.). Oxford: Oxford University Press.

Boukabou, W. R., & Bouridane, A. (2007). An Improved LDA Approach with DFB Preprocessing for Face Recognition. In *Proceedings of IEEE International Symposium on Bio-inspired Learning, and Intelligent Systems for Security*, 106-110.

Caticha, N., Pelado, J. E. P., Lancet, D., & Domany, E. (2002). Computational Capacity of an Odorant Discriminator: The Linear Separability of Curves. *Neural Computation*, *14*(9), 2201–2220. doi:10.1162/089976602320264051

Chen, W., Shan, C., & de Haan, G. (2009). Optimal Regularization Parameter Estimation for Spectral Regression Discriminant Analysis. *IEEE Transactions on Circuits and Systems for Video Technology*, *19*(12), 1921–1926. doi:10.1109/TCSVT.2009.2026953

Dayan, P., & Abbot, L. F. (2001). *Theoretical Neuroscience: Computational and Mathematical Modeling of Neural Systems*. Cambridge, MA: MIT Press.

Efron, B., & Tibshirani, R. (1997). Improvements on Cross-validation: The .632+Bootstrap Method. *Journal of the American Statistical Association*, *92*(438), 548–560. doi:10.2307/2965703

Fisher, R. A. (1936). The Use of Multiple Measurements in Taxonomic Problems. *Annals of Eugenics*, *7*, 179–188.

Fletcher, R., & Reeves, C. M. (1964). Function Minimization by Conjugate Gradients. *The Computer Journal*, *7*, 149–154. doi:10.1093/comjnl/7.2.149

Freeman, J. A., & Skapura, D. M. (1991). *Neural Networks: Algorithms, Applications, and Programming Techniques*. Reading, MA: Addison-Wesley.

Furber, S., & Temple, S. (2007). Neural Systems Engineering. *Journal of the Royal Society, Interface*, *4*, 193–206. doi:10.1098/rsif.2006.0177

Gong, G. (1986). Cross-validation, the Jackknife, and the Bootstrap: Excess Error Estimation in Forward Logistic Regression. *Journal of the American Statistical Association*, *81*(393), 108–113. doi:10.2307/2287975

Griva, I., Nash, S. G., & Sofer, A. (2009). *Linear and Nonlinear Optimization* (2 nd ed.).

Guyon, I., & Elisseeff, A. (2003). An Introduction to Variable and Feature Selection. *Journal of Machine Learning Research*, *3*, 1157–1182. doi:10.1162/153244303322753616

Härdle, W., & Simar, L. (2003). *Applied Multivariate Statistical Analysis*. Berln, Germany: Springer-Verlag.

Hartman, K., Keeler, J. D., & Kowalski, J. M. (1990). Layered Neural Networks with Gaussian Hidden Units as Universal Approximations. *Neural Computation*, *2*, 210–215. doi:10.1162/neco.1990.2.2.210

Haykin, S. (2003). *Neural Networks: A Comprehensive Foundation* (4th ed.). Upper Saddle River, New Jersey: Prentice Hall.

Hebb, D. O. (1949). *The Organization of Behavior: A Neuropsychological Theory*. New York: John Wiley & Sons.

Hodgkin, A. L., & Huxley, A. F. (1952). A Quantitative Description of Membrane Current and its Application to Conduction and Excitation in Nerve. *The Journal of Physiology*, *117*, 500–544.

Jacobs, R. A. (1988). Increased Rates of Convergence Through Learning Rate Adaptation. *Neural Networks*, *1*, 295–307. doi:10.1016/0893-6080(88)90003-2

Kasabov, N. K. (1998). *Foundations of Neural Networks, Fuzzy Systems, and Knowledge Engineering*, (2nd ed.). Cambridge, MA: MIT Press. Philapdelphia: SIAM.

Kneer, S., Personnaz, L., & Dreyfus, G. (1992). Handwritten Digit Recognition by Neural Networks with Single-Layer Training. *IEEE Transactions on Neural Networks*, *3*(6), 962–968. doi:10.1109/72.165597

Kohonen, T. (1982). Self-organized Formation of Topographically Correct Feature Maps. *Biological Cybernetics*, *43*, 59–69. doi:10.1007/BF00337288

Kohonen, T. (1990). Improved Versions of Learning Vector Quantizations. *Proceedings of International Joint Conference on Neural Networks*, *I*, 545–550. doi:10.1109/IJCNN.1990.137622

Kohonen, T. (1990). The Self-organizing Map. *Proceedings of the IEEE*, *78*(9), 1464–1480. doi:10.1109/5.58325

Kohonen, T. (1993). Physiological Interpretation of the Self-organising Map Algorithm. *Neural Networks*, *6*, 895–905.

Kolb, B., & Whishaw, I. Q. (2008). *Fundamentals of Human Neuropsychology. Hampshire*. Macmillan.

Kreiman, G. (2004). Neural Coding: Computational and Biophysical Perspectives. *Physics of Life Reviews*, *1*(2), 71–102. doi:10.1016/j.plrev.2004.06.001

Lee, Y., Oh, S. H., Song, H. K., & Kim, M. W. (1982). Design Rules of Multilayer Perceptron. *Proceedings of SPIE, Science of Artificial Neural Networks,* 1710, 329–339.

Liberati, C., Howe, J. A., & Bozdogan, H. (2009). Data Adaptive Simultaneous Parameter and Kernel Selection in Kernel Discriminant Analysis Using Information Complexity. *Journal of Pattern Recognition*, *4*(1), 119–132.

MacLahlan, G. J. (1992). *Discriminant Analysis and Statistical Pattern Recognition*. New York: Wiley & Sons.

McCulloch, W. S., & Pitts, W. (1943). A Logical Calculus of the Ideas Immanent in Nervous Activity. *Bulletin of Mathematical Biology*, *5*, 115–133.

McDonough, J. (2004). Least Mean Square Error (LMSE) Estimation. *Lecture Notes of Interactive Systems Laboratories Institut für Logik, Komplexitat, und Deduktionssysteme Universitat Karlsruhe.*

Minsky, M. L., & Pappert, S. A. (1969). *Perceptrons*. Cambridge, MA: MIT Press.

Nilsson, N. J. (1965). *Learning Machines: Foundations of Trainable Pattern-Classifying Systems*. New York: McGraw-Hill.

Orna, M. V., & Stock, J. (1989). *Electrochemistry, Past and Present*. Columbus: American Chemical Society.

Osuna, R. G-., & Nagle, H. T. (1999). A Method for Evaluating Data-preprocessing Techniques for Odour Classification with an Array of Gas Sensors. *IEEE Transactions on Systems, Man, and Cybernetics. Part B*, *29*(5), 626–632.

Pandya, A. S., & Macy, R. B. (1995). *Pattern Recognition with Neural Networks in C*. CRC Press.

Pandya, A. S., & Venugopal, P. (1991). A Stochastic Parallel Algorithm for Supervised Learning in Neural Networks. *IEEE Transactions on Information Systems. E (Norwalk, Conn.)*, *77-D*(4), 376–384.

Pardo, M., & Sberveglieri, G. (2004). Feature Evaluation for an Electronic Node. *Proceedings of the IEEE, 2*, 595–596. doi:10.1109/ICSENS.2004.1426235

Perelman, Y., & Ginosar, R. (2008). *The Neuroprocessor: An Integrated Interface to Biological Neural Networks*. Springer-Verlag. Porto, A. B., & Pazos, A. (2006). Neuroglial Behaviour in Computer Science. In Rabuna, J. R., & Dorado, J. (Eds.), *Artificial Neural Networks in Real-life Applications* (pp. 1–21). London: Idea Group Publications.

Potter, S.M (2007). What can AI Get from Neuroscience. *Lecture Notes in Artificial Intelligence*, 174-185.

Rabinowitch, I., & Segev, I. (2008). Two Opposing Plasticity Mechanisms Pulling a Single Synapse. *Trends in Neurosciences, 31*(8), 377–383. doi:10.1016/j.tins.2008.05.005

Riedel, G., Platt, B., & Micheau, J. (2003). Glutamate Receptor Function in Learning and Memory. *Behavioural Brain Research, 140*, 1–47. doi:10.1016/S0166-4328(02)00272-3

Rosenblatt, F. (1958). The Perceptron: A Probabilistic Model for Information Storage and Organization in the Brain. *Psychological Review, 65*, 386–408. doi:10.1037/h0042519

Rosenblatt, F. (1962). *Principles of Neurodynamics*. Washington, DC: Spartan Books.

Roy, A., Steinmetz, P. N., Hsiao, S. S., Johnson, K. O., & Niebur, E. (2007). Synchrony: A Neural Correlate of Somatosensory Attention. *Journal of Neurophysiology, 98*, 1645–1661. doi:10.1152/jn.00522.2006

Sherrington, C. S. (1933). *The Brain and Its Mechanism. New London*. Cambridge University Press.

Soucek, B. (1992). *Fast Learning and Invariant Object Recognition*. New York: John Wiley & Sons.

Srivastava, A. K., Srivastava, S. K., & Shukla, K. K. (1997). On the Design Issue of Intelligent Electronic Nose System. *Proceedings of the International Conference on Industrial Technology, 1*, 243–248.

Temel, T., & Karlik, B. (2007). An improved Odor Recognition System Using Learning Vector Quantization with a New Discriminant Analysis. *Neural Network World, 4*(7), 287–294.

Tsai, S., Hong, P., & Chieu, B. (1992). Handwritten Digit Recognition via OCON Neural Network by Selective Pruning. *Proceedings of the IEEE 11th International Conference on Pattern Recognition*, 656–659.

von Neumann, J. (1958). *The Computer and the Brain*. New Haven: Yale University Press.

Wachowiak, M., Cohen, L. B., Zochowski, M., & Falk, C. X. (2000). The Spatial Representation of Odors by Olfactory Receptor Neuron Input to the Olfactory Bulb is Concentration Invariant. *The Biological Bulletin, 199*(2), 162–163. doi:10.2307/1542876

Wang, H., Hu, Z., & Zhao, Y. (2007). An Efficient Algorithm for Generalized Discriminant Analysis Using Incomplete Cholesky Decomposition. *Pattern Recognition Letters, 28*, 254–259. doi:10.1016/j.patrec.2006.07.008

Wehr, M., & Laurent, G. (1996). Odour Encoding by Temporal Sequences of Firing in Oscillating Neural Assemblies. *Nature, 384*(6605), 162–166. doi:10.1038/384162a0

Werbos, P. J. (1974). *Beyond Regression: New Tools for Prediction and Analysis in the Behavioral Sciences,* Unpublished Ph.D. dissertation: Harvard University.

Widrow, B. & Hoff, M. E. (1960). Adaptive Switching Circuits. *IRE WESCON Convention Record*. 96-104.

Wiener, N. (1948). *Cybernetics: Or, Control and Communication in the Animal and the Machine*. New York: John Wiley & Sons.

Chapter 5
Optimality-Oriented Stabilization for Recurrent Neural Networks

Ziqian Liu
State University of New York Maritime College, USA

ABSTRACT

This chapter presents an approach of how optimality-oriented stabilization is achieved for recurrent neural networks, which includes both the input-to-state stabilization for deterministic recurrent neural networks and the noise-to-state stabilization for stochastic recurrent neural networks. Owing to the difficulty in solving the Hamilton-Jacobi equation for nonlinear systems, optimal regulation seems to be an unachievable goal in control design for recurrent neural networks. However, a methodology proposed in this chapter solves the problem and obtains optimal stabilization by using the knowledge of Lyapunov technique, inverse optimality, and differential game theory. Numerical examples demonstrate the effectiveness of the proposed design.

INTRODUCTION

Inspired by biological neuronal systems, artificial neural networks have demonstrated superior characteristics of learning, adaptation, classification and function-approximation. They have been successfully applied to many areas. However, conventional neural networks are feed-forward networks that move the information in only one direction, forward, from the inputs to the outputs. There are no cycles or loops in the network and no feedback connections are present. Therefore, there are some drawbacks in using those networks.

Since the Hopfield's paper (Hopfield, 1984), recurrent neural networks, also called dynamic neural networks, have emerged to be a highly effective methodology. Because these networks have feedback connections that represent dynamic memory, which make them more suitable for modeling biological intelligence than purely feed-forward neural networks. In addition, within the structure of recurrent neural networks, they have bi-directional data flow. Therefore, they have been used to solve various difficult problems in many

DOI: 10.4018/978-1-60960-018-1.ch005

scientific areas, such as pattern recognition, operational analysis, system identification and control, and content-addressable memory. Moreover, they are easy for VLSI implementation. Motivated by the successful applications of recurrent neural networks, theoretical studies on both stability and controllability of recurrent neural networks have emerged in the last few years, see for example, (Arik, 2000; Ensari & Arik, 2005; Hu & Wang, 2002; Kulawski & Brdys, 2000; Liu, Torres, Patel, & Wang, 2008; Liu, Wang, & Schurz, 2009; Liu & Wang, 2007; Sanchez & Perez, 2003), and references therein. The latest research results, obtained in (Liu, Torres, Patel, & Wang, 2008; Liu, Wang, & Schurz, 2009; Liu & Wang, 2007), solve both the problem of the input-to-state stabilization for deterministic recurrent neural networks and the problem of the noise-to-state stabilization for stochastic recurrent neural networks.

Based on the results in (Liu, Torres, Patel, & Wang, 2008; Liu, Wang, & Schurz, 2009; Liu & Wang, 2007), this chapter provides a rigorous theoretical foundation to the theory and algorithms of optimality-oriented stabilization for recurrent neural networks, which includes both input-to-state stabilization for deterministic recurrent neural networks and noise-to-state stabilization for stochastic recurrent neural networks. In order to achieve the aforementioned goals, the rest of the chapter is organized as follows. Part A presents the theoretical results of input-to-state stabilization for deterministic recurrent neural networks, together with two numerical examples to show the effectiveness. Part B illustrates an approach to achieve noise-to-state stabilization in probability for stochastic recurrent neural networks driven by noise of unknown covariance. In addition, two numerical examples are given. Finally, the main conclusions are reported.

PART-A: INPUT-TO-STATE STABILIZATION FOR DETERMINISTIC RECURRENT NEURAL NETWORKS

This part considers the design of input-to-state stabilization for deterministic recurrent neural networks. This approach is developed by using Lyapunov technique, inverse optimality, and Hamilton-Jacobi-Bellman (HJB) equation. Depending on the dimensions of state and input, two optimal control laws are constructed in order to achieve input-to-state stabilization for the networks. Furthermore, the proposed designs achieve global asymptotic stability and global inverse optimality with respect to some meaningful cost functional. Two numerical examples demonstrate the performance of the approach. The content of this part is based on (Liu, Torres, Patel, & Wang, 2008) and (Liu & Wang, 2007).

Problem Formulation and Mathematical Preliminaries

Based on the formulation of recurrent neural networks, we consider the following deterministic recurrent neural networks.

$$\dot{x}_i(t) = -\lambda x_i(t) + \sum_{k=1}^{n} w_{ik}^1 s(x_k) + \sum_{j=1}^{m} w_{ij}^2 u_j \tag{1}$$

where $i = 1, 2, \ldots, n$. Mathematically, this can be described by the following compact form

$$\dot{x} = -Ax + W_1 S(x) + W_2 u \tag{2}$$

where $x \in R^n$ is the state of recurrent neural networks, $u \in R^m$ is the input, usually $m \neq n$, $A = diag(-\lambda, \cdots, -\lambda) = -\lambda I \in R^{n\times n}$ and $\lambda > 0$, $S(x) = \left[s(x_1), \cdots, s(x_n)\right]^T \in R^n$ is a nonlinear vector-valued activation function with $s(\cdot) =$

tanh(·), $W_1 \in R^{n\times n}$, $W_2 \in R^{n\times m}$ are weight matrices describing the connections of hidden and output layers. If $W_2 = I \in R^{n\times n}$, it is obvious that this neural network becomes the famous Hopfield-type neural network. Therefore, the model of recurrent neural networks, in which the number of the state is different from the number of the input, encompasses a larger class of recurrent neural networks (see e.g. (Kulawski & Brdys, 2000) and (Rovithakis & Christodoulou, 2000)).

Before we develop the main analytical results, let us first introduce the following mathematical notations, mathematical theorems, and the theorem of optimality and stability.

1. Vector and Matrix Norms

The norm $\|x\|$ of a vector x is the Euclidean norm

$$\|x\| = \sqrt{x_1^2 + \cdots + x_n^2} = \sqrt{x^T x} \tag{3}$$

If A is a matrix, then $\|A\|$ denotes the Frobenius matrix norm, defined as

$$\|A\| = \sqrt{\sum_{ij} |a_{ij}|^2} = \sqrt{tr\{A^T A\}} \tag{4}$$

where $tr\{\cdot\}$ denotes the trace of a matrix.

2. Young's Inequality (Hardy, Littlewood, & Polya, 1989)

For any two vectors x and y of the same dimension, the following inequality holds

$$x^T y \le \frac{\|x\|^2}{2} + \frac{\|y\|^2}{2} \tag{5}$$

3. Mean Value Theorem (Khalil, 1996)

If x and y are two distinct points in R^n, then the line segment $L(x, y)$ joining x and y is

$$L(x, y) = \{z \mid z = \theta x + (1-\theta)y, 0 < \theta < 1\} \tag{6}$$

Assuming f: $R^n \rightarrow R$ is continuously differentiable at each point x of an open set $S \subset R^n$, let x and y be two points of S such that the line segment $L(x, y) \subset S$. Then there exists a point ξ of $L(x, y)$ such that

$$f(y) - f(x) = \left.\frac{\partial f}{\partial x}\right|_{x=\xi} (y - x) \tag{7}$$

4. Optimality and Stability (Sepulchre, Jankovic, & Kokotovic, 1997)

It is known that for the following kind of general nonlinear system

$$\dot{x} = F(x) + G(x)u \tag{8}$$

Suppose that there exists a C^1 positive semi-definite function $V(x)$, which satisfies the following Hamilton-Jacobi-Bellman (HJB) equation

$$V_x(x)F(x) - \frac{1}{4}V_x(x)G(x)r^{-1}(x)G^T(x)V_x^T(x) + q(x) = 0 \tag{9}$$

In addition, there is a feedback control

$$u^*(x) = -\frac{1}{2}r^{-1}(x)G^T(x)V_x^T(x) \tag{10}$$

which achieves asymptotic stability of the equilibrium $x = 0$. Then $u^*(x)$ is the optimal stabilizing control, which minimizes the cost functional

$$J = \int_0^{\infty} \left(q(x) + u^T r(x) u \right) dt \qquad (11)$$

where $q(x) \geq 0$ and $r(x) > 0$ for all x and $V(x)$ is the optimal value function.

Main Results

Consider the recurrent neural networks described by the system (2). Let us rewrite it as

$$\dot{x} = -\lambda x + W_1 S(x) + W_2 u \qquad (12)$$

where $\lambda > 0$. We now define a positive semi-definite Lyapunov function V, which is the same as the one given in (Kulawski & Brdys, 2000)

$$V = \frac{1}{2} x^T x = \frac{1}{2} \|x\|^2 \qquad (13)$$

and take the time derivative of it along the trajectory of x

$$\begin{aligned} \dot{V} &= x^T \dot{x} \\ &= x^T(-\lambda x + W_1 S(x) + W_2 u) \\ &= -\lambda x^T x + x^T W_1 S(x) + x^T W_2 u \end{aligned} \qquad (14)$$

For the second term $x^T W_1 S(x)$, let us apply the Young's Inequality to it

$$\begin{aligned} x^T W_1 S(x) &\leq \frac{1}{2} x^T x + \frac{1}{2} \|W_1 S(x)\|^2 \\ &\leq \frac{1}{2} x^T x + \frac{1}{2} \|W_1\|^2 \|S(x)\|^2 \end{aligned} \qquad (15)$$

From the Mean Value Theorem, we have

$$\|S(x)\| - \|S(0)\| = \left. \frac{\partial \{\|S(x)\|\}}{\partial x} \right|_{x=\xi} \cdot (x - 0) \qquad (16)$$

That is

$$\|S(x)\| = \left. \frac{\partial \{\|S(x)\|\}}{\partial x} \right|_{x=\xi} \cdot x \qquad (17)$$

where

$$\left. \frac{\partial \{\|S(x)\|\}}{\partial x} \right|_{x=\xi} = \left[\left. \frac{\partial \{\|S(x)\|\}}{\partial x_1} \right|_{x_1=\xi_1}, \cdots, \left. \frac{\partial \{\|S(x)\|\}}{\partial x_n} \right|_{x_n=\xi_n} \right] \qquad (18)$$

and

$$\frac{\partial \{\|S(x)\|\}}{\partial x_i} = \sqrt{\frac{s^2(x_i)}{s^2(x_1) + \cdots + s^2(x_n)}} \; s'(x_i) \qquad (19)$$

Since

$$s(x_i) = \tanh(x_i) \qquad (20)$$

So

$$s'(x_i) = \sec h^2(x_i) = \frac{1}{\cosh^2(x_i)} \leq 1 \qquad (21)$$

Then

$$\begin{aligned} \|S(x)\| &\leq \left[s'(\xi_1), \cdots, s'(\xi_n) \right] \begin{bmatrix} x_1 \\ \vdots \\ x_n \end{bmatrix} \\ &\leq \sqrt{\left[s'(\xi_1)\right]^2 + \cdots + \left[s'(\xi_n)\right]^2} \cdot \|x\| \\ &\leq \sqrt{n} \|x\| \end{aligned} \qquad (22)$$

From (15), we obtain

$$x^T W_1 S(x) \leq \frac{1}{2} x^T x + \frac{1}{2} n \left\| W_1 \right\|^2 \left\| x \right\|^2 \leq \frac{1}{2} x^T x + \frac{1}{2} n \left\| W_1 \right\|^2 x^T x \leq x^T \left(\frac{1 + n \left\| W_1 \right\|^2}{2} \right) x \tag{23}$$

Substituting (23) into (14), we have

$$\dot{V} = -\lambda x^T x + x^T W_1 S(x) + x^T W_2 u \leq -\lambda x^T x + x^T \left(\frac{1 + n \left\| W_1 \right\|^2}{2} \right) x + x^T W_2 u \tag{24}$$

Depending on the dimensions of state x and input u, we consider two cases.

Case 1

$x \in R^n$, $u \in R^n$, and $W_2 \in R^{n \times n}$.

Based on (24), let us consider

$$x^T \left(\frac{1 + n \left\| W_1 \right\|^2}{2} \right) x + x^T W_2 u = 0 \tag{25}$$

In order to proceed with the following analysis, we consider:

- **Assumption 1:** For the system of recurrent neural networks (12), the weight matrix W_2 is selected to be invertible, that is

$$\left| W_2 \right| \neq 0 \tag{26}$$

With assumption 1, we can determine a control law as

$$u = -\left(W_2 \right)^{-1} \left(\frac{1 + n \left\| W_1 \right\|^2}{2} \right) x \tag{27}$$

Then the inequality of (24) becomes that

$$\dot{V} \leq -\lambda x^T x \leq 0 \tag{28}$$

Therefore, the control law of (27) is a stabilizing control.

For the system of recurrent neural network (12), which has a positive semi-definite Lyapunov function V defined by (13), we are able to get two Lie derivatives (Khalil, 1996)

$$V_x F(x) = -\lambda x^T x + x^T W_1 S(x) \tag{29}$$

$$V_x G(x) = x^T W_2 \tag{30}$$

Then the substitution of the above equations into the HJB equation (9) yields the next relation

$$-\lambda x^T x + x^T W_1 S(x) - \frac{1}{4} x^T W_2 r^{-1}(x) W_2^T x + q(x) = 0 \tag{31}$$

Let us make modification of (27)

$$u = -c \left(W_2 \right)^{-1} \left(\frac{1 + n \left\| W_1 \right\|^2}{2} \right) x = -c \left(W_2 \right)^{-1} \left(\frac{1 + n \left\| W_1 \right\|^2}{2} \right) \left(W_2^T \right)^{-1} \left(W_2^T \right) x = -c \left(W_2^T W_2 \right)^{-1} \left(\frac{1 + n \left\| W_1 \right\|^2}{2} \right) W_2^T x = -\frac{1}{2} c \left(W_2^T W_2 \right)^{-1} \left(1 + n \left\| W_1 \right\|^2 \right) W_2^T x \tag{32}$$

where $c > 2$ is constant.

Substituting (30) into (10) and comparing the result with (32), we find that the function $r(x)$ can be selected as

$$r(x) = c^{-1}W_2^T W_2\left(1 + n\left\|W_1\right\|^2\right)^{-1} \tag{33}$$

Then from the equation of (31), the function $q(x)$ is given by

$$q(x) = \lambda x^T x + \frac{c}{4}\left(1 + n\left\|W_1\right\|^2\right)x^T x - x^T W_1 S(x) \tag{34}$$

Based on the theorem of optimality and stability, for $c > 2$, we get the following result.

Theorem 1
A positive-definite function $q(x)$ defined by (34) and a strictly positive-function $r(x)$ defined by (33) exist, such that the feedback control law

$$u = u^* = -\frac{1}{2}r^{-1}(x)W_2^T x \tag{35}$$

applied to the system (12), achieves global inverse optimality with respect to a cost functional of the form

$$J = \int_0^\infty\left(q(x) + u^T r(x)u\right)dt \tag{36}$$

Also the optimal control law (35) renders the equilibrium $x = 0$ globally asymptotical stability (GAS). Therefore, the input control defined by (35) achieves input-to-state stabilization for the system of recurrent neural networks (12).

Proof

- **Step 1:** By considering the Lyapunov function (13) which is a positive semi-definite function, we take the time derivative of V along the trajectory of x

$$\dot{V} = -\lambda x^T x + x^T W_1 S(x) + x^T W_2 u \tag{37}$$

The substitution of the control law (35) into $\dot{V}$ (37) yields

$$\begin{aligned}\dot{V} &= -\lambda x^T x + x^T W_1 S(x) \\ &\quad -\frac{1}{2}cx^T W_2\left(W_2^T W_2\right)^{-1}\left(1 + n\left\|W_1\right\|^2\right)W_2^T x \\ &= -\lambda x^T x + x^T W_1 S(x) - \frac{1}{2}c\left(1 + n\left\|W_1\right\|^2\right)x^T x\end{aligned} \tag{38}$$

Replacing the second term of (38) by (23), we have

$$\begin{aligned}\dot{V} &\le -\lambda x^T x + \left(\frac{1 + n\left\|W_1\right\|^2}{2}\right)x^T x - \frac{1}{2}c\left(1 + n\left\|W_1\right\|^2\right)x^T x \\ &\le -\lambda x^T x - \left(\frac{c-1}{2}\right)\left(1 + n\left\|W_1\right\|^2\right)x^T x \\ &< 0 \quad \forall x \ne 0\end{aligned} \tag{39}$$

So the feedback control law (29) achieves global asymptotic stability of the equilibrium $x = 0$ and guarantees

$$\lim_{t\to\infty} x = 0 \tag{40}$$

- **Step 2:** Let us consider $q(x)$ and $r(x)$. From the equation of (34)

$$q(x) = \lambda x^T x + \frac{c}{4}(1 + n\left\|W_1\right\|^2)x^T x - x^T W_1 S(x) \tag{41}$$

Appling (23) to the third term of the equation above, we have

$$q(x) \geq \lambda x^T x + \frac{c}{4}(1 + n\|W_1\|^2)x^T x - x^T \left(\frac{1 + n\|W_1\|^2}{2} \right) x$$
$$\geq \lambda x^T x + \left(\frac{c-2}{2} \right) \left(\frac{1 + n\|W_2\|^2}{2} \right) x^T x$$
$$\geq 0 \quad (42)$$

Then $q(x)$ is positive definite and radially unbounded.
From the equation of (33)

$$r(x) = c^{-1} W_2^T W_2 (1 + n\|W_1\|^2)^{-1} \quad (43)$$

If $|W_2| \neq 0$, we know that $r(x) > 0$ since $W_2^T W_2 > 0$
For the choice of $q(x)$ and $r(x)$ represented by (34) and (33), $\dot{V}$ can be evaluated by the following form

$$\dot{V} = -q(x) - u^T r(x) u + (u - u^*)^T r(x)(u - u^*) \quad (44)$$

which can be written as

$$q(x) + u^T r(x) u + \dot{V} = (u - u^*)^T r(x)(u - u^*) \geq 0 \quad (45)$$

Then it is shown from the equation of (45) that the optimal control $u = u^*$ is an optimal solution to J (36), that is, $u = u^*$ satisfies

$$\min_u \left[q(x) + u^T r(x) u + \dot{V} \right] = 0 \quad (46)$$

Also the Lyapunov function $V(x)$ (13) satisfies the HJB equation

$$V_x(x) f(x) - \frac{1}{4} V_x(x) g(x) r^{-1}(x) g^T(x) V_x^T(x) + q(x) = 0 \quad (47)$$

Therefore, $V(x)$ is the value function for the cost functional (36).

Finally, based on the result of paper (Malisoff, Rifford, & Sontag, 2004), it is obvious that the input control defined as (35) achieves input-to-state stabilization for the system (12). This completes the proof.

Case 2

$x \in R^n$, $u \in R^n$, and $W_2 \in R^{n \times m}$, and $m \neq n$ ($m < n$ or $m > n$)

In order to proceed with the following analysis, we consider the following assumption.

- **Assumption 2:** For the system of recurrent neural networks (12), the weight matrix W_2 is selected to satisfy the inequality below

$$W_2 W_2^T > 0 \quad (48)$$

With the assumption above, we do not loss the generality because $W_2 W_2^T$ is always nonnegative definite, that is, $W_2 W_2^T \geq 0$.
From the inequality (24), let us define

$$\psi_1(x) = x^T \left(\frac{1 + n\|W_1\|^2}{2} \right) x \quad (49)$$

$$\psi_2^T(x) = x^T W_2 \quad (50)$$

Similar to Sontag's formula described in (Sontag, 1989), we create a scalar function

$$\varphi(x) = \begin{cases} \dfrac{\psi_1(x) + \sqrt{[\psi_1(x)]^2 + [\psi_2^T(x)\psi_2(x)]^2}}{\psi_2^T(x)\psi_2(x)}, & x \neq 0 \\ 0 & x = 0 \end{cases} \quad (51)$$

- **Remark 1:** With the assumption of (48), we know that

$$\psi_2^T(x)\psi_2(x) = x^T W_2 W_2^T x \neq 0 \quad (\forall x \neq 0) \qquad (52)$$

- **Remark 2:** From the functions of (49) and (50), it is obvious that $\psi_1(x)$ and $\psi_2(x)$ are continues with respect to x. Therefore, the function $\varphi(x)$ defined by (51) is continuous at $x = 0$. A possible singularity of $\varphi(x)$ due to division by $\psi_2^T(x)\psi_2(x)$ is removed with the definition of $\varphi(x) = 0$ at $x = 0$. Interested readers can consult (Sontag, 1989) for details.

  Then let us choose a control signal as the following

$$u = -\varphi(x)\psi_2(x) \qquad (53)$$

  Using (50), this is equivalent to

$$u = -\varphi(x)W_2^T x \qquad (54)$$

- **Remark 3:** With the analysis above, we know that u is continuous for $\forall x$ under the assumption of (48). With respect to the weight value of $W_2 W_2^T$, if it becomes very small, the control u may become very big. Therefore, one has to adjust the weight W_2 to avoid this situation.

  Comparing (54) with (10) and using (30) and (31), we obtain

$$r(x) = \frac{1}{2}\varphi^{-1}(x) \qquad (55)$$

  and

$$q(x) = \frac{1}{4}\psi_2^T(x)r^{-1}(x)\psi_2(x) + \lambda x^T x - x^T W_1 S(x) \qquad (56)$$

With the results above, we now give the following theorem.

Theorem 2

A positive-definite function $q(x)$ (56) and a strictly positive-function $r(x)$ (55) exist, such that the feedback control law

$$u = u^* = -\frac{1}{2}r^{-1}(x)W_2^T x \qquad (57)$$

applied to the system (12), achieves global inverse optimality with respect to a cost functional of the form

$$J = \int_0^\infty \left(q(x) + u^T r(x) u\right) \, dt \qquad (58)$$

and the optimal control law (57) renders the equilibrium $x = 0$ globally asymptotical stability (GAS). Therefore, the input control defined as (57) achieves input-to-state stabilization for the system of recurrent neural networks (12).

Proof

- **Step 1:** By considering the Lyapunov function (13) which is a positive semi-definite function, we take the time derivative of V along the trajectory of x

$$\dot{V} = -\lambda x^T x + x^T W_1 S(x) + x^T W_2 u \qquad (59)$$

  The substitution of the control law (57) into $\dot{V}$ (59) yields

$$\dot{V} = -\lambda x^T x - \sqrt{[\psi_1(x)]^2 + [\psi_2^T(x)\psi_2(x)]^2} < 0, \quad \forall x \neq 0 \qquad (60)$$

  So the feedback control law (57) achieves global asymptotic stability of the equilibrium $x = 0$ and guarantees

$$\lim_{t\to\infty} x = 0 \tag{61}$$

- **Step 2:** Let us consider $q(x)$ and $r(x)$. From the equation of (56)

$$\begin{aligned} q(x) &= \frac{1}{4}\psi_2^T(x)r^{-1}(x)\psi_2(x) + \lambda x^T x - x^T W_1 S(x) \\ &= \frac{1}{4}2\varphi(x)\psi_2^T(x)\psi_2(x) + \lambda x^T x - x^T W_1 S(x) \\ &= \frac{1}{2}\left(\psi_1(x) + \sqrt{[\psi_1(x)]^2 + [\psi_2^T(x)\psi_2(x)]^2}\right) \\ &\quad + \lambda x^T x - x^T W_1 S(x) \end{aligned} \tag{62}$$

Appling (23) to the equation above

$$\begin{aligned} q(x) &\geq \frac{1}{2}\left(\psi_1(x) + \sqrt{[\psi_1(x)]^2 + [\psi_2^T(x)\psi_2(x)]^2}\right) \\ &\quad + \lambda x^T x - x^T \left(\frac{1 + \|W_1\|^2}{2}\right) x \\ &\geq \lambda x^T x + \frac{1}{2}\left(\sqrt{[\psi_1(x)]^2 + [\psi_2^T(x)\psi_2(x)]^2} - \psi_1(x)\right) \\ &\geq 0 \end{aligned} \tag{63}$$

Then we can see that $q(x)$ is positive definite and radially unbounded.
By (55), we have

$$\begin{aligned} r(x) &= \frac{1}{2}\varphi^{-1}(x) \\ &= \frac{1}{2}\left(\frac{\psi_2^T(x)\psi_2(x)}{\psi_1(x) + \sqrt{[\psi_1(x)]^2 + [\psi_2^T(x)\psi_2(x)]^2}}\right) > 0 \end{aligned} \tag{64}$$

For the choice of $q(x)$ and $r(x)$ represented by (56) and (55), $\dot{V}$ can be evaluated by the following form

$$\dot{V} = -q(x) - u^T r(x) u + (u - u^*)^T r(x)(u - u^*) \tag{65}$$

which can be written as

$$q(x) + u^T r(x) u + \dot{V} = (u - u^*)^T r(x)(u - u^*) \geq 0 \tag{66}$$

Then it is shown from (66) that the optimal control $u = u^*$ is an optimal solution to J (58), that is, $u = u^*$ satisfies

$$\min_u \left[q(x) + u^T r(x) u + \dot{V}\right] = 0 \tag{67}$$

Also the Lyapunov function $V(x)$ (13) satisfies the HJB equation

$$V_x(x)f(x) - \frac{1}{4}V_x(x)g(x)r^{-1}(x)g^T(x)V_x^T(x) + q(x) = 0 \tag{68}$$

Therefore $V(x)$ is the value function for the cost functional (58).

The same as before, based on the result of paper (Malisoff, Rifford, & Sontag, 2004), it is obvious that the input control defined as (42) achieves input-to-state stabilization for the system (12). This completes the proof.

Numerical Examples

In order to illustrate the effectiveness of the proposed methodology, we consider the following two examples.

Example 1

The neural network is described by

$$\begin{bmatrix}\dot{x}_1 \\ \dot{x}_2\end{bmatrix} = -\begin{bmatrix}4 & 0 \\ 0 & 4\end{bmatrix}\begin{bmatrix}x_1 \\ x_2\end{bmatrix} + \begin{bmatrix}3 & 4 \\ -7 & 8\end{bmatrix}\begin{bmatrix}\tanh(x_1) \\ \tanh(x_2)\end{bmatrix} + \begin{bmatrix}4 & 0 \\ 0 & 4\end{bmatrix}\begin{bmatrix}u_1 \\ u_2\end{bmatrix} \tag{69}$$

with $x_1(0) = -4$, $x_2(0) = 4$, $m = n = 2$.

Figure1 presents the simulation result of system response for $u = 0$. The neural network is not

Figure 1. System Response (u = 0)

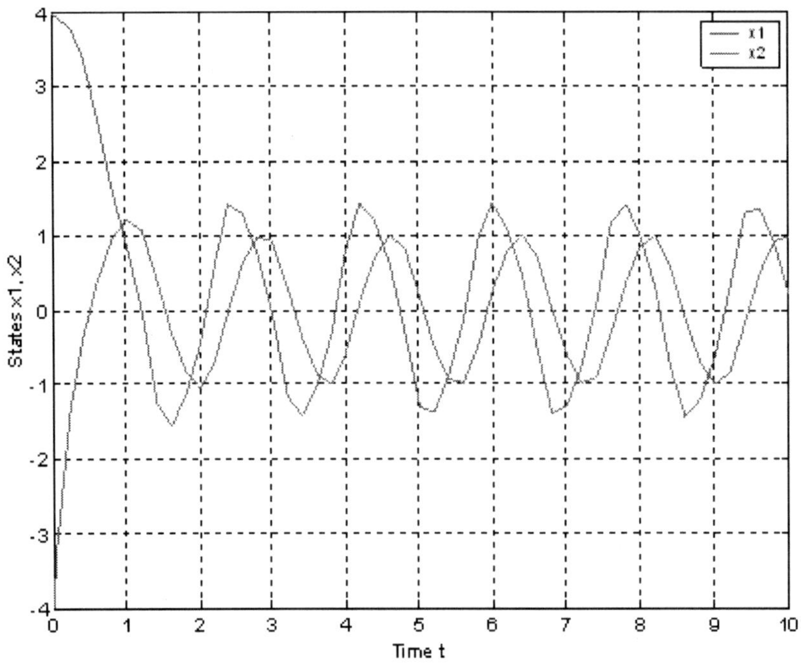

Figure 2. System Response (u = Theorem 1)

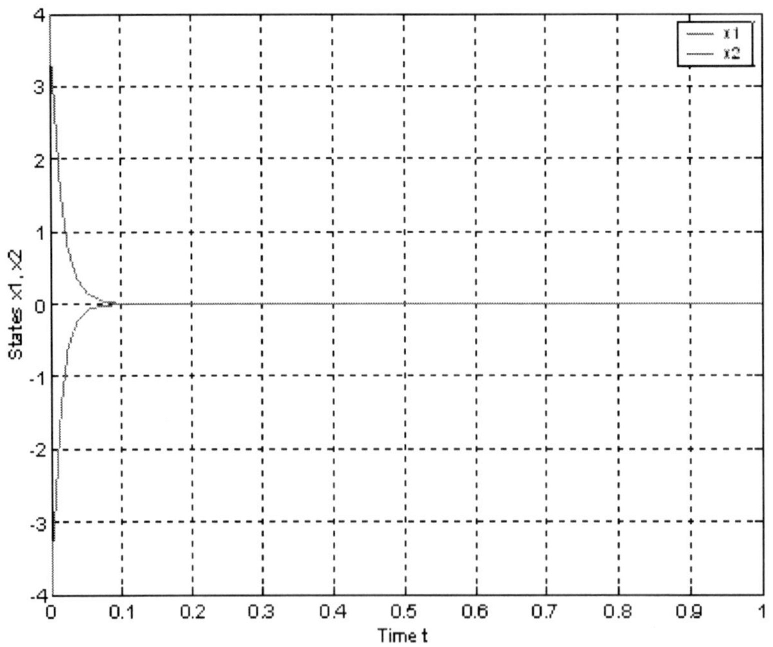

Figure 3. System Response (u = Theorem 2)

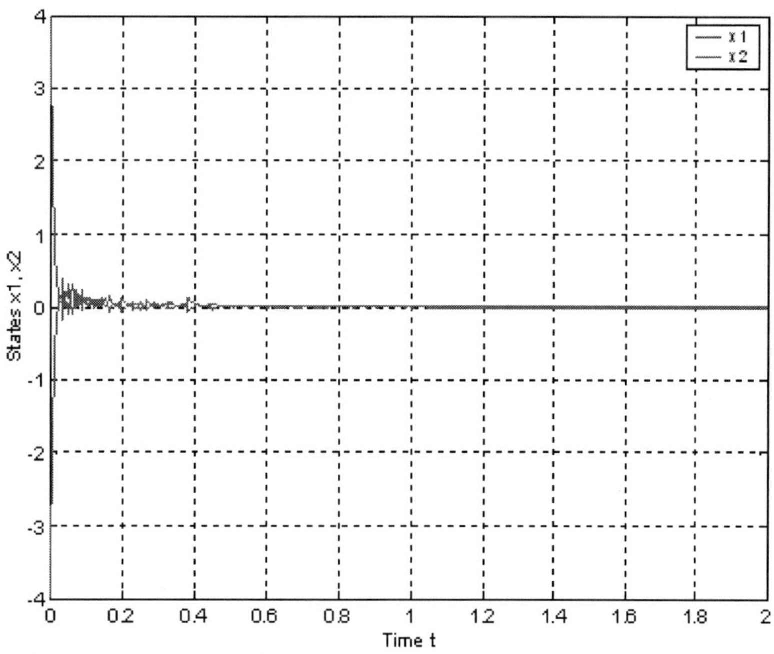

globally asymptotical stability. Then, we apply the control signal that is the input signal given by Theorem 1 to the neural network. The corresponding simulation result is shown in Figure2. From both figures, we know that input-to-state stabilization is achieved. Moreover, the neural network is globally asymptotical stability.

Example 2

The neural network is described by

$$\begin{bmatrix} \dot{x}_1 \\ \dot{x}_2 \end{bmatrix} = -\begin{bmatrix} 4 & 0 \\ 0 & 4 \end{bmatrix}\begin{bmatrix} x_1 \\ x_2 \end{bmatrix} + \begin{bmatrix} 3 & 4 \\ -7 & 8 \end{bmatrix}\begin{bmatrix} \tanh(x_1) \\ \tanh(x_2) \end{bmatrix} + \begin{bmatrix} 4 \\ -4 \end{bmatrix} u \tag{70}$$

with $x_1(0) = 10$, $x_2(0) = -10$, $m = 1$, $n = 2$. This neural network has the same structure as the Example 1 with the only exception of the input.

We apply the control signal given by Theorem 2 to the neural network, the simulation result is presented in Figure3. From the figure, we know that the neural network achieves input-to-state stabilization together with globally asymptotical stability.

All simulation results illustrate and confirm the main theoretical results.

PART-B: NOISE-TO-STATE STABILIZATION FOR STOCHASTIC RECURRENT NEURAL NETWORKS

As a continuation of the work in Part A, this part extends the previous results about the stabilization of recurrent neural networks from the concept of input-to-state stability to noise-to-state stability, and presents a new design to achieve noise-to-state stabilization in probability for stochastic recurrent neural networks driven by noise of unknown covariance. This approach is developed by using Lyapunov technique, inverse optimality, differential game theory, and Hamilton-Jacobi-

Isaacs (HJI) equation. Two numerical examples are given to demonstrate the effectiveness of the proposed approach. The content of this part is based on (Liu, Wang, & Schurz, 2009).

Problem Formulation

Based on the standard formulation of stochastic neural networks (Das & Olurotimi, 1998), we consider the following stochastic recurrent neural network, which is derived from the most common model of deterministic recurrent neural networks defined by (2) plus an additive white noise

$$dx = (-Ax + W_1 S(x) + W_2 u)dt + dW \tag{71}$$

where $x \in R^n$ is the state of stochastic recurrent neural network, $u \in R^m$ is the input, usually $m \neq n$, $A = diag(-\lambda, \cdots, -\lambda) = -\lambda I \in R^{n\times n}$ and $\lambda > 0$, $S(x) = [s(x_1), \cdots, s(x_n)]^T \in R^n$ is a nonlinear vector-valued activation function with $s(\cdot) = \tanh(\cdot)$, $W_1 \in R^{n\times n}$, $W_2 \in R^{n\times m}$ are weight matrices describing the connections of hidden and output layers, W is an n-dimensional independent Wiener process with incremental covariance $\Sigma(t)\Sigma(t)^T dt$, i.e., $E\{dWdW^T\} = \Sigma(t)\Sigma(t)^T dt$ where $\Sigma(t)$ is a unknown bounded function taking values in the set of nonnegative definite matrices.

In order to analyze the system (71) by using differential game theory, let us introduce the following definition.

Definition1: Let us define a nonnegative bounded function $\Delta(t) \in R^{n\times n}$ which will be used as a player opposed to control in order to solve a differential game problem addressed in this chapter. For this function, we define

$$\Delta(t) = \sum(t) \sum(t)^T \tag{72}$$

Main Results

We first rewrite the system of stochastic recurrent neural network (71) as

$$dx = (-Ax + W_1 S(x))dt + dW + W_2 u dt \tag{73}$$

Now let us define a Lyapunov function V, which is the same as the one given in (13)

$$V = \frac{1}{2} x^T x = \frac{1}{2} \|x\|^2 \tag{74}$$

By (Florchinger, 1995) and (Krstic & Deng, 1998), the infinitesimal generator of stochastic differential equation (73) is given as

$$LV = L_f V + \frac{1}{2} T_r \{\sum(t)^T g_1^T \frac{\partial^2 V}{\partial x^2} g_1 \sum(t)\} + L_{g_2} V u \tag{75}$$

where $L_f V = \frac{\partial V}{\partial x}(-Ax + W_1 S(x))$,

$L_{g_2} V u = \frac{\partial V}{\partial x} W_2 u$, $g_1 = I$, $\frac{\partial V}{\partial x} = x^T$, and

$\frac{\partial^2 V}{\partial x^2} = I$.

Thus

$$LV = -\lambda x^T x + x^T W_1 S(x) + x^T W_2 u + \frac{1}{2} T_r \{\sum(t)^T \sum(t)\} \tag{76}$$

For the second term $x^T W_1 S_1(x)$ by using (23), we obtain

$$x^T W_1 S_1(x) \leq x^T \left(\frac{1 + n\|W_1\|^2}{2} \right) x \tag{77}$$

Substituting (77) into (76), we have

$$LV \le -\lambda x^T x + x^T \left(\frac{1 + n\left\|W_1\right\|^2}{2} \right) x + x^T W_2 u + \frac{1}{2} T_r \{\sum(t)^T \sum(t)\} \quad (78)$$

For the further analysis, two cases are considered depending on different structures of stochastic recurrent neural networks.

Case 1

For a stochastic recurrent neural network, the number of inputs is same as the number of states, that is, $x \in R^n$, $u \in R^n$ and $W_2 \in R^{n \times n}$. This structure is the most common one in the literature.

Based on (78), let us consider

$$x^T \left(\frac{1 + n\left\|W_1\right\|^2}{2} \right) x + x^T W_2 u = 0 \quad (79)$$

If square matrix W_2 is invertible, that is $|W_2| \neq 0$, we can determine the stabilizing control law as

$$u = -\left(W_2\right)^{-1} \left(\frac{1 + n\left\|W_1\right\|^2}{2} \right) x \quad (80)$$

Then (78) becomes that

$$LV \le -\lambda x^T x + \frac{1}{2} T_r \{\sum(t)^T \sum(t)\} \quad (81)$$

We see that LV is negative, that is, $LV < 0$ whenever $\left\|x\right\| > \dfrac{(\frac{1}{2} T_r \{\sum(t)^T \sum(t)\})^{1/2}}{\sqrt{\lambda}}$. By the definition of noise-to-state stability (Krstic & Deng, 1998), we conclude that the system (71) is noise-to-state stabilization with the control (80).

Next let us discuss how to find an inverse optimal noise-to-state control for the stochastic recurrent neural network (71). From the concept of inverse optimal noise-to-state stabilization (Krstic & Deng, 1998), it is known for the following general stochastic nonlinear system affined in the noise W and control u

$$dx = f(x)dt + g_1(x)dW + g_2(x)udt \quad (82)$$

If we pursue a differential game problem which uses $\Delta(t)$ defined in *definition2* as a player to oppose the control, and suppose that there exists a positive optimal value function $V(x)$, which satisfies the following HJI equation

$$L_f V + \frac{1}{4}\gamma^{-2} \left\| g_1^T(x) \frac{\partial^2 V}{\partial x^2} g_1(x) \right\|^2 - \frac{1}{4} L_{g_2} V r^{-1}(x) L_{g_2}^T V + q(x) = 0 \quad (83)$$

Then

$$u^*(x) = -\frac{1}{2} r^{-1}(x) L g_2^T V \quad (84)$$

Equation (84) is an optimal stabilizing control which minimizes the cost functional

$$J(u, \Delta) = \lim_{t \to \infty} E\left[V(x(t)) + \int_0^t (q(x) + u^T r(x) u - \gamma^2 \left\|\Delta\right\|^2) d\tau \right] \quad (85)$$

where $\gamma > 0$ is a design parameter, both $q(x) \ge 0$ and $r(x) > 0$ for all x, and the worst case $\Delta^*(t)$ is

$$\Delta^*(t) = \frac{1}{2\gamma^2} \left(g_1^T(x) \frac{\partial^2 V}{\partial x^2} g_1(x) \right) \quad (86)$$

We now take the infinitesimal generator of stochastic differential equation (82)

$$LV = L_f V + \frac{1}{2}T_r\{\sum(t)^T g_1^T \frac{\partial^2 V}{\partial x^2} g_1 \sum(t)\} + L_{g_2} Vu \tag{87}$$

For the model of stochastic recurrent neural networks (71), if the solution V is given by (74), we get the following equations

$$L_f V = -\lambda x^T x + x^T W_1 S_1(x) \tag{88}$$

$$\begin{aligned}&\frac{1}{2}T_r\{\sum(t)^T g_1^T \frac{\partial^2 V}{\partial x^2} g_1 \sum(t)\}\\ &= \frac{1}{2}T_r\{\sum(t)^T \sum(t)\}\end{aligned} \tag{89}$$

$$Lg_2 V = x^T W_2 \tag{90}$$

Then the substitution of the equation (74) into HJI equation (83) yields the next relation

$$\begin{aligned}&-\lambda x^T x + x^T W_1 S_1(x) + \frac{1}{4}\gamma^{-2} n\\ &-\frac{1}{4}x^T W_2 r^{-1}(x) W_2^T x + q(x) = 0\end{aligned} \tag{91}$$

Let us define a new control that is a modification of (80)

$$\begin{aligned}u &= -c(W_2)^{-1}\left[\frac{1+n\|W_1\|^2}{2} + \frac{2}{c}\right]x\\ &= -c(W_2)^{-1}\left[\frac{1+n\|W_1\|^2}{2} + \frac{2}{c}\right](W_2^T)^{-1}(W_2^T)x\\ &= -c(W_2^T W_2)^{-1}\left[\frac{1+n\|W_1\|^2}{2} + \frac{2}{c}\right]W_2^T x\\ &= -\frac{1}{2}c(W_2^T W_2)^{-1}(1+n\|W_1\|^2 + \frac{4}{c})\ W_2^T x\end{aligned} \tag{92}$$

where $c > 2$ is a constant.

Comparing the result with u^* of (84), we find that the function $r(x)$ can be selected as

$$r(x) = c^{-1} W_2^T W_2 (1 + n\|W_1\|^2 + \frac{4}{c})^{-1} \tag{93}$$

and from (91) the function $q(x)$ is given by

$$\begin{aligned}q(x) = \lambda x^T x + \frac{c}{4}(1+n\|W_1\|^2 + \frac{4}{c})x^T x\\ -\frac{1}{4}\gamma^{-2} n - x^T W_1 S_1(x)\end{aligned} \tag{94}$$

Now let us assume

$$\|x\| \geq \max\left\{\frac{\sqrt{n}}{2\gamma}, \frac{\gamma}{\sqrt{\lambda}}\|\Delta\|\right\} \tag{95}$$

With the assumption above, theorem 3 is given as follows.

Theorem 3

For the stochastic recurrent neural network described by (71) with as many inputs as its states, there exist a positive-definite function $q(x)$ (94) and a strictly positive function $r(x)$ (93), such that the feedback control law

$$u = u^* = -\frac{1}{2}r^{-1}(x) W_2^T x \tag{96}$$

achieves both noise-to-state stabilization and inverse optimality with respect to a meaningful cost functional

$$J(u,\Delta) = \lim_{t\to\infty} E\left[V(x(t)) + \int_0^t (q(x) + u^T r(x) u - \gamma^2 \|\Delta(\tau)\|^2) d\tau\right] \tag{97}$$

for the worst case $\Delta(t)$

$$\Delta(t) = \Delta^*(t) = \frac{1}{2\gamma^2} I \qquad (98)$$

Proof

- **Step 1:** By considering the Lyapunov function candidate (74), the infinitesimal generator of the stochastic differential equation (73) is

$$\begin{aligned} LV &= -\lambda x^T x + x^T W_1 S(x) \\ &\quad + x^T W_2 u + \frac{1}{2} T_r\{\textstyle\sum(t)^T \sum(t)\} \end{aligned} \qquad (99)$$

The substitution of the control law (96) into LV (99) yields

$$\begin{aligned} LV &= -\lambda x^T x + x^T W_1 S(x) + \frac{1}{2} Tr\{\Delta(t)\} \\ &\quad - \frac{1}{2} c x^T W_2 (W_2{}^T W_2)^{-1} (1 + n\|W_1\|^2 + \frac{4}{c}) W_2{}^T x \\ &= -\lambda x^T x + x^T W_1 S(x) + \frac{1}{2} T_r\{\Delta(t)\} \\ &\quad - \frac{1}{2} c(1 + n\|W_1\|^2 + \frac{4}{c}) x^T x \end{aligned} \qquad (100)$$

From both (77) and (95), we obtain

$$\begin{aligned} LV &\le -\lambda x^T x + x^T (\frac{1 + n\|W_1\|^2}{2}) x + \frac{1}{2} T_r\{\Delta(t)\} \\ &\quad - \frac{1}{2} c(1 + n\|W_1\|^2 + \frac{4}{c}) x^T x \\ &= -\lambda x^T x - \left[(\frac{c-1}{2})(1 + n\|W_1\|^2) + 1\right] x^T x \\ &\quad - x^T x + \frac{1}{2} T_r\{\Delta(t)\} \\ &\le -\lambda x^T x - \left[(\frac{c-1}{2})(1 + n\|W_1\|^2) + 1\right] x^T x \\ &\quad - \frac{n}{4\gamma^2} + \frac{1}{2} T_r\{\Delta(t)\} \\ &= -\lambda x^T x - \left[(\frac{c-1}{2})(1 + n\|W_1\|^2) + 1\right] x^T x \\ &\quad - T_r\left\{\left(\frac{1}{2\gamma} I - \gamma\Delta(t)\right)^T \left(\frac{1}{2\gamma} I - \gamma\Delta(t)\right)\right\} \\ &\quad + \gamma^2 \|\Delta(t)\|^2 \\ &\le -\lambda x^T x + \gamma^2 \|\Delta(t)\|^2 \end{aligned} \qquad (101)$$

Therefore $LV \le 0$ whenever $\|x\| \ge \frac{\gamma}{\sqrt{\lambda}} \|\Delta(t)\|$

By the definition of (Krstic & Deng, 1998), we know that the system (71) achieves noise-to-state stabilization with the control law (96).

- **Step 2:** Let us consider $q(x)$ and $r(x)$ By (94)

$$\begin{aligned} q(x) &= \lambda x^T x + \frac{c}{4}(1 + n\|W_1\|^2 + \frac{4}{c}) x^T x \\ &\quad - \frac{1}{4}\gamma^{-2} n - x^T W_1 S_1(x) \end{aligned} \qquad (102)$$

From (77), we have

$$-x^T W_1 S_1(x) \ge -x^T (\frac{1 + n\|W_1\|^2}{2}) x \qquad (103)$$

Therefore

$$\begin{aligned} q(x) &\ge \lambda x^T x + \frac{c}{4}(1 + n\|W_1\|^2 + \frac{4}{c}) x^T x \\ &\quad - \frac{1}{4}\gamma^{-2} n - (\frac{1 + n\|W_1\|^2}{2}) x^T x \\ &= \lambda x^T x + (\frac{c-2}{2})(\frac{1 + n\|W_1\|^2}{2}) x^T x \\ &\quad + x^T x - \frac{1}{4}\gamma^{-2} n \\ &\ge \lambda x^T x + (\frac{c-2}{2})(\frac{1 + n\|W_1\|^2}{2}) x^T x \\ &\ge 0 \end{aligned} \qquad (104)$$

Box 1.

$$J(u,\Delta)=\lim_{t\to\infty}E\left[V(x(t))+\int_0^t(q(x)+u^Tr(x)u-\gamma^2\left\|\Delta(\tau)\right\|^2)d\tau\right]$$
$$=\lim_{t\to\infty}E\left[V(x(0))+\int_0^t(LV+q(x)+u^Tr(x)u-\gamma^2\left\|\Delta(\tau)\right\|^2)d\tau\right]$$
$$=E\left[V(x(o)\right]+\lim_{t\to\infty}E\int_0^t\left[(u-u^*)^Tr(x)(u-u^*)-T_r\left\{\left(\frac{1}{2\gamma}I-\gamma\Delta(t)\right)^T\left(\frac{1}{2\gamma}I-\gamma\Delta(t)\right)\right\}\right]d\tau \quad (107)$$

Then $q(x)$ is positive definite and radially unbounded.
By (93)

$$r(x)=c^{-1}W_2^TW_2(1+n\left\|W_1\right\|^2+\frac{4}{c})^{-1} \quad (105)$$

If $|W_2|\neq 0$, we know that $r(x)>0$ since $W_2^TW_2>0$.
With the choice of $q(x)$ and $r(x)$ in (94) and (93), LV can be written as the following form

$$LV=-q(x)-u^Tr(x)u+\gamma^2\left\|\Delta(t)\right\|^2$$
$$-T_r\left\{\left(\frac{1}{2\gamma}I-\gamma\Delta(t)\right)^T\left(\frac{1}{2\gamma}I-\gamma\Delta(t)\right)\right\}$$
$$+(u-u^*)^Tr(x)(u-u^*) \quad (106)$$

According to Dynkin's formula (Krstic & Deng, 1998), we have (see Box 1.)
From the equation above we know that the optimal control $u=u^*$ is an optimal solution to J (97) for the worst disturbance $\Delta(t)=\Delta(t)^*$ and

$$\min_u\max_\Delta J(u,\Delta)=E\left[V(x(o)\right] \quad (108)$$

This completes the proof.

Case 2

Let us consider a more general stochastic recurrent neural network, as described in (71), with arbitrary number of inputs, that is, $x\in R^n$, $u\in R^m$, $W_2S(x)\in R^{n\times m}$ and $m\neq n$. The inequality in (78) is rewritten as

$$LV\leq-\lambda x^Tx+x^T\left(\frac{1+n\left\|W_1\right\|^2}{2}\right)x$$
$$+x^TW_2u+\frac{1}{2}T_r\{\sum(t)^T\sum(t)\}$$
$$=-\lambda x^Tx+x^T\left(\frac{3+n\left\|W_1\right\|^2}{2}\right)x$$
$$+x^TW_2u-x^Tx+\frac{1}{2}T_r\{\Delta(t)\} \quad (109)$$

From (109), we can set up

$$\psi_1(x)=x^T\left(\frac{3+n\left\|W_1\right\|^2}{2}\right)x \quad (110)$$

$$\psi_2^T(x)=x^TW_2 \quad (111)$$

Similar to the equation (51), let us define a scalar function

$$\varphi(x) = \frac{\psi_1(x) + \sqrt{[\psi_1(x)]^2 + [\psi_2^T(x)\psi_2(x)]^2}}{\psi_2^T(x)\psi_2(x)} \quad (112)$$

Then a control signal can be determined as

$$u = -\varphi(x)\psi_2(x) \quad (113)$$

with the assumption of $\psi_2^T(x)\psi_2(x) \neq 0$.

Using the equation (88), this is equivalent to

$$\begin{aligned} u &= -\varphi(x)W_2^T x \\ &= -\varphi(x)L_{g_2}^T V \end{aligned} \quad (114)$$

Comparing (114) with (84) and using (90), (91) and (111), we obtain

$$r(x) = \frac{1}{2}\varphi^{-1}(x) \quad (115)$$

and

$$\begin{aligned} q(x) &= \frac{1}{4}\psi_2^T(x)r^{-1}(x)\psi_2(x) \\ &+ \lambda x^T x - x^T W_1 S(x) - \frac{1}{4}\gamma^{-2} n \end{aligned} \quad (116)$$

Consequently theorem 4 is given below.

Theorem 4

For the system (71), which has arbitrary number of inputs, a positive-definite function $q(x)$ (116) and a strictly positive function $r(x)$, for $x \neq 0$, (115) exist, such that the feedback control law

$$u = u^* = -\frac{1}{2}r^{-1}(x)W_2^T x \quad (117)$$

achieves both noise-to-state stabilization and inverse optimality with respect to a meaningful cost functional

$$J(u,\Delta) = \lim_{t\to\infty} E\left[V(x(t)) + \int_0^t (q(x) + u^T r(x) u - \gamma^2 \|\Delta(\tau)\|^2) d\tau\right] \quad (118)$$

for the worst case $\Delta(t)$

$$\Delta(t) = \Delta^*(t) = \frac{1}{2\gamma^2} I \quad (119)$$

Proof

- **Step 1:** By considering the Lyapunov function candidate (74), the infinitesimal generator of stochastic differential equation (73) is

$$\begin{aligned} LV &= -\lambda x^T x + x^T W_1 S(x) + x^T W_2 u \\ &+ \frac{1}{2} T_r\{\textstyle\sum(t)^T \sum(t)\} \end{aligned} \quad (120)$$

Substituting (77) into (119), we have

$$\begin{aligned} LV &\leq -\lambda x^T x + x^T \left(\frac{1 + n\|W_1\|^2}{2}\right) x \\ &+ x^T W_2 u + \frac{1}{2} T_r\{\textstyle\sum(t)^T \sum(t)\} \\ &= -\lambda x^T x + x^T \left(\frac{3 + n\|W_1\|^2}{2}\right) x \\ &+ x^T W_2 u - x^T x + \frac{1}{2} T_r\{\Delta(t)\} \end{aligned} \quad (121)$$

The substitution of the control law (117) into LV (121) yields

$$\begin{aligned} LV &\leq -\lambda x^T x + x^T \left(\frac{3 + n\|W_1\|^2}{2}\right) x - \psi_1(x) \\ &- \sqrt{[\psi_1(x)]^2 + [\psi_2^T(x)\psi_2(x)]^2} \\ &- x^T x + \frac{1}{2} T_r\{\Delta(t)\} \end{aligned} \quad (122)$$

Using the equation of (110), we obtain

$$LV \leq -\lambda x^T x - \sqrt{[\psi_1(x)]^2 + [\psi_2^T(x)\psi_2(x)]^2} \\ -x^T x + \frac{1}{2} T_r\{\Delta(t)\} \tag{123}$$

With the assumption of (95), we know that

$$x^T x = \|x\|^2 \geq \frac{n}{4\gamma^2} \tag{124}$$

Thus

$$\begin{aligned} LV &\leq -\lambda x^T x - \sqrt{[\psi_1(x)]^2 + [\psi_2^T(x)\psi_2(x)]^2} \\ &\quad -\frac{n}{4\gamma^2} + \frac{1}{2} T_r\{\Delta(t)\} \\ &\leq -\lambda x^T x - \sqrt{[\psi_1(x)]^2 + [\psi_2^T(x)\psi_2(x)]^2} \\ &\quad -T_r\left\{\left(\frac{1}{2\gamma} I - \gamma\Delta(t)\right)^T \left(\frac{1}{2\gamma} I - \gamma\Delta(t)\right)\right\} \\ &\quad +\gamma^2 \|\Delta(t)\|^2 \\ &\leq -\lambda x^T x + \gamma^2 \|\Delta(t)\|^2 \end{aligned} \tag{125}$$

Therefore $LV \leq 0$ whenever $\|x\| \geq \frac{\gamma}{\sqrt{\lambda}} \|\Delta(t)\|$

The above procedures demonstrate that the system (71) achieves noise-to-state stabilization with the control law (117).

- **Step 2:** Using the inequality (103) and relations (115), (112) and (95), the expression $q(x)$ given in (116), can be written as

$$\begin{aligned} q(x) &\geq \frac{1}{2}\left(\psi_1(x) + \sqrt{[\psi_1(x)]^2 + [\psi_2^T(x)\psi_2(x)]^2}\right) \\ &\quad +\lambda x^T x - x^T \left(\frac{3 + n\|W_1\|^2}{2}\right) x + x^T x \\ &\quad -\frac{1}{4}\gamma^{-2} n \\ &\geq \lambda x^T x + \frac{1}{2}\left(\sqrt{[\psi_1(x)]^2 + [\psi_2^T(x)\psi_2(x)]^2} - \psi_1(x)\right) \\ &\geq 0 \end{aligned} \tag{126}$$

This means that $q(x)$ is positive definite, for all $x \neq 0$, and is radially unbounded.

Also, from (115), it can be seen that $r(x) > 0$ when $\psi_2^T(x)\psi_2(x) \neq 0$. That is

$$\begin{aligned} r(x) &= \frac{1}{2}\varphi^{-1}(x) \\ &= \frac{1}{2}\left(\frac{\psi_2^T(x)\psi_2(x)}{\psi_1(x) + \sqrt{[\psi_1(x)]^2 + [\psi_2^T(x)\psi_2(x)]^2}}\right) > 0 \end{aligned} \tag{127}$$

For the choice of $q(x)$ and $r(x)$ in (116) and (115), LV can be written as the following form

$$\begin{aligned} LV &= -q(x) - u^T r(x) u + \gamma^2 \|\Delta(t)\|^2 \\ &\quad -T_r\left\{\left(\frac{1}{2\gamma} I - \gamma\Delta(t)\right)^T \left(\frac{1}{2\gamma} I - \gamma\Delta(t)\right)\right\} \\ &\quad +(u - u^*)^T r(x)(u - u^*) \end{aligned} \tag{128}$$

Similar to the steps in the proof of *Theorem 3*, it can be seen that the optimal control $u = u^*$ is an optimal solution to J (118) for the worst disturbance $\Delta(t) = \Delta(t)^*$ and

$$\min_u \max_\Delta J(u, \Delta) = E\left[V(x(o)\right] \tag{129}$$

This completes the proof.

Finally, the last result is given as follows.

Theorem 5

Under the control of (96) and (117), the state of the system of stochastic recurrent neural networks (71) is globally uniformly bounded in probability.

Proof

Back to the inequality of (101) and the inequality of (125), It is obvious that LV is negative whenever $\|x\| \geq \frac{\gamma}{\sqrt{\lambda}} \|\Delta(t)\|$. Since $\Delta(t)$ is a non-negative bounded function, we conclude that LV is negative outside the compact residual set

Figure 4. System Response (u = 0)

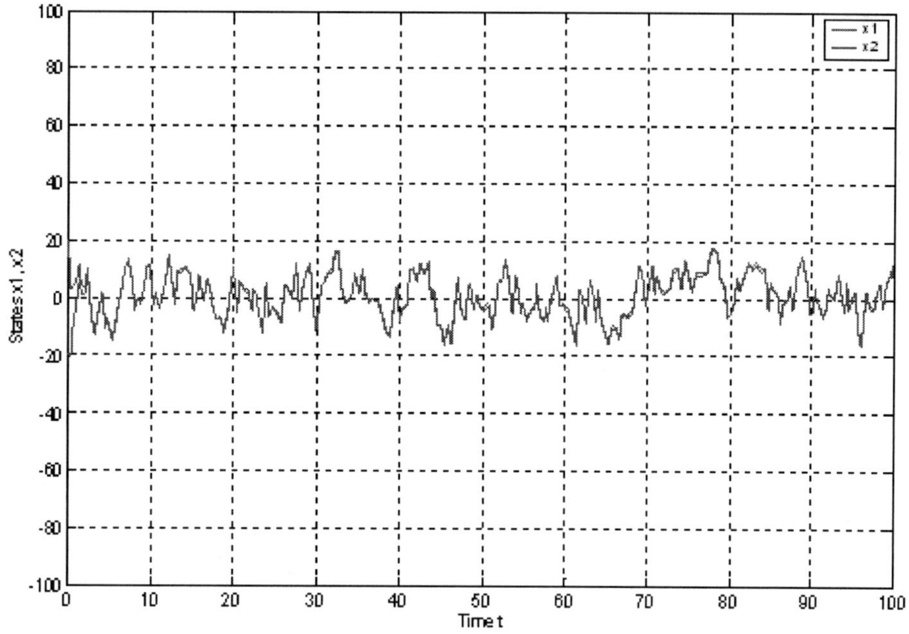

$$R = \left\{ x : \|x\| \le \frac{\gamma}{\sqrt{\lambda}} \|\Delta(t)\| \right\} \quad (130)$$

which ensures that $x(t)$ converges to the compact set R.

Numerical Examples

In order to effectively describe our results, we adopted a recurrent neural network that has the same structure as the one in (Sanchez & Perez, 2003). But the neural network is driven by different noises and inputs. To be consistent with the theoretical discussions, two cases are discussed. In one case, there are same number of inputs and states. In the other case, the number of inputs and states are not the same.

Example 3

The model of stochastic recurrent neural network is given as

$$\begin{bmatrix} dx_1 \\ dx_2 \end{bmatrix} = \left(-\begin{bmatrix} 2 & 0 \\ 0 & 2 \end{bmatrix} \begin{bmatrix} x_1 \\ x_2 \end{bmatrix} + \begin{bmatrix} 1 & 2 \\ -3 & 4 \end{bmatrix} \begin{bmatrix} \tanh(x_1) \\ \tanh(x_2) \end{bmatrix} \right) dt + \begin{bmatrix} dW_1 \\ dW_2 \end{bmatrix} + \left(\begin{bmatrix} 1 & 0 \\ 0 & 1 \end{bmatrix} \begin{bmatrix} u_1 \\ u_2 \end{bmatrix} \right) dt \quad (131)$$

where $x_1(0) = 20$, $x_2(0) = -20$, W_1, W_2 are white noises (uniformly random) with the magnitude of $|W_i| = 40$ $(i = 1, 2)$, and $m = n = 2$.

Figure 4 shows the results of time responses of two states ($x_1(t)$ and $x_2(t)$) for this stochastic recurrent neural network without any control inputs. Figure5 shows the results of time responses of two states when the proposed control law (96) is inputted at $t = 100s$. It can be seen that the system achieves the expected performance given by theoretical analysis in Part B.

Example 4

Given the following model

Figure 5. System Response (u = Theorem 3 at t = 100s)

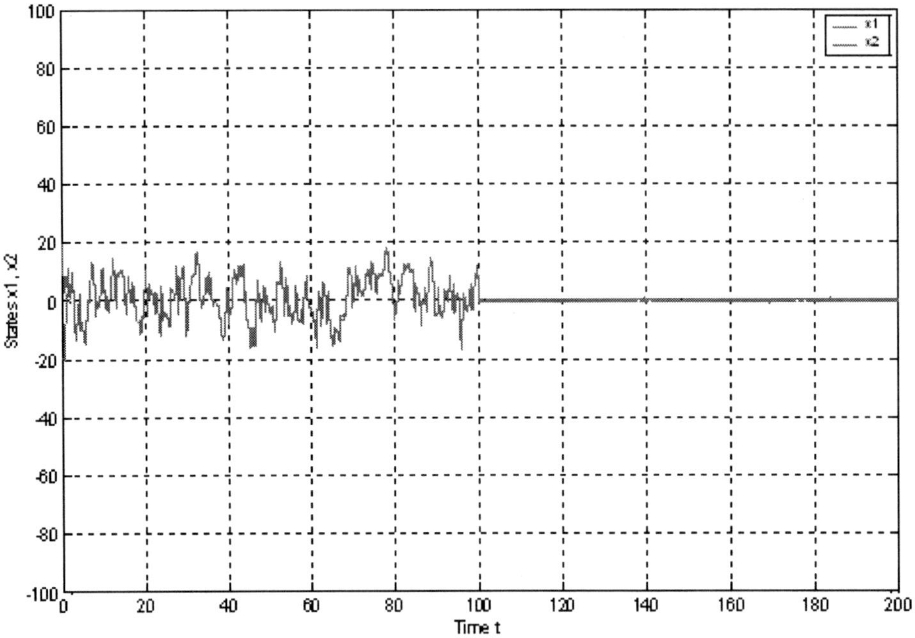

Figure 6. System Response (u = Theorem 4 at t = 100s)

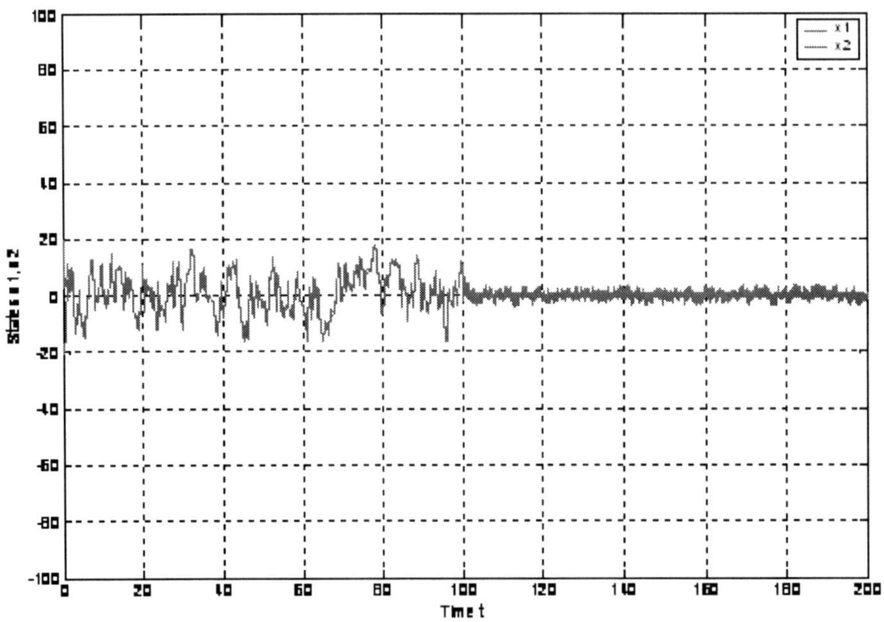

$$\begin{bmatrix} dx_1 \\ dx_2 \end{bmatrix} = \left(-\begin{bmatrix} 2 & 0 \\ 0 & 2 \end{bmatrix}\begin{bmatrix} x_1 \\ x_2 \end{bmatrix} + \begin{bmatrix} 1 & 2 \\ -3 & 4 \end{bmatrix}\begin{bmatrix} \tanh(x_1) \\ \tanh(x_2) \end{bmatrix} \right) dt + \begin{bmatrix} dW_1 \\ dW_2 \end{bmatrix} + \left(\begin{bmatrix} 1 \\ -1 \end{bmatrix} u \right) dt \tag{132}$$

where $x_1(0) = 20$, $x_2(0) = -20$, W_1, W_2 are disturbance noises (uniformly random), $|W_i| = 40$ ($i = 1, 2$), $m = 1$, and $n = 2$. When inputs are not considered, both networks have the same structure. The difference lies on the dimension number of external control.

Figure6 shows the results of time responses of two states ($x_1(t)$ and $x_2(t)$) for this stochastic recurrent neural network when the proposed control law (117) is inputted at $t = 100s$. The system once more demonstrates the expected performance given by theoretical analysis in Part B.

Both numerical examples illustrate and confirm the theoretical findings.

CONCLUSION

This chapter has presented a methodology to achieve optimality-oriented stabilization for recurrent neural networks, which includes both the input-to-state stabilization for deterministic recurrent neural networks and the noise-to-state stabilization for stochastic recurrent neural networks. Due to the difficulty to solve the Hamilton-Jacobi equation, for nonlinear systems, optimal stabilization seems to be an unachievable goal in feedback design. However, an alternative way has been given in this chapter to solve the problem and obtain an optimal feedback controller with respect to a meaningful cost functional with the knowledge of inverse optimality. Using Lyapunov technique, inverse optimality, and Hamilton-Jacobi-Bellman (HJB) equation, the design of optimal input-to-state stabilization has been developed for deterministic recurrent neural networks. With respect to stochastic recurrent neural networks driven by noise of unknown covariance, an approach of optimal noise-to-state stabilization in probability has been established by using Lyapunov technique, inverse optimality, differential game theory, and Hamilton-Jacobi-Isaacs (HJI) equation. It is believed that the design method presented in this chapter would benefit the applications of recurrent neural networks.

REFERENCES

Arik, S. (2000). Global asymptotic stability of a class of dynamic neural networks. *IEEE Transactions on Circuits and Systems I*, *47*(4), 568–571. doi:10.1109/81.841858

Das, S., & Olurotimi, O. (1998). Noisy recurrent neural networks: the continuous-time case. *IEEE Transactions on Neural Networks*, *9*(5), 913–936. doi:10.1109/72.712164

Ensari, T., & Arik, S. (2005). Global stability analysis of neural networks with multiple time varying delays. *IEEE Transactions on Automatic Control*, *50*(11), 1781–1785. doi:10.1109/TAC.2005.858634

Florchinger, P. (1995). Lyapunov-like techniques for stochastic stability. *SIAM Journal on Control and Optimization*, *33*(4), 1151–1169. doi:10.1137/S0363012993252309

Hardy, G., Littlewood, J., & Polya, G. (1989). *Inequalities* (2nd ed.). London: Cambridge University Press.

Hopfield, J. J. (1984). Neurons with graded response have collective computational properties like those of two-state neurons. *Proceedings of the National Academy of Sciences of the United States of America*, *81*(10), 3088–3092. doi:10.1073/pnas.81.10.3088

Hu, S., & Wang, J. (2002). Global asymptotic stability and global exponential stability of continuous-time recurrent neural networks. *IEEE Transactions on Automatic Control*, *47*(5), 802–807. doi:10.1109/TAC.2002.1000277

Khalil, H. (1996). *Nonlinear Systems* (2nd ed.). Upper Saddle River, NJ: Prentice Hall.

Krstic, M., & Deng, H. (1998). *Stabilization of Nonlinear Uncertain Systems*. New York, NY: Springer-Verlag.

Krstic, M., Kanellakopoulos, I., & Kokotovic, P. V. (1995). *Nonlinear and Adaptive Control Design*. New York: John Wiley & Sons.

Kulawski, G. J., & Brdys, M. A. (2000). Stable adaptive control with recurrent networks. *Automatica*, *36*(1), 5–22. doi:10.1016/S0005-1098(99)00092-8

Liu, Z., Torres, R., Patel, N., & Wang, Q. (2008). Further development of input-to-state stabilizing control for dynamic neural network systems. *IEEE Transactions on Systems, Man, and Cybernetics A*, *38*, 1425–1433. doi:10.1109/TSMCA.2008.2003464

Liu, Z., & Wang, Q. (2007). Further result on input-to-state stabilization of dynamic neural network systems. *Proceedings of American Control Conference,* 4798-4803.

Liu, Z., Wang, Q., & Schurz, H. (2009). Inverse optimal noise-to-state stabilization of stochastic recurrent neural networks driven by noise of unknown covariance. *Optimal Control Applications and Methods*, *30*(2), 163–178. doi:10.1002/oca.851

Malisoff, M., Rifford, L., & Sontag, E. D. (2004). Global asymptotic controllability implies input-to-state stabilization. *SIAM Journal on Control and Optimization*, *42*, 2221–2238. doi:10.1137/S0363012903422333

Rovithakis, G. A., & Christodoulou, M. A. (2000). *Adaptive Control with Recurrent High-order Neural Networks*. London: Springer-Verlag.

Sanchez, E. N., & Perez, J. P. (2003). Input-to-state stabilization of dynamic neural networks. *IEEE Transactions on Systems, Man, and Cybernetics A*, *33*(4), 532–536. doi:10.1109/TSMCA.2003.811509

Sepulchre, R., Jankovic, M., & Kokotovic, P. (1997). *Constructive Nonlinear Control*. New York: Springer-Verlag.

Sontag, E. O. (1989). A universal construction of artstein's theorem on nonlinear stabilization. *Systems & Control Letters*, *13*, 117–123. doi:10.1016/0167-6911(89)90028-5

KEY TERMS AND DEFINITIONS

Artificial Neural Networks: A term has been used to refer to a mathematical model or computational model that simulates the structure and functions of biological neural systems with the hope of achieving human-like performance.

Recurrent Neural Networks: A class of neural networks, in which the networks have feedback connections that represent dynamic memory, which make them more suitable for modeling biological intelligence.

Optimality: The property of a system to either minimize or maximize some function called as cost functional under certain given constraints.

Inverse Optimality: A design technique that solves the inverse problem of optimal stabilization, in which a stabilizing feedback is developed first and then modifies it to achieve an optimal control for a cost functional.

Hamilton-Jacobi-Bellman (HJB) Equation: A partial differential equation that provides a sufficient condition in optimal control. Therefore, it is central to optimal control theory.

Input-to-State Stabilization: See the definition of the term on Page 13 (Definition 2.1) in reference (Krstic & Deng, 1998).

Noise-to-State Stabilization: See the definition of the term on Page 78 (Definition 4.1) in reference (Krstic & Deng, 1998).

Chapter 6
Design of Globally Robust Control for Biologically-Inspired Noisy Recurrent Neural Networks

Ziqian Liu
State University of New York Maritime College, USA

ABSTRACT

This chapter presents a theoretical design of how a global robust control is achieved in a class of noisy recurrent neural networks which is a promising method for modeling the behavior of biological motor-sensor systems. The approach is developed by using differential minimax game, inverse optimality, Lyapunov technique, and the Hamilton-Jacobi-Isaacs equation. In order to implement the theory of differential games into neural networks, we consider the vector of external inputs as a player and the vector of internal noises (or disturbances or modeling errors) as an opposing player. The proposed design achieves global inverse optimality with respect to some meaningful cost functional, global disturbance attenuation, as well as global asymptotic stability provided no disturbance. Finally, numerical examples are used to demonstrate the effectiveness of the proposed design.

INTRODUCTION

Recurrent neural networks have become one of the most promising methodologies to solve various difficult problems in different scientific areas, such as system identification and control, pattern recognition, image processing, modeling biological sensor-motor systems, etc. Therefore, theoretical studies on both stability and controllability of recurrent neural networks have received much attention during the last several years, see for example, (Arik, 2000; Ensari & Arik, 2005; Hu & Wang, 2002; Kulawski & Brdys, 2000; Liu, Torres, Patel, & Wang, 2008; Marco, Forti, & Tesi, 2004; Sanchez & Perez, 2003; Sontag & Qiao, 1999; Sontag, 1989), and references therein. However, these studies primarily focused on these mathematical models, which do not consider the noise process that is fraught with signal transmission particularly in biological systems.

On the other hand, Haykin (Haykin, 1999) indicated that the synaptic transmission is a noise

DOI: 10.4018/978-1-60960-018-1.ch006

process in real nervous systems. Therefore, in order to build mathematical specifications for neural networks, which will be used as models of intelligence in the brain, and as highly effective artificial intelligent systems implemented in engineering and computer science, we must consider the noise or disturbance environment (Werbos, 2009). Hence, it is important to analytically explore the characteristics of stabilization and controllability for recurrent neural networks under the influence of noise or disturbance.

Based on our research (Liu, Shih, & Wang, 2009), this chapter provides a groundbreaking nonlinear $\boldsymbol{H}_\infty$ optimal control for deterministic noisy recurrent neural networks to achieve a prescribed level of noise attenuation with stability margins. It is constructed by using differential minimax game, inverse optimality, Lyapunov technique, and the Hamilton-Jacobi-Isaacs equation. In order to realize a minimax equilibrium of differential game, we considered the vector of external inputs as a player and the vector of internal noises (or disturbances or modeling errors) as an opposing player. To complete the aforementioned goals, the rest of the chapter is organized as follows. The following section introduces the problem formulation. Next section shows the main results of a nonlinear $\boldsymbol{H}_\infty$ control design for noisy recurrent neural networks. After that, two numerical examples are given demonstrate the effectiveness of the proposed design. Finally, the main conclusions are reported.

PROBLEM FORMULATION

Consider the class of recurrent neural networks described by the following differential equations

$$\dot{x} = -Ax + W_1 S(x) + W_2 u \qquad (1)$$

where $x \in R^n$ is the state of recurrent neural network, $u \in R^m$ is the input, usually $m \neq n$, $A \in R^{n\times n}$ is a matrix that represents the neuron self-inhibitions, $S(x) = [s(x_1), \ldots, s(x_n)]^T \in R^n$ is a vector function and its component $s(x_i)$ is a sigmoidal function that models the nonlinear input-output activations of the neurons, $W_1 \in R^{n\times n}$, $W_2 \in R^{n\times m}$ are weight matrices. Model (1) encompasses a large class of neural networks, such as the popular Hopfield neural networks, the paradigm of cellular neural networks, and many other recurrent neural network models frequently used in the literature.

In this chapter, we are interested in dealing with recurrent neural networks under the influence of noise or disturbance. Therefore, the model of noisy recurrent neural networks in the deterministic form can be considered as

$$\dot{x} = -Ax + W_1 S(x) + W_2 u + d \qquad (2)$$

where $d \in R^n$ is an unknown n-dimensional internal noise or disturbance or modeling error.

The design objective is to attenuate the noise to a prescribed level with stability margins. This can be achieved by implementing differential minimax game with the consideration of the vector of external inputs as a player and the vector of internal noises as an opposing player, which is equivalent to develop a nonlinear $\boldsymbol{H}_\infty$ optimal control for the system (2). The main difficulty in obtaining the solution is in finding the solution of a Hamilton-Jacobi-Isaacs (HJI) equation. When the system dynamics are nonlinear, solving this HJI equation has presented a great challenge. However, the knowledge of inverse optimality allows us to find an alternative way to solve the problem and obtain optimal feedback controllers. The design procedure will be illustrated in the following section.

GLOBAL ROBUST CONTROL DESIGN

Before we develop the main results, let us first introduce the following definitions and propositions.

Definition 1: The norm $\|x\|$ of a vector x is the Euclidean norm. If A is a matrix, then $\|A\|$ denotes the Frobenius matrix norm, defined as $\|A\| = (T_r\{A^T A\})^{1/2}$, where $T_r\{.\}$ denotes the trace of a matrix.

Definition 2: Without loss of generality, the matrix of neuron self-inhibitions can be defined as a diagonal matrix

$$A = diag(-\lambda, \cdots, -\lambda) = -\lambda I \in R^{n\times n} \tag{3}$$

with $\lambda > \frac{1}{8}\gamma^{-2} > 0$ (γ is a design parameter).

Definition 3: The function of $s(x_i)$ possesses the following properties:

1. $s(x_i)$ is bounded on R;
2. $s(x_i)$ is piecewise analytic and strictly increasing on R, *i.e.*, $0 < \frac{ds(x_i)}{dx_i} < M_i$ and $M_i < \infty$ for all $x_i \in R$;
3. $s(x_i) = 0$ when $x_i = 0$.

Remark: Because of *Definition 3*, it is important to point out that the model (2) is significantly different from the model of the reference (Liu, Shih, & Wang, 2009). The activation function $s(x_i)$ in this chapter represents a class of general nonlinear function, which is not a specific hyperbolic tangent function $\tanh(x_i)$ as (Liu, Shih, & Wang, 2009). Therefore, the model of (2) encompasses a much larger class of systems.

Proposition 1: For any two vectors x and y, the following holds (Hardy, Littlewood, & Polya, 1989)

$$x^T y \le \frac{\|x\|^2}{2} + \frac{\|y\|^2}{2} \tag{4}$$

Proposition 2: If x and y are two distinct points in R^n, then the line segment $L(x, y)$ joining x and y is

$$L(x, y) = \{z \mid z = \theta x + (1-\theta)y, 0 < \theta < 1\} \tag{5}$$

Assume that $f: R^n \to R$ is continuously differentiable at each point x of an open set $S \subset R^n$. Let x and y be two points of S such that the line segment $L(x, y) \subset S$. Then, there exists a point ξ of $L(x, y)$ such that (Khalil, (1996)

$$f(y) - f(x) = \left.\frac{\partial f}{\partial x}\right|_{x=\xi} (y - x) \tag{6}$$

In order to have a solid description, let us briefly discuss the concept of nonlinear $\boldsymbol{H}_\infty$ optimal control. It is known (Basar & Bernhard, 1995) that for the following type of general nonlinear system

$$\dot{x} = f(x) + g_1(x)d + g_2(x)u \tag{7}$$

Suppose that there exists a positive optimal value function $V(x)$, which satisfies the HJI equation

$$\begin{aligned} &V_x(x)f(x) + \frac{1}{4}V_x(x)[\gamma^{-2}g_1(x)g_2^T(x) \\ &-g_2(x)r^{-1}(x)g_2^T(x)]V_x^T(x) + q(x) = 0 \end{aligned} \tag{8}$$

Then

$$u^*(x) = -\frac{1}{2}r^{-1}(x)g_2^T(x)V_x^T(x) \tag{9}$$

is the optimal stabilizing control which minimizes the cost functional

$$J(u,d) = \int_0^{\infty} \left[q(x) + u^T r(x) u - \gamma^2 d^T d \right] dt \tag{10}$$

where $q(x)$ is positive definite and radially unbounded, $r(x)$ is also positive definite, and $\gamma^2 d^T d$ represents the level of disturbance attenuation. In addition, the worst case disturbance $d^*(x)$ is

$$d^*(x) = \frac{1}{2\gamma^2} g_1^T(x) V_x^T(x) \tag{11}$$

that is

$$\min_u \max_d [q(x) + u^T r(x) u - \gamma^2 d^T d + \dot{V}(x)] = 0 \tag{12}$$

It should be pointed out that the control law represented by (9) achieves stability margins which are a nonlinear analog of Kalman's margins for the linear quadratic regulators, that is, the infinite gain margin and the 60° phase margins. As discussed in (Basar & Bernhard, 1995), this nonlinear $\boldsymbol{H}_\infty$ problem is equivalent to the differential game $\min_u \max_d J(u,d)$ for the cost (10) constrained by system (7). Because it is too difficult to solve the formidable HJI equation of (8) in general, the direct $\boldsymbol{H}_\infty$ optimal control problem for general nonlinear systems remains open. However, by using the technique of inverse optimality (Freeman & Kokotovic, 1996), we can circumvent the task of solving the HJI equation and still develop a $\boldsymbol{H}_\infty$ control. The new challenge is to develop a stabilizing control first and then convert this stabilizing control to an optimal control.

We now rewrite the system of noisy recurrent neural networks described by (2) as

$$\dot{x} = -\lambda x + W_1 S(x) + W_2 u + d \tag{13}$$

Then a Lyapunov function E is considered as

$$E = \frac{1}{2} x^T x = \frac{1}{2} \|x\|^2 \tag{14}$$

and take the time derivative of it along the trajectory of x.

$$\begin{aligned} \dot{E} &= x^T \dot{x} \\ &= x^T(-\lambda x + W_1 S(x) + W_2 u + d) \\ &= -\lambda x^T x + x^T W_1 S(x) + x^T W_2 u + x^T d \end{aligned} \tag{15}$$

For the second term $x^T W_1 S(x)$, we apply the inequality (4)

$$\begin{aligned} x^T W_1 S(x) &\le \frac{1}{2} x^T x + \frac{1}{2} \|W_1 S(x)\|^2 \\ &\le \frac{1}{2} x^T x + \frac{1}{2} \|W_1\|^2 \|S(x)\|^2 \end{aligned} \tag{16}$$

From (6), we have

$$\|S(x)\| - \|S(0)\| = \left. \frac{\partial \{\|S(x)\|\}}{\partial x} \right|_{x=\xi} \cdot (x - 0) \tag{17}$$

That is

$$\|S(x)\| = \left. \frac{\partial \{\|S(x)\|\}}{\partial x} \right|_{x=\xi} \cdot x \tag{18}$$

Where

$$\left. \frac{\partial \{\|S(x)\|\}}{\partial x} \right|_{x=\xi} = \left[\left. \frac{\partial \{\|S(x)\|\}}{\partial x_1} \right|_{x=\xi}, \dots, \left. \frac{\partial \{\|S(x)\|\}}{\partial x_n} \right|_{x=\xi} \right] \tag{19}$$

and

$$\frac{\partial\{\|S(x)\|\}}{\partial x_i} = \sqrt{\frac{s^2(x_i)}{s^2(x_1)+\cdots+s^2(x_n)}}\frac{ds(x_i)}{dx_i} \tag{20}$$

From the definition of $s(x_i)$, we have $\frac{ds(x_i)}{dx_i} \le M\left(M = \max\left\{M_i\right\}, i = 1,\cdots,n\right)$.

Therefore

$$\left.\frac{\partial\{\|S(x)\|\}}{\partial x_i}\right|_{x=\xi} \le M \tag{21}$$

Then

$$\begin{aligned}\|S(x)\| &\le \left\|\left.\frac{\partial\{\|S(x)\|\}}{\partial x}\right|_{x=\xi}\right\| \cdot \|x\| \\ &\le \sqrt{M^2+\cdots+M^2}\cdot\|x\| \\ &\le M\sqrt{n}\,\|x\|\end{aligned} \tag{22}$$

From (16), we obtain

$$\begin{aligned}x^T W_1 S(x) &\le \frac{1}{2}x^T x + \frac{1}{2}nM^2\left\|W_1\right\|^2\|x\|^2 \\ &= \frac{1}{2}x^T x + \frac{1}{2}nM^2\left\|W_1\right\|^2 x^T x \\ &= x^T\left(\frac{1+nM^2\left\|W_1\right\|^2}{2}\right)x\end{aligned} \tag{23}$$

For the fourth term $x^T d$, by the inequality (4), we have

$$\begin{aligned}x^T d &\le k^2\|x\|^2 + \frac{1}{4k^2}\|d\|^2 \\ &= k^2 x^T x + \frac{1}{4k^2}d^T d\end{aligned} \tag{24}$$

where k is a design parameter.

Substituting (23) and (24) into (15), we have

$$\begin{aligned}\dot{E} &= -\lambda x^T x + x^T W_1 S(x) + x^T W_2 u + x^T d \\ &\le -\lambda x^T x + x^T\left(\frac{1+nM^2\left\|W_1\right\|^2}{2}\right)x \\ &\quad + x^T W_2 u + k^2 x^T x + \frac{1}{4k^2}d^T d \\ &= -\lambda x^T x + x^T\left(\frac{1+nM^2\left\|W_1\right\|^2+2k^2}{2}\right)x \\ &\quad + x^T W_2 u + \frac{1}{4k^2}d^T d\end{aligned} \tag{25}$$

For further analysis, two cases are considered depending on different structures of noisy recurrent neural networks.

Case 1

For a class of recurrent neural networks, the number of inputs is same as the number of states, that is, $x \in R^n$, $u \in R^n$ and $W_2 \in R^{n\times n}$. This structure is the most common one in the literature.

From (25), let us consider

$$x^T\left(\frac{1+nM^2\left\|W_1\right\|^2+2k^2}{2}\right)x + x^T W_2 u = 0 \tag{26}$$

If the square matrix W_2 is invertible, that is $|W_2| \neq 0$, then we can determine a stabilizing control law as

$$u = -\left(W_2\right)^{-1}\left(\frac{1+nM^2\left\|W_1\right\|^2+2k^2}{2}\right)x \tag{27}$$

Then (25) becomes that

$$\dot{E} \le -\lambda x^T x + \frac{1}{4k^2} d^T d \tag{28}$$

We see that $\dot{E}$ is negative, that is, $\dot{E} \le 0$ whenever $\|x\| \ge \frac{\|d\|}{2k\sqrt{\lambda}}$.

Since the noise d is a bounded signal, we conclude that $\dot{E}$ is negative outside the compact residual set

$$R = \left\{ x : \|x\| \le \frac{\|d\|}{2k\sqrt{\lambda}} \right\} \tag{29}$$

Therefore, we have the following theorem.

Theorem 1

For the system of noisy recurrent neural networks described by (2) with the same number of states and inputs, if the noise d is bounded, then the control

$$u = -(W_2)^{-1} \left[\frac{1 + nM^2 \|W_1\|^2 + 2k^2}{2} \right] x \tag{30}$$

stabilizes the closed-loop system and guarantees that the state x converges to the compact set (29). If, in addition, the noise d converges to zero, the state x will also converge to zero asymptotically.

The proof of the theorem is given in appendix.

Now let us define

$$\gamma^2 = \frac{1}{4k^2} \Rightarrow k^2 = \frac{1}{4\gamma^2} \tag{31}$$

Then

$$\dot{E} \le -\lambda \|x\|^2 + \gamma^2 \|d\|^2 \tag{32}$$

and

$$u = -(W_2)^{-1} \left[\frac{1 + nM^2 \|W_1\|^2}{2} + \frac{1}{4\gamma^2} \right] x \tag{33}$$

With the concept of nonlinear H_∞ optimal control described at the beginning of this section, let us first consider the Lyapunov function E as the optimal value function $V(x)$. Then, we apply the concepts of differential minimax game (Basar & Bernhard, 1995) and inverse optimality (Freeman & Kokotovic, 1996). Regarding the system of (2), we consider the control $u(t)$ as a player to oppose the noise function $d(t)$ in the game of controlling the system (2).

The time derivative of the optimal value function $V(x)$ for the general nonlinear system (7) can be expressed as follows

$$\begin{aligned} \dot{V} &= V_x \dot{x} \\ &= V_x (f(x) + g_1(x) d + g_2(x) u) \\ &= V_x f(x) + V_x g_1(x) d + V_x g_2(x) u \end{aligned} \tag{34}$$

For the model of noisy recurrent neural networks, if the solution V is given by (14), we get the following equations

$$V_x f(x) = -\lambda x^T x + x^T W_1 S(x) \tag{35}$$

$$V_x g_1(x) = x^T \tag{36}$$

$$V_x g_2(x) = x^T W_2 \tag{37}$$

Then the substitution of the solution (14) into HJI equation (8) yields the next relation

$$\begin{aligned} &-\lambda x^T x + x^T W_1 S(x) + \frac{1}{4} \gamma^{-2} x^T x \\ &- \frac{1}{4} x^T W_2 r^{-1}(x) W_2^T x + q(x) = 0 \end{aligned} \tag{38}$$

Let us make modification for (33)

$$\begin{aligned} u &= -c(W_2)^{-1}\left[\frac{1+nM^2\left\|W_1\right\|^2}{2}+\frac{1}{4c\gamma^2}\right]x \\ &= -c(W_2)^{-1}\left[\frac{1+nM^2\left\|W_1\right\|^2}{2}+\frac{1}{4c\gamma^2}\right](W_2^{\,T})^{-1}(W_2^{\,T})x \\ &= -c(W_2^{\,T}W_2)^{-1}\left[\frac{1+nM^2\left\|W_1\right\|^2}{2}+\frac{1}{4c\gamma^2}\right]W_2^{\,T}x \\ &= -\frac{1}{2}c(W_2^{\,T}W_2)^{-1}(1+nM^2\left\|W_1\right\|^2+\frac{1}{2c\gamma^2})W_2^{\,T}x \end{aligned} \tag{39}$$

where $c > 2$ and c is a constant.

Comparing the result with (9) u^*, we find that the function $r(x)$ can be selected as

$$r(x) = c^{-1}W_2^{\,T}W_2(1+nM^2\left\|W_1\right\|^2+\frac{1}{2c\gamma^2})^{-1} \tag{40}$$

and from (38) the function $q(x)$ is given by

$$\begin{aligned} q(x) &= \lambda x^T x + \frac{c}{4}(1+nM^2\left\|W_1\right\|^2 \\ &\quad +\frac{1}{2c\gamma^2})x^T x - \frac{1}{4}\gamma^{-2}x^T x - x^T W_1 S(x) \end{aligned} \tag{41}$$

We now complete the design of a nonlinear $\boldsymbol{H}_\infty$ control law that attenuates the noise to a prescribed level (represented by the parameter of γ) with stability margins. Consequently we give the following theorem. We now have the following theorem.

Theorem 2

For the system of noisy recurrent neural networks described by (2) with the same number of states and inputs, there exist a positive-definite function $q(x)$ (41) and a strictly positive function $r(x)$ (40), such that the feedback control law

$$u = u^* = -\frac{1}{2}r^{-1}(x)W_2^{\,T}x \tag{42}$$

applied to it, achieves global inverse optimality with respect to a meaningful cost functional

$$J = \int_0^\infty \left[q(x) + u^T r(x) u - \gamma^2 d^T d\right] dt \tag{43}$$

for the worst case disturbance

$$d = d^* = \frac{1}{2\gamma^2}x \tag{44}$$

In addition, $x(t) \to 0$ as $t \to \infty$ for all $d(t) \in L_2$, and $x(t) \in L_\infty$ for all $d(t) \in L_\infty$. Without a noise, $d = 0$, the control law (42) makes the equilibrium $x = 0$ global asymptotic stability (GAS). Furthermore, a minimax equilibrium (u^*, d^*) is achieved.

Proof

- **Step 1:** Considering a positive-definite control Lyapunov function $V = \frac{1}{2}\left\|x\right\|^2$, which is the same as (14), the time derivative of V along the trajectory of x results in

$$\dot{V} = -\lambda x^T x + x^T W_1 S(x) + x^T W_2 u + x^T d \tag{45}$$

The substitution of the control law (42) into $\dot{V}$ (45) yields

$$\begin{aligned}\dot{V} &= -\lambda x^T x + x^T W_1 S(x) + x^T d \\ &\quad -\frac{1}{2} c x^T W_2 (W_2^T W_2)^{-1} (1 + nM^2 \|W_1\|^2 \\ &\quad + \frac{1}{2c\gamma^2}) W_2^T x \\ &= -\lambda x^T x + x^T W_1 S(x) + x^T d \\ &\quad -\frac{1}{2} c (1 + nM^2 \|W_1\|^2 + \frac{1}{2c\gamma^2}) x^T x\end{aligned} \tag{46}$$

From (23), we obtain

$$x^T W_1 S(x) \le x^T (\frac{1 + nM^2 \|W_1\|^2}{2}) x \tag{47}$$

So

$$\begin{aligned}\dot{V} &\le -\lambda x^T x + x^T (\frac{1 + nM^2 \|W_1\|^2}{2}) x + x^T d \\ &\quad -\frac{1}{2} c (1 + nM^2 \|W_1\|^2 + \frac{1}{2c\gamma^2}) x^T x \\ &= -\lambda x^T x - (\frac{c-1}{2})(1 + nM^2 \|W_1\|^2) x^T x \\ &\quad -\frac{1}{4\gamma^2} x^T x + x^T d \\ &= -\lambda x^T x - (\frac{c-1}{2})(1 + nM^2 \|W_1\|^2) x^T x \\ &\quad -\gamma^2 \left\| \frac{1}{2\gamma^2} x - d \right\|^2 + \gamma^2 d^T d \\ &\le -\lambda x^T x + \gamma^2 d^T d\end{aligned} \tag{48}$$

Therefore $\dot{V} \le 0$ whenever $\|x\| \ge \frac{\gamma}{\sqrt{\lambda}} \|d\|$.

By (Teel, 1999) and (Krstic, Kanellakopoulos, & Kokotovic, 1995), we know that $x(t) \to 0$ as $t \to \infty$ for all $d(t) \in L_2$, and $x(t) \in L_\infty$ for all $d(t) \in L_\infty$. In the absence of a noise, $d = 0$, the control law (42) renders the equilibrium $x = 0$ global asymptotic stability (GAS).

- **Step 2:** Let us consider $q(x)$ and $r(x)$
  By (41)

$$\begin{aligned}q(x) &= \lambda x^T x + \frac{c}{4}(1 + nM^2 \|W_1\|^2 \\ &\quad + \frac{1}{2c\gamma^2}) x^T x - \frac{1}{4}\gamma^{-2} x^T x - x^T W_1 S_1(x)\end{aligned} \tag{49}$$

From (47), we have

$$-x^T W_1 S(x) \ge -x^T (\frac{1 + nM^2 \|W_1\|^2}{2}) x \tag{50}$$

Therefore

$$\begin{aligned}q(x) &\ge \lambda x^T x + \frac{c}{4}(1 + nM^2 \|W_1\|^2 + \frac{1}{2c\gamma^2}) x^T x \\ &\quad -\frac{1}{4}\gamma^{-2} x^T x - (\frac{1 + nM^2 \|W_1\|^2}{2}) x^T x \\ &= \lambda x^T x + (\frac{c-2}{2})(\frac{1 + nM^2 \|W_1\|^2}{2}) x^T x \\ &\quad -\frac{1}{8}\gamma^{-2} x^T x \\ &= (\lambda - \frac{1}{8}\gamma^{-2}) x^T x + (\frac{c-2}{2})(\frac{1 + nM^2 \|W_1\|^2}{2}) x^T x \\ &\ge 0\end{aligned} \tag{51}$$

Then $q(x)$ is positive definite and radially unbounded.
By (40)

$$r(x) = c^{-1} W_2^T W_2 (1 + nM^2 \|W_1\|^2 + \frac{1}{2c\gamma^2})^{-1} \tag{52}$$

If $|W_2| \neq 0$, we know that $r(x) > 0$ since $W_2^T W_2 > 0$.
For the choice of $q(x)$ and $r(x)$ in (41) and (40), $\dot{V}$ is evaluated in the following form

$$\dot{V} = -q(x) - u^T r(x) u + \gamma^2 d^T d - \gamma^2 \left\| \frac{1}{2\gamma^2} x - d \right\|^2 + (u - u^*)^T r(x)(u - u^*) \quad (53)$$

Then it is shown from (53) that the optimal control $u = u^*$ is an optimal solution to J (43) for the worst disturbance $d = d^*$ and satisfies

$$\min_u \max_d [q(x) + u^T r(x) u - \gamma^2 d^T d + \dot{V}] = 0 \quad (54)$$

Therefore, by considering the control $u(t)$ as a player and the noise $d(t)$ as the opposing player, a minimax equilibrium (u^*, d^*) is achieved (Basar & Bernhard, 1995). In addition, the Lyapunov function $V(x)$ satisfies the HJI equation

$$V_x(x) f(x) + \frac{1}{4} V_x(x) \left[\gamma^2 g_1(x) g_1^T(x) - g_2(x) r^{-1}(x) g_2^T(x) \right] V_x^T(x) + q(x) = 0 \quad (55)$$

Thus, $V(x)$ is the value function for the cost functional (43). This completes the proof.

Case 2

Let us consider a more general recurrent neural network, as described in (2), with arbitrary number of inputs, that is, $x \in R^n$, $u \in R^m$, and $W_2 \in R^{n \times m}$ ($m \neq n$).

The inequality in (25) is rewritten as

$$\dot{E} \leq -\lambda x^T x + x^T \left(\frac{1 + nM^2 \|W_1\|^2 + 2k^2}{2} \right) x + x^T W_2 u + \frac{1}{4k^2} d^T d \quad (56)$$

From (56), we can choose

$$\psi_1(x) = x^T \left(\frac{1 + nM^2 \|W_1\|^2 + 2k^2}{2} \right) x \quad (57)$$

$$\psi_2^T(x) = x^T W_2 \quad (58)$$

Similar to Sontag's formula described in (Krstic, Kanellakopoulos, & Kokotovic, 1995) and (Sontag, 1989), Let us define a scalar function

$$\varphi(x) = \frac{\psi_1(x) + \sqrt{[\psi_1(x)]^2 + [\psi_2^T(x)\psi_2(x)]^2}}{\psi_2^T(x)\psi_2(x)} \quad (59)$$

Then a control signal can be determined as

$$u = -\varphi(x)\psi_2(x) \quad (60)$$

with the assumption of $\psi_2^T(x)\psi_2(x) \neq 0$.

Let us consider the Lyapunov function E as the optimal value function $V(x)$ and apply the concepts of differential minimax game (Basar & Bernhard, 1995) and inverse optimality (Freeman & Kokotovic, 1996) to the system of (2), in which we consider the control $u(t)$ as a player to oppose the noise function $d(t)$ in the game of controlling the system (2).

Using the equation (58), this is equivalent to

$$\begin{aligned} u &= -\varphi(x) W_2^T x \\ &= -\varphi(x) g^T(x) V_x^T(x) \end{aligned} \quad (61)$$

Comparing (61) with (9) and using (37) and (38), we obtain

$$r(x) = \frac{1}{2}\varphi^{-1}(x) \quad (62)$$

and

$$q(x) = \frac{1}{4}\psi_2^T(x) r^{-1}(x) \psi_2(x) + \lambda x^T x - x^T W_1 S(x) \quad (63)$$

Consequently we now give the following theorem.

Theorem 3

For system (2), which has an arbitrary number of inputs, a positive semi-definite function $q(x)$ (63) and a positive function $r(x)$, for $x \neq 0$, (62) exist, such that the feedback control law

$$u = u^* = -\frac{1}{2} r^{-1}(x) W_2^T x \tag{64}$$

when applied to the system, achieves inverse optimality with respect to a cost functional of the form

$$J = \int_0^\infty \left[q(x) + u^T r(x) u - \gamma^2 d^T d \right] dt \tag{65}$$

for the worst case disturbance

$$d = d^* = \frac{1}{2\gamma^2} x \tag{66}$$

In addition, $x(t) \to 0$ as $t \to \infty$ for all $d(t) \in L_2$, and $x(t) \in L_\infty$ for all $d(t) \in L_\infty$. In the absence of a noise, $d = 0$, the control law (64) renders the equilibrium $x = 0$ globally asymptotically stable (GAS). Furthermore, a minimax equilibrium (u^*, d^*) is achieved.

Proof

- **Step 1:** Considering a positive-definite control Lyapunov function $V = \frac{1}{2}\|x\|^2$, which is the same as (14), the time derivative of V along the trajectory of x results in

$$\dot{V} = -\lambda x^T x + x^T W_1 S(x) + x^T W_2 u + x^T d \tag{67}$$

Substitution of the control law (64) into the above $\dot{V}$ yields

$$\begin{aligned} \dot{V} &= -\lambda x^T x + \frac{1}{4k^2} d^T d - \sqrt{[\psi_1(x)]^2 + [\psi_2^T(x)\psi_2(x)]^2} \\ &\leq -\lambda x^T x + \frac{1}{4k^2} d^T d \end{aligned} \tag{68}$$

Therefore $\dot{V} \leq 0$ whenever $\|x\| \geq \frac{\gamma}{\sqrt{\lambda}} \|d\|$

From (Ezal, Pan, & Kokotovic, 2000) and (Teel, 1999), we know that $x(t) \to 0$ as $t \to \infty$ for all $d(t) \in L_2$, and $x(t) \in L_\infty$ for all $d(t) \in L_\infty$. In the absence of a noise, $d = 0$, the control law (64) renders the equilibrium $x = 0$ global asymptotic stability (GAS).

- **Step 2:** Using the inequality (50) and relations (62) and (59), the expression $q(x)$, given in (63), can be written as

$$\begin{aligned} q(x) &\geq \frac{1}{2}\left(\psi_1(x) + \sqrt{[\psi_1(x)]^2 + [\psi_2^T(x)\psi_2(x)]^2} \right) + \lambda x^T x \\ &\quad - x^T \left(\frac{1 + nM^2 \|W_1\|^2 + 2k^2}{2} \right) x \\ &= \lambda x^T x + \frac{1}{2}\left(\sqrt{[\psi_1(x)]^2 + [\psi_2^T(x)\psi_2(x)]^2} - \psi_1(x) \right) \\ &\geq 0 \end{aligned} \tag{69}$$

This means that $q(x)$ is positive definite, for all $x \neq 0$, and is radially unbounded.
Also, from (62), it can be seen that $r(x) > 0$ when $\psi_2^T(x)\psi_2(x) \neq 0$. That is

$$\begin{aligned} r(x) &= \frac{1}{2} \varphi^{-1}(x) \\ &= \frac{1}{2}\left(\frac{\psi_2^T(x)\psi_2(x)}{\psi_1(x) + \sqrt{[\psi_1(x)]^2 + [\psi_2^T(x)\psi_2(x)]^2}} \right) \\ &> 0 \end{aligned} \tag{70}$$

Figure 1. System response (u = 0 and d = 0)

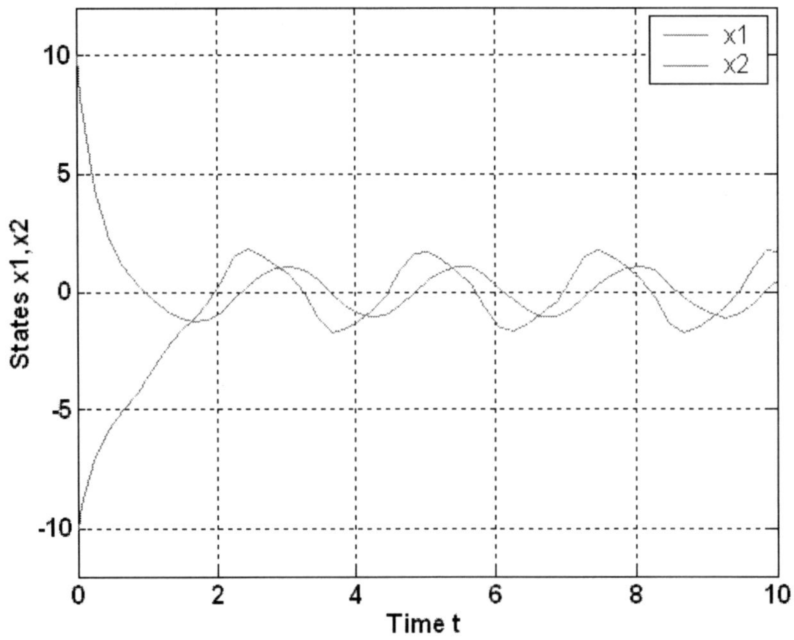

Figure 2. Phase plane (u = 0 and d = 0)

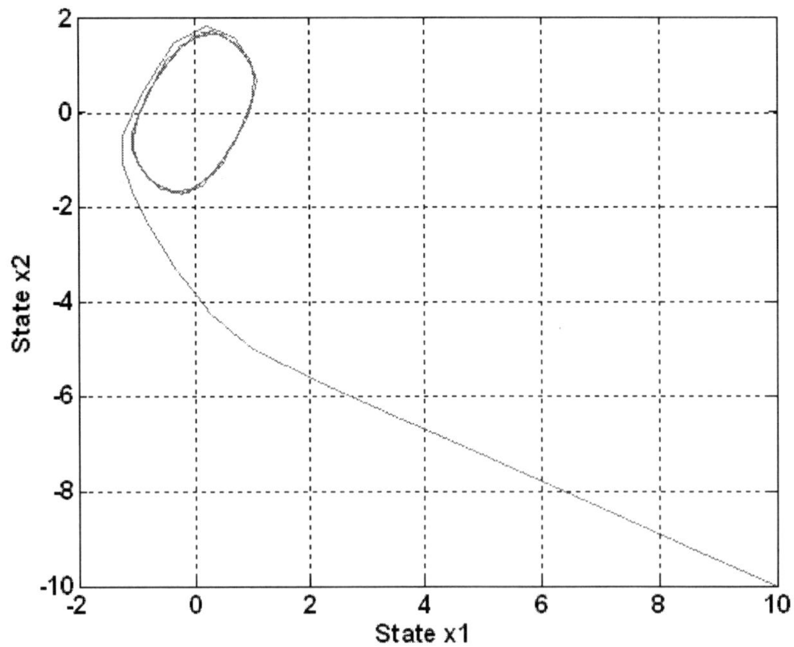

Figure 3. System response (u = 0 but d ≠ 0)

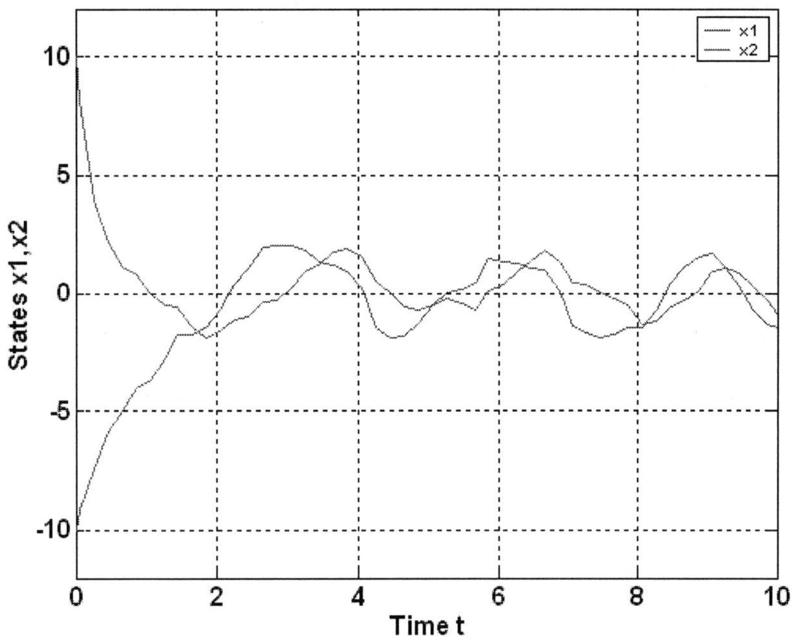

Figure 4. Phase plane (u = 0 but d ≠ 0)

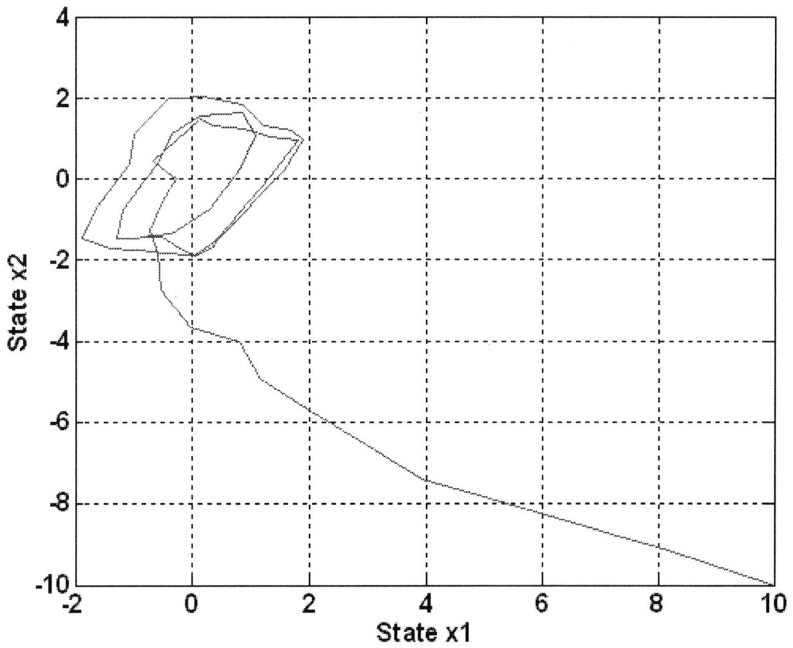

Figure 5. System response with the $\boldsymbol{H}_{\infty}$ *control (u = (42))*

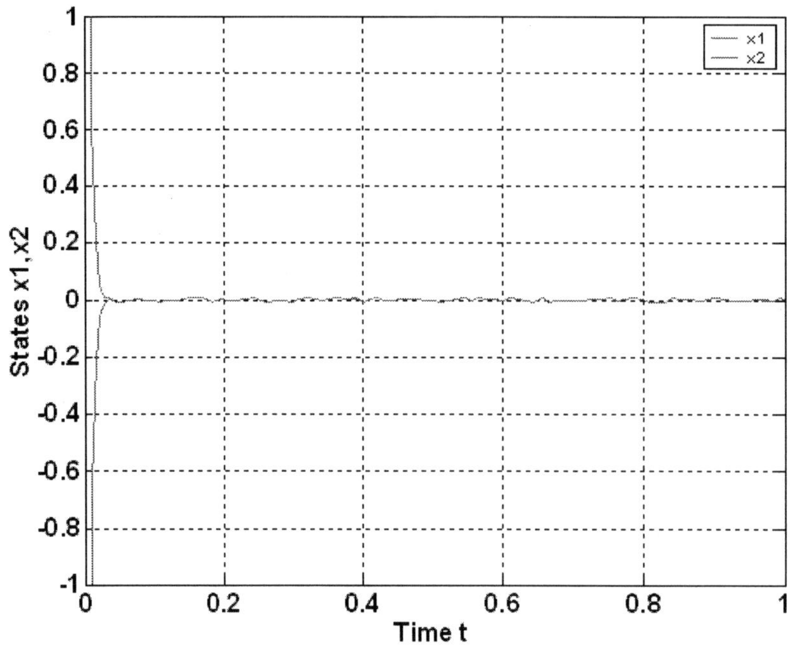

Figure 6. Phase plane with the $\boldsymbol{H}_{\infty}$ *control (u = (42))*

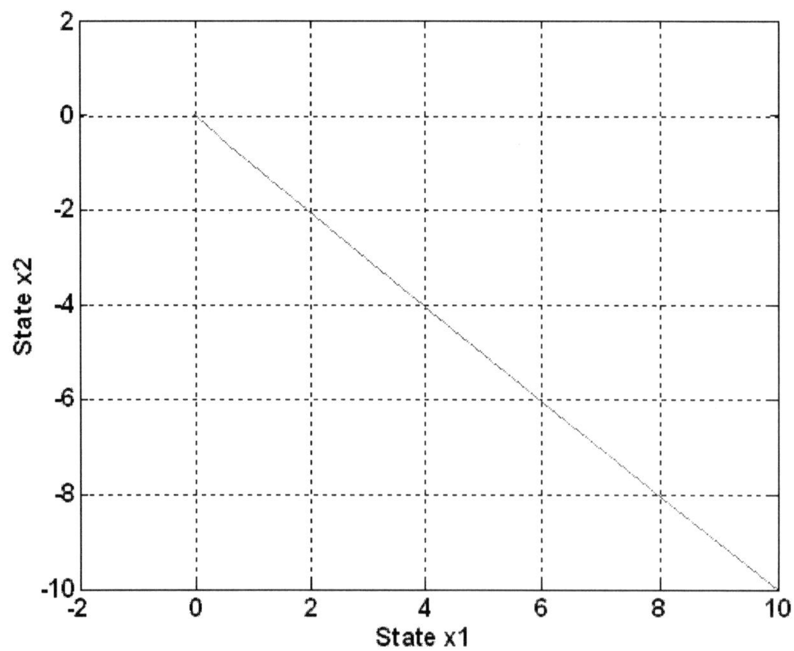

Figure 7. System response with the $\boldsymbol{H}_\infty$ *control (u = (64))*

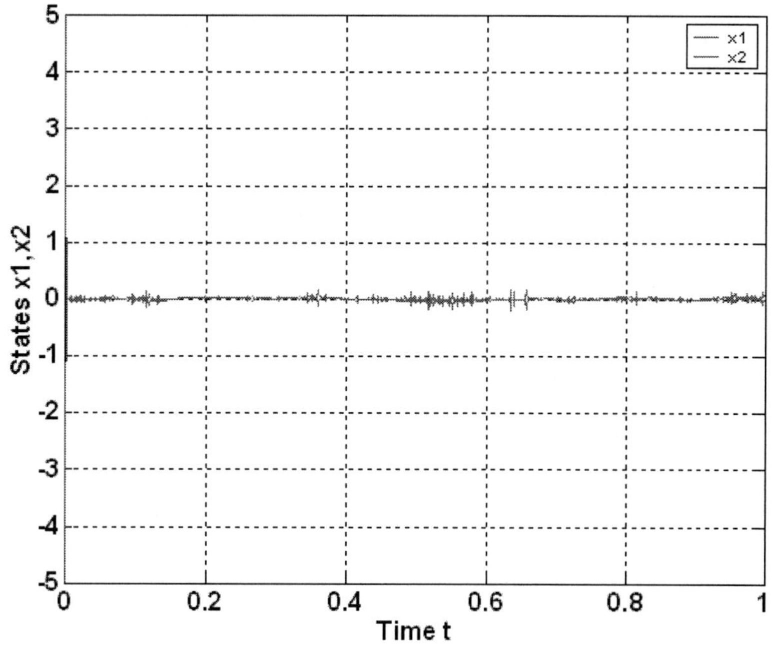

Figure 8. Phase plane with the $\boldsymbol{H}_\infty$ *control (u = (64))*

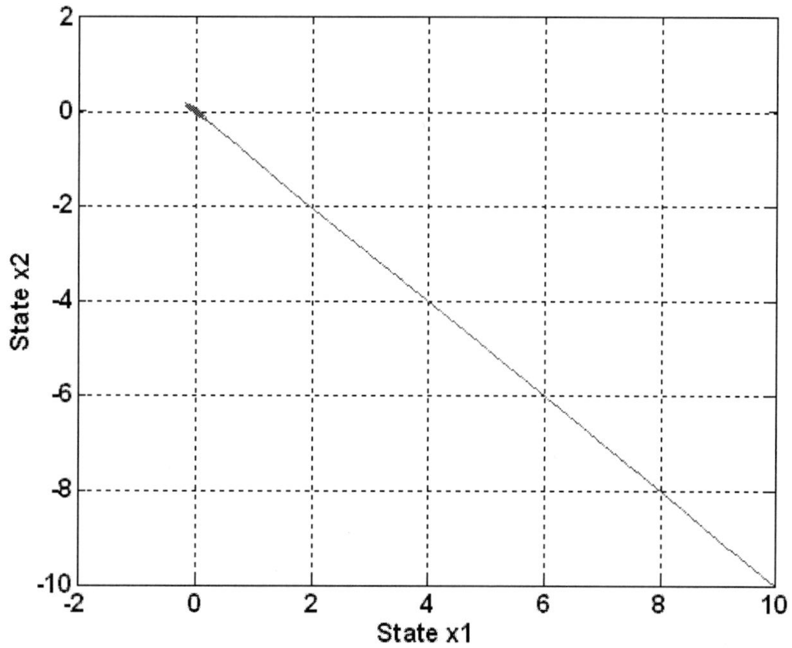

For the choice of $q(x)$ and $r(x)$ in (63) and (62), $\dot{V}$ is evaluated in the following form

$$\dot{V} = -q(x) - u^T r(x) u + \gamma^2 d^T d - \gamma^2 \left\| \frac{1}{2\gamma^2} x - d \right\|^2 + (u - u^*)^T r(x)(u - u^*) \qquad (71)$$

Therefore, it is shown from (71) that the optimal control $u = u^*$ is an optimal solution to J (65) for the worst disturbance $d = d^*$ and satisfies

$$\min_u \max_d [q(x) + u^T r(x) u - \gamma^2 d^T d + \dot{V}] = 0 \qquad (72)$$

Therefore, by considering the control $u(t)$ as a player and the noise $d(t)$ as the opposing player, a minimax equilibrium (u^*, d^*) is achieved (Basar & Bernhard, 1995). In addition, the Lyapunov function $V(x)$ satisfies the HJI equation

$$V_x(x) f(x) + \frac{1}{4} V_x(x)[\gamma^2 g_1(x) g_1^T(x) - g_2(x) r^{-1}(x) g_2^T(x)] V_x^T(x) + q(x) = 0 \qquad (73)$$

Thus, $V(x)$ is the value function for the cost functional (65). This completes the proof.

NUMERICAL EXAMPLES

In order to effectively demonstrate the results of our theoretical findings, two numerical examples adopted from (Liu, Shih, & Wang, 2009) are given as follows.

Example 1

The recurrent neural network is given as

$$\begin{bmatrix} \dot{x}_1 \\ \dot{x}_2 \end{bmatrix} = -\begin{bmatrix} 3 & 0 \\ 0 & 3 \end{bmatrix}\begin{bmatrix} x_1 \\ x_2 \end{bmatrix} + \begin{bmatrix} 2 & 3 \\ -6 & 7 \end{bmatrix}\begin{bmatrix} \tanh(x_1) \\ \tanh(x_2) \end{bmatrix} + \begin{bmatrix} d_1 \\ d_2 \end{bmatrix} + \begin{bmatrix} 2 & 0 \\ 0 & 2 \end{bmatrix}\begin{bmatrix} u_1 \\ u_2 \end{bmatrix} \qquad (74)$$

where $x_1(0) = 10$, $x_2(0) = -10$, d_1, d_2 are disturbance noises (uniformly random functions) with the magnitude of $|d_i| \leq 3$, $(i = 1, 2)$, and $m = n = 2$.

Figure1 and Figure2 show the results of time response and phase plane of this system without both the external control and the disturbance, that is, both $u = 0$ and $d = 0$. This recurrent neural network is not global asymptotic stability (GAS). Figure3 and Figure4 show the results of time response and phase plane of this system with the noise ($d \neq 0$) but without the external control ($u = 0$). The effect of disturbance noises in the system can be seen obviously. After the $\boldsymbol{H}_\infty$ control signal (42) is implemented. The corresponding simulation results are shown in Figure5 and Figure6. One can see, the neural network is GAS, as well as the noises in the system are reduced significantly.

Example 2

Let us look at the second example given

$$\begin{bmatrix} \dot{x}_1 \\ \dot{x}_2 \end{bmatrix} = -\begin{bmatrix} 3 & 0 \\ 0 & 3 \end{bmatrix}\begin{bmatrix} x_1 \\ x_2 \end{bmatrix} + \begin{bmatrix} 2 & 3 \\ -6 & 7 \end{bmatrix}\begin{bmatrix} \tanh(x_1) \\ \tanh(x_2) \end{bmatrix} + \begin{bmatrix} d_1 \\ d_2 \end{bmatrix} + \begin{bmatrix} 1 \\ -1 \end{bmatrix} u \qquad (75)$$

where $x_1(0) = 10$, $x_2(0) = -10$, d_1, d_2 are disturbance noises (uniformly random functions) with the magnitude of $|d_i| \leq 3$, $(i = 1, 2)$, and $m = 1$, $n = 2$. Without considering inputs, both neural networks have the same structure. The only difference is the dimension number of external control.

Figure 7 and Figure 8 show the results of time response and phase plane of this recurrent neural network after the H_∞ control signal (64) is applied. The system achieves the expected performance provided by theoretical results.

CONCLUSION

This chapter has presented an approach to achieve global robust control for deterministic noisy recurrent neural networks, as well as noise attenuation to a prescribed level with stability margins. Owing to the difficulty to solve the Hamilton-Jacobi-Isaacs equation, for nonlinear systems, the design of a nonlinear H_∞ optimal controller seems to be an unachievable goal in feedback design. However, the knowledge of inverse optimality allows us to find an alternative way to solve the problem and obtain an optimal feedback controller with respect to a meaningful cost functional. The controller developed in this chapter achieves the following design objectives: (i) global inverse optimality with respect to a meaningful cost functional (ii) global disturbance attenuation (iii) global asymptotic stability provided no disturbance. It is believed that the new design presented in this chapter would benefit the applications of recurrent neural networks.

REFERENCES

Arik, S. (2000). Global asymptotic stability of a class of dynamic neural networks. *IEEE Transactions on Circuits and Systems I*, *47*, 568–571. doi:10.1109/81.841858

Basar, T., & Bernhard, P. (1995). *Optimal Control and Related Minimax Design Problems: A Dynamic Game Approach* (2nd ed.). Boston: Birkhauser.doi:10.1007/978-0-8176-4757-5

Ensari, T., & Arik, S. (2005). Global stability analysis of neural networks with multiple time varying delays. *IEEE Transactions on Automatic Control*, *50*, 1781–1785. doi:10.1109/TAC.2005.858634

Ezal, K., Pan, Z., & Kokotovic, V. P. (2000). Locally optimal and robust backstepping design. *IEEE Transactions on Automatic Control*, *45*, 260–271. doi:10.1109/9.839948

Freeman, R., & Kokotovic, V. P. (1996). Inverse optimality in robust stabilization. *SIAM Journal on Control and Optimization*, *34*(4), 1365–1391. doi:10.1137/S0363012993258732

Hardy, G., Littlewood, J., & Polya, G. (1989). *Inequalities* (2nd ed.). London: Cambridge University Press.

Haykin, S. (1999). *Neural Networks*. Upper Saddle River, NJ: Prentice-Hall.

Hu, S., & Wang, J. (2002). Global asymptotic stability and global exponential stability of continuous-time recurrent neural networks. *IEEE Transactions on Automatic Control*, *47*, 802–807. doi:10.1109/TAC.2002.1000277

Khalil, H. (1996). *Nonlinear Systems* (2nd ed.). Upper Saddle River, NJ: Prentice Hall.

Krstic, M., Kanellakopoulos, I., & Kokotovic, V. P. (1995). *Nonlinear and Adaptive Control Design*. New York: John Wiley & Sons.

Kulawski, J. G., & Brdys, A. M. (2000). Stable adaptive control with recurrent networks. *Automatica*, *36*, 5–22. doi:10.1016/S0005-1098(99)00092-8

Liu, Z., Shih, S., & Wang, Q. (2009). Global robust stabilizing control for a dynamic neural network system. *IEEE Transactions on Systems, Man, and Cybernetics A*, *39*, 426–436. doi:10.1109/TSMCA.2008.2010749

Liu, Z., Torres, R., Patel, N., & Wang, Q. (2008). Further development of input-to-state stabilizing control for dynamic neural network systems. *IEEE Transactions on Systems, Man, and Cybernetics A*, *38*, 1425–1433. doi:10.1109/TSMCA.2008.2003464

Marco, M., Forti, M., & Tesi, A. (2004). On absolute stability of convergence for nonlinear neural network models. In W. Kang et al. (Eds.), *New Trends in Nonlinear Dynamics and Control and their Applications, Lecture Notes in Control and Information Sciences,* 209-220, Berlin: Springer.

Sanchez, N. E., & Perez, P. J. (2003). Input-to-state stabilization of dynamic neural networks. *IEEE Transactions on Systems, Man, and Cybernetics A*, *33*, 532–536. doi:10.1109/TSMCA.2003.811509

Sontag, D. E. (1989). A universal construction of artstein's theorem on nonlinear stabilization. *Systems & Control Letters*, *13*, 117–123. doi:10.1016/0167-6911(89)90028-5

Sontag, D. E., & Qiao, Y. (1999). Further results on controllability of recurrent neural networks. *Systems & Control Letters*, *36*, 121–129. doi:10.1016/S0167-6911(98)00068-1

Sontag, D. E., & Sussmann, H. (1997). Complete controllability of continuous-time recurrent neural networks. *Systems & Control Letters*, *30*, 177–183. doi:10.1016/S0167-6911(97)00002-9

Teel, A. (1999). Asymptotic convergence from L_p stability. *IEEE Transactions on Automatic Control*, *44*, 2169–2170. doi:10.1109/9.802938

Werbos, P. (2009). Intelligence in the brain: a theory of how it works and how to build it. *Neural Networks*, *22*(3), 200–212. doi:10.1016/j.neunet.2009.03.012

ADDITIONAL READING

Albus, J. (1991). Outline for a theory of intelligence. *IEEE Transactions on Systems, Man, and Cybernetics A*, *21*, 473–509. doi:10.1109/21.97471

Arbib, M. (1995). Schema theory. In Arbib, M. (Ed.), *The Handbook of Brain Theory and Neural Networks*. Cambridge, MA: MIT Press.

Camazine, S., Deneubourg, J., Franks, N., Sneyd, J., Theraulaz, G., & Bonabeau, E. (2003). *Self-organization in Biological Systems*. Princeton, NJ: Princeton Univ. Press.

Delgado, A., Kabhampati, C., & Warwick, K. (1995). Dynamical recurrent neural network for system identification and control. *IEE Proceedings. Control Theory and Applications*, *142*, 307–314. doi:10.1049/ip-cta:19951873

Edwards, D., Heitler, W., & Krasne, F. (1999). Fifty years of a command neuron: the neurobiology of escape behavior in the crayfish. *Trends in Neurosciences*, *22*, 153–161. doi:10.1016/S0166-2236(98)01340-X

Lewis, F. (1986). *Optimal Control*. New York: John Wiley & Sons.

Rovithakis, G., & Christodoulou, M. (1995). Direct adaptive regulation of unknown nonlinear dynamical systems via dynamical neural networks. *IEEE Transactions on Systems, Man, and Cybernetics A*, *25*, 1578–1594. doi:10.1109/21.478444

Tino, P., Horne, B., Giles, C., & Collingwood, P. (1998). Finite state machines and recurrent neural networks – automata and dynamical systems approaches. In Dayhoff, J. and Omidvar, O., (Eds), *Neural Networks and Pattern Recognition*, pages 171–220, Academic Press.

Zhu, R., Chai, T., & Shao, C. (1997). Robust nonlinear adaptive observer design using dynamic recurrent neural networks. *Proceedings of the American Control Conference,* Albuquerque, NM, 1096-1100.

KEY TERMS AND DEFINITIONS

Noisy Recurrent Neural Networks: A class of recurrent neural networks that are under the influence of noise or disturbance.

Differential Minimax Game: It is a design approach that the objective is to develop a control that minimizes a given cost functional under worst possible noises or disturbances, which maximize the same cost functional.

Robust Control: A control methodology that specifically deals with uncertainty in the development of controller design.

Optimal Control: A mathematical optimization method for finding a control law under a certain optimality criterion for a given system.

Hamilton-Jacobi-Isaacs (HJI) Equation: A generalization of the Hamilton-Jacobi-Bellman partial differential equation that provides a sufficient condition in nonlinear optimal control.

Inverse Optimality: A design technique that solves the inverse problem of optimal stabilization, in which a stabilizing feedback is developed first and then modifies it to achieve an optimal control for a cost functional.

APPENDIX

Proof of Theorem 1: From (28), we have

$$\frac{d}{dt}\left(\frac{1}{2}\|x\|^2\right) \leq -\lambda x^T x + \frac{1}{4k^2} d^T d = -\lambda \|x\|^2 + \frac{\|d\|^2}{4k^2} \tag{76}$$

Let us consider the time derivative of $\|x\|^2 e^{2\lambda t}$

$$\frac{d}{dt}\left(\|x\|^2 e^{2\lambda t}\right) = \frac{d}{dt}\left(\|x\|^2\right) \ e^{2\lambda t} + 2\lambda \|x\|^2 e^{2\lambda t} \tag{77}$$

The substitution of (76) into (77) yields

$$\frac{d}{dt}\left(\|x\|^2 e^{2\lambda t}\right) \leq -2\lambda \|x\|^2 e^{2\lambda t} + \frac{\|d\|^2}{2k^2} e^{2\lambda t} + 2\lambda \|x\|^2 e^{2\lambda t} = \frac{\|d\|^2}{2k^2} e^{2\lambda t} \tag{78}$$

Taking the integration of both sides, we have

$$\begin{aligned} \|x\|^2 e^{2\lambda t} &\leq \|x(0)\|^2 + \int_0^t \frac{\|d(\tau)\|^2}{2k^2} e^{2\lambda\tau} d\tau \\ &\leq \|x(0)\|^2 + \frac{1}{2k^2}\left[\sup_{0\leq\tau\leq t} \|d(\tau)\|^2\right] \int_0^t e^{2\lambda\tau} d\tau \\ &\leq \|x(0)\|^2 + \frac{1}{4k^2\lambda}\left[\sup_{0\leq\tau\leq t} \|d(\tau)\|^2\right]\left(e^{2\lambda t} - 1\right) \end{aligned} \tag{79}$$

Let us multiply both sides with $e^{-2\lambda t}$, we obtain

$$\|x\|^2 \leq \|x(0)\|^2 e^{-2\lambda t} + \frac{1}{4k^2\lambda}\left[\sup_{0\leq\tau\leq t} \|d(\tau)\|^2\right]\left(1 - e^{-2\lambda t}\right) \tag{80}$$

$$\sqrt{p^2 + q^2} \leq |p| + |q| \tag{81}$$

$$\begin{aligned}\|x\| &\leq \|x(0)\|\ e^{-\lambda t} + \frac{1}{2k\sqrt{\lambda}}\left[\sup_{0\leq\tau\leq t}\|d(\tau)\|\right]\left(1-e^{-2\lambda t}\right)^{\frac{1}{2}} \\ &\leq \|x(0)\| e^{-\lambda t} + \frac{1}{2k\sqrt{\lambda}}\left[\sup_{0\leq\tau\leq t}\|d(\tau)\|\right] \\ &\leq \|x(0)\| e^{-\lambda t} + \frac{\|d\|_{\infty}}{2k\sqrt{\lambda}}\end{aligned} \tag{82}$$

Therefore we conclude that the control signal described by (30) guarantees convergence of x to the residual set (29), and particularly to zero if d tends to zero. This completes the proof.

Chapter 7
A Biologically Inspired Evolving Spiking Neural Model with Rank-Order Population Coding and a Taste Recognition System Case Study

S. Soltic
Manukau Institute of Technology, New Zealand & Auckland University of Technology, New Zealand

N. Kasabov
Auckland University of Technology, New Zealand

ABSTRACT

The human brain has an amazing ability to recognize hundreds of thousands of different tastes. The question is: can we build artificial systems that can achieve this level of complexity? Such systems would be useful in biosecurity, the chemical and food industry, security, in home automation, etc. The purpose of this chapter is to explore how spiking neurons could be employed for building biologically plausible and efficient taste recognition systems. It presents an approach based on a novel spiking neural network model, the evolving spiking neural network with population coding (ESNN-PC), which is characterized by: (i) adaptive learning, (ii) knowledge discovery and (iii) accurate classification. ESNN-PC is used on a benchmark taste problem where the effectiveness of the information encoding, the quality of extracted rules and the model's adaptive properties are explored. Finally, applications of ESNN-PC in recognition of the increasing interest in robotics and pervasive computing are suggested.

INTRODUCTION

Our sense of taste is a vital part of our existence. It discriminates between foodstuff (such as vegetables, meats, tea, mineral waters), assesses their quality and nutritious content and detects potentially poisonous substances. In sharp contrast to its importance, the taste sensory system is poorly explored compared to other sensory systems such as the visual and olfactory systems. Only recently have studies started to paint a picture of taste biol-

DOI: 10.4018/978-1-60960-018-1.ch007

Figure 1. Block diagram of an artificial taste recognition system. The system comprises an array of sensors modeling the tongue, i.e. an electronic tongue, and a pattern recognition system classifying the tastants

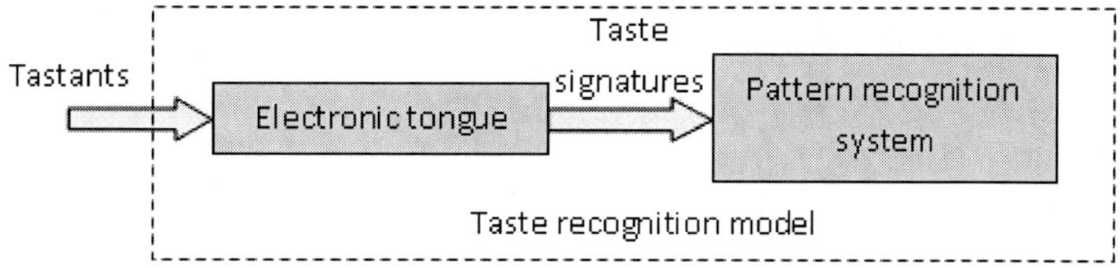

ogy; and exactly how the taste signals are coded and transmitted to the brain is still unknown. For years, two biological models of taste-coding have been favored, namely the 'labeled-line' coding and the 'cross-fiber' coding (Chandrashekar, Hoon, Ryba, & Zuker, 2006; Reed, Tanaka, & McDaniel, 2006, Bradbury, 2004; Dulac, 2000; Margolskee, 1993). In 'labeled-line' coding the taste receptor cells (TRC) are specialized for responding to only one taste modality, either bitter, salty, sour, sweet or umami. In the 'cross-fiber' coding, the TRC are broadly tuned to more than one taste and a pattern of activity across a number of TRC characterizes the taste sensation.

Most taste recognition models use the 'cross-fiber' scenario. In these models broadly tuned TRC are simulated using an array of non-selective sensors with partially overlapping selectivity where the sensors' electrical characteristics, for example capacitance, change under the influence of the chemical composition of a tastant. These arrays of sensors are called 'electronic tongues' (Cortina, Duran, Alegret, & del Valle, 2006; Gallardo *et al.,* 2003; Riul Jr. *et al.*, 2002). An 'electronic tongue' responds differently to different types of tastants forming unique taste signatures, which can be analyzed by a pattern recognition system as shown in Figure 1. The tasting of tastants must not be confused with the chemical analysis of tastants. Taste sensors do not provide a chemical composition of a tastant, *i.e.* what chemicals are present in the tastant, but rather produce responses closely associated with the tastant's chemical composition. The pattern recognition system is usually based on a multilayer perceptron (MLP) neural network (Gutiérrez *et al.*, 2008; Gutés, Ibáñez, Céspedes, Alegret, & del Valle, 2005; Riul Jr. *et al.*, 2004; Gallardo *et al.*, 2003; de Sousa, Carvalho, Riul Jr., & Mattoso, 2002). An electronic tongue together with a pattern recognition system is called an 'artificial tongue' (Riul Jr. *et al.*, 2002).

While MLP have been found to be accurate taste classifiers, a number of difficulties associated with such networks have been reported: the rather limited exploratory capabilities (Varkevisser, 2001) linked to the 'black-box' property of these networks, the problems with tuning network parameters (Stitt, Gaumond, Frazier, & Hanson, 1997) and the problem of finding the appropriate size for the hidden layer (Gutiérrez *et al.*, 2008; Cortina, 2006; Gallardo, 2003; de Sousa, 2002). The knowledge that an MLP acquires is hard or impossible to extract. Moreover, MLP are slow to learn. Training these networks consists of repetitively presenting the network with large training data sets where the number of repetitions (epochs) is usually found by trial-and-error. Furthermore, these networks must be retrained on old and new data every time a new data sample is obtained. In other words, they have a limited ability to learn new tastes as they become available. These problems hinder the MLP network from being an efficient taste classifier. Hence, the objective of this work is to tackle these problems by building a more biologically plausible taste recognition model that:

1. Uses integrate-and-fire neurons capable of modeling the dynamic behavior of real neurons.
2. Encodes data samples using a temporal encoding scheme that models the action potentials occurring in the brain.
3. Has a layer simulating taste cell interactions.
4. Learns quickly, using a one-pass learning algorithm.
5. Learns new tastants without forgetting the ones that it has already learnt. This is a very important feature. Human beings do not forget all the previously learned tastes as they are introduced to new ones.
6. Has knowledge discovery facility and delivers its knowledge in the form of fuzzy rules.
7. Evolves its structure in time to accept new data samples and tastants.

Acknowledging that there are no current spiking neural network (SNN) models for taste recognition, the work presented in this chapter is the first of its kind. It contributes to the promotion of SNN in general and, more specifically, as a new tool for building taste recognition systems.

BACKGROUND

Taste Perception

Taste perception starts in the mouth where chemicals in foods and beverages excite the TRC that are organized in the taste buds which are positioned throughout the mouth cavity. The TRC are connected to the gustatory nucleus of the brain via three types of sensory fibers (Dulac, 2000). However exactly how the taste signals are coded and transmitted to the brain still remains incompletely understood.

It is accepted now that the two previously mentioned models of taste-coding are not enough to explain taste responses (Katz, Nicolelis, & Simon, 2002). First, both models are static. The static nature of taste perception is disputed by empirical evidence that gustatory neural system responses are dynamic. Di Lorenzo and Victor (2003) measured the taste response variability in the nucleus of the solitary tract of a rat while influenced by taste stimuli. The measured responses showed a significant contribution of spike timing to the discrimination of taste stimuli, especially in the initial 2 seconds (20% of the total response time). They also observed that some cells showed more temporal rich responses than others, suggesting that taste coding is indeed very complex. Glendinning, Davis and Rai (2006) are also in favor of temporal coding. Their measurements of the responses of the taste system of an insect to three bitter tastants showed that different bitter compounds generate distinct temporal patterns. Second, both models are unimodal. They assume that taste perception only depends on the taste information processed by the gustatory neurons and is not influenced by any other non-gustatory system, *i.e.* the auditory, olfactory, visual and somatosensory systems. Humans are intrinsically aware that their perception of a meal is governed by more than just taste information. Evidence shows that the smell-taste interaction is particularly significant to the perception of taste (Stein & Stoodley, 2006; Verhagen & Engelen, 2006; Yoshimura *et al.*, 2004; Dulac, 2000). Third, even though the 'cross-fiber' model of taste coding has historically been favored, recent discoveries of highly dedicated taste sensors support the 'labeled-line' model of taste perception (Chandrashekar *et al.*, 2006). Nevertheless, the knowledge of how exactly the taste information is conveyed from the taste receptors to the brain is incomplete and breakthrough findings on taste coding are still to come.

Artificial Taste Recognition Models

The static and unimodal 'cross-fiber' model of taste coding has been used as the backbone to many artificial taste recognition systems. As shown earlier in Figure 1, the system consists of an array of taste sensors mimicking the taste receptor cells and a pattern recognition system modeling the neural activities in the brain. The number and type of utilized sensors in the sensor array differ from model to model. In some cases, features are extracted from the captured responses in order to lower the number of inputs into the pattern recognition system (Ivarsson *et al.,* 2001). The most popular liquid sensing techniques are based on either:

- Potentiometry, where the potential between sensing electrodes and a reference electrode is measured (Gutiérrez *et al.*, 2008).
- Voltammetry, where the current responses of sensing electrodes at different voltage pulses are measured (Krantz-Rülcker, Stenberg, Winquist, & Lundström, 2001).
- Conductometry, where the changes in the conductivity of sensors characterize the tastant (Riul Jr *et al.*, 2002).

Taste sensors are built and evaluated in laboratories. Unfortunately the datasets from those evaluations are typically not provided to the wider research community. In fact, there are no such datasets available in the popular UCI Machine Learning repository (http://archive.ics.uci.edu/ml/datasets.html). The wine dataset that could be downloaded from this repository was the result of a chemical analysis of wines rather than a utilization of an electronic tongue.

As stated earlier, taste signatures are typically classified by a MLP network. MLP networks process rate coded signals, continuous signals with amplitudes that typically fall within a range of 0 and 1. When the dynamic responses are available, the responses must be rate coded before being fed to a MLP (Varkevisser *et al.*, 2001; Stitt *et al.*, 1997). A number of questions could be asked. Should a MLP be used to evaluate dynamic responses? If not, which neural network would do the better job? Is the 'black-box' syndrome a problem when networks are used to perform taste recognition? Could an evolving training algorithm solve the problem of finding an optimal network topology? Could using spiking neural networks improve the biological relevance of computational models of taste recognition? The ESNN-PC model explained within this chapter addresses these questions.

EVOLVING SPIKING NEURAL NETWORK WITH RANK ORDER POPULATION CODING

Recently, spiking neurons and spiking neural networks (SNN) have received a lot of research attention by being biologically more plausible and computationally richer than their predecessors (Maass, 1999). Spiking neurons have been designed to mimic more biologically the spiking activities of real neurons. Hence, the spiking neurons communicate using spikes, *i.e.* discrete voltage events within a continuous time period, which is similar to real neurons. Each incoming spike from a presynaptic neuron causes a change in the membrane potential of the postsynaptic neuron. The change is positive if the spike comes via an excitatory synapse, or negative in the case of an inhibitory synapse. If enough spikes arrive in a short period of time and the membrane potential of the postsynaptic neuron reaches some threshold value PSP_{θ}, the postsynaptic neuron produces a spike itself. All spikes have very similar amplitudes and durations, hence their shapes are considered insignificant in the transfer of information and only the timing of the spikes is thought to be important for information processing.

Evolving Spiking Neural Network Architecture eSNN

Here we explain the use of an evolving spiking neural network (eSNN) for taste recognition. In general, an evolving system changes its structure and/or structural parameters under the influence of its environment. It could start as an empty or simple structure and grow during its operation through creation and insertion of new neurons (Kasabov, 2007). We build neural networks capable of taste recognition using an evolving learning algorithm proposed by Wysoski, Benuskova and Kasabov (2006). In these networks both the size of the network, *i.e.* the number of spiking neurons, and two structural parameters, *i.e.* the values of connection weights and thresholds PSP_{θ}, change under the influence of the input signals. Evolving process consists of three steps, (i) creating and training a new neuron for each new data sample, (ii) comparing this new neuron against pre-existing neurons for the same class of data, and (iii) aggregating the new neuron into an existing neuron if the new and an existing neuron are similar enough. Hence, each time a neuron is created its similarity to other neurons is checked. If the similarity to an existing neuron is greater than a chosen similarity threshold S_{θ}, two neurons are merged and the weights and threshold values set to:

$$W_{aggr} = \frac{W_{new} + n \times W_{similar}}{1 + n} \quad (1)$$

$$PSP_{\theta aggr} = \frac{PSP_{\theta new} + n \times PSP_{\theta similar}}{1 + n} \quad (2)$$

In (1) and (2) W_{new} and $PSP_{\theta new}$ represent the weights/threshold of the new neuron being checked for similarity, $W_{similar}$ and $PSP_{\theta similar}$ represent the weights/threshold of the existing similar neuron and n is the number of samples already being associated (learnt) by the similar neuron. The question could be asked; why a taste recognition model should have an evolving structure? The main reason is that such systems are able to learn new tastants as they become available, without forgetting the ones that has already been learnt. This makes the model more realistic because human beings do not forget all previously learned tastes as they are introduced to new ones. Furthermore, we refer again to the problem of finding an appropriate size for the hidden layer of an MLP network. If the hidden layer is too small or too big, the MLP might become a poor classifier. The evolving neural network resolves this size problem.

The taste recognition system (Figure 2) based on the above explained dynamic structure was first introduced in (Soltic, Wysoski, & Kasabov, 2008). We call this neural network ESNN-PC, recognizing its evolving structure but also the fact that the inputs into the network undergo population encoding. ESNN-PC comprises an electronic tongue, a receptive field layer and two layers of spiking neurons, L1 and L2. The input taste signatures are encoded using a family of equally spaced Gaussian receptive fields and distributed to multiple L1 neurons through delayed synaptic connections. The stronger the input excitation, the earlier L1 fires. Each L1 neuron has a single connection to its input and one weighted excitatory connection to each of the L2 neurons via a weight w_{ij}. The L2 neurons are simple integrate-and-fire neurons whose behavior is defined in (Thorpe, Delorme, & Van Rullen, 2001). The L2 neurons are created over time for each input taste signature. Every newly created L2 neuron is checked for aggregation as explained above. In our taste recognition system each taste signature is presented to the system for tasting only once. During the creation of a L2 layer, clusters of L2 neurons are formed. All L2 neurons in one cluster are trained on the taste signatures sampled from only one tastant. Hence, every L2 neuron in the G_p cluster learns to respond to earlier spikes when presented with taste signatures from C_p.

Population encoding of taste signatures increases the temporal distance between them and

Figure 2. The taste recognition system based on an evolving spiking neural network

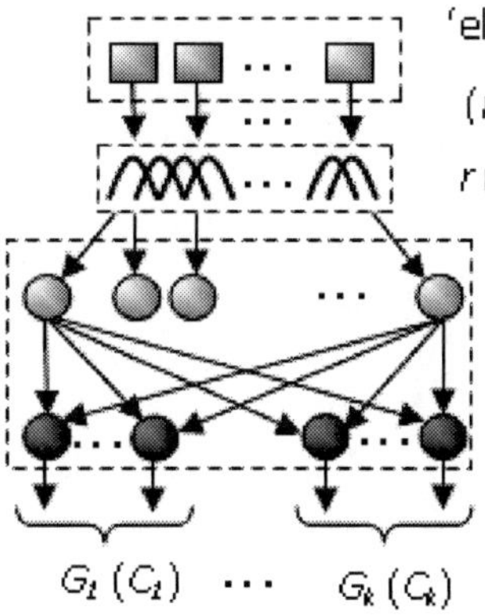

consequently increases the accuracy of the taste recognition system. Furthermore, using this encoding enhances the biological relevance of the model. Recent studies on taste processing reported possible cell interactions within taste buds (Huang *et al*., 2005; Zhao *et al*., 2005; Katz, Nicolelis, & Simon, 2002). In ESNN-PC every taste signature variable is encoded into a set of spiking times. A delay is introduced moving away from the centers of the receptive fields, increasing as the distance from the center increases. Hence, a single value excites a population of L1 neurons which in turn excite the connected L2 neurons to smaller or greater degree. Figure 3 shows the result of encoding 10 taste signatures of tastant 1 and 16 taste signatures of tastant 2 using six Gaussian receptive fields with overlapping sensitivities ($r = 6$). The grayscale levels represent the intensity of the input values. Darker levels are associated with stronger input intensities and the white levels represent the input intensities that do not cause the firings of the L1 neurons and therefore have no effect on the postsynaptic potential of the connected L2 neurons. The left plot shows the temporal distance between taste signatures before the encoding and the plot on the right after the encoding. While the left plot is rather puzzling, there is a visible temporal difference between the excitations of the L1 neurons 'belonging' to different tastants in the right plot. Consequently classification accuracy of the taste recognition system using population encoding improves.

The latency of the L2 neurons' firing is decided by the order ($order_j$) of the incoming spikes (Thorpe, Delorme, & Van Rullen, 2001). Earlier spikes are given a lower rank order (0, 1, ...) and a higher importance:

$$PSP_i(t) = w_{ij} \times m^{order_j} \quad (3)$$

where m is the modulation factor, j is the index for the pre-synaptic L1 neuron spiking at time t and w_{ij} is the synaptic efficacy (weight) of the incoming connection. Both m and w_{ij} are in the range of 0 and 1.

According to (3) each incoming spike from an L1 neuron causes a change in the membrane potential of every L2 neuron. An $L2_i$ neuron fires a post-synaptic spike at its output when its PSP_i reaches a certain threshold value $PSP_{\theta i}$. Immediately after firing the post-synaptic spike, the neuron's PSP_i returns to 0. The synapses between L1 and L2 neurons are created and their w_{ij} values are updated during training. Synapses conveying earlier spikes are given a higher weight change resulting in connection strengthening:

$$\Delta w_{ij} = m^{order_j} \quad (4)$$

with the same convention as in (3). Hence, the synaptic connections conveying earlier spikes become more effective in causing the corresponding L2 neuron to fire in the future. During classification, the processing of spikes stops once the first L2 neuron spikes, signaling that this taste signature has been classified, which results in fast classification. Also, the L2 neurons have dynamic thresholds (Wysoski, Benuskova and Kasabov, 2006) found during the training of the network. These thresholds are set to a proportion of the

Figure 3. The results of encoding taste signatures of two tastants with six receptive fields (r = 6). The left plot shows the temporal distances between signatures before the encoding and the right plot after the encoding. The grayscale levels represent the levels of input intensities. Darker levels are associated with stronger input intensities

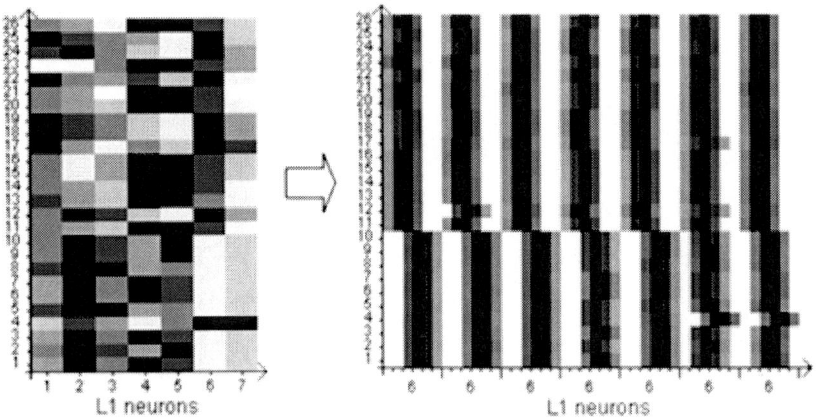

neurons' maximum membrane potential value generated with the propagation of the training taste signatures:

$$PSP_{0_i} = c \times PSP_{\max_i} \tag{5}$$

where c is a constant in the range of 0 to 1 shared by all L2 neurons. Note that neuron weights and thresholds are set once and are not changed unless the neuron aggregates.

Using this type of neuron for taste recognition offers a number of advantages. Firstly, these neurons are capable of modeling spiking neural dynamics and as stated earlier the dynamics of the taste recognition systems are important for taste coding. Secondly, the exact timing of the spikes is not explicitly present in the model, only the order is important. This makes the encoding appropriate for data which lacks a temporal component. Thirdly, these neurons have been proven efficient and effective for modeling the visual system (Thorpe, Delorme, & Van Rullen, 2001) and classifying multimodal audio-visual signals related to person authentication (Wysoski, Benuskova, & Kasabov, 2008). This becomes important when a multimodal approach to taste recognition is explored. Finally, its neural behavior is simple and easy to implement – a very important feature when a hardware implementation is considered.

Knowledge Discovery from ESNN-PC

Most traditional artificial neural networks, such as the MLP network, suffer from the 'black box' syndrome because they do not provide any knowledge extraction facilities or indicate how they make their decisions. The knowledge that such networks acquire is encoded in weights, a format that cannot be easily interpreted (Kolman & Margaliot, 2005). The same is true for the spiking neural networks. Unfortunately only a small amount of research is centered on the issue of knowledge extraction from such networks (Kasabov, 2007; Wu, Bell, & Cai, 2006). Hence, the lack of knowledge representation capability is becoming a major disadvantage to the end users of these networks. Acknowledging that knowledge discovery is a very important feature of intelligent systems we show how knowledge can be extracted from a trained ESNN-PC. The ESNN-PC architecture captures structured information

Figure 4. (a) An example of population encoding of two input one-dimensional data samples v_1 and v_2 ($v_1 < v_2$) using six receptive fields (r = 6); (b) The weights of an ESNN-PC trained using v_1 and v_2

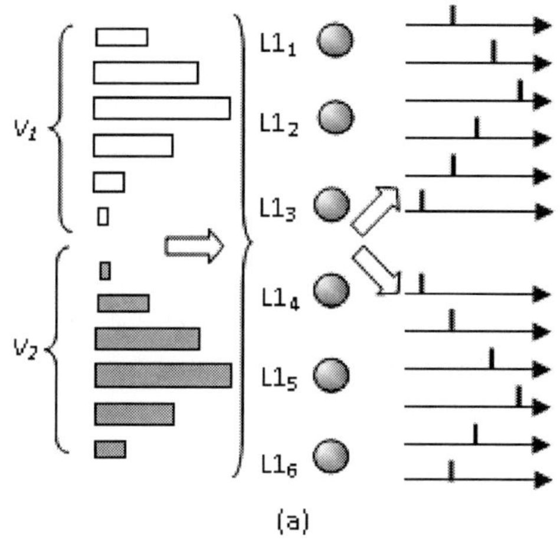

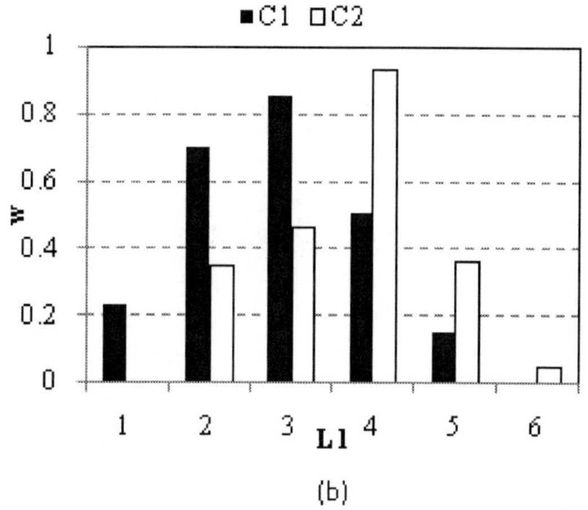

from data that can be represented in the form of zero-order Takagi-Sugeno fuzzy rules:

$$\text{IF } (x_1 \textit{ is } F_1) \text{ AND } (x_i \textit{ is } F_i) \text{ AND } (x_n \textit{ is } F_n) \text{ THEN } y \text{ is } C_k \quad (6)$$

where x_i is an input variable, F_i is a linguistic value represented by its membership function such as SMALL, MEDIUM, LARGE *etc.* and C_j represents a class label. Such knowledge would help us to better understand how taste influences food preferences and aversions and would have, for example, an important role in correcting bad eating habits and fighting the growing epidemic of obesity.

According to (4), the connections conveying earlier spikes strengthen more than those conveying the later ones. We postulate that knowledge about the relationship between input patterns is stored in the synaptic weights of the L2 neurons representing a long-term memory. Hence, based on the weight patterns it is possible to deduce the size of an input value and the contribution of this input value to the modeled output. This is illustrated by the help of Fig. 4. Assume two one dimensional data samples v_1 and v_2 belonging to tastants C_1 and C_2 are used to train an ESNN-PC containing six L1 neurons. Assume that two L2 neurons are created and trained; $L2_1$ has been trained to recognize C_1 samples and $L2_2$ to recognize C_2 samples. The most stimulated L1 neuron fires first ($t^f = 0$) and the least stimulated neuron fires some time later ($t^f = t_{max}$). In Fig. 4 the values of v_1 and v_2 are deliberately chosen so they cause a maximum excitation of two different L1 neurons, *i.e.* two earliest spikes appear at $L1_3$ for v_1 and $L1_4$ for v_2. As a result, two very similar spike patterns occur out of sequence by one L1 neuron. There is a relationship between which L1 neuron spikes first in a set of L1 neurons and the value encoded into this set of L1 neurons. When smaller values are encoded the first neuron to spike tends towards the lower end of the observed set ($L1_1$). When higher values are encoded the first neuron to spike tends towards the higher end of the observed set ($L1_6$ in this example). These two spike patterns are visible in the weight pattern on the right. It can be seen that $L2_1$ (black bars) 'favors' lower input values, *i.e.* a lower input value will cause a bigger ΔPSP_1. The $L2_2$ neuron does the opposite. Hence, the lower values will be classified as C_1 and the higher values as C_2 or:

IF v_i is SMALL THEN C_1

IF v_i is LARGE THEN C_2

Hardware Implementation of Spiking Neural Networks

Without a doubt, the main advantage of building the hardware implementations of artificial neural networks is the speed of these implementations compared to the speeds achieved in software simulation (Himavathi, Anitha, & Muthuramalingam, 2007; Lee & Ko, 2006). To date, the majority of hardware implementations are of MLP networks. Spiking neural networks are most often simulated using custom-built software (Delorme, Gautrais, Van Rullen, & Thorpe, 1999) or off-the-shelf simulating environments that allow for detailed biophysical simulations such as NEURON (http://www.neuron.yale.edu/neuron/) and GENESIS (http://www.genesis-sim.org).

Recently the use of field-programmable gate arrays (FPGA) as the hardware platform for building SNN as well as other artificial neural networks has been explored. The FPGA are high density digital devices that can operate in a parallel manner. This makes them a logical choice for building highly parallel processing systems such as artificial neural networks (Reaz, Islam, Ali, & Sulaiman, 2002). However, FPGA implementations are still rare compared to the number of cases where artificial neural networks are simulated in software. This is due to the fact that the hardware implementations are linked to a number of issues, such as: data representation, precision and reconfiguration time overheads. Moving a neural network from a software simulation to an FPGA-based hardware implementation is not a straightforward exercise, as many features found in the software are not available when using the hardware, for example, precision multiplication, abundance of multipliers and a large memory space. As the FPGA chips become more sophisticated, the lack of suitable SNN learning algorithms is starting to emerge as the main reason for SNN not being hosted in hardware more frequently (Maguire *et al.*, 2007; Burgsteiner, 2006). An on-chip learning mechanism can occupy as much hardware resources as the network itself and this can be impractical for a very large neural network. Thus, the learning is often performed in a simulation and the final weights are then frozen in an FPGA during the programming phase (Schrauwen & Van Campenhout, 2006). This enables higher processing speeds and lower resource costs but comes at a price because the network is unable to retrain in-situ for new data.

Hardware implementations of SNN often target a specific task, for example, a network of spiking neurons was designed for use on mobile robotic devices (Pearson *et al.*, 2007), for image processing (Waldemark, Millberg, Lindblad, Waldemark, & Becanovic, 2000) and for hardware modeling of neuronal ion channel dynamics (Mak, Rachmuth, Lam, & Poon, 2005). A compact and fast hardware implementation of a taste recognition system would open many possibilities for the system's application. For example, it could be used within autonomous robots enabling them to taste liquids and solids, and these intelligent robots could be employed in situations where a human presence is not practical. Therefore, we built an FPGA-based implementation of ESNN-PC and compared it to the software simulations in terms of their processing speed and classification accuracy. The complete ESNN-PC system, including the logic circuitry which controls the evolving of the L2 layer was implemented on a single Altera Cyclone II EP2C35F672C6 FPGA situated on an Altera NIOS II Development Kit. The implementation was based on the concepts of virtual neurons and virtual synapses. Hence, only a single neuron with one synapse was instantiated and all other neurons used the same resources. The problem of limited resources is even more profound when an evolving architecture is considered. While, it would be great to have an FPGA that

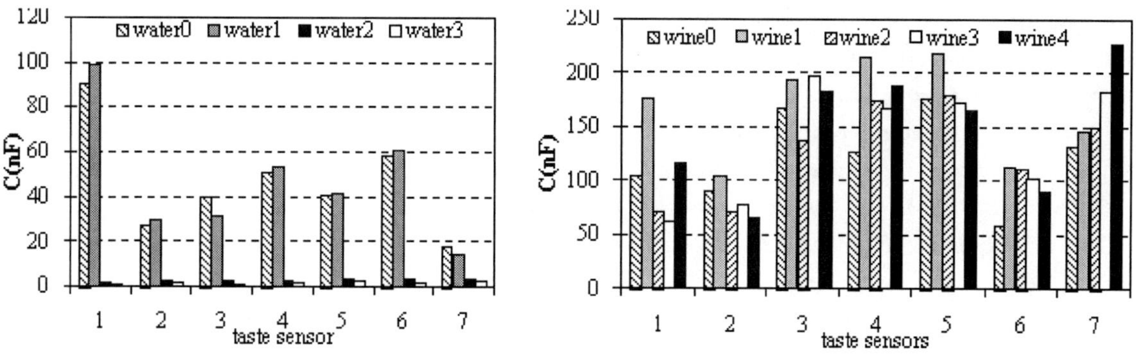

Figure 5. Average values of the water (left) and wine (right) taste signatures

is sufficiently large to allow a network to evolve freely the reality is that this is currently impossible. The particular FPGA chip used within our study was big enough to evolve an ESNN-PC network comprising of 64 neurons with 64 synapses each, *i.e.* a total of 4096 synapses. A detailed description of the FPGA implementation of ESNN-PC is given in (Zuppicich & Soltic 2008) and the details of the fast on-chip learning algorithm in (Soltic & Zuppicich, 2008).

CASE STUDY ON A BENCHMARK TASTE DATASET

Both implementations were validated on a taste dataset that has been previously used by Humberto de Sousa, Antonio Riul Jr. and their teams (de Sousa *et al.*, 2002; Riul Jr. *et al.*, 2004). In their work, the pattern recognition systems were based on MLP networks. The dataset is composed of 799 taste signatures taken from four types of water (49 signatures) and five brands of wine (750 signatures). The taste signatures were generated by an array of seven non-selective sensor units based on conducting polymers (Riul Jr. *et al.*, 2002). Collectively the sensors acquired enough information for the discrimination of the liquids.

Data

The dataset was divided into two subsets, D_1 containing water taste signatures and D_2 containing wine taste signatures. Figure 5 shows the average values of the taste signatures. Two important features characterize D_1: (i) the similarity between $water_0$ and $water_1$ averages as well as between $water_2$ and $water_3$ averages; (ii) the difference between $water_0/water_1$ averages and the $water_2/water_3$ averages. In (de Sousa *et al.*, 2002) conventional neural networks were used for the classification of the water and wine samples. The authors experimented with MLP networks with 5, 10, 15, 20 and 25 hidden neurons trained with four different algorithms (Standard backpropagation, Backpropagation momentum, Quickprop and RPROP). They reported classification accuracy between 85% and 100% for the classification of wines and between 66% and 100% for the classification of water samples. The learning algorithm used to train the networks and the topology of the hidden layer substantially influenced the accuracy of the results.

Experiments

ESNN-PC was tested on various subsets of D_1 and D_2. In each experiment the training datasets (D_{tr}) were obtained by taking random subsets, typically about 50%, of the original data. The remaining samples made up the testing sets (D_t) used to validate the trained network. The optimal values of the network parameters (m, c and S_0) and the number of receptive fields r were chosen empirically to achieve the highest classification accuracy for the particular subset D_{subi} The equally spaced receptive fields with the same width were used in all experiments. Because the order of training data could influence the creation of the network and affect the network's classification accuracy, each experiment was repeated 10 times; each time the data was randomly split, the network was created, evaluated and the average accuracy was calculated. Changing or placing the receptive fields in a different place can affect the performance of ESNN-PC. We observed that more receptive fields were required to discriminate between classes with low inter-class distances. For example, more receptive fields were required for classifying the $water_0$ and $water_1$ signatures ($r=8$) than to classify the $water_0$ and $water_2$ signatures ($r = 6$). This can be ascribed to the fact that the $water_0$ and $water_1$ taste signatures exhibit a higher similarity than the $water_0$ and $water_2$ signatures (as explained by Figure 5).

The software experiments were done in a Java simulation tool specially designed for this investigation. Unfortunately, not all the experiments could be repeated with hardware implementation. As discussed earlier, the size of the network was limited with the size of the FPGA chip. However, for those experiments that could be repeated the accuracies obtained with the FPGA implemented ESNN-PC were comparable to the accuracies achieved with the software simulations. As expected the FPGA implementation was faster than the software simulations, even allowing for the fact that the software simulations were run on a 2 GHz Intel Core 2 host and the FPGA chip was clocked at a much slower frequency of 50 MHz. We must bear in mind that the processing speed of the FPGA implementation was influenced considerably by the delivery of the taste signatures and the processing speed could be increased further by delivering samples via a faster interface. It takes around 20 μs to deliver one taste signature and 1.12 μs to encode it with six receptive fields. A neuron is created after 30 to 70 μs. In total it takes from 40 to 80 μs to create and train one L2 neuron with 56 synapses. This is 10 to 25 times faster than in software simulations for the same network (t_{soft} = 1040 μs). Likewise, the FPGA implementation classifies one taste signature 74 times faster than the software tool. A taste signature is classified within 6 μs by the FPGA implementation while it takes 445 μs by the software.

The accuracy of the ESSN-PC model was consistently above the 90% mark for both the wine and water datasets. The ESNN-PC classified four different water types with 5 training and 5 testing samples per class. The network parameters m and S_0 were kept constant in all ten runs and $r = 6$. On average 4.7 L2 neurons were created and an accuracy of 91% was achieved. On the wine dataset, D_2, the average accuracy over the ten runs was 99.62% ($r = 16$, on average 25.5 L2 neurons). These results show that the ESNN-PC is viable classifier of taste signatures from both small and large datasets.

Table 1 shows the rules derived from the structure of an ESNN-PC evolved on the $water_0$ and $water_1$ taste signatures. Two membership functions were used in the experiment, representing small and large sensor values respectively, only two L2 were created and each learned a different water type. The two rules show how a new unseen $water_0$/$water_1$ taste signature will be classified. The water signatures with smaller s_1, s_3, s_5 and s_6 values will be classified as $water_0$. The opposite is true for the taste signatures of $water_1$. It is interesting to observe that the measurements of the sixth taste sensor, s_6, did not contribute to the process of distinguishing between the water samples. This means that contributions of the spikes caused by corresponding L1 neurons to the post-synaptic potential of L2 neurons were very similar or identical. It is noteworthy that all sensors contribute to the classification of $wine_0$ and

Table 1. Rules extracted from an evolved ESNN-PC on the $water_0$ and $water_1$ taste signatures

Rule 0: IF (s_1 is SMALL) AND (s_2 is LARGE) AND (s_3 is SMALL) AND (s_4 is LARGE) AND (s_5 is SMALL) AND (s_7 is SMALL) THEN $water_0$
Rule 1: IF (s_1 is LARGE) AND (s_2 is SMALL) AND (s_3 is LARGE) AND (s_4 is SMALL) AND (s_5 is LARGE) AND (s_7 is LARGE) THEN $water_1$

Table 2. Rules extracted from an evolved ESNN-PC on the $wine_0$ and $wine_1$ taste signatures

Rule 0: IF (s_1 is SMALL) AND (s_2 is LARGE) AND (s_3 is SMALL) AND (s_4 is SMALL) AND (s_5 is LARGE) AND (s_6 is LARGE) AND (s_7 is SMALL) THEN $wine_0$
Rule 1: IF (s_1 is LARGE) AND (s_2 is SMALL) AND (s_3 is SMALL) AND (s_4 is LARGE) AND (s_5 is LARGE) AND (s_6 is SMALL) AND (s_7 is LARGE) THEN $wine_1$

$wine_1$, including sensor s_6 which was irrelevant in the classification of $water_0$ and $water_1$ (Table 2).

Table 3 shows two sets of rules derived from the structure of an ESNN-PC evolved on D_1. In the first set of rules three membership functions representing small, medium and large sensor values respectively were used. In the second set, the degree of granularity of the fuzzification was increased to four. In both experiments one L2 neuron per water type was created. The second set of rules more accurately captured the data set characteristics. The high variable values that characterize the $water_0$ and $water_1$ taste signatures and their fine differences are described in Rule 0 and Rule 1, while the characteristics of the $water_2$ and $water_3$ values are embedded in Rule 2 and Rule 3.

FUTURE RESEARCH DIRECTIONS

The main strength of the ESNN-PC model is its biologically inspired learning and structure. ESNN-PC is based on biologically inspired

Table 3. Rules extracted from an ESNN-PC evolved on the water taste signatures using: (a) three membership functions; (b) four membership functions

Rule 0: IF (s_1 is 2) AND (s_2 is 3) AND (s_3 is 2) AND (s_4 is 2) AND (s_5 is 2) AND (s_6 is 2) THEN $water_0$
Rule 1: IF (s_1 is 3) AND (s_2 is 2) AND (s_3 is 3) AND (s_4 is 3) AND (s_5 is 3) AND (s_6 is 2) AND (s_7 is 2) THEN $water_1$
Rule 2: IF (s_1 is 1) AND (s_2 is 1) AND (s_3 is 1) AND (s_4 is 2) AND (s_5 is 2) AND (s_7 is 1) THEN $water_2$
Rule 3: IF (s_1 is 2) AND (s_2 is 2) AND (s_3 is 2) AND (s_4 is 1) AND (s_5 is 1) AND (s_6 is 1) AND (s_7 is 2) THEN $water_3$
Rule 0: IF (s_1 is 3) AND (s_2 is 4) AND (s_3 is 3) AND (s_4 is 3) AND (s_5 is 3) AND (s_6 is 2) THEN $water_0$
Rule 1: IF (s_1 is 4) AND (s_2 is 3) AND (s_3 is 4) AND (s_4 is 4) AND (s_5 is 4) AND (s_6 is 3) AND (s_7 is 3) THEN $water_1$
Rule 2: IF (s_1 is 1) AND (s_2 is 1) AND (s_3 is 1) AND (s_4 is 2) AND (s_5 is 2) AND (s_7 is 1) THEN $water_2$
Rule 3: IF (s_1 is 2) AND (s_2 is 2) AND (s_3 is 2) AND (s_4 is 1) AND (s_5 is 1) AND (s_6 is 1) AND (s_7 is 2) THEN $water_3$
Denotation: '1' means membership function VERY SMALL, '2' means membership function SMALL, '3' means membership function MEDIUM and '4' means membership function LARGE

processing units. In keeping with the recent advances in our understanding of the biology of taste, ESNN-PC employs simple spiking neurons capable of modeling neural dynamics which are better at modeling the dynamic behavior of real neurons than the summation units fed with rate coded inputs which are used in traditional neural networks. The introduction of population encoding made the model more biologically realistic. Furthermore, ESNN-PC has biologically inspired architecture which evolves as it learns to recognize new tastants. This evolving results in a new formation of neurons and connections within the model. ESNN-PC learns new tastes by adding new ensembles of L2 neurons when exploring new tastants without losing the knowledge about the previously observed taste signatures. This learning is similar to the process in the biological taste system where new tastes are remembered without forgetting all the previously learned flavors. Another advantage of the ESNN-PC is that it learns quickly, using a one-pass learning algorithm. This type of learning is much faster than the learning used to train traditional neural networks, such as MLP. Finally, ESNN-PC explains what it has learnt about the tastants in the form of easy to understand IF-THEN rules. For example the network could learn to taste a safe drinking water, and then detect when the water becomes undrinkable. This is possible because the network creates conditions for drinkable water and then flags any tastant that does not fit into these conditions. In the basic ESNN-PC the linguistic values are chosen based on the information stored in the synaptic weights. Hence, the knowledge representation in ESNN-PC can be further developed as a quantitative way of mapping the receptive fields to pre-defined fuzzy membership functions where conditions of the input variables will be fuzzy values represented by membership degree to which each variable s_i belongs to the corresponding receptive field (Kasabov, 2007). Next we plan to develop a fuzzy rule extraction procedure for the recently proposed integrative probabilistic evolving spiking neural networks (Kasabov, 2009, 2010), where the fuzzy rules will have additional probability parameters to represent uncertainty in the data and the classification model. Optimization of the network parameters, including the number of receptive fields and fuzzy membership functions, which further improve the accuracy of the classification and the quality of the extracted fuzzy rules, is another future task (Schliebs, Defoin-Platel, & Kasabov, 2009).

The hardware implementation creates new possibilities for the use of ESNN-PC. For instance, one or a number of ESNN-PC modules embedded in a mobile robot, would make the robot suitable for applications where the tasting and classification of tastants is required, *e.g.* hazardous spills. To achieve this goal, two main requirements must be satisfied. Firstly, we need to have quality electronic tongues that are able to operate continuously outside experimental environments. Secondly, we need a robust hardware implementation of the taste recognition system. In the current implementation of taste recognition, taste signatures were collected in advance and fed to the system via a personal computer and an on-chip embedded microprocessor. To avoid this, the sensors would need to be mounted on the robot and measurements fed to the taste module(s). In the cases where the classification speed is a critical requirement the taste signatures will need to be pre-processed in a fast interface module. Initially, the robot could be trained to taste only a few tastants, but would also be able to acquire new tastes during its operational phase. A group of testing robots could communicate wirelessly, forming an autonomous sensor net that could provide continuous monitoring for a large area. Some envisaged applications are in biosecurity, the chemical and food industries, security, the automotive industry, and in home automation. ESNN-PC could be also utilized in distributed sensory systems. For example, ESNN-PC systems could be used to taste (ESNN-PC-TR) or smell (ESNN-PC-O) if beverages and foods have passed their ‘best before’ dates. Also, together with an appropriate set of sensors capable of ‘smelling’ different species, the ESNN-PC could be used to detect the presence of unwanted species. Our design of having the whole system on one chip satisfies the requirement that the pervasive device must have a low price and must be easy to fit into a wide range of deployed infrastructures (Hansmann, Merk, Nicklous, & Stober, 2003). Currently the main obstacle to the creation of such systems is the lack of off-the-shelf sensors. However, as technology evolves this obstacle will hopefully disappear.

Acknowledging that the olfactory and auditory system plays an important role in taste perception (Verhagen & Engelen, 2006), the authors suggest that the biological realism of a taste recognition model could be improved by building a taste-smell-audio model based on ESNN-PC. Ultimately, the resulting system could be implemented in hardware either on one chip or alternatively on a number of separate chips.

CONCLUSION

This chapter shows how spiking neurons can be employed for building more biologically plausible and efficient taste recognition systems. It has provided a brief summary of the current knowledge on taste perception and discussed the shortcomings of using MLP networks, the most often used neural network, for taste recognition. The authors have provided a detailed description of a taste recognition model based on an evolving spiking neural network with rank order population coding, ESNN-PC. The model was validated on a benchmark taste dataset and the results were compared to those of a recent work where traditional neural networks were used on the same datasets. The knowledge learnt from the benchmark dataset was presented and evaluated. Our simulations have shown that ESNN-PC can perform the sophisticated tasks of taste recognition and knowledge discovery from taste data. In addition, the authors have summarized the main challenges of hosting classical and spiking neural networks on FPGA and suggested some possible applications of the FPGA hosted ESNN-PC. Finally, it is worth noting that it is not the aim of this chapter to claim that the presented ESNN-PC represents an accurate model of the gustatory system, but it rather presents a different approach to previously published work on taste recognition. Clearly, a great deal of further work will be required if we are to fully understand the human system and successfully build an artificial replica of it. Furthermore, the evolving neutral network discussed within this chapter is not limited to taste recognition only and we suggest that it can be applied to many other classification problems.

REFERENCES

Bradbury, J. (2004). Taste perception: Cracking the code. *PLOS BIOL., 2*(3). Retrieved September 20, 2008 from http://biology.plosjournals.org

Burgsteiner, H. (2006). Imitation learning with spiking neural networks and real-world devices. *Engineering Applications of Artificial Intelligence, 1*, 741–752. doi:10.1016/j.engappai.2006.05.007

Chandrashekar, J., Hoon, M. A., Ryba, N. J., & Zuker, C. S. (2006). The receptors and cells for mammalian taste. *Nature, 444*, 288–294. doi:10.1038/nature05401

Cortina, M., Duran, A., Alegret, S., & del Valle, M. (2006). A sequential injection electronic tongue employing the transient response from potentiometric sensors for anion multidetermination. *Analytical and Bioanalytical Chemistry, 358*(7), 1186–1194. doi:10.1007/s00216-006-0530-2

de Sousa, H. C., Carvalho, A. C. P. L. F., Riul, A., Jr., & Mattoso, L. H. C. (2002). Using MLP networks to classify red wines and water readings of an artificial tongue. *The VII Brazilian Symposium on Neural Networks SBRN'02*, 13-18.

Delorme, A., Gautrais, J., van Rullen, R., & Thorpe, S. (1999). SpikeNET: A simulator for modelling large networks of integrate and fire neurons. *Neurocomputing, 26-27*, 989–996. doi:10.1016/S0925-2312(99)00095-8

Di Lorenzo, P. M., & Victor, J. D. (2003). Taste response variability and temporal coding in the nucleus of the solitary tract of the rat. *Journal of Neurophysiology, 90*, 1418–1431. doi:10.1152/jn.00177.2003

Dulac, C. (2000). The physiology of taste, vintage 2000. *Cell, 100*, 607–610. doi:10.1016/S0092-8674(00)80697-2

Gallardo, J., Alegret, S., Muñoz, R., De-Román, M., Leija, L., Hernández, P. R., & del Valle, M. (2003). An electronic tongue using potentiometric all-solid-state PVC-membrane sensors for the simultaneous quantification of ammonium and potassium ions in water. *Analytical and Bioanalytical Chemistry*, *377*(2), 248–256. doi:10.1007/s00216-003-2042-7

Glendinning, J. I., Davis, A., & Rai, M. (2006). Temporal coding mediates discrimination of "bitter" taste stimuli by an insect. *The Journal of Neuroscience*, *26*(35), 8900–8908. doi:10.1523/JNEUROSCI.2351-06.2006

Gutés, A., Ibáñez, A. B., Céspedes, F., Alegret, S., & del Valle, M. (2005). Simultaneous determination of phenolic compounds by means of an automated voltammetric electronic tongue. *Analytical and Bioanalytical Chemistry*, *382*, 471–476. doi:10.1007/s00216-005-3201-9

Gutiérrez, M., Gutiérrez, J. M., Alegret, S., Leija, L., Hernández, P. R., & Favari, L. (2008). Remote environmental monitoring employing a potentiometric electronic tongue. *International Journal of Environmental Analytical Chemistry*, *88*, 103–117. doi:10.1080/03067310701441005

Hansmann, U., Merk, L., Nicklous, M. S., & Stober, T. (2003). *Pervasive computing* (2nd ed.). Springer.

Himavathi, S., Anitha, D., & Muthuramalingam, A. (2007). Feedforward neural network implementation in FPGA using layer multiplexing for effective resource utilization. *IEEE Transactions on Neural Networks*, *18*(3), 880–888. doi:10.1109/TNN.2007.891626

Huang, Y. J., Maruyama, Y., Lu, K. S., Pereira, E., & Roper, S. D. (2005). Mouse taste buds release serotonin in response to taste stimuli. *Chemical Senses*, *30*(Supplement 1), i39–i40. doi:10.1093/chemse/bjh102

Ivarsson, P., Kikkawa, Y., Winquist, F., Krantz-Rülcker, C., Höjer, N.-E., & Hayashi, K. (2001). Comparison of a voltmetric electronic tongue and a lipid membrane taste sensors. *Analytica Chimica Acta*, *449*, 59–68. doi:10.1016/S0003-2670(01)01349-6

Kasabov, N. (2007). *Evolving connectionist systems. The knowledge engineering approach.* London: Springer-Verlag London Limited.

Kasabov, N. (2009). Integrative Connectionist Learning Systems Inspired by Nature: Current Models, Future Trends and Challenges. *Natural Computing*, *8*(2), 199–210. doi:10.1007/s11047-008-9066-z

Kasabov, N. (2010). To spike or not to spike: A probabilistic spiking neural model. *Neural Networks*, *23*(1), 16–19. doi:10.1016/j.neunet.2009.08.010

Katz, D. B., Nicolelis, M. A. L., & Simon, S. A. (2002). Gustatory processing is dynamic and distributed. *Current Opinion in Neurobiology*, *12*, 448–454. doi:10.1016/S0959-4388(02)00341-0

Kolman, E., & Margaliot, M. (2005). Are artificial neural networks white boxes? *IEEE Transactions on Neural Networks*, *16*(4), 844–852. doi:10.1109/TNN.2005.849843

Krantz-Rülcker, C., Stenberg, M., Winquist, F., & Lundström, I. (2001). Electronic tongues for environmental monitoring based on sensor arrays and pattern recognition: a review. *Analytica Chimica Acta*, *426*, 217–226. doi:10.1016/S0003-2670(00)00873-4

Lee, Y., & Ko, S.-B. (2006). FPGA implementation of a face detector using neural networks. *IEEE Conference on Electrical and Computer Engineering CCECE/CCGEI*, 1914-1917.

Maass, W. (1999). Computing with spiking neurons. In Maass, W., & Bishop, C. H. (Eds.), *Pulsed Neural Networks*. WA: Bratford Book.

Maguire, L. P., McGinnity, T. M., Glackin, B., Ghani, A., Belatreche, A., & Harkin, J. (2007). Challenges for large-scale implementations of spiking neural networks on FPGAs. *Neurocomputing, 71*(1-3), 13–29. doi:10.1016/j.neucom.2006.11.029

Mak, T. S., Rachmuth, G., Lam, K. P., & Poon, C.-S. (2005). Field programmable gate array implementation of neuronal ion channel dynamics. *The 2th International IEEE EMBS Conference on Neural Engineering*, v-ix.

Margolskee, R. F. (1993). The molecular biology of taste transduction. *BioEssays, 15*(10), 645–650. doi:10.1002/bies.950151003

Pearson, M. J., Pipe, A. G., Mitchinson, B., Gurney, K., C. Melhuish, C., Gilhespy, I. & Nibouche, M. (2007). Implementing spiking neural networks for real-time signal-processing and control applications: a model-validation FPGA approach. *IEEE Transactions on Neural Networks, 18*(5), 1472-1487.

Reaz, M. B. I., Islam, S. Z., Ali, M. A. M., & Sulaiman, M. S. (2002). FPGA realization of backpropagation for stock market prediction. *9th International Conference on Neural Information Proceedings of ICONIP'02. 2*, 960-964.

Reed, D. R., Tanaka, T., & McDaniel, A. H. (2006). Diverse tastes: genetics of sweet and bitter perception. *Physiology & Behavior, 88*(3), 215–226. doi:10.1016/j.physbeh.2006.05.033

Riul, A. Jr, de Sousa, H. C., Malmegrim, R. R., dos Santos, D. S. Jr, Carvalho, A. C. P. L. F., & Fonseca, F. J. (2004). Wine classification by taste sensors made from ultra-thin films and using neural networks. *Sensors and Actuators. B, Chemical, 98*, 77–82. doi:10.1016/j.snb.2003.09.025

Riul, A. Jr, dos Santos, D. S. Jr, Wohnrath, K., Di Tommazo, R., Carvalho, A. C. P. L. F., & Fonseca, F. J. (2002). Artificial taste sensor: efficient combination of sensors made from Langmuir-Blodgett films of conducting polymers and a ruthenium complex and self-assembled films of an Azobenzene-containing polymer. *Langmuir, 18*, 239–245. doi:10.1021/la011017d

Schliebs, S., Defoin-Platel, M., & Kasabov, N. (2009). Integrated feature and parameter optimization for an evolving spiking neural network. In Köppen, M. (Ed.), *ICONIP 2008, Lecture Notes in Computer Science, Part I, 5506* (pp. 1229–1236). Berlin, Heidelberg: Springer-Verlag.

Schrauwen, B., & Van Campenhout, J. (2006). Parallel hardware implementation of a broad class of spiking neurons using serial arithmetic. *European Symposium on Artificial Neural Networks ESANN'2006*, 623-628.

Soltic, S., Wysoski, S. G., & Kasabov, N. (2008), Evolving spiking neural networks for taste recognition. *International Joint Conference on Neural Networks*, 2092-2098.

Soltic, S., & Zuppicich, A. (2008). Comparison between software and FPGA implementation of ESNN in terms of processing speed. *15th Electronics New Zealand Conference ENZCon08*, 56-61.

Stein, J. F., & Stoodley, C. J. (2006). *Neuroscience: an introduction*. John Wiley and sons.

Stitt, J. P., Gaumond, R. P., Frazier, J. L., & Hanson, F. E. (1997). A comparison of neural spike classification techniques. *The 19th International Conference IEEE/EMBS*, 1092-1094.

Thorpe, S., Delorme, A., & Van Rullen, R. (2001). Spike-based strategies for rapid processing. *Neural Networks, 14*, 715–725. doi:10.1016/S0893-6080(01)00083-1

Varkevisser, B., Peterson, D., Ogura, T., & Kinnamon, S. C. (2001). Neural networks distinguish between taste qualities based on receptor cell population responses. *Chemical Senses, 26*, 499–505. doi:10.1093/chemse/26.5.499

Verhagen, J. V., & Engelen, L. (2006). The neurocognitive bases of human multimodal food perception: sensory integration. *Neuroscience and Biobehavioral Reviews, 30*(5), 613–650. doi:10.1016/j.neubiorev.2005.11.003

Waldemark, J., Millberg, M., Lindblad, T., Waldemark, K., & Becanovic, V. (2000). Implementation of a pulse coupled neural network in FPGA. International Journal of Neural Systems. *Special Issue on Hardware Implementations, 10*(3), 171–177.

Wu, Q.-X., Bell, D., & Cai, J. (2006). Knowledge representation and learning mechanism based on network of spiking neurons, *IEEE International Conference on Systems, Man, and Cybernetics*, 2796-2801.

Wysoski, S., Benuskova, L., & Kasabov, N. (2008). Adaptive spiking neural networks for audiovisual pattern recognition. In Ishikawa, M. (Eds.), *ICONIP2007, Lecture Notes in Computer Science, Part II, 4985* (pp. 406–415). Berlin, Heidelberg: Springer-Verlag.

Wysoski, S. G., Benuskova, L., & Kasabov, N. (2006). On-line learning with structural adaptation in a network of spiking neurons for visual pattern recognition. In Kollias, S. (Eds.), *ICANN 2006, Lecture Notes in Computer Science, Part I, 4131* (pp. 61–70). Berlin, Heidelberg: Springer-Verlag.

Yoshimura, H., Kato, N., Sugai, T., Honjo, M., Sato, J., Segami, N., & Onoda, N. (2004). To-and-fro optical voltage signal propagation between the insular gustatory and perietal oral somatosensory areas in rat cortex slices. *Brain Research, 1015*, 114–121. doi:10.1016/j.brainres.2004.04.056

Zhao, F.-I., Shen, T., Kaya, N., Lu, S.-G., Cao, Y., & Herness, S. (2005). Expression, physiological action, and coexpression patterns of neuropeptide Y in rat taste-bud cells. *National Academy of Sciences of the United States of America, 102*(31), 11100–11105. doi:10.1073/pnas.0501988102

Zuppicich, A., & Soltic, S. (2008). FPGA implementation of an evolving spiking neural network. In Köppen, M. (Ed.), *ICONIP 2008, Lecture Notes in Computer Science, Part I, 5506* (pp. 1129–1136). Berlin, Heidelberg: Springer-Verlag.

ADDITIONAL READING

Abbott, L. F., & Nelson, S. B. (2000). Synaptic plasticity: timing the best. *Nature Neuroscience, 3*(supplement), 1178–1183. doi:10.1038/81453

Abeles, M., Bergman, H., Margalit, E., & Vaadia, E. (1993). Spatiotemporal firing patterns in the frontal cortex of behaving monkeys. *Journal of Neurophysiology, 70*(4), 1629–1638.

Andrews, R., Diederich, J., & Tickle, A. B. (1995). Survey and critique of techniques for extracting rules from trained artificial neural networks. *Knowledge-Based Systems, 8*(6), 373–389. doi:10.1016/0950-7051(96)81920-4

Baddeley, R. (1996). An efficient code in V1? *Nature, 381*(6583), 560–561. doi:10.1038/381560a0

Belatreche, A., Maguire, L. P., & McGinnity, M. (2007). Advances in design and application of spiking neural networks. *Soft Computing, 11*, 239–248. doi:10.1007/s00500-006-0065-7

Bishop, C. M. (1995). *Neural networks for pattern recognition*. Oxford: Clarendon Press.

Bonnet, C., Zamora, M. C., Buratti, F., & Guirao, M. (1999). Group and individual gustatory reaction times and Piéron's law. *Physiology & Behavior, 66*(4), 549–558. doi:10.1016/S0031-9384(98)00209-1

Bothe, S. M. (2004). The evidence for neural information processing with precise spike-times: a survey. *Neural Computation*, *3*(2), 1–13.

Bothe, S. M., La Poutré, H., & Kok, J. N. (2002). Unsupervised clustering with spiking neurons by sparse temporal coding and multilayer RBF networks. *IEEE Transactions on Neural Networks*, *13*, 426–435. doi:10.1109/72.991428

Brette, R., Rudolph, M., Carnevale, T., Hines, M., Beeman, D., & Bower, J. M. (2007). Simulation of networks of spiking neurons: A review of tools and strategies. *Journal of Computational Neuroscience*, *23*, 349–398. doi:10.1007/s10827-007-0038-6

Buračas, G. T., Zador, A. M., De Weese, M. R., & Albright, T. D. (1998). Efficient discrimination of temporal patterns by motion-sensitive neurons in primate visual cortex. *Neuron*, *20*, 959–969. doi:10.1016/S0896-6273(00)80477-8

Damak, A., Krid, M., Sellami Masmoudi, D., & Derbel, N. (2006). FPGA implementation of programmable pulse mode neural network with on-chip learning. *International Conference on Design and Test of Integrated Systems in Nanoscale Technology DTIS2006*, 159-164.

Gautrais, J., & Thorpe, S. (1998). Rate coding versus temporal order coding: a theoretical approach. *Bio Systems*, *48*, 57–65. doi:10.1016/S0303-2647(98)00050-1

Gerstner, W., & Kistler, W. M. (2002). *Spiking Neural Models, Single Neurons, Populations, Plasticity*. Cambridge: University Press.

Gilbertson, T. A. (1998). Gustatory mechanisms for the detection of fat. *Current Opinion in Neurobiology*, *8*(4), 447–452. doi:10.1016/S0959-4388(98)80030-5

Glackin, B., McGinnity, T. M., Maguire, L. P., Wu, Q. X., & Belatreche, A. (2005). A novel approach for implementation of large scale spiking neural networks on FPGA hardware. In Cabestany, J., Prieto, A., & Sandoval, D. F. (Eds.), *IWANN 2005, Lecture Notes in Computer Science, 3512* (pp. 552–563). Berlin, Heidelberg: Springer-Verlag.

Glackin, C., McDaid, L., Maguire, L., & Sayers, H. (2008). Implementing fuzzy reasoning on a spiking neural network. In Kůrkova, V. (Eds.), *ICANN 2008, Part II, Lecture Notes in Computer Science, 5164* (pp. 254–267). Berlin, Heidelberg: Springer-Verlag.

Hellmich, H. H., & Klar, H. (2004). An FPGA based simulation acceleration platform for spiking neural networks. *The 47th IEEE International Midwest Symposium on Circuits and Systems*, II 389-II 392.

Hopfield, J. J. (1995). Pattern recognition computation using action potential timing for stimulus representation. *Nature*, *376*(6536), 33–36. doi:10.1038/376033a0

Kasabov, N. (1996). *Foundations of Neural Networks, Fuzzy Systems, and Knowledge Engineering*. MIT.

Kasabov, N. (2001). Evolving Fuzzy Neural network for Supervised/Unsupervised Online Knowledge-based learning. *IEEE Transactions on Systems, Man, and Cybernetics. Part B, Cybernetics*, *31*(6), 902–918. doi:10.1109/3477.969494

Kasabov, N. (2003). *Evolving Connectionist Systems, Methods and applications in Bioinformatics, Brain Study and Intelligent Machines*. Springer-Verlag.

Katz, D. B. (2003). Making time with taste. Focus on "Taste response Taste response variability and temporal coding in the nucleus of the solitary tract of the rat". *Journal of Neurophysiology*, *90*, 1375–1376. doi:10.1152/jn.00435.2003

Labib, R., Audette, F., Fortin, A., & Assadi, R. (2005). Hardware implementation of a new artificial neuron. *International Journal of Neural Systems*, *15*(6), 427–433. doi:10.1142/S0129065705000402

Larkin, D., & Kinane, A. Muresan, V., & O'Connor, N. (2006). An efficient hardware architecture for a neural network activation function generator. In J. Wang *et al.* (Eds.): I*SNN 2006, Lecture Notes in Computer Science*, 3973, pp. 1319-1327, Berlin Heidelberg: Springer-Verlag.

Maass, W. (1997). Fast sigmoidal networks via spiking neurons. *Neural Computation*, *9*, 279–304.

Martinelli, E., D'Amico, A., & Di Natale, C. (2006). Spike encoding of artificial olfactory sensor signals. *Sensors and Actuators. B, Chemical*, *119*, 234–238. doi:10.1016/j.snb.2005.12.029

Mattes, R. D. (2005). Fat taste and lipid metabolism in humans. *Physiology & Behavior*, *86*(5), 691–697. doi:10.1016/j.physbeh.2005.08.058

Merchant, S., Peterson, G. D., Ki Park, S., & Kong, S. G. (2006). FPGA implementation of evolvable block-based neural networks. *IEEE Congress on Evolutionary Computation*, 3129-3136.

Murray, A. F. (1999). Pulse-based computation in VLSI neural networks. In W. Maass & C. M. Bishop (Eds.) *Pulse Neural Networks* (pp. 87-109). London: A Bradford Book, The MIT Press.

Natschläger, T., & Ruf, B. (1998). Spatial and temporal pattern analysis via spiking neurons. *Network (Bristol, England)*, *9*, 319–332. doi:10.1088/0954-898X/9/3/003

Peterson, R. S., Panzeri, S., & Diamond, M, E. (2002). Population coding in somatosensory cortex. *Current Opinion in Neurobiology*, *12*, 441–447. doi:10.1016/S0959-4388(02)00338-0

Reid, D., & Muyeba, M. (2008). Fuzzification of spiked neural networks. *Second UKSIM European Symposium on Computer Modelling and Simulation,* 135-140.

Rojas, R. (1996). *Neural networks, A Systematic Approach*. Berlin: Springer-Verlag.

Sejnowski, T. J. (1995). Pattern recognition. Time for a new neural code? *Nature*, *376*(6535), 21–22. doi:10.1038/376021a0

Ševčik, P. (2005). Implementation design of pulse coded neural network neuron into field programmable gate array device. *Applied Electronics*, *6-7*(Sep), 197–200.

Softky, W. R. (1995). Simple codes versus efficient codes. *Current Opinion in Neurobiology*, *5*, 239–247. doi:10.1016/0959-4388(95)80032-8

Toko, K. (2000). Taste sensor. *Sensors and Actuators. B, Chemical*, *64*, 205–215. doi:10.1016/S0925-4005(99)00508-0

Van Rullen, R., Guyonneau, R., & Thorpe, S. J. (2005). Spike times make sense. *Trends in Neurosciences*, *28*(1), 1–4. doi:10.1016/j.tins.2004.10.010

Wide, P., Winquist, F., Bergsten, P., & Petriu, E. M. (1998). The human-based multisensor fusion method for artificial nose and tongue sensor data. *IEEE Transactions on Instrumentation and Measurement*, *47*(5), 1072–1077. doi:10.1109/19.746559

Wu, Q. X., McGinnity, T. M., Maguire, L. P., Glackin, B., & Belatreche, A. (2006). Learning under weight constrains in networks of temporal encoding spiking neurons. *Neurocomputing*, *69*, 1912–1922. doi:10.1016/j.neucom.2005.11.023

Zhang, K., & Sejnowski, T. J. (1999). Neural tuning: to sharpen or broaden? *Neural Computation*, *11*, 75–84. doi:10.1162/089976699300016809

Zhuang, H., Low, K.-S., & Yau, W.-Y. (2007). A pulse neural network with on-chip learning and its practical applications. *IEEE Transactions on Industrial Electronics*, *54*(1), 34–42. doi:10.1109/TIE.2006.888684

KEY TERMS AND DEFINITIONS

Adaptive Learning: Learning where the system is capable of learning new data patterns without losing knowledge about the previously learnt patterns. Hence, the acquired knowledge is fine-tuned with every newly presented data pattern.

Artificial Tongue: Systems, consisting of an array of taste sensors and a pattern recognition system, capable of modeling taste recognition.

Evolving Spiking Neural Betworks (ESNN): Spiking neural networks that can change either their structure or structural parameters or both under the influence of input data samples.

Field Programmable Gate Arrays (FPGA): High density devices that can operate in a highly parallel manner.

Knowledge Discovery: Process of searching data for patterns that can be considered valuable knowledge.

Spiking Neurons: Models of biological neurons that communicate using spikes, discrete voltage events within a continuous time period.

Spiking Neural Networks (SNN): Biologically inspired computational systems based on spiking neurons. The neurons are trained to respond favorably to the presentation of some inputs and to ignore others.

Tastants: Chemicals that stimulate the sensory cells in taste buds.

Chapter 8
Faster Self-Organizing Fuzzy Neural Network Training and Improved Autonomy with Time-Delayed Synapses for Locally Recurrent Learning

Damien Coyle
University of Ulster, UK

Girijesh Prasad
University of Ulster, UK

Martin McGinnity
University of Ulster, UK

ABSTRACT

This chapter describes a number of modifications to the learning algorithm and architecture of the self-organizing fuzzy neural network (SOFNN) to improve its computational efficiency and learning ability. To improve the SOFNN's computational efficiency, a new method of checking the network structure after it has been modified is proposed. Instead of testing the entire structure every time it has been modified, a record is kept of each neuron's firing strength for all data previously clustered by the network. This record is updated as training progresses and is used to reduce the computational load of checking network structure changes, to ensure performance degradation does not occur, resulting in significantly reduced training times. It is shown that the modified SOFNN compares favorably to other evolving fuzzy systems in terms of accuracy and structural complexity. In addition, a new architecture of the SOFNN is proposed where recurrent feedback connections are added to neurons in layer three of the structure. Recurrent connections allow the network to learn the temporal information from data and, in contrast to pure feed forward architectures which exhibit static input-output behavior in advance, recurrent models are able to store information from the past (e.g., past measurements of the time-series) and are therefore better suited to analyzing dynamic systems. Each recurrent feedback connection includes a weight which must be learned. In this work a learning approach is proposed where the recurrent feedback weight is

DOI: 10.4018/978-1-60960-018-1.ch008

updated online (not iteratively) and proportional to the aggregate firing activity of each fuzzy neuron. It is shown that this modification can significantly improve the performance of the SOFNN's prediction capacity under certain constraints.

INTRODUCTION

Over recent years there has been significant emphasis on developing self-organizing fuzzy systems that continuously evolve and adapt to non-stationary dynamics in complex datasets (Leng et al, 2004; Leng, 2003; Wu & Er, 2000; Kasabov, 2003; Angelov & Filev, 2004; Lughofer & Klement, 2005; Kasabov, 2001; Kasabov & Song, 2002).Many of the developments have been used successfully for applications such as function approximation, system identification and time-series prediction and are often tested on benchmark problems such as the two-input non-linear-sinc problem, Mackey-Glass time-series prediction and others (Leng et al., 2004; Leng, 2003; Wu & Er, 2000; Kasabov, 2003; Jang et al., 1997. An example of a network with an online, self-organizing training algorithm is the self-organizing fuzzy neural network (SOFNN) (Coyle et al., 2006; Coyle et al., 2009; Leng, 2003; Leng et al., 2004; Prasad et al., 2010). The SOFNN is capable of self-organizing its architecture, adding and pruning neurons as required. New neurons are added to cluster new data that the existing neurons are unable to cluster. Inevitably, if the data is highly non-linear and non-stationary, as training progresses and more data are fed to the network, the structure complexity increases and the training efficiency begins to degrade. This is due to the necessity to calculate each neuron's firing strength for a greater number of neurons for all data previously presented to the network, to ensure that changes to the network do not affect the networks ability to optimally cope with older, previously learned data dynamics. This problem occurs if the structure update algorithm depends on information contained in the error derived from the existing network, which is often the case, and is the case with the SOFNN. The problem is amplified if the neurons contain fuzzy membership functions (MFs) which are expensive to compute e.g., the exponential function.

There are algorithms in the literature which have tackled this problem however fuzzy based approaches have a structure which restricts utilization of many of these proposed techniques. For example, the growing and pruning radial basis function network (GAP-RBFN) (Huang et al., 2004) enables determination of the effect of neuron removal on the whole structure by only checking that neuron's contribution to the network. For the fuzzy based approaches such as the SOFNN (Coyle et al. 2009; Leng et al., 2004; Leng, 2003) this method cannot be applied because the fourth layer of the network contains the consequent part of the fuzzy rules in the fuzzy inference system (FIS) which employs a global learning strategy. A single fuzzy rule does not determine system output alone; it works conjunctively with all fuzzy rules in the FIS therefore the SOFNN error cannot be determined by removing a neuron and implementing the same technique described for the GAP-RBFN (Huang et al., 2004). Also, as the fuzzy rules of the SOFNN are based on zero or first order Takagi-Sugeno(TS) models, the linear parameters (consequent parameters of the fuzzy rules) are updated using the recursive least squares estimator (RLSE) however; if the structure is modified during training, the parameters must be estimated using the LSE, therefore the SOFNN is only recursive if the network structure remains unchanged. There have been a number of approaches developed for online recursive estimation of the consequence parameters and local learning rules (Kasabov, 2003; Angelov & Filev, 2004; Lughofer & Klement, 2005; Kasabov, 2001; Kasabov & Song, 2002) although in this study it is shown that these algorithms are not as accurate as the SOFNN, even though they normally evolve complex structures.

To improve the SOFNN's (Leng et al., 2004; Leng, 2003) computational efficiency, a new method of checking the network structure after it has been modified is proposed. Instead of testing the entire structure every time it has been modified, a record is kept of each neuron's firing strength for all data previously clustered by the network. This record is updated as training progresses and is used to reduce the computational load of checking network structure changes, to ensure performance degradation does not occur, resulting in significantly reduced training times.

In addition to these changes and to further enhance the accuracy and autonomy of the SOFNN an extension to the SOFNNs learning process involving the incorporation of local recurrent connections is proposed. The notion of using recurrent models for modeling and predicting dynamic systems and signals has been a popular field of interest in neural network and fuzzy systems research (Budik & Elhanany, 2006; Juang, 2002; Juang & Lin, 1999; Pearlmutter, 1995). Structurally, recurrent models have feedback loops for capturing the dynamic response of a system, and can learn system dynamics without knowing the number of delayed inputs and output in advance, and therefore exhibit particular desired temporal behavior. In contrast to pure feed forward architectures, which exhibit static input-output behavior in advance, recurrent models are able to store information from the past (e.g., past measurements of time-series) and are therefore better suited to analyzing dynamic systems (Juang, 2002). For example, in prediction outputs, the number of delayed outputs, also referred to as the embedding dimension normally has be tuned to ensure maximum prediction performance. This can often be time consuming and suboptimal if the data dynamics are evolving. A new approach currently being investigated for local recurrent connections is proposed in this work where information derived from the aggregate firing strength of the fuzzy neurons is used to adjust the weights of the recurrent feedback connections through an online learning approach.

In summary, this chapter will describe a number of modifications to SOFNN which improve accuracy, increase training speed and improve overall autonomy. The aims of the chapter are to:

1. Describe a new method of checking the network structure after it has been modified to significantly reduce the computational overhead associated with network checking after structural changes. This will improve training speed.
2. Present a thorough comparative analysis of the modified SOFNN and the older version and other state-of-the-art evolving fuzzy methods. The analysis is carried out on a range of benchmark datasets and electroencephalogram (EEG) datasets.
3. Present a new significant structural change to the SOFNN where locally recurrent feedback connections are incorporated to improve accuracy, autonomy and adaptability under certain constraints and make the SOFNN easier applied in dynamic systems applications. To achieve this, a new online learning strategy for recurrent feedback weights is presented and compared with iterative approaches.

BACKGROUND

Fuzzy Logic and Fuzzy Inference Systems

The chapter focuses on describing new developments in the self-organising-fuzzy neural network (SOFNN) therefore it is deemed appropriate to provide some basic background information on fuzzy logic and fuzzy inference systems as well as hybrid fuzzy neural network topologies. In

Figure 1. Typical MFs of linguistic values "young", "middle-aged," and "old" (Figure plotted using the lingmf.m file from Jang et al. 1997)

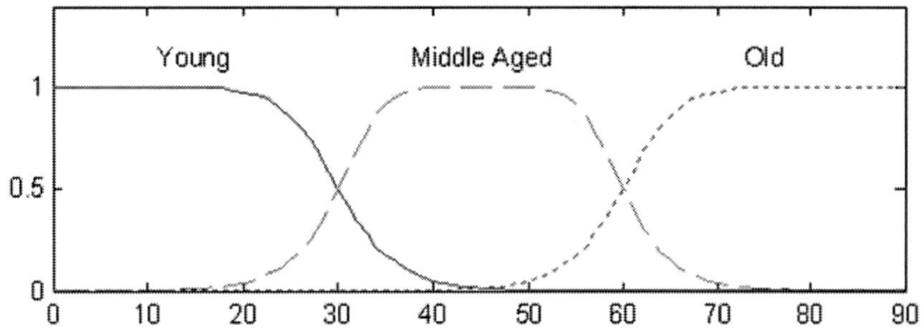

order to effectively handle the complexity and dynamics of real-world problems, there is often the need to model on-line non-linear and time-varying complex systems. Such a need arises in both industrial and biological systems, e.g. models for market forecasts, optimal manufacturing control, and administering anesthesia optimally. The complexity of modeling these systems is exacerbated due to the fact that there is often very little or insufficient expert knowledge available to describe the underlying behavior. Additional common problems that arise in these systems include large dimensions, extensive amounts of data and noisy measurements. In such cases, it is thus an obvious requirement that an appropriate modeling algorithm should have a much higher level of autonomy in the modeling process as well as being capable of providing an interpretation of the resulting model. In order to meet these stringent modeling requirements, an algorithm which has been developed using a hybrid intelligent systems approach is reported in this chapter. The algorithm is basically a fuzzy neural network (FNN) identification procedure, in which fuzzy techniques are used to enhance certain aspects of the neural network's learning and adaptation performance. The term fuzzy stems from within the field of fuzzy logic. Fuzzy logic can be described by contrasting with crisp set theory, for example, a classical set is a set with a crisp boundary. The example given by Jang et al 1997 states that a classical set A of real numbers greater than 6 can be expressed as

$$A = \{x | x > 6\} \tag{1}$$

where there is a clear unambiguous boundary, either x belongs to the set (x is greater than six) or it does not.

In contrast a fuzzy set is a set without crisp boundaries, a class of objects with a continuum of grades of membership to more than one set. Such a set is characterized by a membership function which assigns to each object a grade of membership ranging between zero and one (Zadeh, 1965). In such cases the transition from belonging to one set and not belonging to the set is gradual and smooth. Fuzzy sets have some biological premise in terms of approximate reasoning, and play an important role in human thinking, particularly in the domains of pattern recognition, communication of information and abstraction (Zadeh, 1965). The flexibility of fuzzy sets give rise to easily modeling commonly used linguistic expressions. For example, in a similar way to a variable assuming various values, a linguistic variable "age" can assume different linguistic values, such as "young", "middle-aged" and "old" therefore if "age" assumes the value of "young" then the expression "age is young" is produced and likewise for other values of age. *Figure* 1 shows typical memberships functions for linguistic values associated with age which is based on an example given by Jang et al. 1997. Fuzzy sets and fuzzy set operations are the subjects and verbs of fuzzy logic. *if-then* rule statements are used to formulate the conditional statements that comprises fuzzy logic. A simple fuzzy if-then rule assumes the form

if x is A_1 then y is B_2

where A_1 and B_2 are linguistic variables defined by fuzzy sets on the ranges (i.e., universe of discourse) X and Y, respectively. The *if*-part of the rule 'x is A_1' is called the antecedent or premise and the *then*-part of the rule ' y is B_2 ' is called the consequent. The fuzzy inference system (FIS) is a popular computing framework based on the concepts of fuzzy set theory, fuzzy if-then rules, and fuzzy reasoning. The basic structure of a fuzzy inference system consists of 3 conceptual components which include the rule base consisting of multiple rules in a similar format to that shown above, a database which define the membership function used in the fuzzy rules and a reasoning mechanism which performs the inference procedure based on the information obtained from fuzzy rules and memberships to produce a reasonable output. The output of fuzzy system is normally required to be a crisp output, a value that may be used to perform some operation or control a system. To achieve this, a defuzzification step is performed to extract a crisp output that best represents the fuzzy set. With a crisp input and output, a fuzzy inference system implements a nonlinear mapping from its input space to the output space. There are range of different types of fuzzy inference systems (FIS) including those based on Mandani fuzzy models (Mandani and Assilian, 1975), Sugeno fuzzy models (also known as Takagi-Sugeno-Kang (TSK) fuzzy models) (Takagi and Sugeno, 1993, 1985; Sugeno and Kang, 1988) and Tsukamoto fuzzy models (Tsukamoto, Y. 1979). A detailed description of these can be found in Jang et al, 1997). In this work a brief description of the TSK fuzzy models is provided as this model is used in the SOFNN. A typical fuzzy rule in the TSK fuzzy model has the form

if x is A and y is B then $z = f(x,y)$

where A and B are fuzzy sets in the antecedent, while $z = f(x,y)$ is a crisp function in the consequent. Usually $f(x,y)$ is a first order polynomial and the resulting inference system is called the first order Sugeno fuzzy model. When f is a constant the model is referred to as zero order Sugeno fuzzy model. The Sugeno model is by far the most popular model for data-sample based fuzzy modeling and it provides a very efficient approach to defuzzification compared to other models. Figure 2 below provides a diagrammatic overview of a complete fuzzy inference system with multiple rules. (For a more detailed coverage of Fuzzy Inference Systems see Jang et al., 1997 which provides an excellent introduction and coverage of neuro, fuzzy and hybrid neuro-fuzzy based computing approaches as well as traditional and other intelligent approaches to regression and optimization).

HYBRID FUZZY NEURAL NETWORKS

Fuzzy neural networks (FNNs) are usually represented as multi-layer feedforward networks and are used to learn the fuzzy membership functions in a FIS and explain the rules that are used to make decisions. A good review of FNNs can be found in (Buckley and Hayashi, 1994; Nauck 1997). Some authors make a distinction between FNNs and neuro-fuzzy systems. No differentiation is however made in this chapter. The algorithm which is modified in this work is based on a self-organizing fuzzy neural network approach, in which the FNN is capable of self-organizing its structure along with associated antecedent and consequent parameters. A type of recursive least

Figure 2. Block diagram of a fuzzy inference system with multiple rules

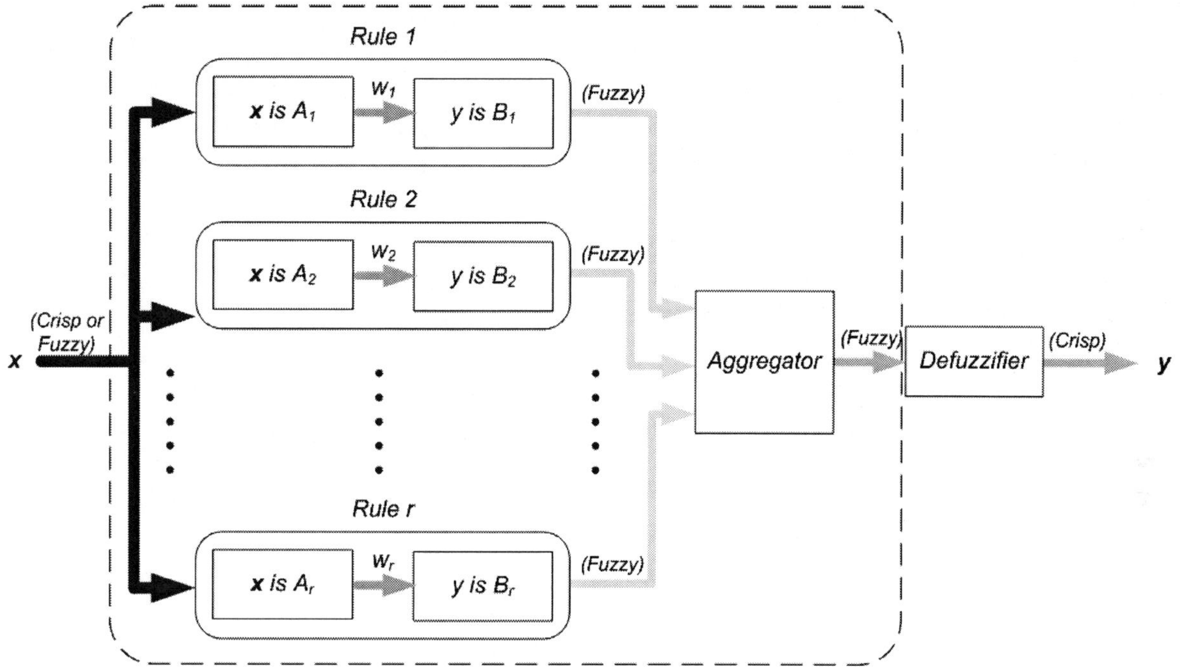

square (RLS) algorithm (Astrom & Wittenmark, 1995) is used to identify the consequent parameters of the Takagi-Sugeno-Kang (TSK) type fuzzy model (Takagi and Sugeno, 1993, 1985; Sugeno and Kang, 1988) described above and forms an integral part of the approach. The main objective of the SOFNN approach is to produce a hybrid fuzzy neural network architecture which self-adapts the fuzzy rules for on-line identification of a TSK fuzzy model for a non-linear time-varying complex system. The algorithm results in a self-organizing neural network which is designed to approximate a fuzzy inference system through the structure of neural networks and thus create a more accurate, efficient and interpretable hybrid neural network model, making effective use of the superior learning ability of neural networks and ease of interpretability of fuzzy systems. The main issues associated with the identification of a TS type fuzzy model are: (1) structure identification involving partitioning the input-output space and thus identifying the number of fuzzy rules for the desired performance and (2) parameter estimation which involves identifying the antecedent and consequent parameters.

There are many supervised training approaches (Mitra & Hayashi, 2000; Wang & Lee, 2001) proposed in the literature for adaptive fuzzy-neural based model identification. The main difference lies in the method adopted for the partitioning of the input-output space during the structure identification procedure. As suggested in (Wang & Lee, 2001), the methods proposed in the literature can be placed into two broad categories: 1. The static adaptation method where the number of input-output partitions are fixed, while their corresponding fuzzy rule configurations are adapted through optimization to obtain the desired performance and 2. The dynamic adaptation method where both the number of input-output space partitions and their corresponding fuzzy rule configurations are simultaneously and concurrently adapted. The main focus of the SOFNN algorithm is the design of an approach for dynamic adaptation of the structure of the hybrid network, so that the underlying behavior of a non-linear time-varying complex system can be captured in a model that is more accurate, compact and interpretable.

For similar performance, the number of fuzzy partitions, and thereby fuzzy rules, can be greatly reduced by cluster-based partitioning of the input-output space (Zadeh, 1994). Therefore, for identifying a more compact structure, input-output space partitioning based on the traditional clustering approaches, such as hard c-means (HCM) and fuzzy c-means (FCM) (Klawonn & Keller, 1998; Wang & Lee, 2001; Gonzalez et al., 2002), has been proposed. The number of partitions, however, needs to be fixed by a priori expert knowledge in many of these approaches. The final configuration of the clusters and the corresponding fuzzy rule parameters are obtained by a non-linear optimization. However, there is no guarantee of convergence to an optimal solution, as the final solution greatly relies on the selection of initial locations of cluster centers. Also, it is difficult and time consuming to visualize the optimal number of partitions required for modeling a complex system, particularly if the underlying structural behavior of the system is time-varying and inadequately known.

Under the dynamic adaptation method, the training may start with only a single fuzzy rule or neuron (Wu & Er, 2000; Wang & Lee, 2001; Rizzi et al., 2002; Er & Wu, 2002; Wu et al., 2001; Kasabov & Song, 2002). During training, the network structure grows and concurrently the parameters of the antecedents and consequents are adapted to obtain the desired modeling accuracy.

A constructive approach for creating an ANFIS-like network is proposed in (Mascioli & Martinelli, 1998; Mascioli et al., 2000; Rizzi et al., 2002) based on Simpson's min-max technique (Simpson, 1992; Simpson, 1993). The input space is partitioned by constructing hyperboxes using the min-max procedure. The hyperbox-based framework facilitates application of different types of fuzzy membership functions. To decrease the complexity of the network, a pruning method, named as the pruning adaptive resolution classifier (PARC), is developed in (Rizzi et al., 2002). This consists of deleting some negligible hyperboxes and a fusion procedure to make actual coverage complete. This constructive approach is however basically developed for batch learning to create a structure-adaptive network with a significantly higher degree of automation.

A dynamic fuzzy neural network (DFNN) architecture reported in (Wu & Er, 2000) and (Er & Wu, 2002) makes use of a hierarchical learning approach and an orthogonal least squares based pruning technique (Chen et al., 1991). In the DFNN architecture, fuzzy rules are represented by RBF neurons in the first hidden layer although the representation is restrictive in the sense that the widths of the membership functions belonging to various inputs that create an RBF neuron in the DFNN have the same value and the widths are not adaptable. An enhanced version of DFNN is the Generalized DFNN (GDFNN) (Wu et al., 2001). It introduces width vectors in the RBF neurons, so that the Gaussian membership functions within a neuron can be assigned appropriate widths separately. The GDFNN also attempts to provide explanations for selecting the values of the width parameter of the Gaussian fuzzy membership functions based on the concept of ε-completeness (Wang, 1992). However, the hierarchical learning approach proposed for training the GDFNN is dependent on the total number of training data patterns. This implies that the GDFNN approach is primarily designed for batch training using a fixed number of training data patterns.

The dynamic evolving neuro-fuzzy system (DENFIS) (Kasabov & Song, 2002) employs a dynamic adaptation method and can be applied for on-line TSK fuzzy model identification. The input space partitioning in DENFIS is accomplished on-line using an evolving clustering method (ECM) that creates new clusters as new data vectors arrive, based on a distance threshold. The fuzzy inference and thereby the consequent parameters are estimated based on only the nearest m fuzzy rules. Although this approach implements the concept of local learning by limiting the learning in a region nearest to the current data vector, it has no provision to ensure that network size remains compact while ensuring higher generalization accuracy. The algorithm is compared in detail in the work presented in this chapter.

In order to model a time-varying non-linear system, a truly on-line training algorithm is required so that the desired accuracy as well as network size can be achieved and maintained. Ensuring convergence of the network parameters and the estimation error is also essential for an on-line training algorithm. Based on the dynamic adaptation method, this chapter presents an algorithm for creating a self-organizing fuzzy neural network (SOFNN) that identifies a singleton or TS type fuzzy model on-line. A modified recursive least squares (RLS) algorithm derived to guarantee the convergence of the estimation error and the linear network parameters is used for estimating consequent parameters. For structure learning, the algorithm makes use of a procedure to decide how to create a new ellipsoidal basis function (EBF) neuron with a center vector and a width vector. The EBF neuron represents a fuzzy rule formed by AND logic (or T-norm) operating on Gaussian fuzzy membership functions. The parameters of the center vector and width vector of the EBF neurons are the centers and widths of the Gaussian membership functions. The structure learning approach consists of a combination of system error and firing strength based criterion for adding new EBF neurons using the concepts from statistical theory and the ε-completeness of fuzzy rules (Lee, 1990). This ensures that the membership functions have the capacity to cluster more data. The SOFNN approach uses a pruning method based on the optimal brain surgeon (OBS) approach (Hassibi & Stork, 1993; Leung et al., 2001). This method is computationally efficient for on-line implementation, as it does not involve any significant additional computation, instead making direct use of the Hermitian matrix obtained as a part of the RLS algorithm however the necessity to use error information based on current and past input examples reduces computational speed. This chapter will describe recent modifications to the structure learning procedure to improve computational efficiency. The capacity to add and prune neurons automatically during training provides the SOFNN with an adaptive structure to model nonlinear and time-varying systems on-line. The structure learning and parameter learning methods are very simple and more efficient and yield a fuzzy neural model with a high accuracy and compact structure.

The remaining sections of the chapter will describe in more detail how the SOFNN achieves this and a number of recent modifications which improve the overall performance, automaticity and learning speed of the SOFNN. Results on a range of different datasets presented and the SOFNN is benchmarked against a range of state-of-the-art methods.

METHODOLOGY

The Architecture of the SOFNN

The SOFNN is a five-layer fuzzy NN and has the ability to self-organize its neurons in the learning process for implementing TSK fuzzy models (Takagi & Sugeno, 1983) (cf. Figure 3). In the EBF layer, each neuron is a T-norm of Gaussian fuzzy MFs belonging to the inputs of the network. Every MF thus has a distinct centre and width, therefore every neuron has a centre and a width vector. Figure 4 illustrates the internal structure of the j-th neuron, where the input vector is $\boldsymbol{x} = [x_1 x_2 \ldots x_r]$, $\boldsymbol{c}_j = [c_{1j}\, c_{1j} \ldots c_{rj}]$ is the vector of centers in the jth neuron, and $\boldsymbol{\sigma}_j = [\sigma_{1j}\, \sigma_{2j} \ldots \sigma_{rj}]$ is the vector of widths in the j-th neuron. Layer 1 is the input layer with r neurons, x_i, i=1,2,…,r. Layer 2 is the EBF layer. Each neuron in this layer represents a premise part of a fuzzy rule. The outputs of (EBF) neurons are computed by products of the grades

Figure 3. Self-organizing fuzzy neural network

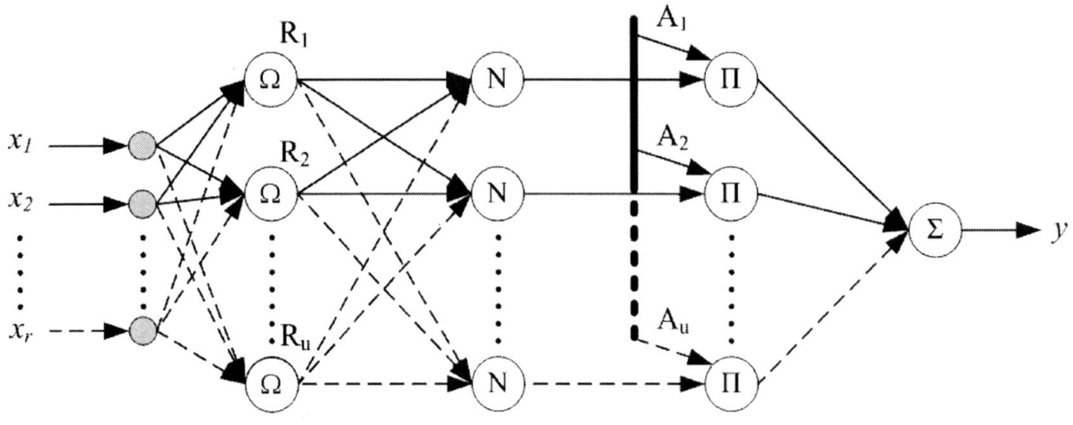

Figure 4. Structure of the jth neuron R_j within the EBF layer

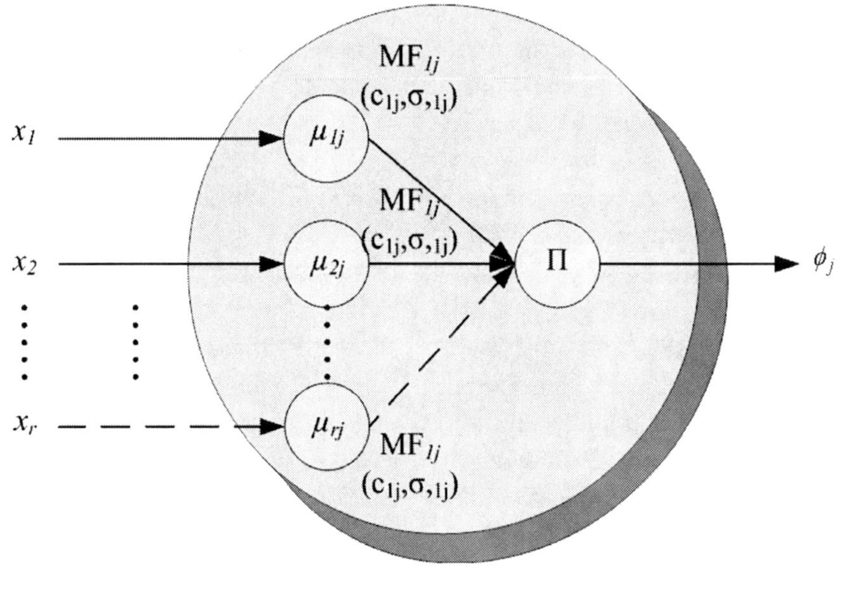

of MFs. Each MF is in the form of a Gaussian function:

$$\mu_{ij} = \exp\left[-(x_i - c_{ij})^2 / 2\sigma_{ij}^2\right] \qquad j = 1, 2, \cdots, u \tag{2}$$

where, μ_{ij} is the i-th MF in the j-th neuron; c_{ij} is the centre of the i-th MF in the j-th neuron; σ_{ij} is the width of the i-th MF in the j-th neuron; r is the number of input variables; u is the number of EBF neurons.

For the jth neuron, the output is

$$\phi_j = \exp\left[-\sum_{i=1}^{r}\left((x_i - c_{ij})^2 / 2\sigma_{ij}^2\right)\right] \qquad j = 1, 2, \cdots, u. \tag{3}$$

Layer 3 is the normalized layer. The number of neurons in this layer is equal to that of layer 2. The output of the *j*th neuron in this layer is

$$\psi_j = \phi_j \Big/ \sum_{k=1}^{u} \phi_k \qquad j = 1, 2, \cdots, u. \tag{4}$$

Layer 4 is the weighted layer. Each neuron in this layer has two inputs and the product of these inputs as its output. One of the inputs is the output of the related neuron in the layer 3 and the other is the weighted bias w_{2j}. For the TS model (Takagi & Sugeno, 1983), the bias $\mathbf{B}=[1, x_1, x_2, \ldots, x_r]^T$ and $\mathbf{A}_j=[a_{j0}, a_{j1}, a_{j2}, \ldots, a_{jr}]$ represents the set of parameters corresponding to the consequent of the fuzzy rule *j* which are obtained using the least square estimator or recursive LSE (RLSE). The weighted bias w_{2j} is

$$w_{2j} = \mathbf{A}_j.\mathbf{B} = a_{j0} + a_{j1}x_1 + \cdots + a_{jr}x_r \qquad j = 1, 2, \cdots, u. \tag{5}$$

This is the consequent part of the *j*th fuzzy rule of the fuzzy model. The output of each neuron is $f_j = w_{2j}\psi_j$.

Layer 5 is the output layer where the incoming signals from layer 4 are summed, as shown in (6)

$$y(\mathbf{x}) = \sum_{j=1}^{u} f_j \tag{6}$$

where, *y* is the value of an output variable. If *u* neurons are generated from *n* training exemplars then the output of the network can be written as

$$\mathbf{Y} = \mathbf{W}_2 \boldsymbol{\Psi}. \tag{7}$$

where for the TS model

$$\mathbf{Y} = [y_1 \quad y_2 \quad \cdots \quad y_n], \tag{8}$$

$$\boldsymbol{\Psi} = \begin{bmatrix} \psi_{11} & \cdots & \psi_{1n} \\ \psi_{11}x_{11} & \cdots & \psi_{1n}x_{1n} \\ \vdots & \vdots & \vdots \\ \psi_{11}x_{r1} & \cdots & \psi_{1n}x_{rn} \\ \vdots & \vdots & \vdots \\ \psi_{u1} & \cdots & \psi_{un} \\ \psi_{u1}x_{11} & \cdots & \psi_{un}x_{1n} \\ \vdots & \vdots & \vdots \\ \psi_{u1}x_{r1} & \cdots & \psi_{un}x_{rn} \end{bmatrix}, \tag{9}$$

and

$$\mathbf{W}_2 = [a_{10} \quad a_{11} \quad \cdots \quad a_{1r} \quad \cdots \quad a_{u0} \quad a_{u1} \quad \cdots \quad a_{ur}]. \tag{10}$$

$\mathbf{W}_2$ is the parameter matrix and ψ_{jt} is the output of the *j*th neuron in the normalized layer for the *t*th training exemplar.

MODIFICATIONS TO THE SOFNN LEARNING ALGORITHM AND ARCHITECTURE

The SOFNN Learning Algorithm

The learning process of the SOFNN includes structure learning and parameter learning. The structure learning process attempts to achieve an economical network size by dynamically modifying, adding and/or pruning neurons. There are two criteria to judge whether or not to generate a new EBF neuron – the system error criterion and the if-part criterion. The *error* criterion considers the generalization performance of the overall network. The *if-part* criterion evaluates whether existing fuzzy rules or EBF neurons can cluster the current input vector suitably. The SOFNN pruning strategy is based on the optimal brain surgeon (OBS) approach (Hassibi & Stork, 1993). Basically, the idea is to use second derivative information to find the least important neuron. If the performance of the entire network is accepted when the least important neuron is pruned, the new structure of the network is maintained.

This section only provides a basic outline of the structure learning process, the complete structure and weight learning algorithm for the SOFNN is detailed in (Leng, 2003; Leng et al., 2004; Prasad et al., 2010). It must be noted that the neuron modifying, adding and pruning procedures are fully dependent upon determining the network error as the structure changes therefore a significant amount of network testing is necessary – to either update the structure based on finalized neuron changes or simply to check if a temporarily deleted neuron is significant. This can be computationally demanding and therefore an alternative approach which minimizes the computational cost of error checking during the learning process is described below.

A Faster SOFNN Structure Learning Procedure

Updating the structure requires updating the matrix **Ψ**, as shown in (8), after which the linear parameters are estimated using the recursive least squares estimator (LSE) i.e., non-recursively after structure changes only. As can be seen from (3) and (8), the **Ψ** matrix requires that all neuron outputs are calculated for every input exemplar that has already entered the network. The time required is therefore of the order $O(nUM^2)$, where n is the number of training data which have already entered the network, U is the number of times the structure needs to be updated, and $M=u.(r+1)$, where r is the number of input variables and u is the number of EBF neurons in the network structure. In small training sets ($n<2000$), with a relatively small input training dimension (r<7), the number of neurons added may not be large (depending on data complexity) therefore $O(nUM^2)$ is normally low and tolerable. However, real-world data sets can often exhibit complex dynamics and are inherently large. In the case of EEG datasets n is large and can thus result in long training times therefore there is necessity to reduce some of the other variables in $O(nUM^2)$.

In this work it is proposed to reduce the training time by reducing the time required to perform tests on the structure when updating the structure and evaluating the importance of neurons. To do this, as training progresses, a record of intermediate network responses can be stored, which contains each EBF neuron's most recent firing strength, denoted as $\Phi \in R^{u \times n}$, and the normalization factor for each input which previously entered the network, denoted as $\xi \in R^{1 \times n}$ i.e., the outputs from each neuron in layer 2 and the sum of the outputs from all neurons in layer 2 are stored. Then, when checking structural modifications during training, instead of calculating the firing strength for all neurons in layer 2, for all previously entered inputs, only those neurons which have been changed should be checked. However, there is an implication in doing this. As can be seen from (3), ψ_j, the output of each neuron in layer 3, depends on the normalization factor which is the sum of the firing strength for all neurons for each input exemplar. Therefore, if any neuron is modified, added or deleted, the normalization factor for all inputs previously entered into the network is changed and therefore all historical data becomes invalid. To overcome this problem, if a neuron e.g., q is changed, then that neuron's previous firing strength is obtained from the stored data and deducted from the saved normalization factor for each of the previously entered inputs. Then the firing strength for neuron q for all inputs is recalculated. The new firing strength is stored in place of the old firing strength and added to the normalization factor. Subsequently, the output from layer 3 can be obtained by dividing all the saved firing strengths by the respective normalization factor for all previously clustered data. To demonstrate this, consider n data exemplars have entered the network and u neurons have been created, then Φ is a $u \times n$ matrix containing the firing strength of each neuron for all previously entered data and ξ is a $1 \times n$ vector containing the normalization factor for all previously clustered data.

1. *Neuron modifying*: If neuron q has been modified then, firstly, its contribution to the normalization factor is excluded using (11)

$$\xi_{i_{new}} = \xi_{i_{old}} - \Phi_{qi} \qquad i = 1, 2, \ldots, n \qquad (11)$$

   and the firing strength for the q-th neuron for the i-th input exemplar, ς_i, is calculated using (2) and (3). This is carried out for all previously entered data (i.e., $i = 1,2,\ldots,n$). The q-th row of the saved firing strength matrix, Φ, is subsequently updated using (11) and the normalization factor is updated using (12) (note: equation (10) must be calculated prior to (12) after which ξ_{inew} obtained using (10) becomes ξ_{iold} in (12).

$$\Phi_{qi} = \varsigma_i \qquad i = 1, 2, \ldots, n \qquad (12)$$

$$\xi_{i_{new}} = \xi_{i_{old}} + \varsigma_i \qquad i = 1, 2, \ldots, n \qquad (13)$$

2. *Neuron adding:* If a new neuron, q, has been added to the structure then the firing strength, ς_i, of that neuron for all data previously entered into the structure is calculated after which Φ is updated using (11) and ξ is obtained using (12).
3. *Neuron deleting*: If the q-th neuron has been deleted ξ is updated using (10) afterwhich the q-th row of Φ is removed.

Subsequent to any network changes and respective changes to the data stored in Φ and ξ, the normalized firing strength for all data and all neurons (output of layer 3) is simply and efficiently calculated by dividing each row of Φ by ξ.

Adding Time-Delayed Synapses for Locally Recurrent Learning in the SOFNN

As outlined in the previous subsection the firing strength for each neuron for all previously learned data exemplars are stored in Φ to speed up the learning process. This section will outline an extra advantage associated with storing this information and how it can be used to facilitate training the weights of locally recurrent synapses which can be added to layer 3 of the SOFNN presented in Figure 3 as shown in Figure 5.

Incorporating recurrent connection through feedback loops (or synapses) can be used to automatically capture the dynamic response of a system, and can learn system dynamics without knowing the number of delayed inputs and outputs in advance. Recurrent neural networks and self organizing fuzzy neural networks are widely acknowledged as an effective tool that can be used by a wide range of applications that store and process temporal sequences (Budik & Elhanany, 2006). For example, in standard time series prediction tasks, the time-series data are structured so that the signal measurements from sample indices t to t-$(\Delta$-$1)\tau$ are used to make a prediction of the signal at sample index $t+\pi$. The parameter Δ is the embedding dimension and

$$\hat{x}(t+\pi) = f\left\langle x(t), \ldots, x(t-(\Delta-1)\tau)\right\rangle \qquad (14)$$

where τ is the time delay, π is the prediction horizon, $f\langle.\rangle$ is the SOFNN model, x is the signal or time series and $\hat{x}$ is the predicted signal. The embedding dimension Δ and the time delay τ are often very important parameters in the prediction task and careful selection can significantly influence the prediction performance, whereas poor selection and/or limited incorporation of temporal information in a dynamic prediction task can result in poor prediction performance. There are many techniques used for selecting the best values

Figure 5. A modified SOFNN architecture with locally recurrent synapses incorporated in layer 3

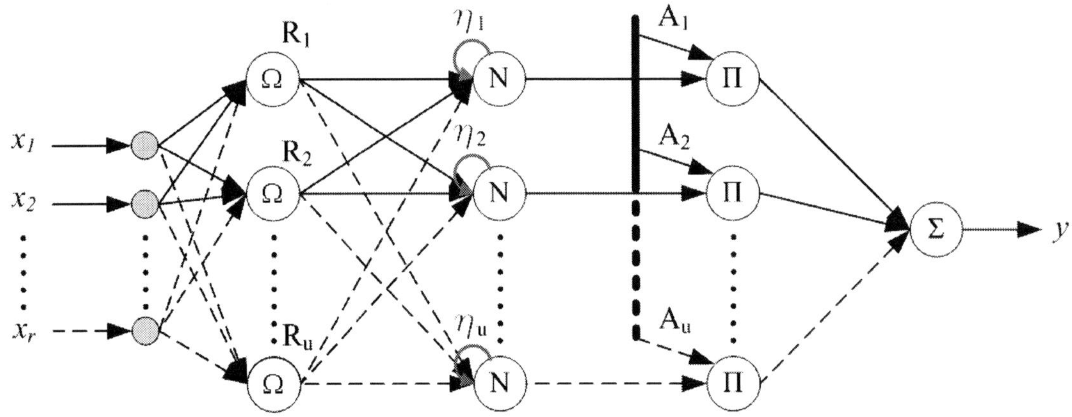

for Δ and τ Williams, G. P. (1997) with an iterative or information theoretic approach often preferred however, this study was not concerned with selecting the optimal Δ and τ values. The objectives here was to incorporate temporal information through the above described modification to the SOFNN architecture where each neurons has feedback weight η. η_j, where $0 \leq \eta_j \leq 1$, is used to govern the percentage of the previous firing strength of neuron j in the 3rd layer that is fed back to neuron j and which subsequently contributes to the current firing strength. This feedback allows the network to discover temporal information in the data and lead to overall performance enhancement, particularly when the data to the network at time instant, t, does not contain any or limited temporal information e.g., when the Δ has been set to 1 or has not been optimized. To achieve this recurrent connection in the SOFNN algorithm (3) is modified as shown in (15).

$$\begin{aligned} \psi_j &= (1-\eta_j)\phi_j \Big/ \sum_{k=1}^{u} \phi_k + \eta_j \phi_j(t-1) \Big/ \sum_{k=1}^{u} \phi_k(t-1) \\ &= (1-\eta_j)\phi_j \Big/ \sum_{k=1}^{u} \phi_k + \eta_j \Phi_{ji} \Big/ \sum_{k=1}^{u} \Phi_{ki} \\ &= (1-\eta_j)\phi_j \Big/ \sum_{k=1}^{u} \phi_k + \eta_j \Phi_{ji} / \xi_i \qquad j = 1,2,\cdots,u. \end{aligned} \tag{15}$$

In (14) Φ_{ji} contains the firing strength of j-th neuron in layer 2 and ξ_i contains the normalization factor for layer 3 at time t-1. As can be seen from (15), the firing strength for the current data exemplar without the feedback contribution is reduced by a factor of hand summed with the contribution of the previous firing strength therefore; the feedback weight η for each neuron determines the ratio of the current and previous inputs firing strengths to the output of neurons in layer 3 and therefore the overall network output. In this sense it becomes obvious that the choice of the weight, η, for each neuron is critical to overall performance and thus must to tuned accordingly.

Many techniques for tuning the feedback weights in recurrent networks have been explored (Budik & Elhanany, 2006; Juang, 2002; Juang & Lin, 1999; Pearlmutter, 1995). For fuzzy neural networks such as the SOFNN which employ online incremental learning, iterative or offline backpropagation based learning approaches to updating the recurrent feedback weights are not satisfactory and, additionally, the consequent part and weights of the fuzzy systems make it difficult to feedback directly error related performance information to update the weights during online training. In some cases the structure is evolved or learned before the weights of the network are updated. To overcome this problem a new approach to updating the recurrent weights is proposed in this chapter.

Given that the firing strength of the neurons in layer 2 for all previously processed input data are saved in the new structure learning process proposed in the previous subsection and the normalized firing strength in layer 3 can be easily calculated using the saved normalization factor information for layer 3 for all previously processed data, the dynamics of the firing activity for each neuron can be easily assessed and determined in an online learning situation i.e., neurons can be ranked in terms of the level or strength of their firing activity over all previously processed data or over a window of previously processed data. Using this information it was hypothesized that, if a particular neuron is dominating the firing activity, then this neuron is contributing more to the network output and is most suited to cluster the majority of the data dynamics in the current time window and therefore this neuron could benefit if the feedback weight was proportional to the strength of its firing activity over a period of time, whilst neurons which have a weaker firing strength should have weaker recurrent connections but again proportional to the strength of their aggregate firing activity over a time window. In such cases the recurrent feedback weights for each neuron could be easily determined and updated in an online situation using the saved firing strength information as shown in (16)

$$\eta_j = \sum_{i=1}^{n} \Phi_{ji} \Big/ \sum_{k=1}^{u} \sum_{i=1}^{n} \Phi_{ki} \qquad j = 1,2,\cdots,u. \tag{16}$$

where η for each neuron is calculated each time Φ is updated and is the normalized aggregate of the firing strength of all previously processed inputs for each neuron. This process is simple and can be updated online easily and can result in the feedback weights being updated effectively to determine an appropriate amount of feedback to apply for each neuron that has been added to the structure in layer 3.

The following section provides information and results on a range of tests that were carried out to show that the modified training process can provide significant speedup to the SOFNN. The SOFNN has already been proven to outperform other well-known fuzzy neural network approaches (Leng et al., 2004; Leng, 2003) and further comparisons are provided here. Results from a range of tests carried out to determine the efficacy of the new SOFNN structure incorporating locally recurrent synaptic connections and the proposed novel synaptic weight learning process are also presented and discussed.

RESULTS & DISCUSSION

EEG Data Acquisition

One of the benchmark tests used in this work is EEG time series prediction. The EEG data used was recorded from 1 person in a timed recording procedure (Pfurtscheller et al., 1998; Schlogl & Pfurtscheller, 2005). All signals were sampled at 125Hz and filtered between 0.5 and 30Hz. Two bipolar EEG channels were measured using two electrodes positioned 2.5cm posterior and anterior to position C3 and C4 according to the international standard (10/20 system) (Fisch, 1999). Data were recorded during brain-computer interface (BCI) based virtual reality feedback and gaming experiments, where the task was to control and perform decisions in various types of virtual environments or control the horizontal position of a ball falling from the top to the bottom of the PC monitor using motor imagery (cf. (Schlogl & Pfurtscheller, 2005) for details). Each trial lasts ~10s, of which 4-5 seconds is related to left/right hand movement imagination i.e., event-related. There are four different time-series' recorded during the experiments described above i.e., left

(C3 and C4) and right (C3 and C4). These will be referred to as l3, l4 and r3, r4.

The Optimized SOFNN Training Algorithm

The computational effort involved in data analysis provided by the optimized SOFNN training algorithms benefited significantly from a reduction in training times inherited from the modified SOFNN learning approach introduced in this work. To demonstrate the speedup, a comparative analysis on ten benchmark datasets was carried out with the older version of the SOFNN and the modified version, using a 3.6GHz Intel Dual Xeon CPU with 4GB of RAM. Error and network complexity results for these benchmarks were presented in (Leng et al., 2004; Leng, 2003) where comparisons to well known algorithms such as the Adaptive Neuro Fuzzy Inference System (ANFIS), the Radial Basis Fuzzy Neural Network (RBFNN), Dynamic Fuzzy Neural network (DFNN), the generalized DFNN (GDFNN) (Jang, 1993; Jang et al., 1997, Wu & Er, 2000) and others were detailed, showing that the SOFNN outperformed these algorithms. For the current tests, as was expected, neuron numbers and training RMSE for the old and new networks were equivalent. Columns 5 and 6 of Table I show the training times for the old and new versions of the SOFNN. In all cases the newer version trained quicker than the older version although datasets 8 and 9 show explicitly the differentiation in training times when more neurons are recruited by the SOFNN to cluster larger datasets.

The results in bold shown in Table 1 are for tests performed on a EEG dataset where the SOFNN was trained on 6000 samples of motor imagery EEG signals recorded from the C3 electrode during imagination of left hand movement. The data was taken from sixteen randomly chosen trials and consists of three second segments of the most separable, event-related portion of each of the trials (to help illustrate how the SOFNN structure adapts to different data, two tests were performed on EEG datasets i.e., each dataset randomly selected but having different complexity and referred to as sEEG (simple) and cEEG (complex)). The SOFNN was trained to perform one-step-ahead-prediction with an embedding dimension 6 and time lag 1. The parameters were stringently selected so that the network would attempt to evolve for maximum performance in terms of accuracy and thus was likely to add a significant number of neurons. Again, the both versions of the SOFNN produce identical results as expected, i.e., both converged on the same minimum error and the same number of neurons pruned and added. However, the elapsed time, ranging from the initiation of the training to completion, was significantly different for each version of the SOFNN. For the sEEG the elapsed time for the old version was approximately 18.4min whereas the elapsed time for the modified SOFNN was ~5.3 min. This is a ~71% reduction in the training duration. Only thirteen neurons were added which shows the compactness of the network but still good performance (RMSE=0.009 which was the target). Conversely, for the more complex EEG dataset (cEEG), 20 neurons were added to maintain the desired prediction accuracy and the training duration was significantly increased, taking approximately 47 minutes for the old SOFNN and 15 minutes for the new SOFNN. Again, the speedup provided by the modifications to the SOFNN is illustrated, circa 68% in this case. It must be noted that these times are greater than normally required. As outlined previously, for these tests and for illustrative purposes, the SOFNN parameters were selected to ensure that accuracy was maximized regardless of the structural complexity.

These tests clearly show the significance of the speedup when working on larger data sets. When learning these larger EEG datasets, any occasion a neuron was added or deleted, only that portion of the network was rechecked using historical records of the firing strengths and simple data manipulations involving subtractions and division (cf. methodology section). In the older

Table 1. Time enhancements by SOFNN modifications with accuracy and complexity performance

D*	N*	Train Error [RMSE]	Test Error [RMSE}	Old Time [s]	New Time [s]
1	4	0.362	-	0.20	0.17
2	8	0.210	-	0.48	0.38
3	4	0.311	1.197	0.22	0.19
4	5	0.016	0.017	2.02	1.95
5	5	0.005	0.004	0.13	0.13
6	10	0.212	0.295	0.31	0.25
7	11	0.069	0.101	0.19	0.11
8	25	0.027	0.018	168	112
9	11	0.027	0.027	124	15.4
10	8	0.006	0.007	1.27	0.33
✧	**13**	**0.009**	**0.009**	**1108**	**322**
✧	**Test Time = 1.01s 618KB**				
⅄	**20**	**0.009**	**0.009**	**2877**	**926**
⅄	**Test Time = 1.50s 928KB**				

*Data type ★Neuron Numbers ✧ sEEG simple ⅄ cEEG complex (See Table 2 for details)

version, after structure changes, if there were 6 inputs, with 6 neurons in the structure and 5,000 past data exemplars then, as described in section IV, there are $O(nUM^2)$ = 5,000.(1)(42^2) = 8,820,000 calculations, involving the exponential function, required to estimate the firing strengths of all the neurons for all past data. With the modified version only the firing strengths for the neuron which has been modified needs to be updated therefore the number of calculations $O(nUM^2)$ = 5,000.(1) (7^2) = 245,000. Differences in structure updating complexity are illustrated in this example which verifies how the improved performance is acquired and the significance of the computational efficiency instilled by the modifications to the SOFNN presented in this work. There is not a large cost in terms of memory required to facilitate the modified structure learning procedure. For example, in the cEEG example, where 6,000 sets of firing strength for 20 neurons are stored, the dimensionality of the firing strength matrix, Φ, is 6,000,320 and the normalization factor vector, ξ, has a dimension of 600,031. Together Φ and ξ requires circa 928KB of memory therefore the modified approach does not have a large memory overhead, unless the structure grows significantly, in which case the computations may become intractable, or the datasets are very large. In such cases various techniques can be employed to alleviate a memory problem, the simplest approach being to only consider data within a predefined window, forgetting data which has been clustered in the distant past. Figures 6 and 7 show the training performance information, neuron growth during training and the membership functions for each input in the sEEG and cEEG datasets. Table 2 provides fuzzy rules for the sEEG dataset.

In summary, the results presented in this section illustrate that the proposed modification to the SOFNN learning algorithms can significantly improve performance without any trade-off in performance and a negligible additional memory requirement.

Comparative Analysis with Other Evolving Fuzzy Systems

It may be argued that the proposed modifications to the SOFNN are essential and should be an inherent part of the learning algorithm however, no other fuzzy neural network approaches in the literature have employed this approach to structure checking which was based on the growing and pruning radial basis function network (GAP-RBFN) developed by Huang et al. (2004). Many of the evolving fuzzy systems approaches (Kasabov, 2003; Angelov & Filev, 2004; Lughofer & Klement, 2005; Kasabov, 2001; Kasabov & Song, 2002) do not check the network using passed input data because the structure and parameters updating procedure employed in evolving fuzzy approaches are based on current input data only and recursive estimation techniques however; it has been observed that these approaches may

Figure 7. Plots showing target and predicted outputs (6 steps ahead) for the Mackey-Glass data using (a) no recurrent connection with Δ=6 and τ=1 (b) locally recurrent connections with Δ=1 (c) no recurrent connections with Δ=1

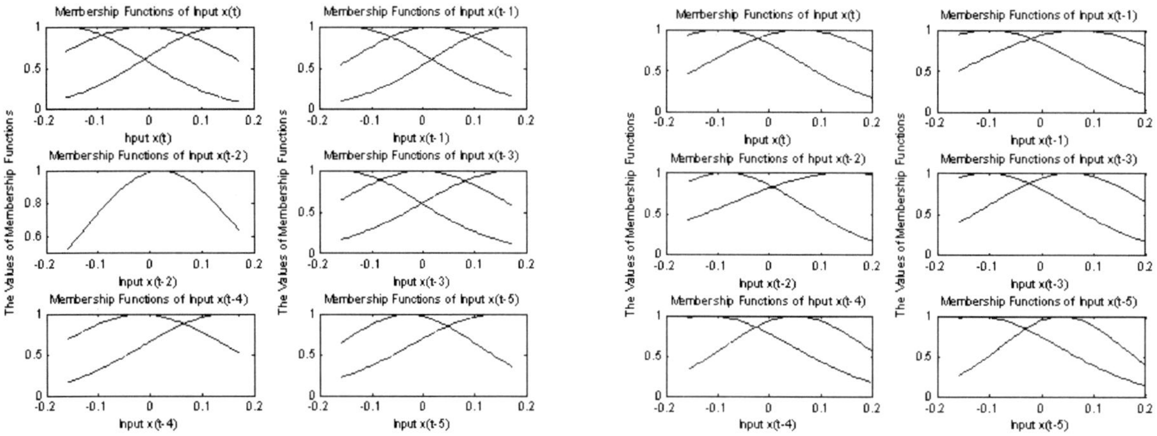

Table 2. Bench mark dataset details (Columns 2 and 3 show the training and testing dataset sizes

Benchmark dataset	Train	Test
1. Box Jenkins Furnace -2 input -	296	-
2. Box Jenkins Furnace -6 input	296	-
3. The heating system	300	500
4. Mackey-Glass Time series prediction	1000	1000
5. Nonlinear Dynamic System Identification.	200	200
6. Three-Input Nonlinear Function	216	125
7. Two-Input Nonlinear Sinc Function	121	121
8. Currency exchange rate prediction	3000	1281
9. The pH neutralization process	1300	1300
10. Static Function Approximation-1 input	200	200
See Gang (2003) and Gang et al., (2004) and references therein for details		
✧⅄ 1-step ahead EEG Prediction (2 tests)	6000	10500

not maintain good accuracy and low structural complexity in applications where this is required. To verify how techniques referred to as *evolving fuzzy* approaches compare to the SOFNN, the well known Evolving Fuzzy Neural Network (EFuNN) (Kasabov, 2003; Kasabov, 2001; Kasabov & Song, 2002) was tested on all the benchmark datasets introduced above. Two versions of the EFuNN (the parameter self tuning version (Kasabov, 2001) and Takagi-Sugeno version (Kasabov & Song, 2002) – Dynamic Evolving Neuro Fuzzy Inference System (DENFIS)) are compared with the SOFNN. The EFuNN and DENFIS methods have been shown to outperform many other evolving and non-evolving approaches. The results are presented in Tables 3, 4 and 5 (Information from Table 1 is reproduced here (as Table 3) for ease of comparison with the SOFNN results – refer to Table IA for data set information). It can be seen that in the ten standard benchmark cases, for both versions of the EFuNN, the structural complexity, in terms of the number of neurons added, is significantly higher than the number obtained with the SOFNN, and yet all the training and testing errors are higher than those obtained with the SOFNN. In terms of training speed, the new version of the SOFNN trains quicker for the first 7 (smaller) datasets and trains quicker than the self-tuning EFuNN on dataset 10 but is slower than the TS-based EFuNN. For datasets 8 and 9 the SOFNN is significantly slower than both versions of the EFuNN. This is due to these being larger datasets that require a greater number of neurons than the other datasets. In these situations the SOFNN algorithm training duration is the longest, due to the necessity to check the structure using more past samples more often (more neurons and more data). The problem does not occur in the EFuNN because it employs a recursive updating procedure however the EFuNN performs much more poorly in terms of accuracy and structural complexity and therefore there is a significant trade-off between speed and accuracy when using the EFuNN.

The main ethos of evolving based approaches is the potential for more rapid evolution of the structure however this advantage does require a substantive tradeoff between performance and training speed. Often, when large datasets are being processed, evolving fuzzy systems have unbounded structural growth and fail to ensure errors are minimized whereas the SOFNN does not exhibit these problems. The SOFNN algorithm employs a global learning approach and uses past data to ensure optimal performance. These methods are more computationally demanding than local learning approaches involving continuous recursive parameter estimates such as those employed in the EFuNN and the Evolving TS approach (Angelov & Filev, 2004, Kasabov, 2001) however it is clear that the best performance in terms of accuracy and structural complexity is

Table 3. (Table 1 reproduced). Modified SOFNN accuracy, complexity and training times

D*	N*	Train Error [RMSE]	Test Error [RMSE]	New Time [s]
1	4	0.362	-	0.17
2	8	0.210	-	0.38
3	4	0.311	1.197	0.19
4	5	0.016	0.017	1.95
5	5	0.005	0.004	0.13
6	10	0.212	0.295	0.25
7	11	0.069	0.101	0.11
8	25	0.027	0.018	112
9	11	0.027	0.027	15.4
10	8	0.006	0.007	0.33
✧	**13**	**0.009**	**0.009**	**322**
✧	**Test Time = 1.01s**			
⅄	**20**	**0.009**	**0.009**	**926**
⅄	**Test Time = 1.50s**			

*Data type ★Neuron Numbers ✧ sEEG simple ⅄ cEEG complex See Table 2 for details

Table 4. Evolving fuzzy neural network with parameter self-tuning

D*	N*	Train Error [RMSE]	Test Error [RMSE]	Train Time [s]
1	107	0.633	-	0.69
2	179	1.025	-	1.03
3	29	3.494	11.25	0.39
4	306	0.038	0.022	5.98
5	74	0.291	0.010	0.50
6	204	1.497	0.827	0.73
7	91	0.113	0.070	0.23
8	535	0.029	0.024	30.33
9	80	0.177	0.108	2.70
10	50	0.305	0.088	0.42
✧	**1581**	**0.018**	**0.017**	**218**
✧	**Test Time = 789**			
⅄	**1628**	**0.020**	**0.017**	**220**
⅄	**Test Time = 779**			

*Data type ★Neuron Numbers ✧ sEEG simple ⅄ cEEG complex See Table 2 for details

Table 5. Evolving fuzzy neural network Takagi Sugeno

D*	N#	Train Error [RMSE]	Test Error [RMSE]	Train Time [s]
1	85	0.438	-	0.64
2	147	0.483	-	1.08
3	29	3.494	11.25	0.38
4	232	0.021	0.009	5.55
5	24	0.120	0.092	0.27
6	165	0.908	0.330	0.77
7	59	0.123	0.095	0.20
8	931	0.065	0.046	53.75
9	33	0.124	0.099	1.52
10	38	0.279	0.098	0.28
✧	**1811**	**0.017**	**0.016**	**240**
✧	**Test Time = 562**			
⅄	**1794**	**0.018**	**0.017**	**238**
⅄	**Test Time = 500**			

*Data type ★Neuron Numbers ✧ sEEG simple ⅄cEEG complex See Table 2 for details

not ensured with local learning and continuous recursive update of the consequent parameters. The question must be posed – is the issue of online training speed critically important? Obviously this depends on the application but it is unlikely that many applications have such fast changing dynamics that require algorithms to be updated on every sample and within the sampling interval. To investigate the implications of training speed, the EEG datasets with 6000 training exemplars and 10,500 testing exemplars were employed.

As can be seen from Tables 3, 4 and 5 both versions of the EFuNN evolve a substantial number of neurons to cluster this dataset even though the error level is significantly higher than the SOFNN i.e., an order of magnitude higher for both the training and testing datasets. This performance differentiation can be attributed to the recursive nature of the algorithm which does result in faster training in some cases, as can be seen from Table 3, 4, and 5 but has shortcomings when robustly ensuring accuracy and structural complexity are optimal. It must be noted that, for the EEG dataset, the SOFNN requires an average of 323s/6,000≈54ms to organize the structure after each exemplar enters the network during training for the SOFNN whereas the TS-based EFuNN requires ~37ms to update the structure. If either algorithm had to adapt to the EEG signal at the rate of the sampling interval which is 8ms (125 Hz sampling), then both would be incapable. The above timings are based on MATLAB® m-files (Matlab, 2009) and therefore could be improved dramatically by encoding the algorithm in C or C-mex using MATLAB Simulink as described in (Coyle, 2006; Guger, 1999) or writing code so that it can be distributed across multiple computing cores..

Notably however, there is a significant issue in relation to the testing of the EFuNN when between 1,500 and 1,800 neurons are added and the dataset is large – the EFuNN requires ~8–10min to process the test data whereas the SOFNN requires 1-1.5s. This is a significant difference and the main cause of the EFuNNs time overhead is the structural complexity – for every exemplar of testing data the distance between each data exemplar and the 1628 clusters for the self-tuning EFuNN (1,794 clusters for the TS based–EFuNN)(cEEG dataset) must be calculated using a Euclidean metric. This is done to determine which local cluster the exemplar belongs to and require a lot of calculations. In the SOFNN the firing strength of each Gaussian MF neuron is calculated using multiplicative and summation terms for each of the 20 neurons added for each data exemplar and is therefore much more efficient in this respect. Based on the above figures, the Self Tuning–EFuNN would require (~13min)/10,500≈74ms to process one data exemplar which is a considerable duration for network testing. Again, however, the problem may be alleviated using more efficient programming languages but this analysis does illustrate a shortcoming with local recursive learning and unbounded structural complexity.

To summarize, this section presents results that show the accuracy and structural complexity of the SOFNN compares favorably to other evolving fuzzy system approaches although there is trade-off in training speed however; the results demonstrate that this trade-off is justified.

Time-Delayed Synapses for Locally Recurrent Learning

To determine if the time time-delayed synapses that were added to the architecture of the SOFNN for locally recurrent learning improved overall performance in certain conditions the following tests were performed:

1. Predicting the Mackey-Glass and the Currency exchange rate prediction data using only one input at time t *i.e.,* $\hat{x}(t+\pi)=f(x(t))$. Results using the SOFNN with and without recurrent synapses are compared and results are analyzed for the case where 4 past inputs with time lags of 6 sample instances are used to predict the Mackey-Glass data 6 steps ahead (Δ=4, τ=6, π =6 in (13)) and for the currency data Δ=4, τ=1 and π =6 .
2. Using the cEEG set described above, 1 step ahead prediction tests were carried out on all four channels (C3 and C4, left and right motor imagery) referred to as l3, l4, r3 and r4 with Δ=1 and π =1 (cf. EEG Data Acquisition section). The training set contained 600 training exemplars for each signal and the test set contained 10500 testing exemplars. To ensure that the newly proposed learning procedure for training the feedback weights is in fact finding a good estimate for the feedback weights, a range of tests were carried out where η was standardized across all neurons and an iterative search was conducted with η incremented by 0.01 for each check in the range 0-1. The iteration that produced the best performance was benchmarked against accuracy obtained using the SOFNN without recurrent synapses and with recurrent synapses where the firing strength aggregation method for updating the recurrent synapse weights is used.

The results for the currency exchange data and Mackey-Glass data are presented in Table 5.The results for the currency data indicate that there is no real benefit in employing a recurrent connection for this data in terms of overall accuracy or structural compactness, even when only one input is being used i.e., the training and testing errors with and without recurrent connections are more or less equal. However, it is also shown that when using Δ=6 and τ=1 the result on the training data is only marginally better, the testing result is significantly worse and there are 11 neurons added to the network. This indicates that this data is overfitted using Δ=6 and τ=1 and this could be due the hyperparameters of the network being selected incorrectly or that the embedding dimension and lag chosen for this are not suitable. Nevertheless, the purpose of this analysis was to determine if the SOFNN with recurrent connections could provide better accuracy at Δ=1 and in this case it is no worse or better that the SOFNN without recurrent connections.

For the Mackey-Glass data which is significantly more complex that the currency data there is clear benefit in employing the recurrent connections when Δ=1 where the training and testing errors are an order of magnitude lower than performance obtained with no recurrent connections. The structural complexity is increased by 2 neurons. This is a significant indication that the recurrent connections updated using the aggregate firing information can significantly improve performance when the embedding Δ dimension is not tuned, and in this case the task is to predict 6 steps ahead. Using Δ=1 the

SOFNN with recurrent connections does not however match the performance of a carefully chosen Δ=4 and τ=6 for this prediction task although this choice of setup needs to be determined

Table 5. The accuracy and complexity of the SOFNN with/without recurrent synapses for the currency and Mackey-Glass data using 1 input. Results using the standard setup with no recurrent connections are also reproduced here for comparison

Setup	N*	Train Error [RMSE]	Test Error [RMSE]	Train Time [s]
Currency Data				
woRecur	3	0.028	0.018	97.81
wRecur	3	0.028	0.018	86.56
Δ=6, τ=1*	11	0.027	0.027	212.19
Mackey-Glass Data				
woRecur	7	0.172	0.175	180.86
wRecur	9	0.083	0.088	179.39
Δ=4, τ=6*	5	0.016	0.017	7.86

✧ η was optimized iteratively using a single weight value for all neurons η=0.32, 0.33, 0.35, 0.09 for l3, l4, r3, and r4, respectively *Neurons *Without Recurrent Connections

based on error tolerance and constraints. For example, considering the plots of test performance for each of the three setups shown in Figure 6(a) it can be seen that the predictions using the standard setup with no recurrent connections are very accurate. In Figure 6(b) it can be seen that the prediction accuracy with recurrent connection and Δ=1 the prediction accuracy is poorer although the dynamics of the signals are tracked and depending on the objectives of the application the error may be tolerable. From Figure 6(c) it can be seen that the SOFNN with no recurrent connections is unable to predict the highest and lowest amplitude signal dynamics using Δ=1. This type of error may not be tolerable and emphasizes the importance of the newly incorporated recurrent synapses in the SOFNN and the proposed learning strategy for updating the synaptic weights when it is desirable not to spend time selecting embedding, Δ, and time delay, τ, parameters to suit the data. It must be noted the training times here are presented for consistency but in these analysis the new code for incorporating the recurrent synapses was not optimized (different setups where coded altogether with flag checks to determine which setup would be tested on a particular run) and many tests were running concurrently therefore the training times do not truly reflect the performance for the SOFNN with recurrent synapses.

The results obtained for the EEG using the SOFNN with and without recurrent connections are presented in Table 6 where 4 different EEG time series where predicted 1 step ahead using Δ=1 with and without recurrent synapses. It can be clearly seen that there is an improvement in the prediction performance for all time series when the recurrent modification is utilized. In some cases the improvement is marginal whilst in other cases there is a significant gain, particularly for the r4 data. This again is evidence that the recurrent synapse and training method is a significant advancement to the SOFNN algorithm.

As outlined, to ensure that the proposed recurrent weight learning approach was in fact improving the performance to the network by optimizing the weights and the results are not simply an enhancement given by the feedback structure i.e., that could be attained by random weights or iteratively selected weights, results from a range of iterative tests were analyzed. The results for the best performing η for each of the 4 EEG times series when η is selected uniformly for all neurons are also presented in Table 6. The results clearly show that the performance with the automated online recurrent weight learning process based on aggregate neuron firing strengths produced identical results to the iterative search of the training data, and produced a better average generalization performance on the test data (0.062 vs 0.07). This indicates that the proposed learning procedure is an effective approach for learning the feedback weights. It must also be noted that the iterative learning procedure requires multiple

Table 6. The accuracy and complexity of SOFNN with/without recurrent synapses for the EEG data using 1 input. Results from the newly proposed aggregated firing strength update method are shown along with an iterative test for comparison

EEG	N*	Train Error [RMSE]	Test Error [RMSE]	Train Time [s]
SOFNN without Recurrent Synapses				
l3	2	0.016	0.015	548
l4	2	0.013	0.013	385
r3	2	0.015	0.014	412
r4	3	0.015	0.071	439
SOFNN with Recurrent Synapses Aggregate Firing Strength Updating				
l3	2	0.014	0.013	800
l4	2	0.012	0.012	583
r3	2	0.013	0.014	657
r4	3	0.012	0.023	734
SOFNN with Recurrent Synapses Iterative Search Updating				
l3✧	2	0.014	0.013	346
l4	2	0.012	0.011	192
r3	2	0.013	0.013	169
r4	3	0.012	0.033	183
✧ η was optimized iteratively using a single weight value for all neurons η=0.32, 0.33, 0.35, 0.09 for l3, l4, r3, and r4, respectively, *Neurons				

runs through the data in batch mode and is not suitable for online training therefore; would not be appositely suited to the characteristics of the online learning and self-organizing characteristics of the SOFNN algorithm. This iterative tests was used here for comparative and verification purposes only.

FUTURE RESEARCH DIRECTIONS

A modified learning algorithm which involves storing the most recent neuron firing strength information for previously clustered input data and using this information to check the network more efficiently as training progresses has been shown to significantly enhance the computational efficiency of the SOFNN. The results show that the processing times are reduced by more than 70% for EEG data and significant training time reductions can also be observed on ten different well known benchmark tests. The SOFNN compares favorably to many other fuzzy neural network algorithms in terms of performance and structural complexity. To reduce the training times further, different local learning and recursive based updating strategies will be investigated. The SOFNN employs a global learning strategy however, if a local learning strategy was employed, the consequent parameters of each rule/neuron could be trained separately from the others. Methods such as those described in (Angelov & Filev, 2004; Birattari et al., 2009; Kasabov, 2001; Kasabov & Song, 2002; Kasabov, 2003; Lughofer & Klement, 2005; may be employed for local learning however, as shown in this study, even though recursive and local learning methods can be trained faster, they do lack in performance and can result in increased structural complexity therefore, when accuracy is paramount, the global semi-recursive learning algorithm of the SOFNN may be the best approach.

In terms of the new recurrent feedback synapses which have been added to the SOFNN architectures, the results have clearly demonstrated the benefits of this addition when working under certain data constraints. For example, if there is need to deploy the algorithms to a prediction task without knowing the optimal embedding dimension or time delay a priori or in the case where the dynamics of the data change and thus the optimal embedding dimension and time lag are non-stationary, these recurrent connections in the SOFNN can significantly improve performance. Even though it has been shown and observed that choosing the optimal embedding dimension and lag, perhaps using an iterative approach, would provide the most accurate predictions, normally, there is a significant advantage in incorporating temporal behavior in the SOFNN. Further work will involve improving this recurrent architecture and online recurrent weight leaning approach to accommodate possibly more delayed connections for each neuron and/or determining if the performance using a standard embedding dimension and time delay for a particular dataset can be improved using additional information provided by the recurrent feedback connections. It is unclear if the proposed aggregate firing strength approach to feedback weights learning would produce better performance in this situation but these are topic of future research. It must also be noted that the recurrent weight learning approach may suffer from some shortcomings such as, when the number of neurons grows, the feedback synapses get weaker for an individual neuron whilst when there are only a low number of neurons the feedback connections will be strong. This is due to the normalization process. This could possibly be improved by introducing another weighting parameter which provides further scaling of the weights so that feedback connections remain reasonably consistent throughout the learning process yet proportional to the firing strength of each neuron.

For further improvement, if it was necessary or desirable to make the feedback synapse more reactive to local data than data in the distant past then η could be updated using only firing strength information from a local window of past data. Both these options would introduce additional hyperparameters into the SOFNN algorithm and structure which is undesirable however these options may have some potential to enhance performance and will be investigated. In addition, a sensitivity analysis of the SOFNN hyperparameters such as that described in (Coyle et al., 2006; 2009; Rizzi et al., 2006) will be conducted in conjunction with modified recurrent feedback structure. In Rizzi et al., (2006) a method to measure the automaticity of an algorithm by relying on its sensitivity to the training parameters is described i.e., a sensitivity analysis. The goal is to find how sensitive the performance is to changes in the predefined parameters. For example, if a slight change in a parameter, θ_i, results in a significant change in the prediction error and/or structural complexity, then this parameter is critical and requires considered selection. The five SOFNN parameters that can be predefined are the error tolerance (δ), the desired training RMSE of the network (k_{rmse}), the distance threshold vector (k_d), the initial width vector (σ_0) and the error tolerance multiplier (λ). All these parameters are standard among many evolving fuzzy algorithms and in many cases are not analyzed in great detail. The selection of these types of parameters is often carried out arbitrarily or expert knowledge is used and therefore these parameters are often neglected or not identified as predefined. Although, results from a sensitivity analysis have been utilized to determine a good set of parameters for predicting motor imagery altered EEG signals using the SOFNN algorithms, the hyperparameters were not tuned during specific test of the modified recurrent feedback structure. This could have a significant impact on performance. Further work will involve ensuring that the hyperparameters of the SOFNN, which govern accuracy and structural complexity, (including any additional parameters introduced due to new modifications such as those proposed above) are analyzed in line with specific modifications however, the results presented here show that even without detailed analysis of the hyperparameters after the recurrent structure modification, the SOFNN still performs well indicating its potential to learn and self-organize in an autonomous fashion.

In this sense the topic of research presented in this chapter is specifically aligned with the motivations for this book and in thematic areas such as learning analogies for neural systems, sensing-acting-learning aspects of biological systems and biologically-inspired learning and intelligent system modeling. The work is biologically inspired in some sense and in terms of biological plausibility the newly proposed structure learning approach may be more apposite because neurons in the brain may not be presented with the same data twice but biological characteristics in the neuron store information related to firing strength for stimuli which initially inherited that neuron for processing i.e., analogous to firing strength memorization in the SOFNN. Self-organization occurs at many levels in the nervous system and recurrent synapses and connections are highly likely to perform an important role in the learning and self-organizing process of the brain (Bubic et al., (2010) therefore the addition of recurrent synapses in the SOFNN is a logical step towards enhancing its self-organizing and learning capacity and therefore, on a high level the SOFNN exhibits some characteristics of the biological brain but the finer details are far from being biologically plausible. The general definition of self-organization is the process by which the internal organization of a system increases in complexity without being guided or managed by an outside source. The system can, and must, receive external signals (inputs and queues), but the management of the system, based on those signals, is totally internal. This work has shown that the SOFNN conforms to this definition of a self-organizing system and that the proposed modifications have enhanced its potential for improved autonomy.Further work will involve investigating the biological processes which equip the human brain with it's unique capacity to sense, perceive and learn in its environment, autonomously, and drawing inspiration from this to inform new developments in the SOFNN.

CONCLUSION

This chapter clearly shows the approximation power of the self-organizing fuzzy neural network (SOFNN) in a range of prediction and function approximation applications. The SOFNN has been previously shown to outperform other well known fuzzy neural networks and this work has illustrated its capacity to outperform an Evolving Fuzzy Neural Network which has previously been proved to perform better than range of other evolving fuzzy approaches in the literature. The main emphasis of this work was to show that a newly proposed learning approach involving the storing of firing strength information can be used to enhance the network training speed and that the online learning of recurrent feedback weights which have been newly introduced to the SOFNN learning structure can improve the automaticity of the algorithm. The results show that these modifications to the SOFNN do impact on training speed and that the learning algorithm for the recurrent feedback weights can be used to train the new structure and improve network performance and autonomy. A range of directions for future research have been identified to improve the SOFNN further.

REFERENCES

Angelov, P. P., & Filev, D. (2004). An approach to online identification of Takagi-Sugeno fuzzy models, *IEEE Trans. on Systems, Man and Cybernetics*, part B, *34*(1), 484-498.

Astrom, K. J., & Wittenmark, B. (1995). *Adaptive Control* (2nd ed.). Reading, MA: Addison-Wesley.

Birattari, M., Bontempi, G., & Bersini, H. (1999). *Lazy learning meets the recursive least-squares algorithm, Advances in Neural Information Processing Systems 11* (Kearns, M. S., Solla, S. A., & Cohn, D. A., Eds.). Cambridge: MIT Press.

Bubic, A., von Cramon, D. Y., & Schubotz, R. I. (2010), Prediction, cognition and the brain, *Frontiersin Journal, 4, 12 pages*

Buckley, J. J., & Hayashi. (1994). Fuzzy Neural Networks: A survey. *Fuzzy Sets and Systems*, *66*, 1–13. doi:10.1016/0165-0114(94)90297-6

Budik, D., & Elhanany, I. (2006, August). TRTRL: A localized resource efficient learning algorithm for recurrent neural networks. In *Proc. IEEE Midwest Symp. Circuits Syst.*, (pp. 371–374).

Coyle, D. (2006). *Intelligent Preprocessing and Feature Extraction Techniques for a Brain Computer Interface*, Unpublished Doctoral Dissertation, University of Ulster, UK.

Coyle, D. (2009). Neural network based auto association and time-series prediction for biosignal processing in brain-computer interfaces. *IEEE Computational Intelligence Magazine*, *4*(4), 47–59. doi:10.1109/MCI.2009.934560

Coyle, D., Prasad, G., & McGinnity (2006). Enhancing autonomy and computational efficiency of the self-organizing fuzzy neural network for a brain-computer interface, *FUZZ-IEEE, World Congress on Computational Intelligence*, pp. 10485-10492. Coyle et al., 2006

Coyle, D., Prasad, G., & McGinnity, T. M. (2009). Faster self-organizing fuzzy neural network training and a hyperparameter analysis for a brain-computer interface [Part B]. *IEEE Transactions on Systems, Man, and Cybernetics*, *39*(6), 1458–1471. doi:10.1109/TSMCB.2009.2018469

Er, M. J., & Wu, S. (2002). A fast learning algorithm for parsimonious fuzzy neural systems. *Fuzzy Sets and Systems*, *126*, 337–351. doi:10.1016/S0165-0114(01)00034-3

Fisch, B. J. (1999). *Fisch & Spellmann's EEG Primer: Basic principles of digital and analog EEG*. New York: Elsevier.

Gonzalez, J., Rojas, I., Pomares, H., Ortega, J., & Prieto, A. (2002). A new clustering technique for function approximation. *IEEE Transactions on Neural Networks*, *13*, 132–142. doi:10.1109/72.977289

Guger, C. (1999). *Real-time Data Processing Under Windows for an EEG-based Brain-Computer Interface*, Unpublished Doctoral Dissertation, Technical University Graz, Austria

Hassibi, B., & Stork, D. G. (1993). Second order derivatives for network pruning: Optimal brain surgeon. *Advances in Neural Information Processing Systems*, *4*, 164–171.

Huang, G. B., Saratchandran, P., & Sundararajan, N. (n.d.). An efficient sequential learning algorithm for growing and pruning RBFNs, *IEEE Transactions on Systems, Man and Cybernetics, Part B*, *34*(6).

Jang, J.-S. R. (1993). ANFIS: Adaptive-network-based fuzzy inference system. *IEEE Transactions on Systems, Man, and Cybernetics*, *23*, 665–685. doi:10.1109/21.256541

Jang, J.-S. R., Sun, C.-T., & Mizutani, E. (1997). *Neuro-Fuzzy & Soft Computing*. Upper-Saddle River, NJ: Prentice Hall.

Juang, C. F. (2002). A TSK-type recurrent fuzzy network for dynamic systems processing by neural network and genetic algorithms. *IEEE Transactions on Fuzzy Systems*, *10*(2), 155–170. doi:10.1109/91.995118

Juang, C. F., & Hsieh, C. D, (In Press). A locally recurrent fuzzy neural network with support vector regression for dynamic system modelling, *IEEE Transactions on Fuzzy Systems*, Kasabov, N. K. (2001). Evolving Fuzzy Neural Networks for Supervised/Unsupervised Online Knowledge-Based Learning, *IEEE Transactions on Systems, Man, and Cybernetics, 31*(6), 902-918.

Juang, C. F., & Lin, C. T. (1999). A recurrent self-organising neural fuzzy inference network. *IEEE Transactions on Neural Networks*, *10*(4), 829–845.

Kasabov, N. K. (2003). *Evolving connectionist systems: methods and applications in bioinformatics*. New York: Springer.

Kasabov, N. K., & Song, Q. (2002). DENFIS: Dynamic evolving neural-fuzzy inference system and its application for time-series prediction. *IEEE Transactions on Fuzzy Systems*, *10*(2), 144–154. doi:10.1109/91.995117

Klawonn, F., & Keller, A. (1998). Grid clustering for generating fuzzy rules. *European Congress on Intelligent Techniques and Soft Computing*, 1365-1369.

Lee, C. C. (1990). Fuzzy logic in control systems: Fuzzy logic controller – Part I and II. *IEEE Transactions on Systems, Man, and Cybernetics*, *20*, 404–435. doi:10.1109/21.52551

Leng, G. (2003). *Algorithmic Developments for Self-Organizing Fuzzy Neural Networks*, (Unpublished doctoral dissertation), University of Ulster, UK.

Leng, G., Prasad, G., & McGinnity, T. M. (2004). An on-line algorithm for creating self-organising fuzzy neural networks. *Neural Networks*, *17*(10), 1477–1493. doi:10.1016/j.neunet.2004.07.009

Leung, C. S., Wong, K. W., Sum, P. F., & Chan, L. W. (2001). A pruning method for the recursive least squared algorithm. *Neural Networks*, *14*, 147–174. doi:10.1016/S0893-6080(00)00093-9

Lughofer, E., & Klement, E. P. (2005). FLEXFIS: A Variant for Incremental Learning of Takagi-Sugeno Fuzzy Systems. In. *Proceedings of FUZZ-IEEE, 2005*, 915–920.

Mamdani, E. H., & S. Assilian. (2008). An experiment in linguistic synthesis with a fuzzy logic controller. *International Journal of Man-Machine Studies, 7*(1), 1:13

Mascioli, F. M. F., & Martinelli, G. (1998). A constructive approach to neuro-fuzzy networks. *Signal Processing*, *64*, 347–358. doi:10.1016/S0165-1684(97)00200-4

Mascioli, F. M. F., Rizzi, A., Panella, M., & Martinelli, G. (2000). Scale-based approach to hierarchical fuzzy clustering. *Signal Processing*, *80*, 1001–1016. doi:10.1016/S0165-1684(00)00016-5

Matlab, (2009), *The Mathworks website*. Retrieved August 15, 2009 from http://www.mathworks.com

Mitra, S., & Hayashi, Y. (2000). Neuro-fuzzy rule generation: Survey in soft computing framework. *IEEE Transactions on Neural Networks*, *11*, 748–768. doi:10.1109/72.846746

Nauck, D. (1997). Neuro-fuzzy systems: Review and prospects. In *Proc. Fifth European Congress on Intelligent Techniques and Soft Computing*, 1044-1053.

Nauck, D., & Kruse, R. (1999). Neuro-fuzzy systems for function approximation. *Fuzzy Sets and Systems*, *101*, 261–271. doi:10.1016/S0165-0114(98)00169-9

Pearlmutter, B. A. (1995). Gradient calculations for dynamic recurrent neural networks: A survey. *IEEE Transactions on Neural Networks*, *6*, 1212–1228. doi:10.1109/72.410363

Pfurtscheller, G., Neuper, C., Schlogl, A., & Lugger, K. (1998). Separability of EEG signals recorded during right and left motor imagery using adaptive autoregressive parameters. *IEEE Transactions on Rehabilitation Engineering*, *6*(3), 316–324. doi:10.1109/86.712230

Prasad, G., McGinnity, T. M., Leng, G., & Coyle, D. (2010). On-line identification of self-organizing fuzzy neural networks for modelling time-varying complex systems. In Plamen, (Eds.), *Evolving Intelligent Systems* (pp. 302–324). New York: John Wiley. doi:10.1002/9780470569962.ch9

Rizzi, A., Panella, M., & Maxioli, F. M. F. (2002). Adaptive resolution of min-max classifiers. *IEEE Transactions on Neural Networks*, *13*(2), 402–414. doi:10.1109/72.991426

Schlogl, A., & Pfurtscheller, G. (2005). *Graz dataset IIIb description for the BCI 2005 data classification competition*. Retrieved October 14, 2005 from http://ida.first.fhg.de/projects/bci/competition_iii/desc_IIIb.pdf

Simpson, P. K. (1992). Fuzzy min-max neural networks-Part 1: Classification. *IEEE Transactions on Neural Networks*, *3*, 776–786. doi:10.1109/72.159066

Simpson, P. K. (1993). Fuzzy min-max neural networks-Part 1: Clustering. *IEEE Transactions on Fuzzy Systems*, *1*, 32–45. doi:10.1109/TFUZZ.1993.390282

Sugeno, M., & Kang, G. T. (1988). Structure identification of fuzzy model. *Fuzzy Sets and Systems*, *28*(15), 33.

Takagi, T., & Sugeno, M. (1983). Derivation of fuzzy control rules from human operator's control action, *Proc. of the IFAC Symp. on Fuzzy Info., Knowledge Rep. and Decision Analysis*, (pp. 55-60).

Takagi, T., & Sugeno, M. (1985). Fuzzy identification of systems and its applications to modeling and control. *IEEE Transactions on Systems, Man, and Cybernetics*, *15*, 116–132.

Tsukamoto, Y. (1979). An approach to fuzzy reasoning method. In Gupta, M. M., Ragade, R. K., & Yager, R. R. (Eds.), *Advances in Fuzzy Set Theory and Applications* (pp. 137–149). Amsterdam: North-Holland.

Wang, J. S., & Lee, C. S. G. (2001). Efficient neuro-fuzzy control systems for autonomous underwater vehicle control. *Proc. of 2001 IEEE Int'l Conf. on Robotics and Automation*, 2986-2991.

Wang, L. X. (1992). Fuzzy systems are universal approximators. In *Proc. Int. Conf. Fuzzy Syst.*, 1163-1170, 1992.

Wang, W. J. (1997). New similarity measures on fuzzy sets and on elements. *Fuzzy Sets and Systems*, *85*, 305–309. doi:10.1016/0165-0114(95)00365-7

Williams, G. P. (1997). *Chaos Theory Tamed*. London: Taylor and Francis.

Wu, S., & Er, M. J. (2000). Dynamic fuzzy neural networks-a novel approach to function approximation. *IEEE Transactions on Systems, Man, and Cybernetics. Part B, Cybernetics*, *30*(2), 358–364. doi:10.1109/3477.836384

Wu, S., Er, M. J., & Gao, Y. (2001). A fast approach for automatic generation of fuzzy rules by generalized dynamic fuzzy neural networks. *IEEE Transactions on Fuzzy Systems*, *9*, 578–594. doi:10.1109/91.940970

Zadeh, L. A. (1965). Fuzzy sets. *Information and Control*, *8*, 338–353. doi:10.1016/S0019-9958(65)90241-X

Zadeh, L. A. (1994). *Soft computing and fuzzy logic*. IEEE Soft.

KEY TERMS AND DEFINITIONS

SOFNN: Self-organizing fuzzy neural network.

Recurrent Feedback Connection: Self connected neuron, one recurrent synapse with one feedback weight.

Electroencephalogram (EEG): Electrical potential of the brain measured using electrodes placed on the scalp.

FIS: Fuzzy inference system.

Takagi-Sugeno-Kang (TSK) Fuzzy Models: Most common type of fuzzy inference system time series - a sequence of numbers collected at regular intervals over a period of time.

Embedding Dimension: The number of past samples plus the current sample used in time series prediction.

Time Lag: The delay between samples used for prediction in a time series prediction.

Time-Series Prediction: The use of a model to predict future events based on known past events: to predict future data points before they are measured.

Recursive LSE: Least squared which can be updated online recursively as new data sammples become available.

Optimal Brain Surgeon (OBS): A technique used to check the significance of a neuron based on 2nd derivative information, if the neuron's contribution to the network is found to be insignificant it can be deleted.

Hybrid Fuzzy Neural Network (FNN): A neural network which is designed to approximate a fuzzy inference systems through the structure of neural networks and thus create a more accurate, efficient and interpretable hybrid neural network model, making effective use of the superior learning ability of neural networks and ease of interpretability of fuzzy systems.

Chapter 9
Biologically-Inspired Learning and Intelligence:
Analog Circuit Design with Fuzzy Inference

Turgay Temel
Bahcesehir University, Istanbul, Turkey

ABSTRACT

Since biologically-inspired intelligent systems with learning and decision-making capabilities vastly act upon comparison among inputs, the ability to select those inputs which satisfy certain conditions is of great significance in realization of such systems. Moreover intelligent systems need to operate with concurrency so as to reflect inherited capability of their biological counterparts like human. Due to difficulties in programmability, storage and design complexities, the analog implementation has been considerably less favored in most computational information processing systems. However, in the case of biologically-inspired computation, their suitability for concurrency, accuracy and capability in simulating the natural behavior of biological signals, analog neural information processing is regarded an attractive solution. Benefiting the full advantage involves comprehensive understanding and knowledge of what trade-offs can be established with design topologies available and theoretical necessities. On the other hand, fuzzy reasoning offers rule-based inferential manipulation on inputs where it expresses the input-output relationship in terms of clauses. Considering a nonlinear operation carried out by artificial neural networks based on experience, realization of rule-based clauses is much easier. This chapter introduces fundamental notions of fuzzy reasoning, and fuzzy-based analog design approaches. Rather than resorting on analytical derivation for the architecture of interest, the main focus is directed at suitability for use, which is expected to indicate possibility toward developing complex intelligent systems. It should be noted that the circuits having selectivity property in deciding maximum and/or minimum on inputs demonstrate their use in much broader field than inference, thus they have great importance in realization of information processing systems. The chapter presents a very compact selectivity circuit as decision maker for the minimum of its inputs. Further to it, a considerably simple yet elaborate membership structure is introduced. The circuit simplifies the fuzzy controller design. Since mostly decision making is performed on a (dis)similarity measure between inputs, e.g. the input and label patterns for

DOI: 10.4018/978-1-60960-018-1.ch009

respective categories, it is convenient to express the proximity in terms of a metric. The chapter also introduces important designs proposed for assessing the similarity in the Euclidean distance.

INTRODUCTION

Vast information processing capability of biological structures consists in immense parallelism and high-level of adaptability. The artificial systems and circuits which mimic such diversity obviously should rely on their natural counterparts so that most possible sources can be learned and identified appropriately. It is also this diversity which makes the mimicking difficult in implementation. Despite considerable progress in research on theoretical aspects of neural information processing, the implementation of biologically-inspired systems is not moving forward at the same pace and it is still undergoing design shortcomings.

Despite programmability, easy maintenance and continuously increasing speed of information processing with digital realization, efficiency for biological inspiration still needs better parallel processing capability for commuting between experiential knowledge, (Bezdek, Keller, Krisnapuram, & Pal, 2005; Kasabov, 2009). In most digital implementations, decision-making among a number of choices mainly relies on successive sub-operations, which is not coherent with adaptivity and intelligence. Such an objective can be accomplished with analog paradigm rather than pursuing sequential algorithms in digital computation. Furthermore, analog design has the capability in mimicking biological stimuli more inherently and naturally than digital approach.

Nevertheless, analog circuit realization for decision–making with processing stimuli has two major drawbacks: design difficulties and representation of compound features embedded in the quantity to be dealt with, (Toumazou, Ligey, & Haigh, 1990). The former involves consideration of design nonlinearities with active components while the latter requires complicated structures to be projected onto highly nonlinear interconnected blocks, (Gottarredona, & Barranco, 2006). Major decision-making circuit blocks can be efficiently implemented in analog approach with almost predictable electrical and physical performance characteristics. Depending on the design quantity, i.e. current or voltage, design difficulties can be overcome significantly, which makes it suitable for attaining highly parallel decision-making operation.

Fuzzy logic (FL) or reasoning is an expert system approach which envisages human thinking and reasoning rather than being nonlinear analytical derivation. The rule-based inferential approach taken up by FL can be regarded a very handy tool to tackle major shortcomings concerning programmability and accuracy. Thus, FL has a considerable precedence to most other biologically-inspired design approaches. Thus, it can play a significant role in realization and implementation of intelligent systems combined with prominence of analog design availabilities.

Considerable studies on design of analog decision-making and associative inference fall into category in evaluating the membership of the input to certain pattern groups, (Lin, & Shi, 1999). Fuzzy-associative rules and membership functions are solid means of expressing possible association in terms of simple reasoning mechanism similar to human thinking. Thus, analog fuzzy design is an attractive candidate to develop systems operating intelligently. Analog inferential circuit design studies based on FL descriptions diversify in representing the design quantity, i.e. voltage or current. The current-mode design as will be shown brings in superiority compared to voltage-mode. With current-mode design, it is possible consider larger number of class labels to be attributed to concurrent (possibly sensory input) stimuli as well as design simplicity and suitability to merge nonlinearity to desired characteristics,

(Shirai, Ueno, & Inoue, 2007). If suitable *rule-mapping* between input and output quantities (even of large dimensionality) is formed it will be possible to implement complicated classifiers in simple and compact circuits, (Temel, 2009; Panella, & Martinelli, 2007).

Since membership refers to similarity to stationary characteristics of ensembles such as first-order statistics of stochastic variables of interest the circuits associated to computing it also need to be investigated in terms of pre-specified metrics. In most cases, (Euclidean) distance is used for assessing the similarity metric. Depending on the design quantity, especially in current-mode, compact and suitable metric-based designs for large number of inputs are possible, (Popa, 2005).

In this chapter, well-known analog voltage and current-mode fuzzy reasoning and metric circuits are presented. They are evaluated for their performance. Their pros and cons in realizing the desired functionality, such as fuzzification and/or defuzzification, and decision-making operations are pointed out. A recent, compact looser-take-all MINIMUM (LTA-MIN) circuit proposed in (Temel, 2008, 2) is also presented. The circuit requires only two transistors per input depending on the adopted configuration. It is shown to be an exact dual of the Lazzaro's well-known winner-take-all MAXIMUM (WTA-MAX) circuit, (Lazzaro, Rykebusch, Mahowald, & Mead, 1989). By combining both, it is possible to develop highly versatile architectures including a compact membership circuit, (Temel, 2009). They are compared to previous designs. The proposed *membership function circuit* (MFC) is utilized in a fuzzy classification structure for seven labels. It should be noted that the circuits provided are also applicable to other neural information processing schemes. In addition to inference circuits, some important distance circuit blocks are also discussed to complete fundamental neural information processing topologies in analog design.

BASIC DEFINITIONS

Expert systems are descriptive algorithms for manipulating *inference rules* with *logical implications* which associate *actions* to *conditions* by means of *symbolic representations*. Symbols represent *thinking* or *short-term memory* whereas the relation between symbols models the *long-term memory*. Contrary to learning involving a non-linear dynamics by experience performed by *artificial neural networks*, (ANN), expert systems encompass pre-programmed human thinking (Kosko, 92; Verleysen, 1992). Moreover, where the symbols are not suitable for mathematical treatment, they need to be codified for hardware implementation (Dualibe, Verleysen, & Jespers, 2003). When applied with implications inference rules imply imprecision and uncertainty in a *knowledge base*. In expert systems, the knowledge base simply refers to a dictionary composed of relationships between data, operations, and the rules. For example it is not convenient to categorize measurements of temperature/humidity etc. subject to certain boundaries since they may be interpreted subjectively. Despite the fact that exact categorization may be especially suited to binary-logic circuit implementation, decision-making with labeled categories is not. A possibility to overcome this shortcoming, it will be appropriate to extend the set axioms valid for binary-logic operators to higher-level descriptions with FL notions under the supervision of an expert system. Therefore, as a generalization to well-known binary logic, FL is a supervised technique which processes information with uncertainty-based reasoning, (Zadeh, 1973; Zadeh, 1965).

FL-based systems rely on human reasoning with encoded '*if-then*' rules expressing fuzzy clauses. Each fuzzy clause is composed of a set of rules while each fuzzy rule represents an *action* to be executed when a *condition* is met. Therefore, fuzzy system is a model-free approximation for categorizing input by using a knowledge base with uncertainties represented by *codified labels*.

It is the concept of *fuzzy set theory* which allows numerical processing of information and estimating the source-relevant results with uncertainties. Fuzzy set theory concern itself with *fuzzy sets, fuzzy operators, linguistic variables, fuzzy propositions, linguistic rules,* which leads to *approximate reasoning* to be treated in detail in the following sections.

Fuzzy Sets and Operations

A *set* is a collection of countable or uncountable and discernible objects. The collectivity property of the set determines how to express it. For example the set $A=\{1,3,5,7\}$ can be expressed in terms of characteristic property as $A=\{x| \; x$ is odd integer and $1\leq x\leq 7\}$. The *membership* relation between an object x and a given set A is expressed as $x\in A$ or $x\notin A$. In case an object is described as a member of a set U such that $U=\{x|x\in\exists A_i$ and $\forall A_i\subseteq U\}$ then U is called the *super set* or *universe of discourse*. It is therefore convenient to define a *characteristic function* which assigns x to a subset A_i of U as

$$\mu_{A_i}(x) = \begin{cases} 1 & \text{if } x \in A_i \\ 0 & \text{otherwise} \end{cases} \quad (1)$$

where the function $\mu_{A1}(.)$ is called the *membership function* (MF) in Fuzzy Set Theory. A set with members whose MF is expressed as in Equation (1) is called a *crisp set.*

Besides the crisp set description above, an important aspect of the set theory is the operations on sets and their associated membership functions. Given crisp sets $A_i, A_j \subseteq U$, the following axiomatic operations are defined:

1. *Complement*:
   $\overline{A_i} = \{x \mid x \notin A_i\}, \; \mu_{\overline{A_i}}(x) = 1 - \mu_{A_i}(x)$
2. *Intersection*:
   $A_i \cap A_j = \{x \mid x \in A_i \text{ and } x \in A_j\},$
   $\mu_{A_i \cap A_j}(x) = \min\{\mu_{A_i}(x), \mu_{Aj}(x)\}$
3. *Union*:
   $A_i \cup A_j = \{x \mid x \in A_i \text{ or } x \in A_j\},$
   $\mu_{A_i \cup A_j}(x) = \max\{\mu_{A_i}(x), \mu_{Aj}(x)\}$

Depending on the context, '$\sim A_i$' for complement of A_i, '∧' for '∩' and '∨' for '∪' will be used interchangeably. Above binary operations, i.e. intersection and union, are *commutative, associative, distributive* and also satisfy *DeMorgan's Laws.*

Consider a set $X\subseteq U$ of x, then a *fuzzy set F* is defined on X as a set of pairs $F = \{(x, \mu_F(x) | x \in U)\}$ where $\mu_F: U\rightarrow[0,1]$ is the *fuzzy membership function* (FMF) of x in fuzzy set F, which for every element $x\in X$ assigns a *membership* $\mu_F(x)\in[0,1]$. As can be seen, fuzzy set is a generalized crisp set with softer membership. Similar to those for crisp sets, it is possible to define set-theory axiomatic operations which can then be associated to membership functions as follows:

1. *Complement*: The unary *complement* or *C-norm* of a fuzzy set F defined in U and membership function is given by

$$\overline{F} = \{(x, \mu_{\overline{F}}(x)) \mid x \in U\}$$
$$\text{and } \mu_{\overline{F}}(x) = \neg(\mu_F(x)) = 1 - \mu_F(x) \quad (2)$$

   where '¬' denotes the *fuzzy negation* of a membership function.
2. *Intersection*: For fuzzy sets F_i and F_j defined in U with membership functions $\mu_{Fi}(x)$ and $\mu_{Fj}(x)$, respectively, their *triangular* or *T-norm* intersection fuzzy set and corresponding membership function are given by

$$F_i \cap F_j = \{(x, \mu_{F_i \cap F_j}(x)) \mid x \in U\}$$
$$\text{and } \mu_{F_i \cap F_j(x) =} \mu_{F_i}(x) \wedge \mu_{F_j}(x) \quad (3)$$

where the symbol '∧' denotes fuzzy intersection or 'fuzzy AND'. As it is shown and detailed in (Chen, & Pham, 2001), *T*-norm operators satisfy following conditions:

a. $T(0,1)=T(1,0)=T(0,0)=0$, $T(1,1)=1$
b. $T(x,1)=x$, $\forall x \in [0,1]$
c. $T(x,y)=T(y,x)$, $\forall x, y \in [0,1]$
d. $T(x_1,y) \leq T(x_2,y)$, $\forall x_1, x_2, y \in [0,1]$ and $x_1 \leq x_2$.

where properties (2) through (4) refer to well-known idempotency, commutativity and monotonicity, respectively while (i) is in compliance with Boolean AND in propositional logic. By attributing to interval algebra, it can be shown that Gödel's *T*-norm as $\min(x,y)$, Larsen's *T*-norm as product $x.y$, and Lukasiewicz's *T*-norm in the form of *bounded difference* defined as $\max(x+y-1,0)$ satisfy the above conditions. The resulting membership function for each *T*-norm also preserves respective operator property, i.e. for example for Gödel's min *T*-norm satisfies

$$\mu_{F_i \cap F_j}(x) = \mu_{F_i}(x) \wedge \mu_{Fj}(x) = \min(\mu_{F_i}(x), \mu_{Fj}(x)) \tag{4}$$

and so on.

3. *Union*: Set theoretic dual of the intersection is the union and corresponding norm is called *T-conorm* or *S-norm*. Given fuzzy sets F_i and F_j defined in U with membership functions $\mu_{Fi}(x)$ and $\mu_{Fj}(x)$, their binary *S*-norm fuzzy union set and its membership function are given by

$$F_i \cup F_j = \{(x, \mu_{F_i \cup F_j}(x)) \mid x \in U\} \text{ and } \mu_{F_i \cup F_j(x)} = \mu_{F_i}(x) \vee \mu_{F_j}(x) \tag{5}$$

where the symbol '∨' denotes fuzzy union or 'fuzzy OR'. The properties of a *S*-norm operator can be deduced from *DeMorgan's duality* with respect to its *T*-norm counterpart. By attributing to interval algebra, it can be shown that the Gödel's *T*-conorm, which is defined as $\max(x,y)$, and Lukasiewicz *T*-conorm, which is based on *bounded sum* and defined as $\min(x+y,1)$ satisfy the above conditions. Therefore, similar to *T*-norm, the resulting membership function for each *S*-norm operator also preserves respective operator property. For example considering Gödel's max *S*-norm it holds

$$\mu_{F_i \cup F_j}(x) = \mu_{F_i}(x) \vee \mu_{F_j}(x) = \max(\mu_{F_i}(x), \mu_{F_j}(x)) \tag{6}$$

and so on.

The duality between *T*- and its conorm is expressed as $S(x,y)=N\{T(N(x),N(y))$ and vice-versa where $N(x)=1-x$ is the Zadeh's fuzzy negation of x. However, duality may not hold for some complement definitions, such as the Yager's negation $N(x) = \left(1 - x^p\right)^{1/p}$ defined for $p>0$ and Sugeno's negation $N(x) = \frac{1-x}{1+px}$ defined for $p>-1$. Besides the duality, these norms are associative, i.e. $T(x,T(y,z))=T(T(x,y),z)$ and $S(x,S(y,z))=S(S(x,y),z)$ while distributiveness is similarly derived, (Chen, & Pham, 2001).

Representation of Fuzzy Sets and Membership Functions

In case the universal set U set is countable with discrete members, the membership of $x \in X \subseteq U$ to F is simply given as a pair $(x, \mu_F(x))$ for instance $(a, 0.35)$. However, in continuous case, the membership is expressed in terms of a predefined analytical FMF. Some well-known FMFs are defined below and their typical shapes are given in Figure 1.

1. *Singleton Membership Function*: Singleton is a membership function taking value 1 only at a particular point x^* of the universe of discourse U and 0 otherwise

Figure 1. Membership functions, (a) singleton, (b) Gaussian, (c) generalized-bell, (d) sigmoidal, (e) triangular, and (f) trapezoidal

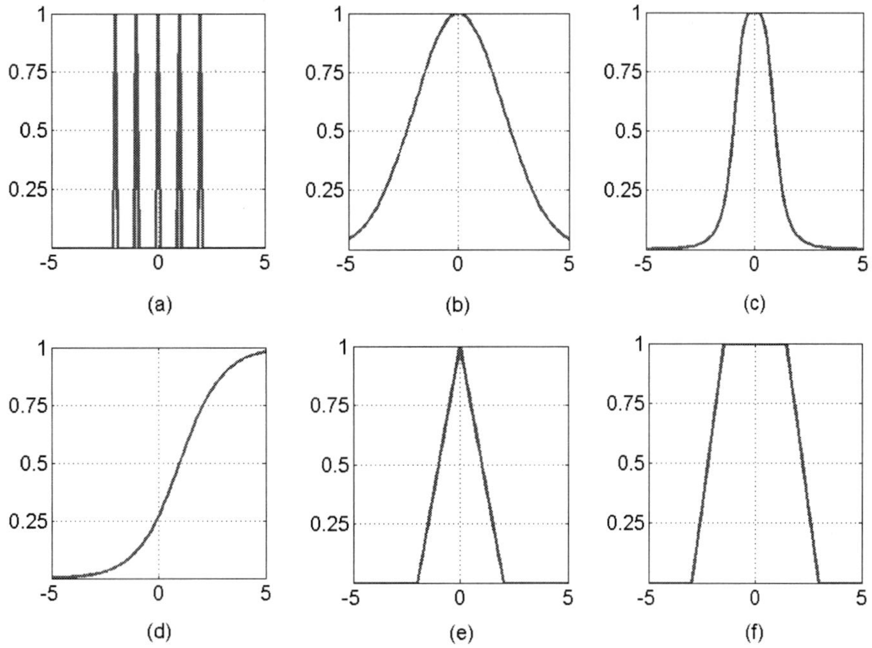

$$\mu_{\sin g}(x) = \begin{cases} 1 & \text{if } x = x^* \\ 0 & \text{otherwise} \end{cases} \tag{7}$$

2. *Gaussian Membership Function*: A Gaussian membership function centered at μ with σ-width is given by

$$\mu_{\text{Gauss}}(x) = \exp\left(-\left(\frac{x-\mu}{\sigma}\right)^2\right) \tag{8}$$

3. *Generalized Bell Membership Function*: A generalized-bell membership function centered at μ with σ-width and λ-slope is given by

$$\mu_{\text{Bell}}(x) = \frac{1}{1 + \left|\frac{x-\mu}{\sigma}\right|^{2\lambda}} \tag{9}$$

4. *Sigmoidal Membership Function*: A sigmoidal membership function with λ-slope at crossover point $x=c$,

$$\mu_{\text{Sigm}}(x) = \frac{1}{1+\exp[-a(x-c)]} \tag{10}$$

5. *Triangular Membership Function*: A triangular membership function is fully described by three parameters $\{a,b,c\}$, with $a < b < c$
6. The *complementary fuzzy membership function* (CFMF) is obtained via DeMorgan's law to each predefined FMF in a given fuzzy rule.

$$\mu_{\text{Triangle}}(x) = \begin{cases} 0 & x \le a \\ \dfrac{x-a}{b-a} & a \le x \le b \\ \dfrac{c-x}{c-b} & b \le x \le c \\ 0 & c \le x \end{cases} \quad \text{or}$$

$$\mu_{\text{Triangle}}(x) = \max\left(\min\left(\frac{x-a}{b-a}, \frac{c-a}{c-b}\right), 0\right) \quad (11)$$

7. *Trapezoidal Membership Function*: A trapezoidal membership function is fully described by four parameters $\{a,b,c,d\}$, $a < b < c < d$

$$\mu_{\text{Trap}}(x) = \begin{cases} 0 & x \le a \\ \dfrac{x-a}{b-a} & a \le x \le b \\ 1 & b \le x \le c \text{ or} \\ \dfrac{d-x}{d-c} & c \le x \le d \\ 0 & d \le x \end{cases}$$

$$\mu_{\text{Trap}} = \max\left(\min\left(\frac{x-a}{b-a}, 1, \frac{d-x}{d-c}\right), 0\right) \quad (12)$$

FUZZY REASONING AND CONTROLLER

A fuzzy inference rule describes a composition of a fuzzy set and a *fuzzy relation*. A simple fuzzy rule or implication can be given in the form

IF x is A THEN y is B (13)

where x and y are so-called input and output *linguistic variables,* respectively, while A and B are the *linguistic values*. Since a fuzzy rule is an expression with uncertainty, a conclusive relationship between rules should be based on *premises*. Now consider the premise: $\{x$ is $A'\}$. Then, if an *implication* is given as {IF x is A THEN y is B}, based on this premise, the conclusion will be of $\{y$ is $B'\}$. In this regard, a fuzzy relation Γ is a subset of the *cartesian product* AxB. The fuzzy reasoning output B' is then to be determined *assuming* the existence of a relation Γ and it is be expressed as $B'=A'\text{o}\Gamma$ where 'o' refers to the *sup-T composition* of A' given the relation Γ, (Rutkowski, 2004; Chen, & Pham, 2001). The membership of y in B', then, can be defined as

$$\mu_{B'}(y) = \mu_{A'oR}(y) = \max_{y \in B}\left(\min\left(\mu_{A'}(x), \mu_R(x,y)\right)\right) \quad (14)$$

Above it is assumed that the membership of $\mu_R(x,y)=\mu_{A\to B}(x,y)$ is unknown and it is to be determined based on the knowledge of $\mu_A(x)$ and $\mu_B(y)$ related to each other as $\mu_{A\to B}(x,y)=I\{\mu_A(x),\mu_B(y)\}$ where $I(\cdot)$ is a fuzzy implication. A fuzzy implication is a function $I{:}[0,1]^2 \to [0,1]$ satisfying following conditions:

1. If $x_1 \le x_3$ then $I(x_1,x_2) \ge I(x_1,x_3)$ for all x_1, x_2, & $x_3 \in [0,1]$,
2. $I[0,x_2]=1$ for all $x_2 \in [0,1]$ (falsity implies anything),
3. $I[x_1,1]=1$ for all $x_1 \in [0,1]$ (anything implies tautology),
4. $I[1,0]=0$ (Booleanity).

Some well-known implications are the Zadeh's $\max\{\min(a,b),1-a\}$, Kleene-Dienes' $\max(1-x,y)$, Yager's $\begin{cases} 1 & \text{if } x=0 \\ x^y & \text{if } x>0 \end{cases}$, Lukasiewic'z $\min(1,1-a+b)$, Fodor's $\begin{cases} 1 & \text{if } x \le y \\ \max(1-x,y) & \text{if } x>y \end{cases}$. Zadeh's implication is in the form of $I(x,y)=S\{N(x),T(x,y)\}$ while Klee-Dienes', Fodor's and Lukasiewicz's implications satisfy $I(x,y)=S(1-x,y)$ where $x,y \in [0,1]$, (Chen, & Pham, 2001).

Each fuzzy rule or implication is simply composed of two parts. Considering the example with *rule* 'IF x_1 is A_1 and x_2 is A_2 THEN y_1 is B_1 and y_2 is B_2', then the following parts are identified:

1. *Input conditioning* or *antecedents*: IF x_1 is A_1 and x_2 is A_2

2. *Output* or *consequent*: THEN y_1 is B_1 and y_2 is B_2

Having defined fuzzy inference and relations, it is convenient to describe well-known fuzzy inference and reasoning models:

Mamdani's Model

In this approach, rules are connected or aggregated with OR to form the *compound rule R* as

$$R_k : \text{IF } \underbrace{\left\{\bigcap_i x_i \text{ is } A_{ki}\right\}}_{Q_k} \text{ THEN } \underbrace{\left\{\bigcap_j y_j \text{ is } B_{kj}\right\}}_{P_k} = I(Q_k, P_k)$$

$$R = \bigcup_k R_k \tag{15}$$

where each implication $I(.,.)$ is interpreted as a min T-norm operator. Considering $\mathbf{x}=[x_1,x_2,\ldots x_n]$, $\mathbf{y}=[y_1,y_2,\ldots y_m]$, the membership of output R given crisp/instance input $\mathbf{x}^0$ is

$$\mu_R(\mathrm{x}^0,\mathrm{y}) = \max_k(\min(\mu_{Q_k}(\mathrm{x}^0),\mu_{P_k}(\mathrm{y}))) \tag{16}$$

where it is seen that once the membership of linguistic variables at crisp values have been determined it is possible to identify the crisp output ($\mathbf{y}$) through its membership, (Mamdani, 1977).

Takagi-Sugeno's Model

In Takagi-Sugeno's rules model (Takagi, & Sugeno, 1985; Sugeno, & Yasukawa, 1993) the antecedent part is the same as Mamdani's approach while each consequent variable is expressed as a *linear combination* of linguistic input variables

$$R_k : \text{IF } \underbrace{\left\{\bigcap_i x_i \text{ is } A_{ki}\right\}}_{Q_k} \text{ THEN } \underbrace{\left\{\bigcap_j y_j \text{ is } B_{kj}\right\}}_{P_k} = I(Q_k, P_k) \tag{17}$$

where $y_j = \alpha_{j0} + \sum_i \alpha_{ji} x_i$, i=1,2,..., n and j=1,2,...m. If $\alpha_0 \neq 0$ while $\alpha_{i\neq 0}=0$ then the zero-order; otherwise the first-order Takagi-Sugeno model is obtained. The first-order Takagi-Sugeno model involves determining the coefficients in the corresponding n-dimensional hyperplane, which may be thought of as neural network known *Adaptive Network-based Fuzzy Inference System* (ANFIS) (Jang, 1992). The output of each rule is then weighted by its corresponding rule membership called *firing degree*. The overall reasoning output is obtained by normalizing the algebraic sum of the linearly weighted rule outputs with respect to weighting factors. It should be noted that the firing degrees of antecedent parts for each rule are identically evaluated by using the min operator. Figure 2 illustrates both the Mamdani and Takagi-Sugeno algorithms.

For inspecting the fuzzy inference by two approaches, consider a two-rule case with crisp inputs x_{10} and x_{20} and corresponding consequent outputs y_1 and y_2. Suppose two rules with firing degrees $w_1 = \mu_{B_1^*}(y) = \min(\mu_{A_{11}}(x_{10}),\mu_{A_{12}}(x_{20}))$ $w_2 = \mu_{B_2^*}(y) = \min(\mu_{A_{21}}(x_{10}),\mu_{A_{22}}(x_{20}))$, respectively. The *fuzzy inference* is carried out as follows:

1. In Mamdani's approach, clipped fuzzy sets at the consequent part of the rules B_{1*} and B_{2*} are connected with the max (union) operator as $B_{1*} \cup B_{2*}$. On the other hand, in Takagi-Sugeno's approach, all weighted consequent part linear expressions are algebraically, e.g. $w_1y_1+w_2y_2$.

Figure 2. Illustration of Mamdani and Takagi-Sugeno reasoning methods for two-rule with two inputs and one output. Adapted from Web: http://lsiwww.epfl.ch/LSI2001/teaching/webcourse/ch09/fuzzy.html

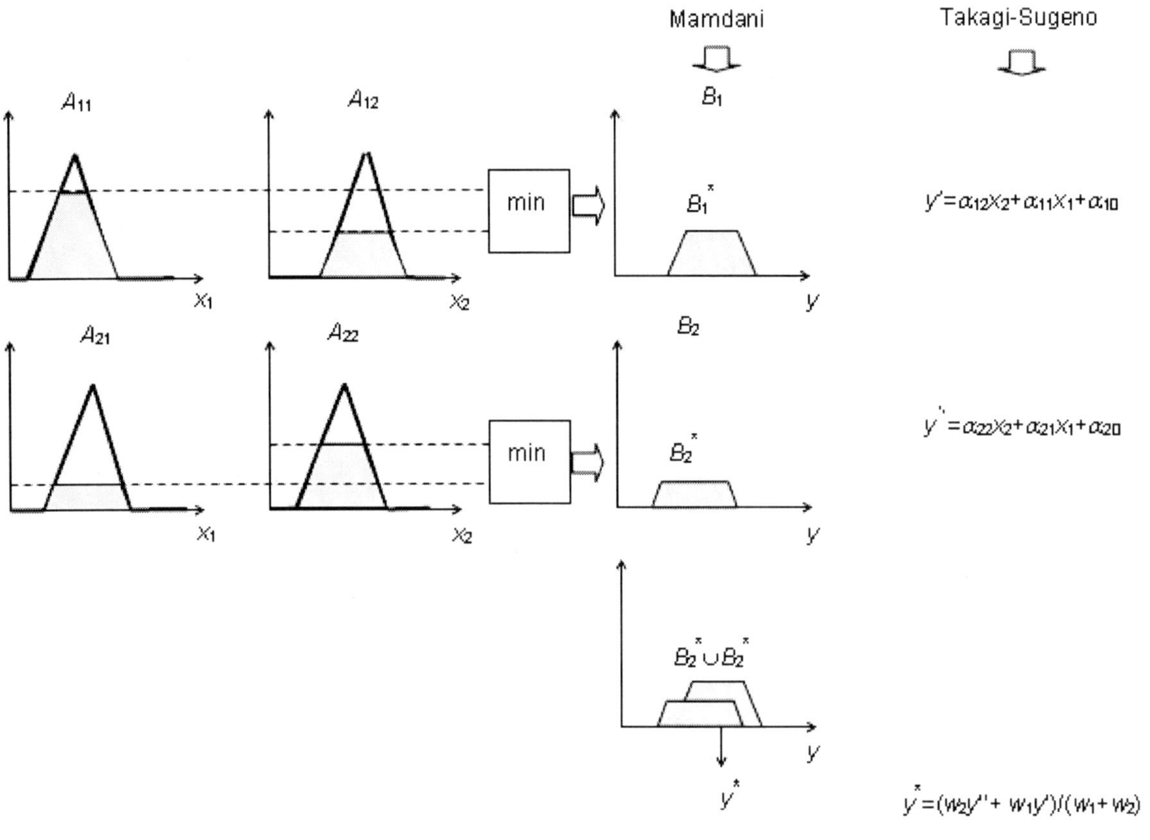

2. In either approach, the *crisp* output y^* is chosen as the best representative of *aggregation* in respective output fuzzy sets. In Mamdani's approach, y^* is obtained by applying the *center of gravity* (COG) to the output fuzzy set $B_{1*} \cup B_{2*}$ with respect to rule output firing degrees while in Takagi-Sugeno's approach, algebraic mean of respective output fuzzy set with respect to consequent weights, (Montero, Lopez, & Gomez, 2007).

Above approaches can also be generalized to construct higher-dimension input space by using fuzzy *rules-map*. A detailed description on how rules-map is formed and they can be applied to problem solving in fuzzy inferences can be found in (Perfiliva, 2007).

Fuzzy Controller

A *fuzzy controller* is a system/algorithm which issues a decision based on fuzzy inference. Therefore, a fuzzy controller maintains relationship between the input, controller state and output all being termed linguistic variables. The operation performed by a fuzzy controller consists of *fuzzification* and *defuzzification* through *controller states* and expressed in terms of linguistic rules, Figure 3.

It should be noted that the fuzzy-rule implementation and evaluation block needs to be provided with appropriate *rule-base* and *data-base*, both of which can be manipulated and stored in a *knowledge-base*. The system learns and operates under the supervision of an *expert*. The expert is

Figure 3. Fuzzy controller architecture with functional blocks

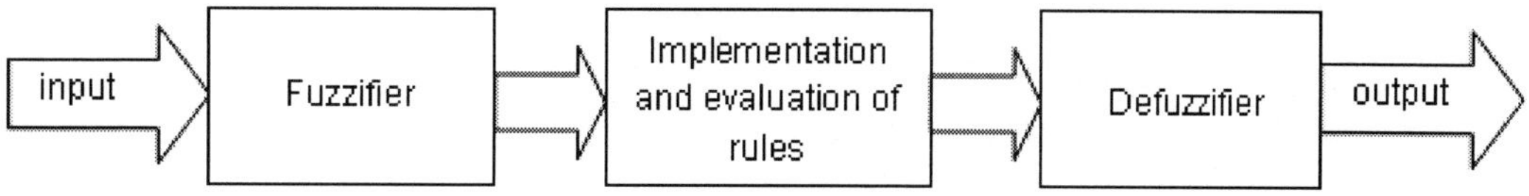

also responsible for updates on data and rules. It also provides overall management of the system in which the controller resides, (Cho, Park, & Park, 2002).

The main function of the *fuzzifier* is to assign respective antecedent and consequential memberships. Simply it extracts item-wise outputs to be assessed and implemented by the succeeding block called *rule evaluator*. In this block, memberships are organized for simulative action so that if the controller needs to be updated with new rules and data by the knowledge-base it would be possible to adapt the input and output quantities adaptively. The *defuzzifier* transforms the rule-based memberships into crisp set of outputs. Therefore, an overall fuzzy controller is a system block which partitions the input space into decision regions based on adaptable rules evaluated on uncertainties.

Analog Fuzzy-Reasoning Circuit Design

From the previous discussions, it is possible to subdivide overall fuzzy logic and inference system into membership, possibly normalization, and defuzzifier blocks. However a consequent block is also necessary because of the algebraic manipulation involved in Takagi-Sugeno approach (Driankov, Hellendoorn, & Reinfrank, 1993). A possible implementation of a fuzzy controller which is supposed to issue a crisp output as decision needs to comply with uncertainties expressed for rules.

As will be shown in the next sections, due to inherent parallelism and suitability to represent inputs in linguistic variables, fuzzy system implementation is mostly given in analog approach, (Panella, & Martinelli, 2007). However, analog design is inherently prone to design shortcomings and irregularities. Particularly the current-mode approach, which is adopted for most fuzzy system implementations, with intense use of mirrors is subject to deviations from the ideal behavior. The first group of deviation known as *systematic errors* arises as non-idealities, such as *Early* and *body-bias* effects, etc. assuming nominal design parameters. Depending on the model used for transistors, systematic errors can be determined up to a certain extent. Since these second-order effects are also related to circuit topology, it is possible to remedy systematic errors with improved designs.

Another group of discrepancies, which is mostly named as *mismatch errors*, is due to random fluctuations in technological model parameters of MOS transistor, e.g. zero body-bias threshold voltage, (VTO), and device transconductance, β. The mismatch errors depend on how transistors are arranged on a silicon wafer, e.g. the distance between them and their area etc. They are given in terms of measurement statistics. Total mismatch error in quantities of interest is derived from analytical expression relating it to those parameters. A detailed analysis of major design irregularities and remedial issues can be found in (Dualibe, Verleysen, & Jespers, 2003).

ANALOG FUZZIFIER IMPLEMENTATIONS

Fuzzification of a given input can be realized by establishing an adequate MFC given a particular fuzzy rule. By appropriately arranging MFCs, it is possible attain an implementation of compound rules. An analog MFC can be implemented in various forms depending on the quantity of interest; voltage-mode (Yamakawa, 1993), current-mode (Baturone, Huertas, Barriga, & Solano, 1994; Kettner, Heite, & Schumacher, 1993) or their mixture, mostly those based on *operational transconductor amplifier* (OTA), (Chen, Chen, & Tsao, 1992; Azeem, & Baig, 2007). OTA-based MFCs are not considered since the fundamental building block of OTAs, i.e. differential stage is discussed distinctly in this chapter.

Voltage-Mode Fuzzification

Most voltage-mode MFC implementations rely on well-known *differential-pair* as the main block, Figure 4.

DC transfer characteristic of the circuits is expressed as

$$I_{out} = I_1 - I_2 = \begin{cases} \sqrt{\beta I_{bias}}(V_{in} - V_k)\sqrt{1 - (V_{in} - V_k)^2 \frac{\beta}{4I_{bias}}} & |V_{in} - V_k| \leq \sqrt{\frac{2I_{bias}}{\beta}} \\ I_{bias}\,\mathrm{sgn}(V_{in} - V_k) & |V_{in} - V_k| \geq \sqrt{\frac{2I_{bias}}{\beta}} \end{cases} \quad (18)$$

where β=KP.(W/L) is the device transconductance with KP, W and L being the *intrinsic technological conductance* parameter, transistor width and length, respectively. It is apparent that the circuit functions as a voltage-controlled current-mode switch. By appropriately adjusting the bias current to be switched between fuzzy categories or levels, similarity or membership measures can be associated to corresponding to circuit DC transfer characteristics. Figure 5 illustrates such a fuzzifier and its expected DC transfer characteristics constructed with stacked differential pairs proposed by (Wilamowski, Jaeger, & Kaynak, 1999). The circuit performs four-level operation where the current I_i refers to fuzzified output in current-mode for the *i*-th level. The circuit yields two Gaussian- or bell-like fuzzy membership functions at the center regions, while at the boundaries two sigmoidal-like membership functions are realized.

Figure 4. Differential-pair circuit with MOS transistors

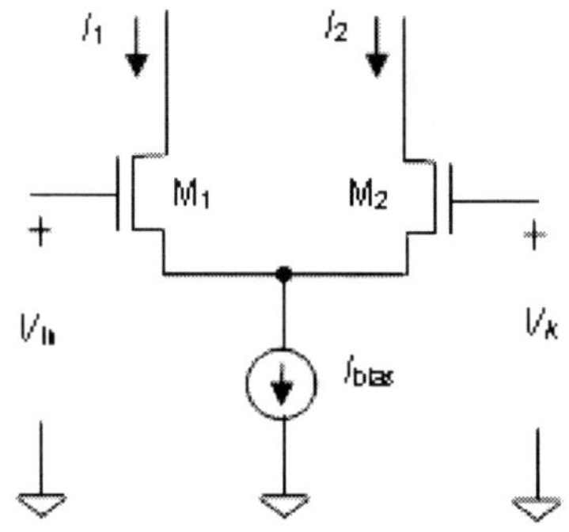

The operational characteristics of a fuzzifier which utilizes differential stage will depend on the behavior of the circuit across the fuzzy transition regions and the number of such regions. Therefore, the switching performance between the levels is mainly determined by I_{bias} and transconductance of the symmetric input transistors M_1 and M_2, which is outlined as follows:

1. If the number of successive stages to be switched is large, the size of the input transistors will be prohibitively large for desired transconductance given an I_{bias}.
2. The transient response of a stage with larger transistors will degrade due to increased input capacitance seen at the gate of input transistors.
3. As the number of stages increases, the necessary input voltage range to switch the same I_{bias} will also increase. It should be noted that the slope between the MF regions corresponding to *transconductance gain* of the stage is determined by the I_{bias}. The supply voltage or the voltage headroom necessary to switch the transistor would be larger, which is in fact limited by the supply voltage. Hence, in case of using fixed supply voltage,

Figure 5. (a) Generation of four fuzzy membership functions with stacked differential-pair based circuit, and (b) its expected DC transfer characteristics

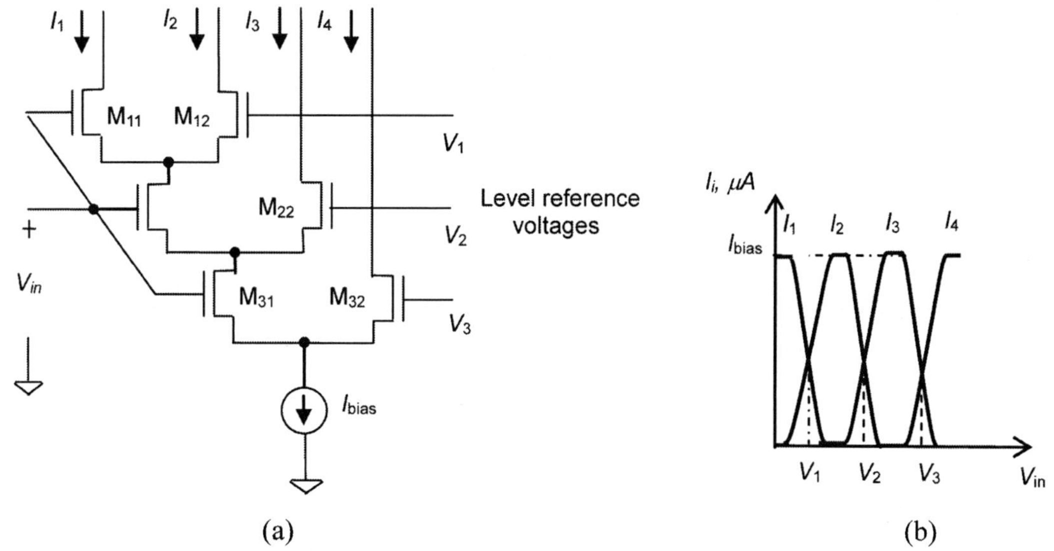

the available voltage headroom with desired slope control will be restricted.

A major solution to above shortcomings is to operate input transistors in the triode region for fast transient response with programmable slopes. The triode-region operation with desired slope control can be achieved with use of *regulated-cascode triode transconductance* structure proposed in (Bult, & Geelen, 1990) shown in Figure 6 with DC transfer response.

In the circuit, DA refers to *differential-amplifier* with buffered- or non-buffered-output. In this configuration, drain-to-source voltage of M_1 and M_2 is kept almost constant through the offset voltages of DA1 and DA2 and gain-boosting transistors M_{C1} and M_{C2}. Since the offset voltages are smaller than the drain-to-source saturation voltages of M1 and M2, input transistors are driven into triode region. Transconductance of a transistor operating in triode region is given by

$$g_m = \frac{\partial I}{\partial V_{gs}} = \beta . V_{ds} \tag{19}$$

It is seen that the slope is proportional to input transistor conductance, hence it is straightforwardly controllable with transistor dimensions. Hence, desired slope is easily achieved with appropriate transistor dimensions.

Moreover, use of nonsymmetrical PMOS differential stage within the DA block also allows both larger controllable range in V_{in}. The slope of the DC transfer characteristic is programmable with V_s. With symmetrical input transistors M_1 and M_2 operating in triode region with $\beta_{M1}=\beta_{M2}=\beta$, $g_{m,M1}=g_{m,M2}=g_m$ and $V_{ds,M1}=V_{ds,M2}=V_{ds}$, by taking V_k as the parametric threshold, it can be shown that

$$I_1 \approx \begin{cases} \frac{g_m}{2} V_{in} & \text{if } V_k - \frac{I_{bias}}{g_m} \leq V_{in} \leq V_k + \frac{I_{bias}}{g_m} \\ 0 & \text{otherwise} \end{cases} \tag{20}$$

and $I_2=I_{bias}-I_1$. However, the circuit has the following shortcomings:

1. Discrepancy from the linearity occurs mainly when the input transistor of the active input

Figure 6. Differential regulated-cascode triode transconductor: (a) circuit schematics with differential amplifiers, and (b) its expected DC transfer characteristics

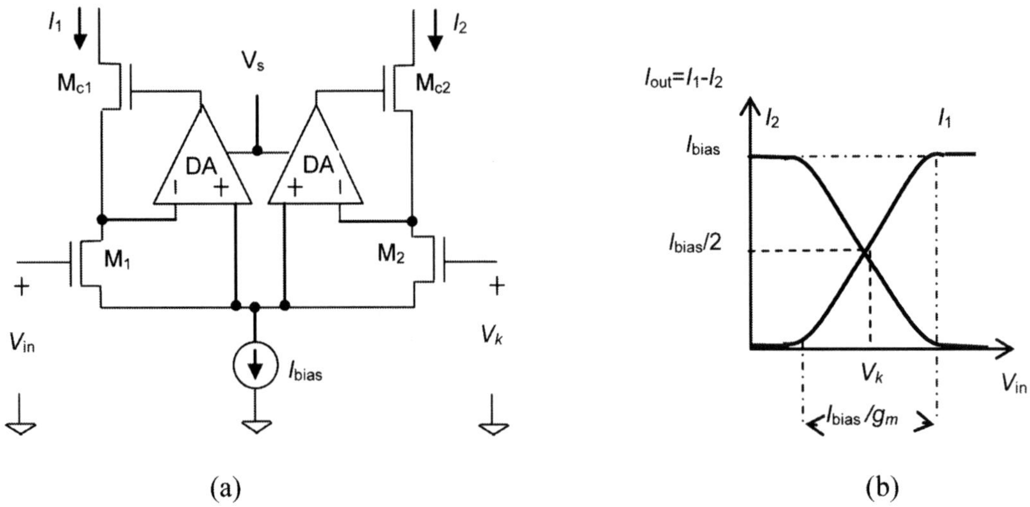

branch of DA enters the saturation region with current value of either zero or I_{bias}. This nonlinearity can be remedied by the regulatory loop consisting of M_C and DA of the active branch.

2. In differential regulated-cascode transconductor, use of two DAs consumes considerably large silicon area. Moreover DC performance is affected by offset voltage variations of DAs. Therefore, the resulting tuning performance will be poor.

One of the DAs can be replaced with a large-size transistor for maintaining almost invariant threshold voltage reference at the common source node. The circuit configuration obtained as such is called *single regulated-cascode triode transconductor*, (Dualibe, Verleysen, & Jespers, 2003). New configuration consumes significantly reduced silicon area.

Transconductors described above can be modified for building up their respective *complementary* version with use of constant current source to provide negation.

Figure 7 depicts a four-label fuzzy partition or fuzzifier circuit based on the differential regulated-cascode transconductor topology, (Dualibe, Verleysen, & Jespers, 2003). The circuit remedies the shortcomings in operating low-voltage levels due to totem pole architecture in Figure 7.

The circuit was shown to exhibit better slope control. The slopes of the FMFs are electrically programmable by voltages $V_{s1} \ldots V_{s3}$ while the voltages $V_1 \ldots V_3$ are the crossover points between the contiguous fuzzy labels similar to previous MFC. However, compared to previous design, the circuit requires larger number of transistors, differential stages and current mirrors. Particularly the current mirrors which act as bias current sources cause mismatch and systematic errors. Due to current conveying between adjacent levels, the error terms are cumulated and the circuit exhibits degraded transient response.

Current-Mode Fuzzification

For a reconfigurable and programmable fuzzy system, e.g. controller, it is desirable to accommodate as many distinct independent fuzzy levels as

Figure 7. Use of differential regulated-cascode triode transconductors for generating four fuzzy membership functions

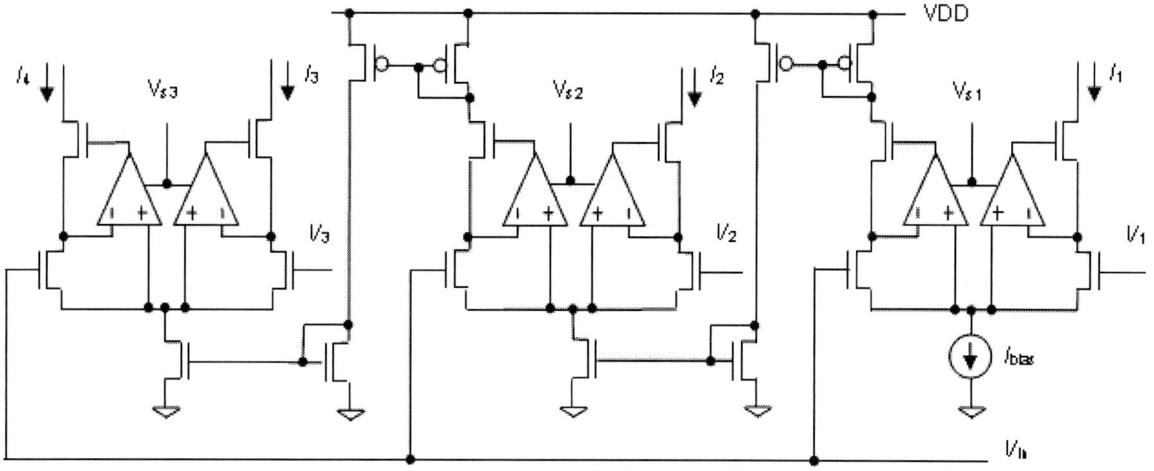

possible for each input while attaining maximum number of inputs. However, fuzzifiers built with voltage-mode input (and possibly internal current-mode operation), and discussed so far have the following shortcomings:

1. They need high-voltage swing at the input, i.e. larger than a threshold value with body-bias effect. The input voltage headroom available will be very limited in case the maximum input voltage is the supply voltage, which is the usual case.
2. Each stage can only be activated if preceding stage has not activated yet due to reference current shift between them. The dependency between successive stages makes designs highly technological-parameter dependent due to body-bias effect.
3. Transition regions between successive FMFs are not easy to adjust and involve complicated circuitries for improvement on each successive stage.

The above design restrictions can be significantly alleviated with use of current-mode design. As outlined in (Toumazou, Ligey, & Haigh, 1990), current-mode design has the advantage of reduced lower switching voltage operation up to the maximum frequency available with the technology used. Simplicity it brings out allows versatile solutions to come about in circuit design. Following sections outline major current-mode FMC designs which can be employed in implementation of fuzzy inference systems. Due to intense use of current mirrors, approaches for piece-wise linear synthesis, e.g. (Thayse, & Deschamps, 1977), are not included in this study.

Multi-valued logic (MVL) is an approach to express switching functions in a higher radix-r, $r>2$. There is a close resemblance between FL and MVL, (Moraga, Trillas, & Guadarrama, 2003) except that in fuzzy-logic a linguistic variable is associated to a number of categories with firing degrees or membership ranging between 0 and 1 while in MVL the quantities take discrete values from a so-called universal set $R=\{0,1,\ldots, r-1\}$. It is possible to form a mapping between $x\in R$ and its membership value as

$$\{x \in R \rightarrow \mu_{A_i}(x) \in [0,1] \mid 0 \rightarrow [0,\ 1/r),\ 1 \rightarrow [1/r,\ 2/r), \ldots, r-1 \rightarrow [(r-1)/r,\ 1)\} \tag{21}$$

Figure 8. Multi-valued logic implementation based trapezoidal-like fuzzy membership functions, (a) circuit, and (b) expected DC transfer characteristics

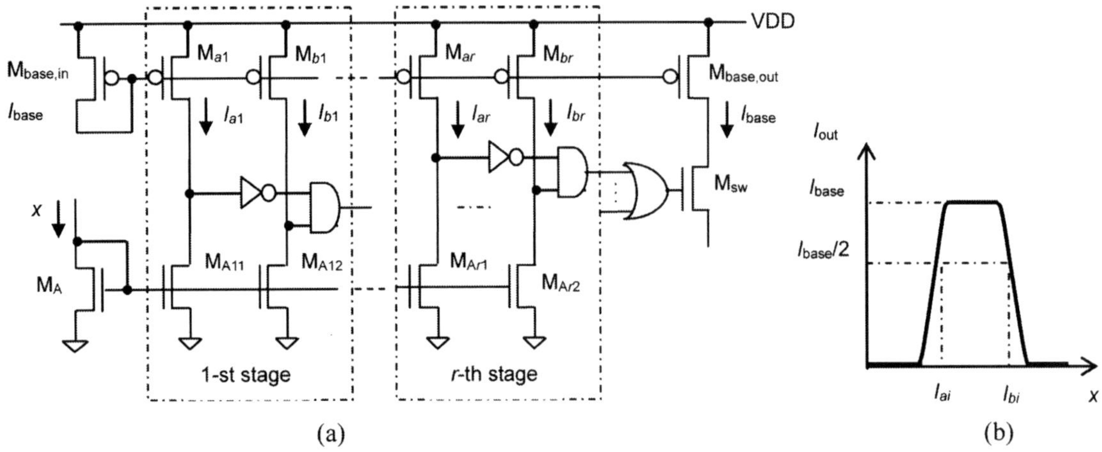

where '→' refers to assignment between the quantities of interest. In current-mode MVL, each logic level $l \in R$ corresponds to a continuous current range $[(l\text{-}0.5)I_{base}, (l\text{+}0.5)I_{base})$ where I_{base} is a *base current.*

Above mapping makes it possible to interpret MVL-*literal* operator defined as, (Moraga, Trillas, & Guadarrama, 2003),

$$L(a,b) = \begin{cases} r-1 & \text{if } a \le x \le b \\ 0 & \text{otherwise} \end{cases} \tag{22}$$

where $a, b \in R$ with $a = b\text{-}1$, as a trapezoidal fuzzy MF for the b-th level centered at b/r. Therefore a trapezoidal FMC can be easily obtained from the MVL-literal circuit with slight modification to that proposed by (Jain, Bolton, & Abd-El Barr, 1993) shown in Figure 8. In the circuit n-type mirrors composed of M_A transistors. The p-type mirror composed of $M_{base,in}$ and $M_{base,out}$ have mirroring factor of 1:1. The circuit exploits the *current-comparator* presented in (Freitas, & Current, 1983). In the circuit I_{base} corresponds to $\mu_{A_i}(x) = 1$ while $I_{ai} = (a_i\text{-}0.5)I_{base}/r$ and $I_{bi} = (b_i\text{+}0.5)I_{base}/r$. It is possible to stack more stages by ORing the outputs of AND gates for producing a simple or compound rule with large number of levels. Overall operational range and the number of levels are controlled with M_{sw}, (Temel, 2004). An obvious advantage of the literal-based MF realization compared to previously presented voltage-mode MFC is seen from the circuit: Given an input x normalized to r, its corresponding rule membership can be established concurrently, i.e. an individual stage does not depend on the preceding stages.

Theoretically, the circuit behavior allows versatile slope control with adjustment of the individual stage gains. However, since usually the gain of stages is high, the slope control is restricted. Moreover, abrupt rail-to-rail digital signal variation at the gate of switching transistor M_{sw} causes spurious transient behavior at the output.

An alternative current-mode realization of the literal with much better control capability and transient behavior is presented in (Temel, 2007). The circuit makes use of *truncated* (or bounded) *difference* and *positive-feedback threshold* circuits. These circuits perform the corresponding operations defined as follows:

Figure 9. Circuit, block representation and expected DC transfer characteristic of main sub-blocks to be used in implementation of membership function circuit based on multi-valued logic literal operation: (a) Truncated-difference, and (b) lower-threshold operation

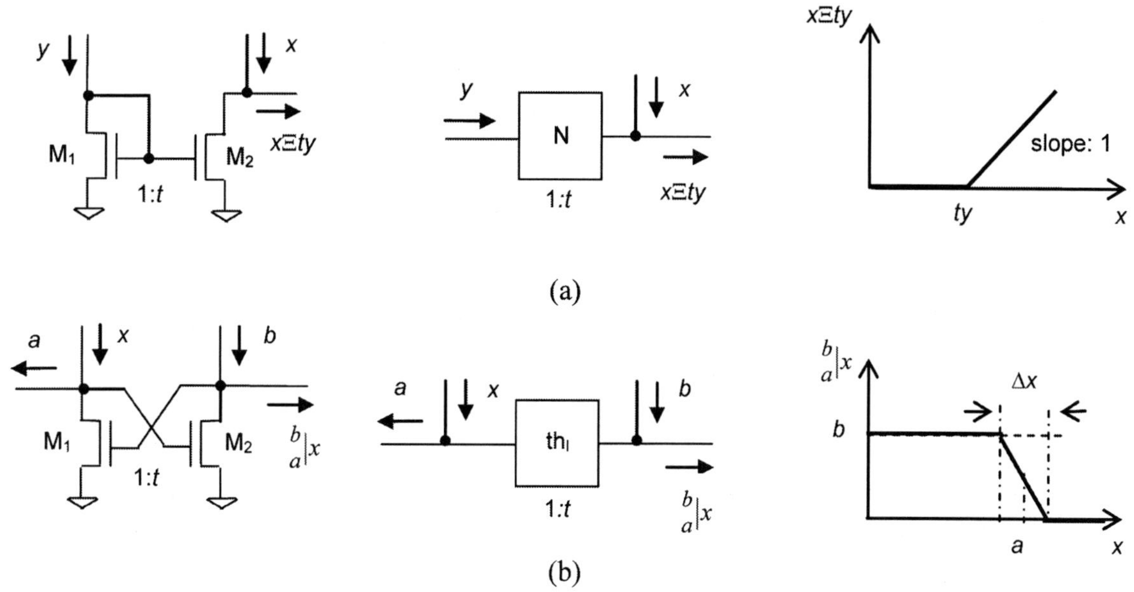

$$\text{truncated difference}: \quad x \boxminus ty = \begin{cases} x - ty & \text{if } x \geq ty \\ 0 & \text{otherwise} \end{cases}$$

$$\text{lower - threshold} \quad (th_l): \quad {}^{b}_{a}|x = \begin{cases} b & \text{if } x \leq a \\ 0 & \text{otherwise} \end{cases}$$

$$\text{upper - threshold} \quad (th_u): \quad x|^{b}_{a} = \begin{cases} b & \text{if } x \geq a \\ 0 & \text{otherwise} \end{cases} \tag{23}$$

respectively. Figure 9 (a) and (b) depict circuit realization, block representation and DC-transfer characteristic of the truncated difference and lower-threshold operations, respectively.

Implementation of the upper-threshold operation, th_u, is obtained by interchanging x and a in the th_l circuit. For threshold circuits the transition region width Δx is adjusted by the parameter $t>1$, i.e. the larger the t is the steeper the transition region goes through. Considering biasing, hence operational condition of p-type mirrors sourcing the input currents and the second-order effects, the threshold circuits exhibit diverse switching behavior depending on the value of t as a parameter, (Baker, Li, & Boyce, 1998).

It can be shown that the literal operation given in Equation (22) can algebraically be expressed as, (Temel, 2007)

$$L(a,b) = \left({}^{x}_{b}|x \right)\Big|^{r-1}_{a} = {}^{r-1}_{b}\Big|\left(x|^{x}_{a} \right) \tag{24}$$

Simultaneous realization of the literal and its complement, i.e. *complementary literal* (CL), is shown in Figure 10, (Temel, 2007), where r-1 stands for the I_{base} while other quantities are obtained as previously. In (Temel, 2007), it was also shown that the new circuit(s) exhibit much better electrical performance and design characteristics compared to previous counterparts. The reader is referred to it for detailed operation and design aspects of the circuit.

Figure 10. Fully current-mode implementation of fuzzy membership function and its complement as multi-valued logic literal operation

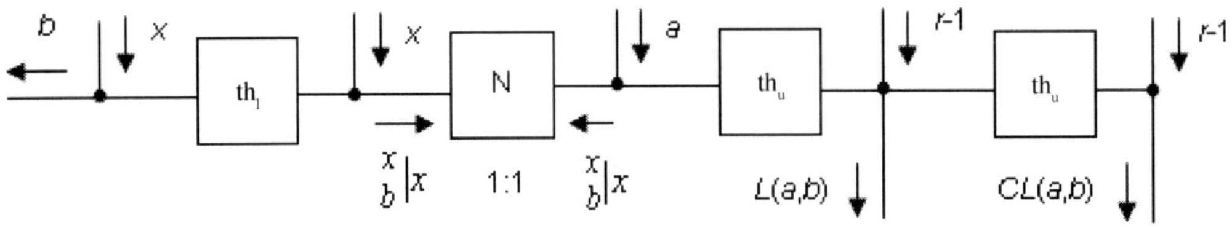

T- and S-Norm Operators

Having defined the membership notion and pointed out some of the relevant circuits for fuzzification, linguistic rule-based designs are to be investigated in this section. As previously mentioned, through the duality, *T*-norm (min) and *S*-norm or *T*-conorm (max) operators are easily obtained from each other via complement and association. An obvious advantage of fuzzy controllers realized with *T*-conorm canonic-form linguistic fuzzy rules is that each *T*-conorm is associated to one rule expressed by *N* fuzzy membership function outputs, where *N* is the number of inputs.

Despite some mixed-mode designs, (Caravajal, Angulo, & Tombs, 2000), owing to larger dynamic range and suitability to linear operation with improved performance current is the most widely used design quantity for realization of *T*-(co)norm operators.

It can be shown that min *T*-norm and max *S*-norm operations can be algebraically expressed in terms of truncated difference which was previously described, (Sasaki, Inoue, Shirai, & Ueno, 1990; Temel, 2004). Therefore, in case of more than two inputs the compound rule output is to be realized by cascading these operators. The resulting circuit implementation will consist of large number of successively cascaded n-type and p-type mirrors. Besides reduced dynamic range due to intense mismatch involved with use of mirrors, the circuit *complexity* is of $O(N^2)$, which makes it almost obsolete in applications for processing large number of inputs. In this section, such designs will not be dealt with. A *T*-(co)norm design should seek high-level of parallelism for a complexity as a linear function of the number of inputs, *N*, and *input transparency* without dependency on it, (Dualibe, Verleysen, & Jespers, 2003).

In this section, major current-mode implementations of *T*-(co)norm operations will be presented. In literature, most current-mode *T*-(co) norm realizations have been given for the MAX, while due to lack of a direct or consistent design scheme T-norm MIN has generally been realized indirectly. However, a recent design in (Temel, 2008) allows a direct implementation of MIN with only two or three transistors for each input. Compared to previous MIN designs, the circuit has improved time-domain response with reduced complexity.

S-norm or T-(co)norm Circuits

Well-known Lazzaro's *winner-take-all* MAX, (WTA-MAX), circuit (Lazzaro, Rykebusch, Mahowald, & Mead, 1989) of *N* identical parallel cell is shown in Figure 11(a). Each cell formed with transistors M_A and M_B is structured as a current-controlled voltage source where M_As are assumed to match the output transistor M_O with 1:1. Assume that cell transistors operating in strong inversion. In this configuration, the source voltages of M_Bs compete to impose their own value at the common node. The cell with the highest value imposes its own voltage and forces M_B transistors of other cells to switch off. The winner cell operates as Wilson current mirror, which replicates its own

Figure 11. (a) CMOS realization Lazzaro's winner-take-all based MAXIMUM circuit, and (b) its improved version with cascoded mirrors

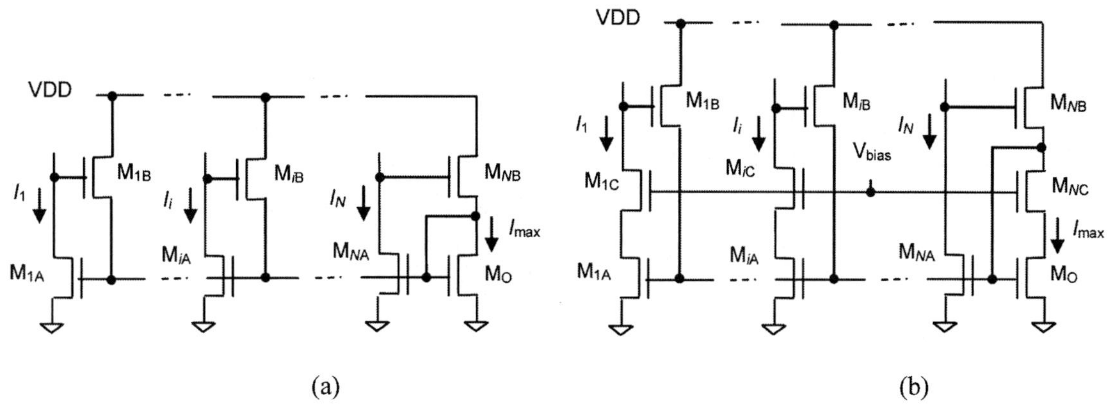

controlling current across M_O while M_Bs of other cells enter triode region.

It is possible to further modify the Lazzaro's WTA-MAX circuit for improved accuracy by converting Wilson current mirror into cascoded mirror, Figure 11(b), with a bias voltage V_{bias} to ensure saturated operation of cell transistors. However, the new circuit consumes larger area and it requires a suitable adjustment of biasing voltage level. Furthermore, increased capacitance at the common node will deteriorate the transient response, (Vida, 1996).

Lazzaro's WTA-MAX and its derivatives, e.g. (Baturone, Huertas, Barriga, & Solano, 1994; Huang, & Liu, 1994) usually have poor frequency response caused by large voltage swings to charge or discharge the parasitic capacitance of replicating transistors. This disadvantage can be overcome by using *flipped-voltage follower* (FVF) topology, (Carvajal, Angulo, & Martin, 2005; Angulo, Acevedo, Carvajal, & Martin, 2005), Figure 12 (a).

Circuit operation consists in comparing the input current with the current generated by gate-to-source voltage (V_1-V_2) of M_{iB} hence making it possible low-voltage operation. The output voltage of the comparison is utilized as a feed-back to drive the sensing transistor M_A.

The operational speed of FVF-based MAX circuit is mainly affected by the voltage swing at the input, hence the voltage at the drains of M_{iA}s. Therefore, time-response performance of an FVF-based MAX circuit will be determined by the feedback gain of the sensing transistors. In case of injecting the input currents through p-type mirrors, which limits the input level (Temel, 2004), the voltage at the drain of winning M_B will reach almost the supply voltage. The drain voltages of loser M_As will cause spikes at the output current due to feedback. which causes overall transient response of FVF architecture to be spurious.

Time response of FVF design can be improved by combining its low-switching voltage operation capability with low-impedance-node driving capability of traditional WTA design as shown in Figure 12 (b), (Temel, 2008, 1). Added transistor M_{iC} operates as a compensator for voltage variations at the drain of winning M_B, hence stabilizing the output waveform. Overall operation speed will further increase due to feed-forward connection. The circuit also allows processing larger input current range while preserving the input voltage swing conditions.

T-norm Circuits

Previously cited current comparator scheme can be exploited as a means for realizing T-norm operators in the form of *looser-take-all* MIN, (LTA-MIN),

Figure 12. (a) Current-mode flipped voltage-follower winner-take-all MAX circuit, and (b) its improved version

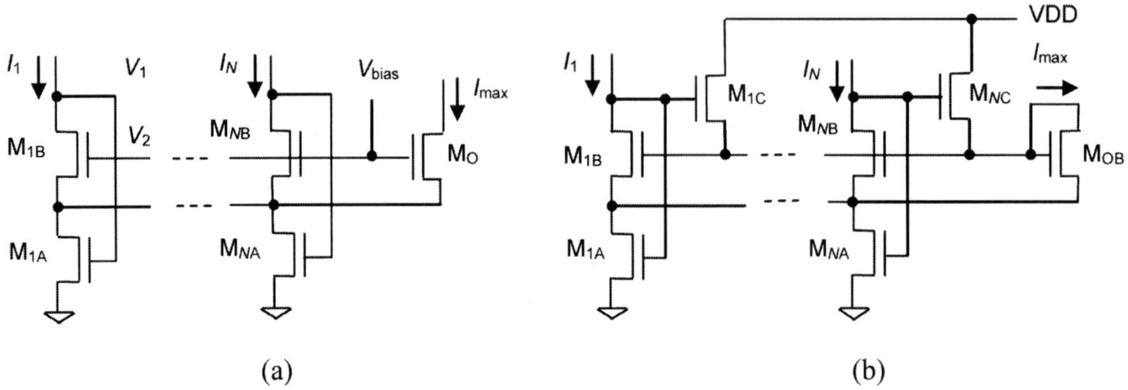

(Dualibe, Jespers, & Verleysen, 2001), as shown in Figure 13(a). The circuit has a complexity of O(N^2). In the circuit p-type mirror circuits match and operate with 1:1. The authors also presented a less-complexity version of the circuit in the same study. For the following reasons the circuit is not preferable in realization of min operator:

1. Due to cascoded operation it is not suitable for large number of inputs. Moreover, due to the lack of symmetry, the circuit is not input-transparent.
2. As the number of inputs increases the cascode architecture at the output branch will dominate the frequency and transient responses with highly reduced bandwidth.
3. The circuit will not be able to provide symmetrical input-output relationship for a certain number of inputs.
4. Parallelism is limited.

The above shortcomings design can be overcome by restraining whole input-output relationship with cell-based approach so that parallelism is achieved with less complexity, e.g. O(N), or regardless of the number of inputs, (Donckers, Dualibe, & Verleysen, 2000). Such a design is given in Figure 13(b) where the circuit employs a voltage-mode feedback controlled by variation of respective input current within each cell. The current sources $I_{\text{bias,p}}$ and $I_{\text{bias,n}}$ are used as connection to between the remaining circuit and relevant terminals, i.e. VDD and GND, respectively.

In each cell the loop consisting of M_B, M_C and M_D acts as current-controlled voltage source at the gate of M_B which is switched on or off depending on the respective cell input current. The drain voltage of M_C drives the gate of M_D which operates as a source follower. The lowest voltage becomes the winner at common node N_C. If PMOS transistor is adequately chosen such that M_B is kept at saturation then the voltage $V_{i,\text{out}}$ can be adjusted so as to exhibit almost digital levels. The reader is referred to (Dualibe, Verleysen, & Jespers, 2003) for detailed descriptions the circuits.

A NEW COMPACT HIGH-PERFORMANCE LTA-MIN CIRCUIT

sMost approaches toward implementing the MIN operation tackle the design problem by exploiting the WTA paradigm within a reverse activation loop to yield a response corresponding to the minimum of the inputs. Designs given by (Donckers, Dualibe, & Verleysen, 2000) employ current-controlled voltage-feedback to achieve this objective while the architecture in (Asloni,

Figure 13. (a) Current-comparator based cascode, and (b) voltage-feedback, cell-based parallel looser-take-all MIN circuits

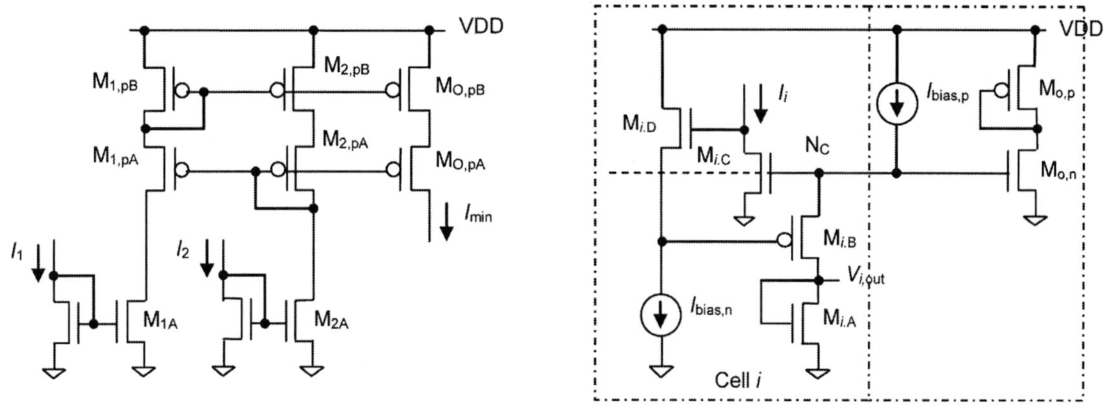

(a) (b)

Khoei, & Hadidi, 2006) relies on comparison of successive inputs providing a feedback signal to drive a WTA circuit. The implementation presented in (Huang, Wang, & Liu, 1996) converts input currents into respective intermediate voltages which will then be applied to a WTA circuit. The main advantage of this group of designs is concurrent processing of inputs and modularity. However, the overall performance usually depends on the feedback structure (Donckers, Dualibe, & Verleysen, 2000; Asloni, Khoei, & Hadidi, 2006) and the gain/conversion factor on input currents as in (Huang, Wang, & Liu, 1996) and output loop to reproduce the minimum of the inputs. Another group, e.g. (Dualibe, Jespers, & Verleysen, 2001), embarks on comparing currents of stacked inputs and coding the consequent output voltages for LTA-MIN operation. The major shortcoming of this approach is the restriction on the number of inputs limited by supply voltage and increased complexity as the number of inputs increases.

The recent multi-input, current-mode CMOS LTA-MIN circuit shown in Figure 14 proposed by (Temel, 2008, 2) has a very modular, compact structure and it requires only three transistors per input. Moreover it should be noted that M_B transistor can be removed, which yields the exact dual of Lazzaro's WTA-MAX circuit with only two transistors per cell.

In the circuit, node N_C is common to gates of transistors M_{iB}s and M_{OB}. Current source I_{bias} is used to provide a path between VDD and N_C. Transistor M_{OC} functions as a voltage-controlled current source and its source is biased by M_{OA} which also biases the gate of transistor M_{iA} in input cells. In each cell, M_{iA} converts the respective input current into a voltage at its drain. Source-to-gate voltages of M_{iC}s compete at node N_C at which the maximum one corresponding to smallest input current is selected as the winner. It should be noted that due to the source follower operation at node N_C the voltage variation at the drain of M_{iA} is shifted toward that of node N_C, which forces the M_{iB}s in loser cells to enter the triode region while the winner-cell M_{iC} to take over I_{bias}. The voltage shift at node N_C reduces the saturation voltage of M_{OB} by almost the same amount and forcing it to enter the triode region where it functions as a linear current source controlled by voltage at node N_C, because its source and drain are at kept almost fixed values. Therefore, the output current will follow the winning input current. Linearity in the transfer characteristics between output and inputs is determined by

Figure 14. New n-input parallel looser-take-all MINIMUM circuit. Dimensions are given for TSMC 0.25 μm HSPICE (level-49) parameters in full post-layout extraction with 1.8V supply voltage

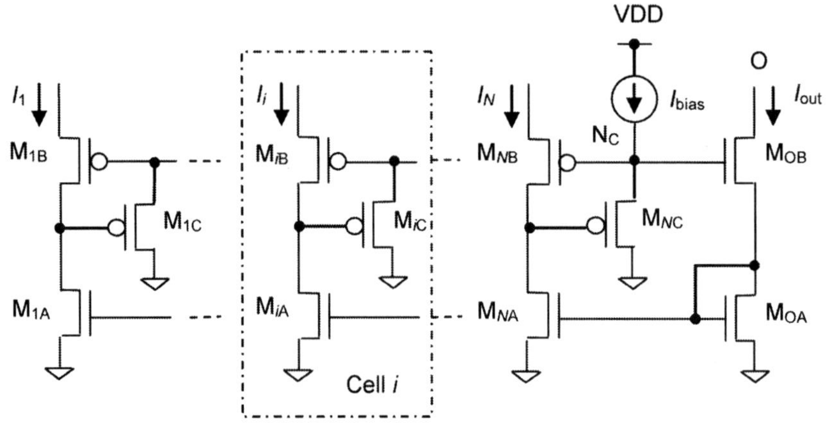

Transistor	M_{iA}	M_{iB}	M_{iC}	M_{OA}	M_{OB}
W(μm)/L(μm)	1.32/0.24	0.6/0.24	2.16/0.24	1.44/0.24	2.44/0.24

M_{iC} of the winner cell and the value of I_{bias}. Transistor M_{iC} in each cell is sized such that it operates with a small saturation voltage for a given I_{bias} so that the output adapts itself to minimum input as closely and fast as possible. The output current can be taken out via either a p-type mirror between O and VDD or M_{OA} can be mirrored while node O is tied up to VDD.

In order to show the performance improvement of the new circuit (Temel, 2008) compared to well- known previous counterparts, employing *bounded-difference* operation in (Sasaki, Inoue, Shirai, & Ueno, 1990), and LTA (Donckers, Dualibe, & Verleysen, 2000; Dualibe, Jespers, & Verleysen, 2001) respectively. The circuits were designed and simulated as three-input circuits for comparison by using TSMC 0.25 μm HSPICE (level-49) parameters in full post-layout extraction with 1.8V supply voltage. In all designs, body-biased effects were included and transistors were sized for an optimum DC transfer characteristics. The bias currents, e.g. I_{bias}, for this study and (Huang, Wang, & Liu, 1996), I_0 and I_p for the improved version in (Asloni, Khoei, & Hadidi, 2006) were all set to the same value with suitable diode-connected transistors. Input currents were reproduced and directed as sourcing, if necessary, by using appropriate mirror circuits.

In proposed design, the inputs were reproduced and sourced by using simple p-type mirrors having aspect ratio of W(μm)/L(μm)=1.44/0.24 while a diode-connected PMOS transistor with aspect ratio of W(μm)/L(μm)=1.44/0.24 was utilized between node O and VDD. The bias current I_b was kept at 1 μA and it was obtained by a diode-connected PMOS transistor between VDD and node N_C with aspect ratio W(μm)/L(μm)=0.36/1.08. Post-layout HSPICE transient simulation results are illustrated in Figure 15 where the output is depicted in solid lines.

In (Temel, 2008) previously proposed well-known LTA-MIN designs as well as the new architecture were also examined in terms of design discrepancies for three inputs, I_1, I_2 and I_3. As stated previously, random variations in transistor parameters such as aspect ratios (W/L) and zero body-bias threshold voltage (VTO) are the main factors which cause deviation from the expected DC operation. In simulations, I_1 was incremented from 20 μA to 60 μA by 20 μA while I_2 and I_3

Figure 15. Transient simulation results of proposed LTA-MIN circuit for three inputs

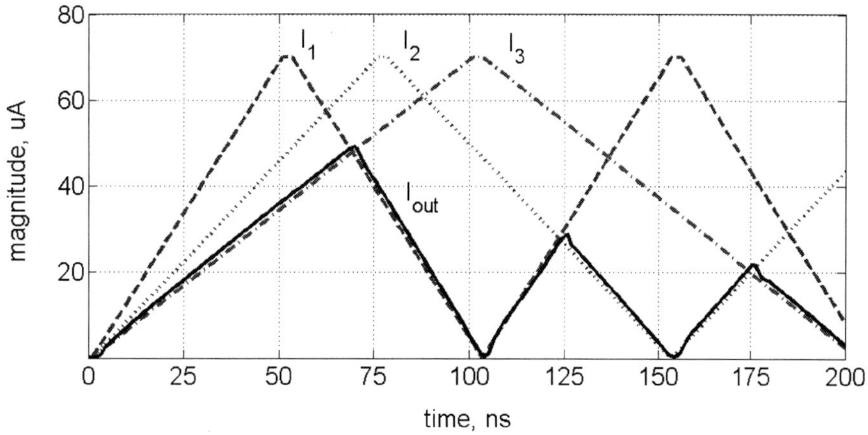

were both held at 70 μA. For each value of I_1, 100-iteration Monte-Carlo DC simulation using normal-Gaussian distribution which represents the relative variations in aspect ratios (W/L) with standard deviation $\sigma_{\Delta W/W, \Delta L/L}$=5% and variations in no- body-bias threshold voltages (VTO) with standard deviation $\sigma_{\Delta VTO}$=25 mV, respectively, was performed. Given a value of I_1 for each design, standard deviation of the maximum value of absolute relative difference, $\delta=\max(|I_{out}-I_{min}|/I_{min})$, where $I_{min}=\min(I_1, I_2, I_3)$, found at each iteration was calculated as an evaluation quantity. Results of the error analysis and some important characteristics of transient simulations are shown in Table 1 where the column '# of transistors' does not regard input reproduction transistors unless necessary in relevant design.

A NEW CURRENT-MODE MEMBERSHIP FUNCTION CIRCUIT AND ITS APPLICATION TO FUZZY CLASSIFICATION

Previously various voltage- and current-mode MFCs along with their advantages and disadvantages were discussed. It was emphasized that the current-mode approach offers such superiorities as high-speed operation with low-switching voltage and design simplicity over voltage-mode designs, (Baturone, Solano, & Huertas, 1994).

Considerable research on current-mode MFC has resorted on *piece-wise linear* (PWL) approximation due to immediate simplicity of current summation/subtraction at nodes, which makes it possible to achieve switching for a given linguistic fuzzy rule: For example, the designs in (Baturone, Solano, & Huertas, 1994; Kashtiban, Khoei, & Hadidi, 2007) explicitly or implicitly exploit truncated (or bounded) difference operation with pre-specified slopes in linearity. However, they have the following pitfalls:

1. They are highly dependent on design quantities, i.e. reference currents and biasing voltages.
2. Successive wired-arithmetic operations in the form of current summation/subtraction limit the maximum dynamic range of the input and the output.
3. Intense use of current-mirrors makes design discrepancies a serious issue; choice of mirror type, e.g. cascoded, can limit the range of the input current given a supply voltage at the expense of lower voltage headroom for operation and larger chip area.

Table 1. Performance and design characteristics of three-input MIN circuits

Design	# of Trans.	Av. Delay (ns)	Av. Power Diss. (mW)	Layout Area, (μm)²	σ_δ (%) (I_1=20/40/60 μA)
Temel, 2008	13	1.7	0.19	3.8	2.8/2.4/2.3
Sasaki, Inoue, Shirai, & Ueno, 1990	21	2.6	0.30	5.3	3.8/3.4/2.9
Donckers, Dualibe, & Verleysen, 2000	18	2.4	0.26	5.1	3.4/2.9/2.6
Asloni, Khoei, & Hadidi, 2006	18	2.5	0.23	5.0	3.4/3.1/2.7
Huang, Wang, & Liu, 1996	14	2.2	0.23	4.6	3.2/2.8/2.5
Dualibe, Jespers, & Verleysen, 2001	19	2.6	0.25	5.3	3.6/3.3/3.0

4. MFC descriptions involve two or more constant current-mode parametric inputs that refer to the main input at which the output is expected to switch. Even there is no input applied, these currents flow through their branches, thereby causing excessive static power dissipation.
5. They usually utilize the voltage as an intermediate controlling variable to switch the output current, which causes spurious transient response.

A current-mode MFC design should be able to adaptively provide an approximate DC transfer characteristic between input and output with least number of inputs as well as remedying the above shortcomings.

In this section, for achieving above objectives, a new current-mode MFC recently described in (Temel, 2009) is presented. The circuit adequately combines both WTA-MAX and LTA-MIN topologies previously introduced. New MFC is very compact and it needs only one parametric reference input current as representing the center of a bell- or Gaussian-like MF. The circuit and its previous counterparts are investigated in terms of important design and performance measures. As an application, a fuzzy classifier is designed with the new circuit.

Description of New MFC

New current-mode MFC shown in Figure 16(a) is based on the concurrent comparison of input current I_{in} to a reference current representing the k-th antecedent label in a fuzzy rule, $I_k=kI_{base}$, where I_{base} is a base current, which is supposed to be the distance between the centers of MFs. In the circuit, current source I_{bias}, transistors M_A, M_C, M_{sw}, M_{OA} and M_l constitute a modified version of the LTA-MIN circuit given in (Temel, 2008, 2) while transistors M_A, M_B, M_{OA} and M_h form well-known WTA-MAX circuit, (Lazzaro, Rykebusch, Mahowald, & Mead, 1989). Transistor M_C in each cell is sized such that it operates with a small saturation voltage for a given I_s so that the output current $I_{k,out}=I_{k,l}$ follows the minimum of the inputs I_{in} and I_k as rapidly and closely as possible. It is seen that $I_{k,h}=\max(I_k,I_{in})$, and $I_{k,l}=\min(I_k,I_{in})$. The output current $I_{k,l}$ flows only when $I_{k,h}=I_{k,l}$ hence $I_{k,out}=I_k$ when $I_{in}=I_k$ otherwise $I_{k,out}=0$, which is normally a singleton membership function behavior. However, due to device and design properties, $I_{k,out}$ ($m_{in,k}$) will spread as nonlinear transition regions around I_k (k) for respective fuzzy set clause as shown in Figure 16(b) to yield a bell-like membership function. The shape of regions around the reference current can be further adjusted with $M_{B'C}$ and the value of I_{bias} such that neighboring respective $m_{in,k}$s intersect at a particular value of $m_{in,k}$, e.g. 0.5. Because membership lies between 0 and 1, (a normalized) membership of the input

Figure 16. (a) Proposed MFC cell for the k-th fuzzy level where dimensions are given for TSMC 0.25 μm HSPICE (level-49) parameters in full post-layout extraction with 1.8V supply voltage, (b) its expected DC transfer characteristics and block representation, and (c) MFC block representation

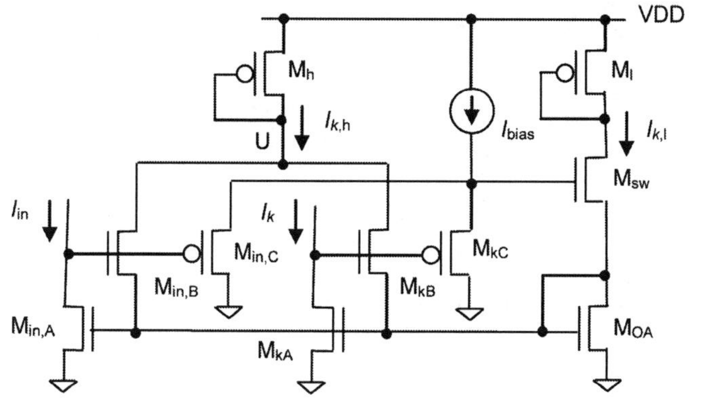

Transistor	Ml-h	MB-C	MAO	Msw
W(μm) /L(μm)	2.4/0.48	2.64/0.24	0.6/0.36	2.88/0.24

(a)

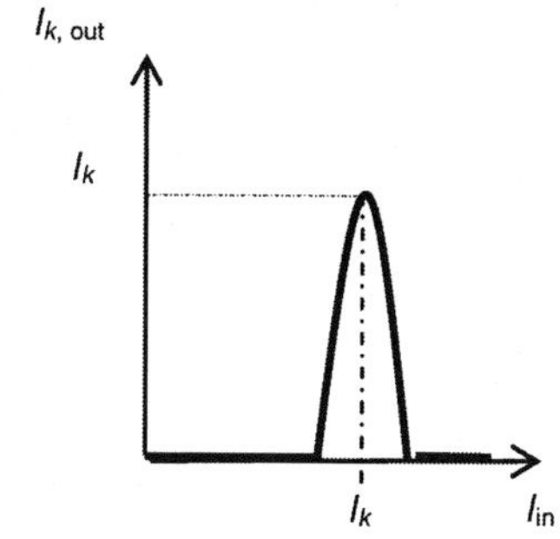

(b)

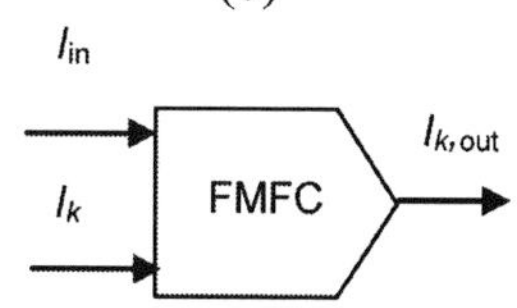

(c)

for the k-th fuzzy label level can be defined as $m_{in,k}=I_{k,out}/I_k$ which could be produced by mirroring $I_{k,out}$ by a factor of $1/k$. It should be noted that transistor M_h can be removed from the circuit and node U can be directly tied up to power supply (VDD) due to selective feature of MAX circuit.

New MFC and its predecessors in (Baturone, Solano, & Huertas, 1994; Kashtiban, Khoei, & Hadidi, 2007; Mesgarzadeh, 2004; Amirkhanzadeh, Khoei, & Hadidi, 2005) which use PWL method were designed and simulated for seven-label membership. Simulations were performed by using TSMC 0.25μm HSPICE (level-49) parameters in full post-layout extraction with 1.8V supply voltage. In all designs, body-biased effects were included and transistors were sized for optimum DC and transient characteristics with input current range of 0 through 70μA. Bias voltages V_{bn} and V_{pn} in (Baturone, Solano, & Huertas, 1994) were obtained by using adequate voltage reference circuits formed with diode-connected PMOS and NMOS transistors. The base current I_{base} for new MFC, reference current I_{ref} in (Baturone, Solano, & Huertas, 1994; Mesgarzadeh, 2004; Amirkhanzadeh, Khoei, & Hadidi, 2005) and the modal norm current I_{norm} used in (Kashtiban, Khoei, & Hadidi, 2007) were taken 10μA and raised to respective label levels for comparison with use of appropriate mirrors. The circuits being compared to new circuit were adjusted such that linear membership functions of neighboring sets intersect at almost 0.5 with transition slope of 1 at rising and falling edges. The output of each design was conditioned on a diode-connected NMOS transistor with dimensional aspect ratio of W(μm)/L(μm)=0.6/0.24. All inputs were chosen as sourcing and they were reproduced, if necessary, by using appropriate mirror circuits. For new MFC, sourcing inputs were reproduced and directed to input nodes by using p-type current mirrors with transistors of dimensional aspect ratio of W(μm)/L(μm)=1.44/0.24. Bias current I_{bias} was taken 1 μA for all labels and it was produced by a diode-connected PMOS transistor with

Figure 17. HSPICE DC simulation results for the new membership-function circuit for seven fuzzy regions

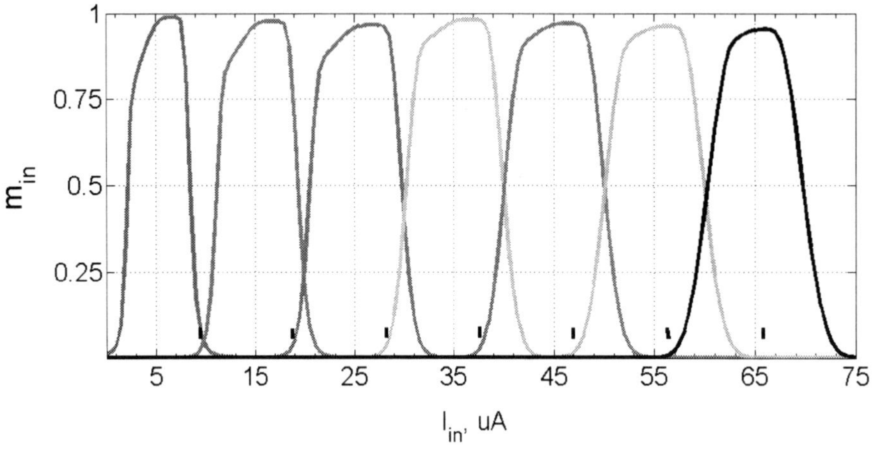

aspect ratio of W(μm)/L(μm)=0.36/1.08. Figure 17 illustrates DC simulation results for generic membership function m_{in} versus I_{in} where each curve represents $m_{in,k}$ centered at respective reference current kI_{base}.

The designed MFCs were also examined concerning relative discrepancies to assess their robustness to parametric variations and design errors. For this objective, I_{in} was varied between 0 and 70μA while I_k was kept at 20μA, 40μA and 60 μA for k=2, 4 and 6, respectively. A set of 100-iteration Monte-Carlo DC simulation analysis using normal-Gaussian distribution which represents the relative variations in aspect ratios (W/L) with standard deviation $\sigma_{\Delta W/W, \Delta L/L}$=5% and variations in zero-body-bias threshold voltages (VTO) with standard deviation $\sigma_{\Delta VTO}$=25mV, respectively, was carried out. In each experiment of analysis, the quantity $\Delta m_{in,k}=(I_{k,out}-I_k)/I_k$ where $I_{k,out}$ is the output current with supplied design parameters of variation is computed. Table 2 presents some important characteristics of MFCs examined: number of transistors, layout area, results of error analysis in terms of standard deviation in per-cent, $\sigma_{\Delta m,k}$ (%), of $\Delta m_{in,k}$ as well as average power drawn from VDD, and delay τ_k for the input waveform I_1 indicated in Figure 15.

Design of Fuzzy Classifier

As an application of new MFC, a single-input, x, is designed for a seven-level fuzzy classifier with output y representing the class label to which x belongs to. The classifier satisfies the following compound rule

R: IF x is A_1 THEN y is B_1 OR IF x is A_2 THEN y is B_2 ... IF x is A_7 THEN y is B_7 (25)

Since each antecedent part consists of single rule, each consequent will be of a single term. Thus the classifier output membership function can be written as

$$\mu_B^*(y)= \max(\mu_{B1}(y), \mu_{B2}(y), \ldots\mu_{B7}(y)) \quad (26)$$

It is clear that since the MF of the new circuit exhibits almost steep transition across the fuzzy regions it can be assumed to be a singleton. Therefore the fuzzy compound rule in Equation (26) can be rewritten as

$$\mu_B^*(y)= \max(\mu_{A1}(x), \mu_{A2}(x), \ldots\mu_{A7}(x)) \quad (27)$$

The overall realization of the classifier is shown as a block diagram shown in Figure 18. Due to approximated singleton characteristics of

Table 2. Design characteristics of MFCs and their transient performance measures for input waveform I_1 varying linearly between 0 through 70μA and other two inputs fixed as indicated

Design	# of Trans.	Layout area $(\mu m)^2$	$\sigma_{\Delta m,k}$ (%)-Average(τ_k (ns))			Av. Power Diss. (mW)
			k=2	k=4	k=6	
Temel, 2009	12	4.0	2.4-1.5	2.7-1.2	2.8-1.0	1.6
Baturone, Solano, & Huertas, 1994	16	5.1	3.0-2.1	3.4-1.9	3.6-1.5	2.9
Kashtiban, Khoei, & Hadidi, 2007	28	16.6	3.6-2.7	4.2-2.3	4.5-2.1	4.0
Mesgerzadeh, 2004	26	13.4	3.6-2.3	4.0-2.0	4.3-1.9	3.5
Amirkhanzadeh, Khoei, & Hadidi, 2005	32	18.3	3.8-2.7	4.5-2.4	4.7-2.1	4.2

the membership function, the class label of the input, k_{in} is obtained as $k_{in}=\lceil \max(I_{k,out})/I_{base}\rceil$ simply by MAXing all $I_{k,out}$ (or $m_{in,k}$ in case of normalised output) terms as shown in Figure 2 where N is the number of fuzzy inputs and $\lceil . \rceil$ refers to the nearest greater integer.

Figure 19 illustrates transient simulation results of the designed classifier for class labels k=2, 4 and 6, i.e. class reference currents were applied at only these levels while reference inputs of other antecedents were left open.

Designed classifier occupied layout area of 31 $(\mu m)^2$ with 91 transistors, had delays of 2.4, 2.0, and 1.8 in ns for k=2, k=4 and 6, respectively, while the average power drawn from VDD was found to be 6.1 mW for the same input waveforms.

CIRCUITS USING ALGEBRAIC FORMS FOR SIMILARITY ASSESSMENT

System design inspired from biological inference does not generally operate on categorical selection of the raw stimuli, (Kolb, & Whishaw, 2008). For example, learning and decision-making with (particularly) *self-organizing mapping* (SOM), (Kohonen, 1988), is an ongoing process where learner (system/model etc.) adjusts itself to input characteristics expressed in terms of a *proximity/distance* measure. In fact most MFs can be expressed in terms of distance, e.g. Gaussian. Therefore, one of the major tasks fulfilled by an intelligent system is to judge how similar a given input pattern is to certain group of labels or other inputs, which is termed *proximity* or *(dis)similarity*. In order to quantify these measures, mostly used *metric* is given in terms of distance.

There have been various distance metric definitions based on respective *norm*, (Soucek, 1992). *Euclidean* distance is a widely adopted distance metric concerning 2-nd order norm between samples. It assumes that the ranges of input features are comparable. Assuming two pattern vectors **x** and **y** in an n-dimensional input space the Euclidean distance between them is given by $d(\mathbf{x},\mathbf{y}) = \sqrt{\sum_{\forall i}\left(x_i - y_i\right)^2}$ with x_i and y_i being the i-th (spatial) attribute or feature of **x** and **y**, respectively.

Analog design provides similar benefits, e.g. parallelism, accuracy in assessing proximity between inputs as it does for categorization, e.g. MFC, or selection, e.g. MAX and MIN. As can be seen from the distance metric expression, major operations in realizing above distance measure are *squaring* and *square-rooting*.

In (Gopalan, & Titus, 2003), two *differential stages* as *transconductor-amplifier*, each of which encodes the difference between voltage-mode inputs, are utilized to derive a quadratic relationship. The overall structure also contains an *absolute-value circuit* for bidirectional operation in voltage-mode difference. Despite modularity

Figure 18. Fuzzy classifier with new FMFC

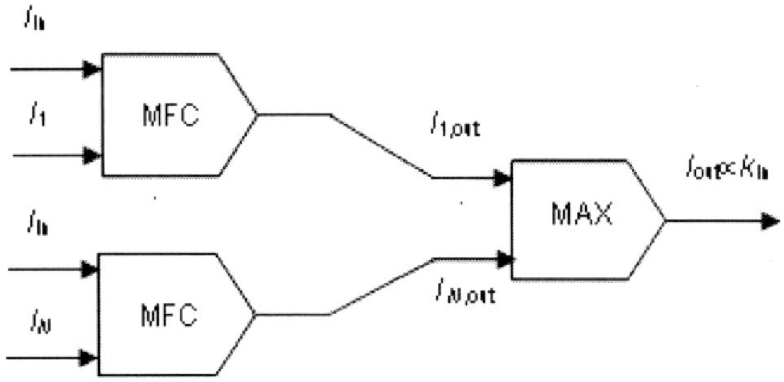

Figure 19. Transient simulation results of the designed classifier for k=2, 4 and 6

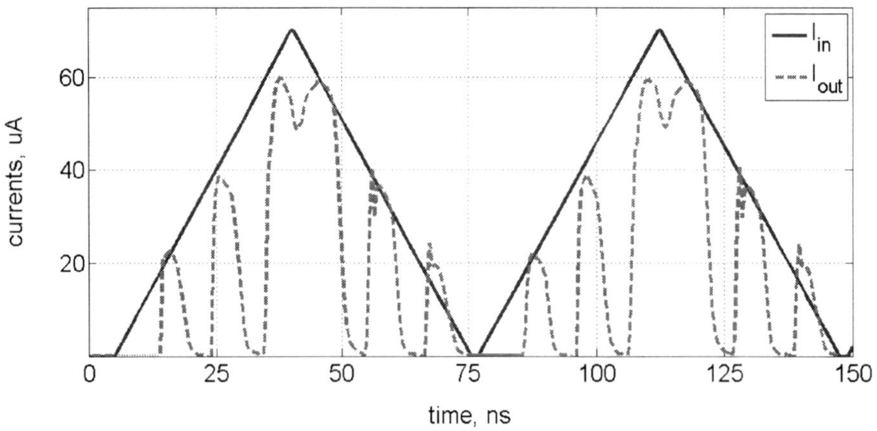

and comprehensiveness the disadvantages which hold for previously discussed voltage-mode circuits employing differential stages are also valid for the circuit. Furthermore linear term involved in the relationship limits the operational capability.

A direct current-mode Euclidean-distance realization can be given by exploiting the principle of *translinear loop* composed of MOS transistors operating in strong-inversion mode, (Toumazou, Ligey, & Haigh, 1990). Figure 20 depicts a current-mode squaring and square-rooting circuits, proposed in (Popa, 2005). The squaring circuit is slightly improved version of the architecture described by (Bult, & Wallinga, 1987). It should be noted that the current source I_{ref} is common to whole processing block into which the circuit resides as well as the blocks illustrated in the figure.

For the squaring circuit, $I_{b,i} = I_{in,i} + I_{a,i}$ and by using the gate-to-source voltage within the loop consisting of M_1, M_2, M_5 and M_4, it can be found that, (Popa, 2005),

$$I_{a,i} = I_{\text{ref}} - \frac{I_{in,i}}{2} + \frac{I_{in,i}^2}{16 I_{\text{ref}}}; \qquad I_{b,i} = I_{\text{ref}} + \frac{I_{in,i}}{2} + \frac{I_{in,i}^2}{16 I_{\text{ref}}} \tag{28}$$

Assuming $I_{\text{out},i} = I_{a,i} + I_{b,i}$ then $I_{out,i} = 2I_{\text{ref}} + \frac{I_{in,i}^2}{8I_{\text{ref}}}$. If $I_{\text{in},i} = | I_{x,i} - I_{y,i} |$ and it has been formed through *bidirectional current mirrors* or *current conveyors*, (Toumazou, Ligey, &

Figure 20. (a) Square, and (b) square-rooting circuits which can be used in the Euclidean-distance circuit

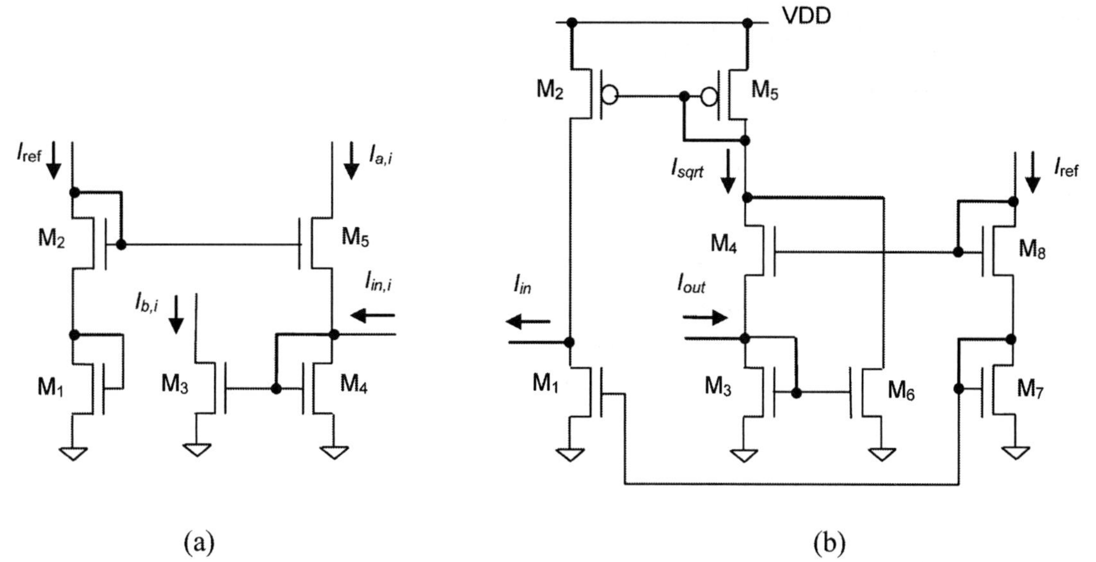

Haigh, 1990), then it is possible to realize Euclidean-distance between the inputs representing the quantities of **x** and **y**. The implementation for compatibility with the exact definition of the square-rooting can be assured by using the square-rooting circuit shown in the Figure 20(b) whose current-mode DC transfer relationship is given by $I_{out} = \sqrt{8I_{\text{ref}}I_{in}}$ (Popa, 2005).

Owing to generality of the translinear-loop principle, it should be noted that both strong inversion and weak inversion region designs are almost the same with minor modifications. In fact both square-law and exponential relationships equivalently and straightforwardly yield almost the identical results. Since in this study we are primarily concerned with design principles both designs can be adapted for needs of interest.

CONCLUSION

In this chapter, as a means of intelligent system realization with decision-making capability fuzzy logic approach was described based on set theoretic axioms. Fuzzy logic relieves the intelligent system design problem with its rule-based nature. Each rule was shown to be expressed in terms simple constituents called the antecedents and the consequents. The fundamental concept for establishing relationship between them is the notion of membership. Membership assignment called the fuzzification is the mechanism which relays the measurement of uncertainty to the quantity under consideration given a rule. As a reverse process, defuzzification is applied to produce a crisp output which best represents the fuzzy inference outcome given a compound rule. Fuzzy controller is a reasoning scheme which performs fuzzification and defuzzification with respect to rule and data bases under the supervision of an expert. As well-known fuzzy reasoning models, namely Mamdani's and Takagi-Sugeno's fuzzy approaches, were also discussed to complete fuzzy inferential system design.

Fuzzy reasoning was shown to be adequately fulfilled with analog circuit design in voltage- and current-mode or their mixture. Current-mode design was shown to be preferred for realization of fuzzy controllers. Major *T*- and *S*-norm-circuits were discussed in terms of their pros and cons.

A new looser-take-all circuit was described to implement *T*-norm min operation. Its performance comparison to previous designs was also presented. Based on the new *T*-norm circuit, a new membership circuit was also presented. It was also shown to outperform previously described current-mode counterparts. As an application of the new membership function circuit a fuzzy classifier was described and designed. In sequel, the chapter introduced some recent current-mode distance circuits as a means of similarity assignment between quantities of interest.

REFERENCES

Angulo, J. R., Acevedo, G. D., Carvajal, R. G., & Martin, A. L. (2005). Low-voltage High-performance Current-mode WTA Circuits Based on Flipped-voltage Followers. *IEEE Transactions on Circuits and Wystems. II, Express Briefs*, *52*(7), 420–423. doi:10.1109/TCSII.2005.850433

Asloni, M., Khoei, A., & Hadidi, K. (2006). Design of Analog Current-mode Looser-take-all Circuit. *IEICE Transactions on Electronics. E (Norwalk, Conn.)*, *89-C*(6), 819–822.

Azeem, M. F., & Baig, A. (2007). Design and Fabrication of Basic Building Blocks for Analog Implementation of Programmable Fuzzy Logic Controller. *Proceedings of IEEE Information Reuse and Integration*, 563-569.

Baker, R. J., Li, H. W., & Boyce, D. E. (1998). *CMOS Circuit Design, Layout, and Simulation*. New York: IEEE Press.

Baturone, I., Huertas, J. L., Barriga, A., & Solano, S.-S. (1994). Current-Mode Multiple-input MAX Circuit, *IEE. Electronics Letters*, *30*(9), 678–680. doi:10.1049/el:19940510

Baturone, I., Solano, S. S., & Huertas, J. L. (1994). Current-mode Singleton Fuzzy Controller. In *Proceedings of the 3rd International Conference on Fuzzy Logic, Neural Networks and Soft Computing*, IIZUKA, 647-648.

Bezdek, J. C., Keller, J., Krisnapuram, R., & Pal, N. R. (2005). *Fuzzy Models and Algorithms for Pattern Recognition and Image Processing*. New York: Springer.

Bult, K., & Geelen, G. J. G. M. (1990). A Fast-Settling CMOS Operational Amplifier for SC Circuits with 90-dB DC Gain. *IEEE Journal of Solid-state Circuits*, *25*(6), 1379–1384. doi:10.1109/4.62165

Bult, K., & Wallinga, H. (1987). A Class of Analog CMOS Circuits Based on the Square-law Characteristic of an MOS Transistor in Saturation. *IEEE Journal of Solid-state Circuits*, *SC-22*(3), 357–365. doi:10.1109/JSSC.1987.1052733

Carvajal, R., Angulo, J. R., & Tombs, J. (2000). High-Speed High-Precision Voltage-mode MIN/MAX Circuits in CMOS Technology. In. *Proceedings of IEEE International Symposium on Circuits and Systems*, *V*, 13–16.

Carvajal, R. G., Angulo, J. R., & Martin, A. J. L. (2005). The Flipped-voltage Follower: A Useful Cell for Low-voltage Low-power Circuit Design. *IEEE Transactions on Circuits and Systems II*, *52*(7), 1276–1291. doi:10.1109/TCSI.2005.851387

Chen, G., & Pham, T. T. (2001). *Introduction to Fuzzy Sets, Fuzzy Logic, and Fuzzy Control Systems*. Boca Raton, FL: CRC Press.

Chen, J. -J., Chen, Chen, C. -C., & Tsao, H. -W. (1992). Tunable Membership Function Circuit for Fuzzy Control Systems Using CMOS Technology. *IEE Electronics Letters*, *28*(22), 2101-2103.

Cho, J. –W., park. C., -W., & Park, M. (2002). An Indirect Model Reference Adaptive Fuzzy Control for SISO Takagi–Sugeno Model. *Fuzzy Sets and Systems*, *131*, 197–215. doi:10.1016/S0165-0114(02)00105-7

Circuits. *Springer-Lecture Notes in Computer Science*, 4578/2007, 237-244.

Controllers. *IEE Electronics Letters*, 30(23), 1924-1925.

Donckers, N., Dualibe, C., & Verleysen, M. (2000). A Current-mode CMOS Loser-take-all with Minimum Function for Neural Computations. In. *Proceedings of IEEE International Symposium on Circuits and Systems*, *I*, 415–418.

Driankov, D., Hellendoorn, H., & Reinfrank, M. (1993). *An Introduction to Fuzzy Control*. Berlin Heidelberg, Germany: Springer-Verlag.

Dualibe, C., Jespers, P., & Verleysen, M. (2001). Embedded Fuzzy Control for Automatic Channel Equalization After Digital Transmissions. In. *Proceedings of IEEE International Symposium on Circuits and Systems*, *III*, 73–176.

Dualibe, C., Verleysen, M., & Jespers, P. G. A. (2003). *Design of Analog Fuzzy Logic Controllers in CMOS Technologies: Implementation, Test and Application*. Dordrecht: Springer.

Freitas, D. A., & Current, K. W. (1983). CMOS Current Comparator Circuit. *IEE Electronics Letters*, *19*(17), 695–697. doi:10.1049/el:19830474

Gopalan, A., & Titus, A. H. (2003). A New Wide Range Euclidean Distance Circuit for Neural Network Hardware Implementations. *IEEE Transactions on Neural Networks*, *14*(5), 1176–1186. doi:10.1109/TNN.2003.816034

Gottarredona, S., & Barranco, B.-L. (2006). A Low-Power Current Mode Fuzzy-ART Cell. *IEEE Transactions on Neural Networks*, *17*(6), 1666–1673. doi:10.1109/TNN.2006.883725

Huang, C. Y., Wang, C. J., & Liu, B. D. (1996). Modular Current-mode Multiple Input Minimum Circuit for Fuzzy Logic Controllers'. *IEE Electronics Letters*, *32*(12), 1067–1069. doi:10.1049/el:19960728

Huang, C. -Y, & Liu, B. -D. (1994). Current-mode Multiple Input Maximum Circuit for Fuzzy Logic

Inoue, T., Ueno, F., Motomura, R. M., & Setoguchi, O. (1991). Analysis and Design of Analog CMOS Building Blocks For Integrated Fuzzy Inference Circuits. *Proceedings of IEEE International Symposium on Circuits and Systems*, *4*, 2024–2027.

Jain, A. K., Bolton, R. J., & Abd-El-Barr, M. (1993). CMOS Multiple-valued Logic Design, Part I and II. *IEEE Transactions on Circuits and Systems-Fundamental Theory and Applications*, *40*(8), 503–522. doi:10.1109/81.242320

Jang, R. (1992). Self-Learning Fuzzy Controllers Based on Temporal Back Propagation. *IEEE Transactions on Neural Networks*, *3*(5), 714–723. doi:10.1109/72.159060

Kasabov, N. (2009). Integrative Connectionist Learning Systems Inspired by Nature: Current Models, Future Trends and Challenges. *Natural Computing*, *8*(2), 199–210. doi:10.1007/s11047-008-9066-z

Kashtiban, M. M-., Khoei, A., & Hadidi, K. (2007). A Current-mode, First-order Takagi-Sugeno-Kang Fuzzy Logic Controller, Supporting Rational-powered Membership Functions. *IEICE Transactions on Electronics. E (Norwalk, Conn.)*, *90-C*(6), 1258–1266.

Kettner, T., Heite, C., & Schumacher, K. (1993). Analog CMOS Realization of Fuzzy Logic Membership Functions. *IEEE Journal of Solid-state Circuits*, *28*(7), 857–861. doi:10.1109/4.222189

Kolb, B., & Whishaw, I. Q. (2008). *Fundamentals of Human Neuropsychology. Hampshire*. Macmillan.

Kosko, K. (1992). *Neural Networks and Fuzzy Systems*. Upper Saddle River, NJ: Prentice-Hall.

Landolt, O., Vittoz, E., & Heim, P. (1992). CMOS Self-biased Euclidean Distance Computing Circuit with High Dynamic Range, *IEE. Electronics Letters*, *28*(4), 352–354. doi:10.1049/el:19920220

Lazzaro, J., Rykebusch, R., Mahowald, A., & Mead, C. (1989). Winner-take-all Networks of O(n) Complexity. In Touretzky, D. (Ed.), *Advances in Neural Information Processing Systems I* (pp. 703–711). San Francisco: Morgan Kaufmann.

Lin, G., & Shi, B. (1999). A Multi-input Current-mode Fuzzy Integrated Circuit for Pattern Recognition. In *Proceedings of IEEE 2nd International Conference on Intelligent Processing and Manufacturing of Materials,* 1, 687-693.

Mamdani, E. H. (1977). Application of Fuzzy Logic to Approximate Reasoning Using Linguistic Synthesis. *IEEE Transactions on Computers*, *C-26*(12), 1182–1191. doi:10.1109/TC.1977.1674779

Montero, J., Lopez, V., & Gomez, D. (2007). The Role of Fuzziness in Decision Making. In Wang, D. P., Ruan, D., & Kerre, E. E. (Eds.), *Fuzzy Logic: A Spectrum of Theoretical & Practical Issues* (pp. 337–350). New York: Springer.

Moraga, C., Trillas, E., & Guadarrama, S. (2003). Multiple-valued Logic and Artificial Intelligence Fundamentals of Fuzzy Control Revisited. *Kluwer-Artificial Intelligence Review*, *20*(3-4), 169–197. doi:10.1023/B:AIRE.0000006610.94970.1d

Panella, M. (2007). *Martinelly, Giuseppe*. Binary Neuro-Fuzzy Classifiers Trained by Nonlinear Quantum.

Perfiliva, I. (2007). Analytical Theory of Fuzzy IF-THEN Rules with Compositional Rule of Inference. In Wang, D. P., Ruan, D., & Kerre, E. E. (Eds.), *Fuzzy Logic: A Spectrum of Theoretical & Practical Issues* (pp. 173–192). New York: Springer.

Popa, C. (2005). Current-mode Euclidean Distance Circuit Independent Technological Parameters. *Proceedings of IEEE Semiconductor Conference*, *2*, 459–462.

Rutkowski, L. (2004). *Flexible Neuro-fuzzy Systems: Structures, Learning and Performance Evaluation*. Boston: Kluwer.

Sasaki, M., Inoue, T., Shirai, Y., & Ueno, F. (1990). Fuzzy Multiple-input Maximum and Minimum Circuits in Current-mode and Their Analyses Using Bounded Difference Equations. *IEEE Transactions on Computers*, *39*(6), 768–774. doi:10.1109/12.53598

Shirai, Y., Ueno, F., & Inoue, T. (2007). Configuration of Fuzzy Membership Function Circuits Using Current-mode. *Wiley Interscience Electronics and Communications in Japan*, *70*(8), 59–67.

Soucek, B. (1992). *Fast Learning and Invariant Object Recognition*. New York: John Wiley & Sons.

Sugeno, M., & Yasukawa, T. (1993). A Fuzzy Logic Based Approach to Qualitative Modeling. *IEEE Transactions on Fuzzy Systems*, *1*(1), 7–31. doi:10.1109/TFUZZ.1993.390281

Takagi, T., & Sugeno, M. (1985). Fuzzy Identification of Systems and Its Application to Modeling and Control. *IEEE Transactions on Systems, Man, and Cybernetics*, *20*(2), 116–132.

Temel, T. (2007). High-performance Current-mode CMOS Simultaneous Implementation of Window-literal Operations for Multi-valued Logic. *IET ElectronicsLetters*, *43*(15), 785–786. doi:10.1049/el:20070434

Temel, T., (2008, 1). Technical Report no: 3, Project no: 107E059 for Turkish Scientific and Technical Research, 2008.

Temel, T. (2008). 2). A New, High-performance Current-mode Loser-take-all Minimum Circuit. *IET Electronics Letters*, *44*(12), 718–719. doi:10.1049/el:20081174

Temel, T. (2009). Technical Report no: 4, Project no: 107E059 for Turkish Scientific and Technical Research, 2009.

Temel, T., & Morgul, A. (2004). Implementation of Multi-Valued Logic Gates Using Full Current-mode CMOS Circuits. *Kluwer. Analog Integrated Circuits and Signal Processing*, *39*, 191–204. doi:10.1023/B:ALOG.0000024066.66847.89

Thayse, A., & Deschamps, J. P. (1977). Logic Properties of Unate Discrete and Switching Functions. *IEEE Transactions on Computers*, *C-26*(12), 1020–1212. doi:10.1109/TC.1977.1674781

Toumazou, C., Ligey, F. J., & Haigh, D. G. (1990). *Analogue IC Design: The Current-mode Approach*. Herts, UK: Peregrinus Cop.

Verleysen, M. (1992). *Neural Networks and Content-Addressable Memories for Vision: From Theory to VLSI*. PhD Dissertation: UCL.

Vida, V. F. (1996). *Design of Mixed-Signal CMOS Neuro-Fuzzy Controllers*. (PhD Dissertation).

Wilamowski, B., Jaeger, R. C., & Kaynak, O. (1999). Neuro-fuzzy Architecture for CMOS Implementation. *IEEE Transactions on Industrial Electronics*, *46*(6), 1132–1136. doi:10.1109/41.808001

Yamakawa, T. (1993). A Fuzzy Inference Engine in Nonlinear Analog Mode and Its Application to a Fuzzy Logic Control. *IEEE Transactions on Neural Networks*, *4*(3), 496–522. doi:10.1109/72.217192

Zadeh, L. (1973). Outline of a New Approach to the Analysis of Complex Systems and Decision Processes. *IEEE Transactions on Systems, Man, and Cybernetics*, *3*(1), 28–44.

Zadeh, L. A. (1965). Fuzzy Sets. *Information and Control*, *8*, 94–102. doi:10.1016/S0019-9958(65)90241-X

Chapter 10
A Biomimetic Adaptive Algorithm and Micropower Circuit Architecture for Implantable Neural Decoders

Benjamin I. Rapoport
Massachusetts Institute of Technology, USA & Harvard Medical School, USA

Rahul Sarpeshkar
Massachusetts Institute of Technology, USA

ABSTRACT

Algorithmically and energetically efficient computational architectures that operate in real time are essential for clinically useful neural prosthetic devices. Such architectures decode raw neural data to obtain direct motor control signals for external devices. They can also perform data compression and vastly reduce the bandwidth and consequently power expended in wireless transmission of raw data from implantable brain–machine interfaces. We describe a biomimetic algorithm and micropower analog circuit architecture for decoding neural cell ensemble signals. The decoding algorithm implements a continuous-time artificial neural network, using a bank of adaptive linear filters with kernels that emulate synaptic dynamics. The filters transform neural signal inputs into control-parameter outputs, and can be tuned automatically in an on-line learning process. We demonstrate that the algorithm is suitable for decoding both local field potentials and mean spike rates. We also provide experimental validation of our system, decoding discrete reaching decisions from neuronal activity in the macaque parietal cortex, and decoding continuous head direction trajectories from cell ensemble activity in the rat thalamus. We further describe a method of mapping the algorithm to a highly parallel circuit architecture capable of continuous learning and real-time operation. Circuit simulations of a subthreshold analog CMOS instantiation of the architecture reveal that its performance is comparable to the predicted performance of our decoding algorithm for a system decoding three control parameters from 100 neural input channels at microwatt levels of power consumption. While the algorithm and decoding architecture are suitable for analog or digital implementation, we indicate how a micropower analog system trades some algorithmic programmability for reductions in power and area consumption that could facilitate implantation of a

DOI: 10.4018/978-1-60960-018-1.ch010

neural decoder within the brain. We also indicate how our system can compress neural data more than 100,000-fold, greatly reducing the power needed for wireless telemetry of neural data.

INTRODUCTION

Brain–machine interfaces have proven capable of decoding neuronal population activity in real time to derive instantaneous control signals for prosthetics and other devices. All of the decoding systems demonstrated to date have operated by analyzing digitized neural data (Chapin, Moxon, Markowitz, & Nicolelis, 1999; Hochberg et al., 2006; Jackson, Mavoori, & Fetz, 2006; Musallam, Corneil, Greger, Scherberger, & Andersen, 2004; Santhanam, Ryu, Yu, Afshar, & Shenoy, 2006; Taylor, Tillery, & Schwartz, 2002; Wessberg et al., 2000). Clinically viable neural prosthetics are an eagerly anticipated advance in the field of rehabilitation medicine, and development of brain–machine interfaces that wirelessly transmit neural data to external devices will represent an important step toward clinical viability. The general model for such devices has two components: a brain–implanted unit directly connected to a multielectrode array collecting raw neural data; and a unit outside the body for data processing, decoding, and control. Data transmission between the two units is wireless. A 100-channel, 12-bit-precise digitization of raw neural waveforms sampled at 30 kHz generates 36 Mbs^{-1} of data; the power costs in digitization, wireless communication, and population signal decoding all scale with this high data rate. Consequences of this scaling, as seen for example in cochlear-implant systems, include unwanted heat dissipation in the brain, decreased longevity of batteries, and increased size of the implanted unit. Recent designs for system components have addressed these issues in several ways, including micropower neural amplification (Holleman & Otis, 2007; Wattanapanitch, Fee, & Sarpeshkar, 2007); adaptive power biasing to reduce recording power in multielectrode arrays (Sarpeshkar et al., 2008); low-power data telemetry (Ghovanloo & Atluri, 2007; Mandal & Sarpeshkar, 2007, 2008; Mohseni, Najafi, Eliades, & Wang, 2005); ultra-low-power analog-to-digital conversion (Yang & Sarpeshkar, 2006); low-power neural stimulation (Theogarajan et al., 2004); energy-efficient wireless recharging (Baker & Sarpeshkar, 2007); and low-power circuits and system designs for brain–machine interfaces (Sarpeshkar et al., 2008; Sarpeshkar et al., 2007). Power-conserving schemes for compressing neural data before transmission have also been proposed (Olsson III & Wise, 2005). However, almost no work has been done in the area of power-efficient neural decoding (Rapoport et al., 2009).

Direct and power-efficient analysis and decoding of analog neural data within the implanted unit of a brain–machine interface could facilitate extremely high data compression ratios. For example, the 36 Mbs^{-1} required to transmit raw neural data from 100 channels could be compressed more than 100,000-fold to 300 bs^{-1} of 3-channel motor-output information updated with 10-bit precision at 10 Hz. Such dramatic compression brings concomitant reductions in the power required for communication and digitization of neural data. Ultra-low-power analog preprocessing prior to digitization of neural signals could thus be beneficial in some applications. Related considerations arise in the design of cochlear implants, and prior work in that field has demonstrated that power-efficient, analog preprocessing before digitization can be used to achieve high data compression ratios, leading to order-of-magnitude reductions in power consumption relative to fully digital data-processing schemes (Sarpeshkar, Baker et al., 2005; Sarpeshkar, Salthouse et al., 2005). Such power savings have been achieved while preserving programmability, as well as robustness to multiple sources of noise and transistor mismatch. Importantly, a processor based on this low-power design paradigm functioned successfully in a deaf patient, enabling her to understand speech on her very first attempt (Sarpeshkar, 2006).

In this chapter we describe an approach to neural decoding using low-power analog preprocessing methods that can handle large quantities of high-bandwidth analog data, processing neural input signals in a slow-and-parallel fashion to generate low-bandwidth control outputs. Parallel architectures for data compression constitute an area in which analog systems perform especially well relative to digital systems, as has been demonstrated analytically (Sarpeshkar, 1998), and as exemplified by biological systems such as the retina and the cochlea (Mead, 1989; Sarpeshkar, 2006).

Multiple approaches to neural signal decoding have been implemented successfully by a number of research groups, as mentioned in the section entitled "Implementation of the Decoding Algorithm in Analog Circuitry." All of these have employed highly programmable, discrete-time, digital algorithms, implemented in software or microprocessors located outside the brain. We are unaware of any work on continuous-time analog decoders or analog circuit architectures for neural decoding (Rapoport et al., 2009). The neural signal decoder we present here is designed to complement and integrate with existing approaches. Optimized for implementation in micropower analog circuitry, it sacrifices some algorithmic programmability to reduce the power consumption and physical size of the neural decoder, facilitating use as a component of a unit implanted within the brain.

We demonstrate a method of designing highly power-efficient adaptive circuit architectures for neural decoding in two stages. We first generalize a discrete-time algorithm for adaptive-filter decoding to a continuous-time analog decoder. We then provide an approach to translating this decoder into a circuit architecture.

In this chapter we show that our algorithm and analog architecture offer good performance when learning to interpret real neural cell ensemble codes in the rat thalamus, from which we decode continuous head direction trajectories, and the macaque monkey parietal cortex, from which we decode discrete reach decisions. We further show that the system is sufficiently flexible to accept local field potentials or mean spike rates as inputs. Circuit simulations of a subthreshold analog CMOS implementation of our circuit architecture suggest that a spike processor and decoder with 100 input channels and 3 output control parameters could be built with a total power budget of approximately 42 μW; this would reduce the power expended in wireless telemetry to approximately 300 nW and the total power consumption of the implanted unit would be under 43 μW.

Our decoding scheme sacrifices the flexibility of a general-purpose digital system for the efficiency of a special-purpose analog system. This tradeoff may be undesirable in some neural prosthetic devices. Therefore, our proposed decoder is meant to be used not as a substitute for digital signal processors but rather as an adjunct to digital hardware, in ways that synergistically fuse the efficiency of embedded analog preprocessing options with the flexibility of a general-purpose external digital processor. The schematic for such a combined system is shown in Figure 1. First, an external digital processor transiently analyzes raw, high-bandwidth neural data to determine spike thresholds and DAC-programmable analog parameters for the implanted analog decoder. Such parameters could control which input channels are turned on or off, set filter time constants for converting spikes to mean firing rates, and establish amplitude thresholds that ensure optimal spike sorting. Such analysis requires a great deal of flexible programmability and so is best done digitally, by an external processor, taking into account all available raw neural data. The analysis generates configuration settings that can be downloaded over a low-bandwidth link to reconfigure the implanted unit, including a low-power analog decoder, digitally. The analog system then learns, decodes, and outputs low-bandwidth informa-

Figure 1. Schematic diagram of a brain–machine interface system incorporating an implantable analog neural decoder

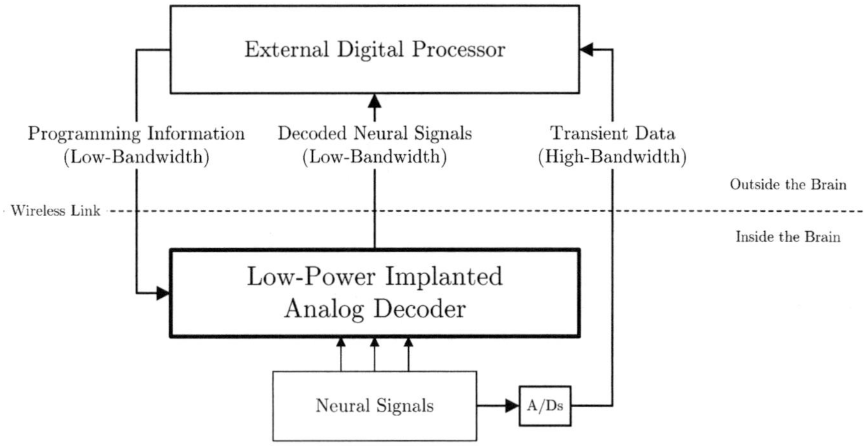

tion in a low-power fashion for most of the time that the brain–machine interface is operational. Digital analysis and recalibration of the analog system may be done infrequently (perhaps once a day, as in early reports of a clinically useful brain–machine interface (Hochberg et al., 2006)) so that the average power consumption is always low even though transient power consumption of the external digital system may be relatively high during recalibration. The architecture of Figure 1 permits exploration of other decoding algorithms in the external unit, allowing high-power operation when necessary to achieve sufficient programmability.

For clinical neural prosthetic devices, the necessity of highly sophisticated decoding algorithms remains open to question, since both animal (Carmena et al., 2003; Musallam et al., 2004; Taylor et al., 2002; Velliste, Perel, Spalding, Whitford, & Schwartz, 2008) and human (Hochberg et al., 2006) users of even first-generation neural prosthetic systems have proven capable of rapidly adapting to the particular rules governing the control of their brain–machine interfaces. In the present work we focus on an architecture to implement a simple, continuous-time analog linear (convolutional) decoding algorithm. The approach we present here can be generalized to implement analog-circuit architectures of more general Bayesian algorithms; examples of related systems include analog probabilistic decoding circuit architectures used in speech recognition and error correcting codes (Lazzaro, Wawrzynek, & Lippmann, 1997; Loeliger, Tarköy, Lustenberger, & Helfenstein, 1999). Related architectures can be adapted through our mathematical approach to design circuits for Bayesian neural decoding.

This chapter is organized as follows: The section entitled "Methods of Designing and Testing a Micropower Neural Decoding System" begins by presenting a derivation of our adaptive-kernel decoder; a corresponding description of an example instantiation in subthreshold micropower analog VLSI is presented in the subsection "Implementation of the Decoding Algorithm in Analog Circuitry." "Methods of Testing the Neural Signal Decoding System" describes methods for testing the algorithm and corresponding circuit architecture in several decoding tasks: continuous trajectory decoding from simulated local field potential (LFP) input signals, continuous head-direction trajectory decoding from spike-train inputs recorded from the thalamus of a freely moving rat, and discrete arm-reach intentions decoded from spike-train inputs recorded from the parietal cortex of a macaque monkey. The results of these tests are subsequently presented in the section entitled "Evaluating the Performance of the Neural Decoding System." The following section, "Evaluating Design Tradeoffs in the Construction of an Implantable Neural Decoder," discusses the simulated performance characteristics of our decoding system and alternative digital implementations from the perspectives of reducing power consumption for implantable brain–machine interfaces. The chapter concludes with a summary of our work and anticipated directions for future research in the field of neural decoding in the context of brain–machine interfaces.

METHODS OF DESIGNING AND TESTING A MICROPOWER NEURAL DECODING SYSTEM

An Algorithm for Adaptive Convolutional Decoding of Neural Cell Ensemble Signals

The function of neuronal population decoding is to map neural signals onto higher-level cognitive processes to which they correspond. This section presents the mathematical foundations of an adaptive convolutional decoder whose kernels can be modified according to a gradient-descent–based learning algorithm that optimizes decoding performance in an on-line, real-time fashion.

In convolutional decoding of neural cell ensemble signals, the decoding operation takes the form

$$\vec{M}(t) = \mathbf{W}(t) \circ \vec{N}(t)$$
$$M_i(t) = \sum_{j=1}^{n} W_{ij}(t) \circ N_j(t) \tag{1.1}$$

where $i \in \{1,\ldots,m\}$; $\vec{N}(t)$ is an n-dimensional vector containing the neural signal (n input channels of neuronal firing rates, analog signal values, or local field potentials, for example) at time t; $\vec{M}(t)$ is a corresponding m-dimensional vector containing the decoder output signal (which in the examples presented here corresponds to motor control parameters, but could correspond as well to limb or joint kinematic parameters or to characteristics or states of nonmotor cognitive processes); $\mathbf{W}$ is a matrix of convolution kernels $W_{ij}(t)$ (formally analogous to a matrix of dynamic synaptic weights), each of which depends on a set of p modifiable parameters, W_{ij}^{k}, $k \in \{1,\ldots,p\}$; and $\circ$ indicates convolution. Accurate decoding requires first choosing an appropriate functional form for the kernels and then optimizing the kernel parameters to achieve maximal decoding accuracy. Since the optimization process is generalizable to any choice of kernels that are differentiable functions of the tuning parameters, we discuss the general process first. We then explain our biophysical motivations for selecting particular functional forms for the decoding kernels; appropriately chosen kernels enable the neural decoder to emulate the real-time encoding and decoding processes performed by biological neurons.

Our algorithm for optimizing the decoding kernels uses a gradient-descent approach to minimize decoding error in a least-squares sense during a learning phase of decoder operation. During this phase the correct output $\hat{\vec{M}}(t)$, and hence the decoder error $\vec{e}(t) = \vec{M}(t) - \hat{\vec{M}}(t)$, is available to the decoder for feedback-based learning. We design the optimization algorithm to evolve $\mathbf{W}(t)$ in a manner that reduces the squared decoder error on a timescale set by the parameter τ, where the squared error is defined as

$$E\left(W\left(t\right),\tau\right) = \int_{t-\tau}^{t} \left|\vec{e}\left(u\right)\right|^{2} du$$
$$= \sum_{i=1}^{m} \int_{t-\tau}^{t} \left|e_{i}\left(u\right)\right|^{2} du \qquad (1.2)$$
$$\equiv \sum_{i=1}^{m} E_{i},$$

and the independence of each of the m terms in Equation (1.2) is due to the independence of the m sets of $n \times p$ parameters W_{ij}^{k}, $j \in \{1,\ldots,n\}$, $k \in \{1,\ldots,p\}$ associated with generating each component $M_i(t)$ of the output. Our strategy for optimizing the matrix of decoder kernels is to modify each of the kernel parameters W_{ij}^{k} continuously and in parallel, on a timescale set by τ, in proportion to the negative gradient of $E(\mathbf{W}(t),\tau)$ with respect to each parameter:

$$-\vec{\nabla}_{ij}^{k} E\left(\mathbf{W}\left(t\right),\tau\right) \equiv -\frac{\partial E}{\partial W_{ij}^{k}}$$
$$= -\int_{t-\tau}^{t} du \left\{ 2\left(M_{i}\left(u\right) - \sum_{j=1}^{n} W_{ij}\left(u\right) \circ N_{j}\left(u\right) \right) \times \left(-\frac{\partial W_{ij}\left(u\right)}{\partial W_{ij}^{k}} \circ N_{j}\left(u\right) \right) \right\}$$
$$= 2\int_{t-\tau}^{t} e_{i}\left(u\right) \left(\frac{\partial W_{ij}\left(u\right)}{\partial W_{ij}^{k}} \circ N_{j}\left(u\right) \right) du. \qquad (1.3)$$

The learning algorithm refines $\mathbf{W}$ in a continuous-time fashion, using $-\vec{\nabla}E\left(t\right)$ as an error feedback signal to modify $\mathbf{W}(t)$, and incrementing each of the parameters $W_{ij}^{k}\left(t\right)$ in continuous time by a term proportional to $-\vec{\nabla}_{ij}^{k}E\left(\mathbf{W}\left(t\right)\right)$ (the proportionality constant, ε, must be large enough to ensure quick learning but small enough to ensure learning stability). If $\mathbf{W}(t)$ is viewed as an array of linear filters operating on the neural input signal, the quantity $-\vec{\nabla}_{ij}^{k}E\left(\mathbf{W}\left(t\right),\tau\right)$ used to increment each filter parameter can be described as the product, averaged over a time interval of length τ, of the error in the filter output and a secondarily filtered version of the filter input. The error term is identical for the parameters of all filters contributing to a given component of the output, $M_i(t)$. The secondarily filtered version of the input is generated by a secondary convolution kernel, $-\dfrac{\partial W_{ij}\left(u\right)}{\partial W_{ij}^{k}}$, which depends on the functional form of each primary filter kernel and in general differs for each filter parameter. Figure 2 shows a block diagram for an analog circuit architecture that implements our decoding and optimization algorithm.

Many functional forms for the convolution kernels are both theoretically possible and practical to implement using low-power analog circuitry. Our approach has been to emulate biological neural systems by choosing a biophysically inspired kernel whose impulse response approximates the postsynaptic currents biological neurons integrate when encoding and decoding neural signals *in vivo* (Arenz, Silver, Schaefer, & Margrie, 2008). Combining our decoding architecture with the choice of a first-order low-pass decoder kernel enables our low-power neural decoder to implement a biomimetic, continuous-time artificial neural network. Numerical experiments have also indicated that decoding using such biomimetic kernels can yield results comparable to those obtained using optimal linear decoders (Eliasmith & Anderson, 2003). But in contrast with our on-line optimization scheme, optimal linear decoders are computed off-line after all training data have been collected. We have found that this simple choice of kernel offers effective performance in practice, and so we confine the present analysis to that kernel.

We also offer a heuristic justification for using first-order low-pass kernels. Kernels for decoding continuous trajectories should be designed to anticipate low-frequency variation in the input and output signals. Two-parameter first-order low-pass filter kernels account for trajectory continuity by exponentially weighting the history of neural inputs:

Figure 2. Block diagram of an analog circuit architecture for linear convolutional decoding and learning

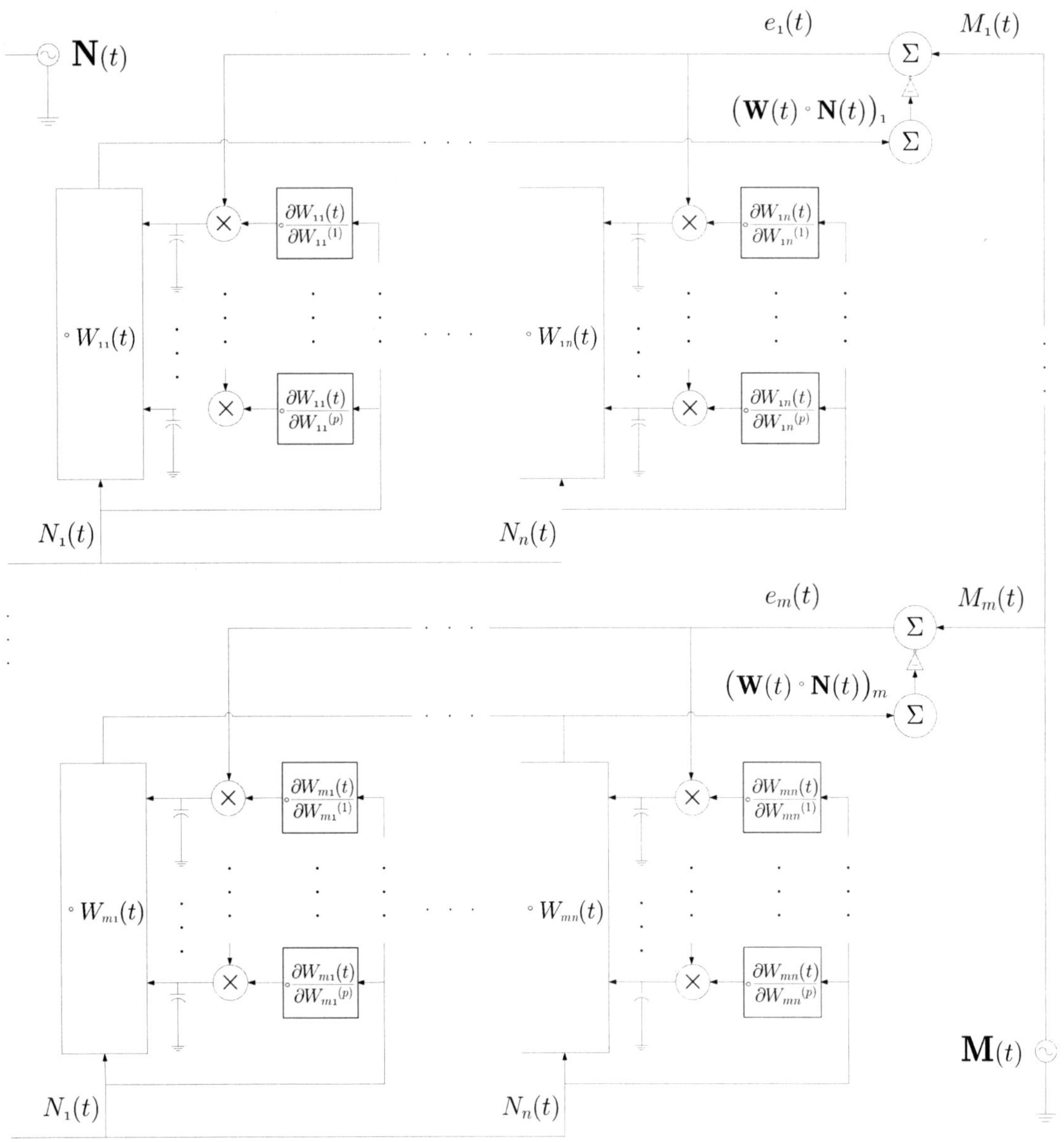

$$W_{ij} = \frac{A_{ij}}{\tau_{ij}} e^{-\frac{t}{\tau_{ij}}}, \tag{1.4}$$

where the two tunable kernel parameters are $W_{ij}^{k=1} = A_{ij}$, the low-pass filter gain, and $W_{ij}^{k=2} = \tau_{ij}$, the decay time over which past inputs $\vec{N}(t')$, $t' < t$, influence the present output estimate $\vec{M}(t) = \mathbf{W} \circ \vec{N}(t)$. The filters used to tune the low-pass filter kernel parameters can be implemented using simple and compact analog circuitry. The gain parameters are tuned using low-pass filter kernels of the form

$$\frac{\partial W_{ij}\left(t\right)}{\partial W_{ij}^{k=1}} = \frac{1}{\tau_{ij}} e^{-\frac{t}{\tau_{ij}}}, \tag{1.5}$$

while the time-constant parameters are tuned using band-pass filter kernels:

$$\frac{\partial W_{ij}\left(t\right)}{\partial W_{ij}^{k=2}} = \frac{A_{ij}}{\tau_{ij}^{2}} e^{-\frac{t}{\tau_{ij}}} \left(\frac{t}{\tau_{ij}} - 1\right). \tag{1.6}$$

When decoding discontinuous trajectories, such as sequences of discrete decisions, we use the limiting case of this kernel as $\tau_{ij} \rightarrow 0$:

$$W_{ij}\left(t\right) = W_{ij}^{k=1}\delta\left(t\right) = A_{ij}\delta\left(t\right). \tag{1.7}$$

Such a decoding system, in which each kernel is a zeroth-order filter characterized by a single tunable constant, performs instantaneous linear decoding, which has successfully been used by others to decode neuronal population signals in the context of neural prosthetics (Hochberg et al., 2006; Wessberg & Nicolelis, 2004). With kernels of this form, $\mathbf{W}(t)$ is analogous to matrices of synaptic weights encountered in artificial neural networks, and our optimization algorithm resembles a 'delta-rule' learning procedure (Haykin, 1999).

Implementation of the Decoding Algorithm in Analog Circuitry

In this section we describe the implementation of our adaptive decoder in an analog circuit architecture. This approach represents a divergence from conventional approaches to neural signal decoding. The ease of implementing sophisticated algorithms in digital systems has led to a proliferation of effective approaches to decoding and learning. Some of the most popular such algorithms in the context of neural decoding involve construction of optimal linear filters (Serruya, Hatsopoulos, Fellows, Paninski, & Donoghue, 2003; Warland, Reinagel, & Meister, 1997); training of artificial neural networks (Sanchez, Erdogmus, Principe, Wessberg, & Nicolelis, 2005); use of Kalman filters (Wu, Black et al., 2004; Wu, Gao, Bienenstock, Donoghue, & Black, 2006; Wu, Shaikhouni, Donoghue, & Black, 2004) and adaptive Kalman filters (Wu & Hatsopoulos, 2008); estimation based on Bayesian inference techniques (Brockwell, Rojas, & Kass, 2004; Srinivasan, Eden, Mitter, & Brown, 2007) and point-process models (Eden, Frank, Barbieri, Solo, & Brown, 2004); and decoding on the basis of frequency-domain data (such as the spectral content of local field potentials) (Musallam et al., 2004; Pesaran, Pezaris, Sahani, Mitra, & Andersen, 2002; Shenoy et al., 2003) or wavelet decompositions of neural signals (Musallam et al., 2004). However, to our knowledge the present work represents the first description of an analog circuit architecture for neural signal decoding.

We separate the present discussion into three parts. The first part treats the preprocessing of the two principal classes of neural input signals, local field potentials (LFPs) and action potentials ('spikes'). We then address the decoding architecture itself. Finally, we describe our estimates of power consumption by each module of the decoder architecture. Figure 3 is a diagram of the circuit modules required to implement a single adaptive kernel of the decoder. These modules fall into six functional classes: (1) Adaptive filters corresponding to the kernels $W_{ij}(t)$; (2) Parameter-learning filters to tune the $\left\{W_{ij}^{(k)}\right\} = \left\{A_{ij}, \tau_{ij}\right\}$; (3) Biasing circuits for the parameter-learning filters; (4) Multipliers; (5) Adders and subtracters; and (6) Memory units for storing learned parameter values. The second part of this section presents the design for each functional subunit of our decoding architecture in turn.

Note that the descriptions given here correspond to an unoptimized, proof-of-concept circuit implementation. Current-mode techniques, circuit optimizations not described here, and noise-robust

Figure 3. Block diagram indicating the functional component circuits required to implement a single adaptive kernel of the convolutional decoder

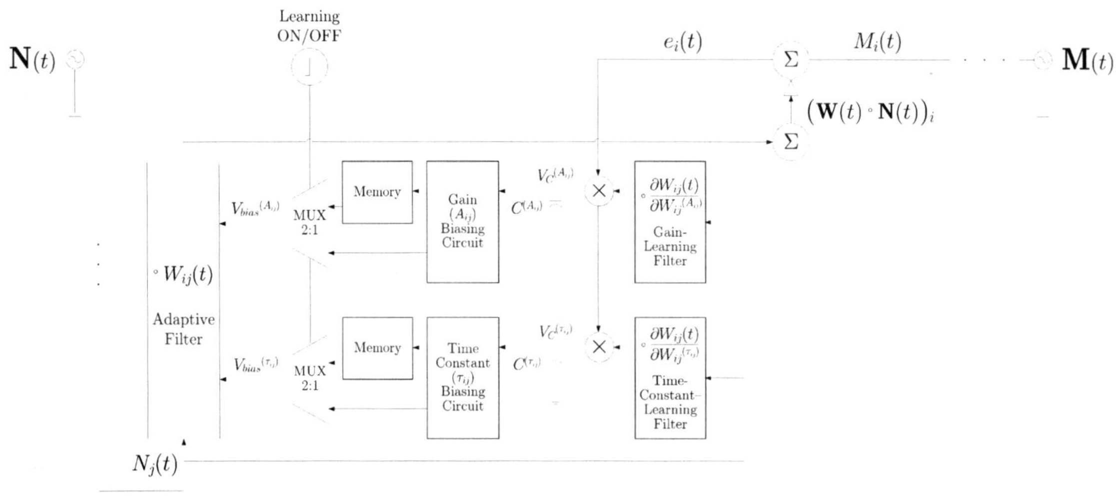

analog biasing techniques such as those described in (Sarpeshkar, Salthouse et al., 2005) will be necessary to ensure robust, programmable, and efficient operation in a practical implementation.

Input Signals for the Neural Decoder

Local-Field-Potential–based decoding

Local field potentials encode information about well defined cognitive states and can also be used as control signals for neural prostheses. Furthermore, it has been found that particular classes of information are encoded in distinct frequency bands of the LFP power spectrum (Pesaran et al., 2002). Information encoded in this manner can be extracted from the LFP by passing the raw LFP signal through a band-pass amplifier tuned to the spectral band of interest, rectifying the output of the band-pass filter, and passing the result through a peak-detection circuit to generate an envelope waveform. Prior work solved this design problem in the context of ultra-low-power bionic-ear (cochlear implant) processors (Sarpeshkar, Baker et al., 2005; Sarpeshkar, Salthouse et al., 2005) for which micropower band-pass amplifier (Salthouse & Sarpeshkar, 2003) and envelope detector circuits (Zhak, Baker, & Sarpeshkar, 2003) were built that can be employed to process neural signals at lower frequencies.

Spike–Based Decoding

Neuronal action potential voltage spikes typically have widths on the order of 1 ms, corresponding to frequencies in the kilohertz range. Spike-based inputs are transformed to lower-frequency signals (of order 1–10 Hz) through time-domain averaging and the resulting spike rates are used as input signals for the decoder. Such averaging can be implemented by low-pass interpolation filters. The simplest such filter is a first-order low-pass filter with frequency-domain transfer function $H_1(s) = \dfrac{1}{1+\tau_1 s}$, and cutoff frequency $f_c = (2\pi\tau_1)^{-1}$ Hz. Smoother interpolation can be obtained by cascading first-order filters. The analog implementation of such filters can be achieved using a G_m–C design: G_m refers to the transconductance of an operational transconductance amplifier (OTA) component, while C denotes a filter capacitance. In such a filter $f_c = \frac{1}{2\pi}\frac{G_m}{C}$, so a low cutoff frequency requires C to be large or G_m to be small. Circuit layout area restrictions will constrain the maximum value of C to approximately 4 pF, so a low f_c requires G_m to be small. Wide-linear-range transconductors with subthreshold bias currents (Sarpeshkar, Lyon, & Mead, 1997) allow G_m to be small enough to achieve such low corner frequencies in a reliable fashion. We convert raw neural input waveforms into smooth time-averaged spike rates (Figure 5) using the circuitry shown in Figure 4, which uses dual thresholding to detect action potentials on each input channel and then smoothens the resulting spike trains to generate mean firing rate input signals. Circuit simulations indicate that the charge pump and smoothing filter modules consume approximately 1.1 nW and 40 pW of power from a 1 V supply in 0.18 μm CMOS technology, respectively. As a result, power consumption of the preprocessing stages will be dominated by the requirements of the comparator; a comparator of the kind described in (Yang & Sarpeshkar, 2006), operating at 30 kHz, requires approximately 240 nW.

Functional Circuit Subunits of the Decoder Architecture

Primary Adaptive Filters

Each of the $m \times n$ tunable kernels used to implement our decoding architecture can be understood as an adaptive filter whose frequency-domain transfer function is obtained from the Laplace transform of the time-domain kernel in Equation (1.4):

$$\overline{W}_{ij}(s) = \frac{A_{ij}}{1+\tau_{ij}} \tag{1.8}$$

where the gain A_{ij} can be positive or negative. This transfer function can be obtained from a filter having the topology shown in Figure 6, which contains four standard, nine-transistor wide-range operational transconductance amplifiers (OTAs) of the form described in (Mead, 1989).

Every OTA is operated subthreshold such that its transconductance is linear in its bias current. The gain of the filter is determined by the three OTAs, $G_{m+}^{(A_{ij})}$, $G_{m-}^{(A_{ij})}$, and $G_{m}^{(R_{ij})}$, which have transconductances $\frac{\kappa I_{+}^{(A_{ij})}}{V_T}$, $\frac{\kappa I_{-}^{(A_{ij})}}{V_T}$, and $\frac{\kappa I^{(R_{ij})}}{V_T}$, respectively, where κ denotes the gate-coupling coefficient of the MOS transistor, and in this analysis $\kappa = 0.7$ is assumed for all transistors; and $V_T = kT/q$, where k denotes the Boltzmann constant, q denotes the electron charge, and T denotes the Kelvin temperature. By applying Kirchoff's Current Law (KCL) at node V_x, we obtain the voltage gain from V_{in} to V_x as

$$\begin{aligned}\frac{V_x}{V_{in}} &= \frac{G_{m+}^{(A_{ij})} - G_{m-}^{(A_{ij})}}{G_{m}^{(R_{ij})}} \\ &= \frac{I_{+}^{(A_{ij})} - I_{-}^{(A_{ij})}}{I^{(R_{ij})}}.\end{aligned} \tag{1.9}$$

If we set the sum of $I_{+}^{(A_{ij})}$ and $I_{-}^{(A_{ij})}$ equal to a constant current $I_{tot}^{(A_{ij})}$, the expression in Equation (1.9) can be reduced to

$$\frac{V_x}{V_{in}} = \frac{2I_{+}^{(A_{ij})} - I_{tot}^{(A_{ij})}}{I^{(R_{ij})}}. \tag{1.10}$$

The transfer function from V_x to V_{out} can be expressed as

Figure 4. Analog preprocessing circuitry for converting raw neural signals into smooth analog inputs for an analog decoder

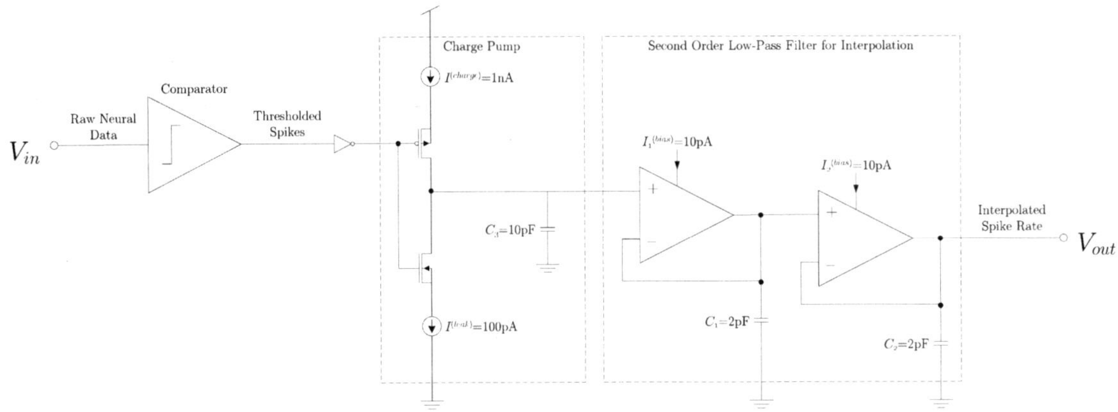

Figure 5. Analog preprocessing of raw neural signals to generate smooth analog inputs to an implantable analog decoder. The raw neural signal (top trace) is thresholded to generate a spike train (middle trace), which is converted to a smooth time-averaged spike rate (bottom trace) using a second-order low-pass filter

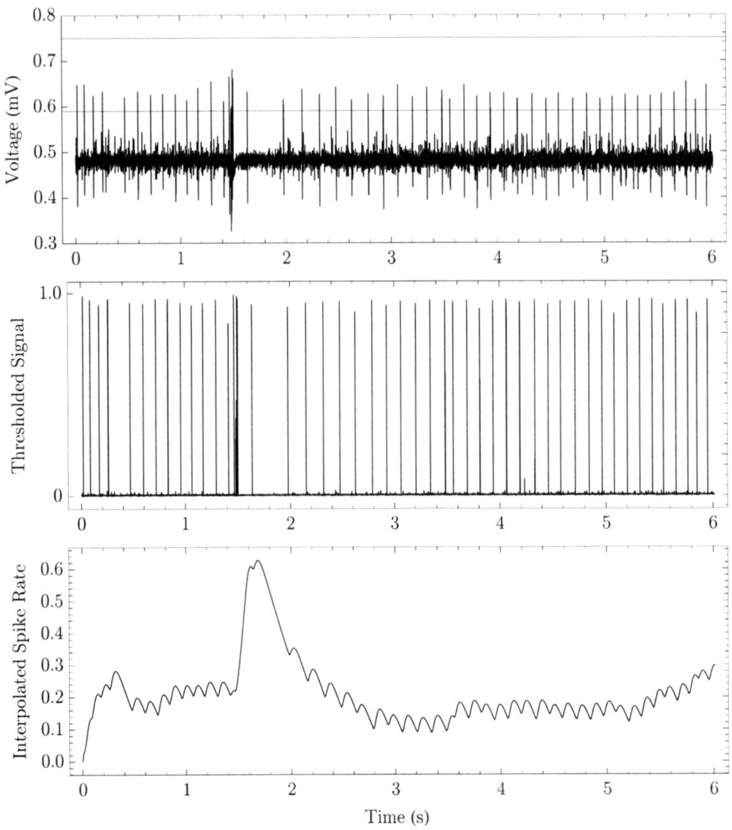

Figure 6. Adaptive filter with tunable parameters for learning the optimal convolution kernels for neural signal decoding

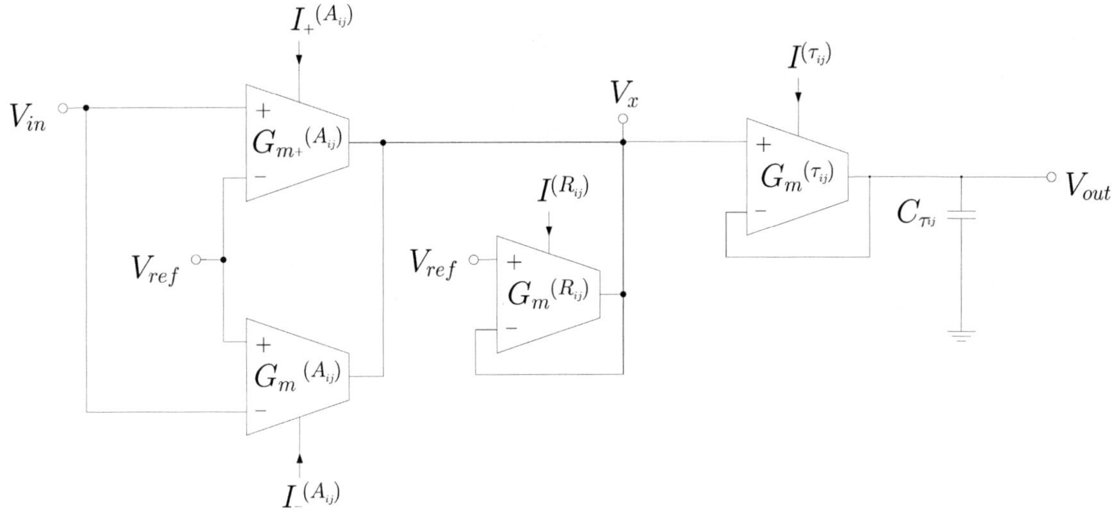

$$\frac{V_{out}}{V_x}\left(s\right) = \frac{1}{1 + s\frac{C_{\tau_{ij}}}{G_m^{\tau_{ij}}}}. \tag{1.11}$$

As a result, we can express the overall transfer function from V_{in} to V_{out} as

$$\frac{V_{out}}{V_{in}}\left(s\right) = \frac{2I_+^{\left(A_{ij}\right)} - I_{tot}^{\left(A_{ij}\right)}}{I^{\left(R_{ij}\right)}} \frac{1}{1 + s\frac{C_{\tau_{ij}}}{G_m^{\tau_{ij}}}}. \tag{1.12}$$

Comparing Equation (1.12) to Equation (1.8), we obtain expressions for the gain and time constant parameters:

$$A_{ij} = \frac{2I_+^{\left(A_{ij}\right)} - I_{tot}^{\left(A_{ij}\right)}}{I^{\left(R_{ij}\right)}} \qquad \tau_{ij} = \frac{C_{\tau_{ij}}}{G_m^{\left(\tau_{ij}\right)}}. \tag{1.13}$$

Since $I_+^{\left(A_{ij}\right)}$ can be adjusted from 0 to $I_{tot}^{\left(A_{ij}\right)}$, A_{ij} can vary from $-I_{tot}^{\left(A_{ij}\right)} / I^{\left(R_{ij}\right)}$ to $I_{tot}^{\left(A_{ij}\right)} / I^{\left(R_{ij}\right)}$. The time constant τ_{ij} can be adjusted by tuning the bias current in $G_m^{\left(\tau_{ij}\right)}$.

Secondary Parameter Tuning Filters

Real-time gradient-descent–based optimization of the convolution kernels can be achieved through tuning the filter parameters $\left\{W_{ij}^{(k)}\right\} = \left\{A_{ij}, \tau_{ij}\right\}$ using signals proportional to $-\vec{\nabla}_{ij}^{(k)}E$. Construction of such signals requires convolution kernels proportional to $\frac{\partial W_{ij}\left(t\right)}{\partial W_{ij}^{(k)}}$. These convolution kernels can be implemented by 'parameter-learning filters' of the kind shown in Figure 7. Figure 7(a) shows a first-order low-pass G_m–C filter with transfer function $W_{ij}^{A_{ij}}\left(s\right) = \frac{1}{1 + \tau_{ij}s}$ to be used as a 'gain-learning filter.' Figure 7(b) shows a second-order band-pass G_m–C filter with transfer

Figure 7. Parameter-learning filters for tuning adaptive filter parameters based on error-signal feedback. (a) A first-order low-pass G_m–C filter with transfer function $W_{ij}^{A_{ij}}(s) = \frac{1}{1+\tau_{ij}s}$ to be used as a 'gain-learning filter.' (b) A second-order band-pass G_m–C filter with transfer function $W_{ij}^{\tau_{ij}}(s) = \frac{\tau_{ij}s}{(1+\tau_{ij}s)^2}$ to be used as a 'time-constant–learning filter'

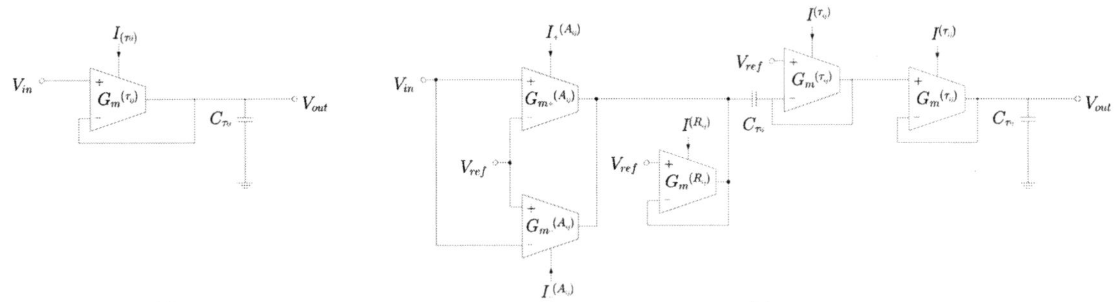

function $W_{ij}^{\tau_{ij}}(s) = \frac{\tau_{ij}s}{(1+\tau_{ij}s)^2}$ to be used as a 'time-constant–learning filter.' The time constant $\tau_{ij} = \frac{C_{\tau_{ij}}}{G_m^{(\tau_{ij})}}$ for the two parameter-learning filters is identical to that of the adaptive filter, as described in the section entitled "Primary adaptive filters." Correspondingly, the bias currents and therefore the transconductances $G_m^{(\tau_{ij})}$ in all three types of filter are identical, so the time constants of all filters in the learning architecture are updated simultaneously. Note that the actual transfer function of the time-constant–learning filter need only be proportional to $W_{ij}^{\tau_{ij}}(s)$, so the factor of τ_{ij}/A_{ij} between the transfer function of Equation (1.8) and the filter shown in Figure 7(b) is acceptable. Implementation of the negation required to adapt the time constants is addressed in the section entitled "Multipliers."

Multipliers

The multipliers that perform the operations $e_i(t) \times \frac{\partial W_{ij}(t)}{\partial W_{ij}^{(k)}}$ required by the gradient-descent algorithm, denoted by the symbol × in Figure 2 and Figure 3, can be implemented using wide-range four-quadrant Gilbert multipliers of the kind described in (Mead, 1989), which accept four voltage inputs $V_i, i \in \{1,2,3,4\}$ and a bias current I_b, and generate an output current; low-power performance can be obtained by operating the multiplier circuit with all transistors in the sub-threshold regime. The input-output characteristic of the Gilbert multiplier is given by

$$\begin{aligned} I_{out} &= I_b \tanh \frac{\kappa(V_1 - V_2)}{2V_T} \tanh \frac{\kappa(V_3 - V_4)}{2V_T} \\ &\approx I_b \left(\frac{\kappa}{2V_T}\right)^2 (V_1 - V_2)(V_3 - V_4), \end{aligned} \tag{1.14}$$

where the approximation of Equation (1.14) is valid in the intended operating region, where V_1

$\approx V_2$ and $V_3 \approx V_4$. Noninverting multiplication, as required for adapting the A_{ij}, can be implemented by feeding e_i into V_1, $\frac{\partial W_{ij}(t)}{\partial W_{ij}^{(A_{ij})}}$ into V_3, and setting V_2 and V_4 to a constant reference voltage. On the other hand, inverting multiplication, as required for adapting the τ_{ij}, can be implemented by interchanging the roles of V_3 and V_4, feeding $\frac{\partial W_{ij}(t)}{\partial W_{ij}^{(\tau_{ij})}}$ into V_4, and setting V_3 to a constant reference voltage.

The output of each multiplier is a current, I_{out}, so the integrations required in Equation (1.3) for updating the parameters $\left\{W_{ij}^{(k)}\right\} = \left\{A_{ij}, \tau_{ij}\right\}$ are conveniently implemented by linear capacitors, as indicated in Figure 3. The voltages $V_C^{\left(W_{ij}^{(k)}\right)}$ on the capacitors $C^{\left(W_{ij}^{(k)}\right)}$ and used in adapting the parameter values $W_{ij}^{(k)}$ are therefore given by

$$V_C^{\left(W_{ij}^{(k)}\right)} = \frac{I_b}{C^{\left(W_{ij}^{(k)}\right)}} \frac{\kappa^2}{4V_T^2} \int_{u=0}^{t} e_i(u) \left(\frac{\partial W_{ij}(u)}{\partial W_{ij}^{(k)}} \circ N_j(u) \right) du \tag{1.15}$$

which has the form required by Equation (1.3). The filter parameters therefore vary continuously in time, and the time variation of the control voltages can be obtained by differentiating Equation (1.15).

Biasing Circuits

As discussed in the section entitled "Multipliers," the filter parameters A_{ij} and τ_{ij} defining the transfer function of adaptive filter W_{ij} are stored on the capacitors $C^{(A_{ij})}$ and $C^{(\tau_{ij})}$, respectively. Furthermore, as indicated in the section entitled "Primary adaptive filters," the values of the filter parameters can be tuned by adjusting the bias currents that determine $G_m^{(A_{ij})}$ and $G_m^{(\tau_{ij})}$. Since the gain A_{ij} depends on $\frac{I_{(A_{ij})}}{I_{(R_{ij})}} \propto I_{(A_{ij})}$, while the time constant τ_{ij} depends on $\frac{C_{\tau_{ij}}}{G_m^{(\tau_{ij})}} \propto \frac{1}{I_{(\tau_{ij})}}$, real-time adaptive parameter tuning requires a scheme for modifying $I_{(A_{ij})}$ in proportion to $V_C^{(A_{ij})}$ and $I_{(\tau_{ij})}$ in inverse proportion to $V_C^{(\tau_{ij})}$.

Tuning $I_{(A_{ij})}$ in proportion to variations in the capacitor voltage $V_C^{(A_{ij})}$ can be accomplished by converting $V_C^{(A_{ij})}$ into a current proportional to $V_C^{(A_{ij})}$ and then using a current mirror to generate a copy of that current that is in turn used to set the transconductance $G_m^{(A_{ij})}$ of the adaptive filter. The conversion of $V_C^{(A_{ij})}$ into a current proportional to $V_C^{(A_{ij})}$ can be performed by a wide-linear-range transconductance amplifier (WLR) of the form described in (Sarpeshkar et al., 1997). Figure 8(a) shows a schematic of the gain-biasing circuit used to generate $I_{(A_{ij})} \propto V_C^{(A_{ij})}$. This biasing circuit is intended to make $I_+^{(A_{ij})} + I_-^{(A_{ij})} = I_{tot}^{(A_{ij})}$. Assuming that all of the NMOS transistors are well matched, the current in M_3 must be equal to that in M_2, which is $I_+^{A_{ij}}$. Using KCL at the drain of M_3, the current in M_4 is thus $I_{tot}^{(A_{ij})} - I_+^{(A_{ij})}$, which is equal to the current in M_5, so $I_-^{(A_{ij})} = I_{tot}^{(A_{ij})} - I_+^{(A_{ij})}$ as required.

Tuning $I_{(\tau_{ij})}$ in inverse proportion to variations in the capacitor voltage $V_C^{(\tau_{ij})}$ can be accomplished using the circuit shown in Figure 8(b), which operates as follows. First, $V_C^{(\tau_{ij})}$ is converted into a proportional current $I_{(\tau_{ij})}^p$ as in the gain-biasing circuit. A translinear circuit, formed by the four

Figure 8. Circuits for setting the bias currents and transconductances that determine the adaptive filter parameters: (a) Bias-current–setting circuit for filter gains, (b) Bias-current–setting circuit for filter time constants

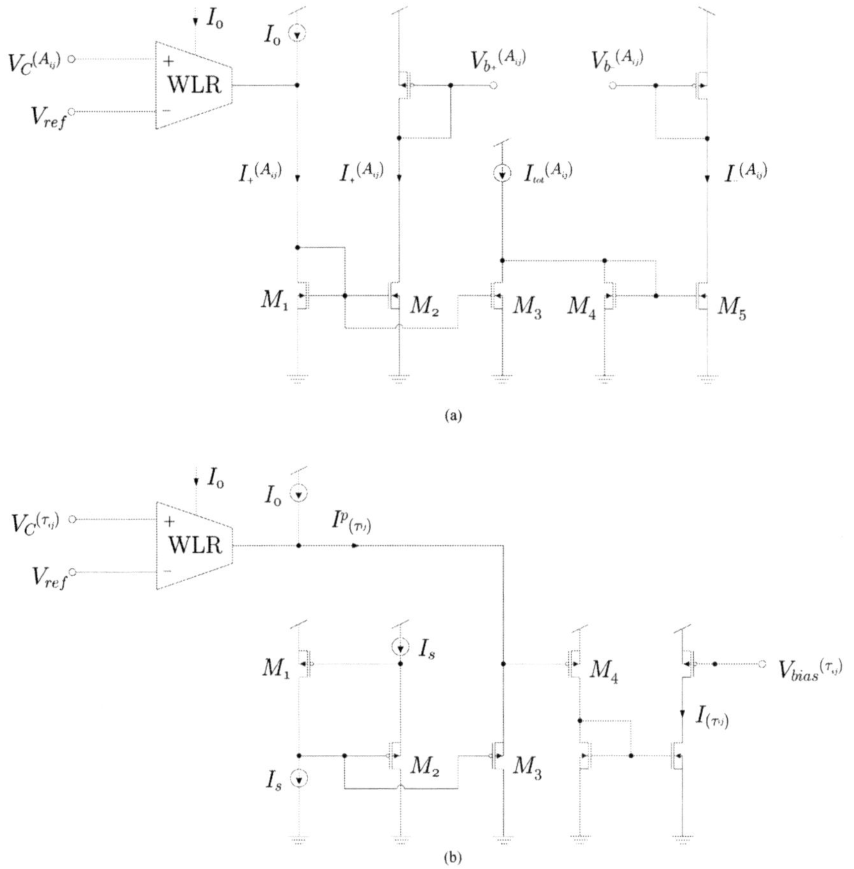

well matched MOS transistors M_1–M_4, is then used to invert $I^p_{(\tau_{ij})}$, producing $I_{(\tau_{ij})} = \frac{I_s^2}{I^p_{(\tau_{ij})}}$, where I_s is a current reference that scales the inversion. A mirror copy of $I_{(\tau_{ij})}$ is then used as the bias current that sets transconductance $G_m^{(\tau_{ij})}$.

Adders and Subtracters

Each adder, denoted by the symbol Σ in Figure 2 and Figure 3, sums the n outputs of each set $\{W_{ij}\}$, $j \in \{1, \ldots, n\}$ of adaptive filters contributing to $\left(\mathbf{W}(t) \circ \mathbf{N}(t)\right)_i = \hat{M}_i(t)$. The adders can be implemented using a follower-aggregation circuit of the kind described in (Mead, 1989). The corresponding error signal, $e_i(t)$, is generated by performing the subtraction $M_i(t) - \hat{M}_i(t)$. This operation can be implemented by another adder, with a unity-gain inverting amplifier negating the adder input from $\hat{M}_i(t)$.

Parameter Memory

A completely analog implementation of our decoder could include analog memory units for storing parameter values when learning ends. Such units could consist of analog memory elements operating in a switched sample-and-hold scheme to permit memoryless adaptation during the learning phase and parameter storage as soon as learning terminates. Analog memory circuits with 8-bit hold times of 3.9 hours and 12-bit hold times of 14.5 minutes have been developed (O'Halloran & Sarpeshkar, 2004, 2006) and could be used in this context. Output from the memory and biasing circuits could be multiplexed onto the adaptive filter nodes whose voltages correspond to the adaptive filter parameters, using a CMOS transmission gate. This scheme is indicated in Figure 3. However, even using digital memory elements does not increase total power consumption significantly, since the termination of a learning phase is a rare event and therefore writing to memory, with its associated power cost, occurs only infrequently.

Power Consumption of the Decoder

Table 1 shows an estimate of the power consumed by each circuit block needed to implement our neural decoder, based on a SPICE simulation of the decoder, the performance of which is shown in Figure 11. The supply voltage of the entire system is 1 V. The bias current of each module is chosen so that the circuit has enough bandwidth to process input signals band-limited to 1 kHz (note that this choice of input signal bandwidth is more than sufficient because the bandwidth of mean-firing-rate changes is typically much smaller than the reciprocal of a refractory period. As indicated in Table 1, the total power consumption of one decoding module is approximately 54 nW.

In order to ensure robust, stable decoding, the learned (optimized) filter parameters for the neural decoder will be programmed using digital-to-analog converters (DACs) as indicated in the "Introduction" section. These DACs do not appreciably increase system power consumption. One DAC is required per filter parameter to set the bias current for each filter constant, so a system decoding 3 motor parameters from 100 neural input channels would require 600 current DACs. The static current in a current DAC is approximately equal to that of a transistor whose gate is connected to the associated capacitors in Figure 3, which is approximately 100 pA. The total power consumed by all 600 DACs, when operated from a 1.8-V supply, is therefore only approximately 110 nW.

Table 1. Power consumption in decoder circuit modules

Portion of Channel	Power Consumption (nW)
Tunable Decoding Filter	16
Gain-Learning Filter	2
Time-Constant–Learning Filter	2
Multipliers (2)	2
Gain Biasing Circuit	10
Time Constant Biasing Circuit	10
Analog Memories (2)	5
Total (One Decoder Module)	54 nW

Methods of Testing the Neural Signal Decoding System

In this section we describe three approaches to testing the ability of our system to decode neural signals. The first experiment is based on a simulation of local field potential input signals, which are used to decode continuous-time motor trajectories. The second experiment involves continuous-time decoding of head direction from spike train data recorded from a small set of neurons in the thalamus of an awake, behaving rat. In the third experiment we decode discrete arm-reach intentions from spike train data recorded using a multielectrode array in the posterior parietal cortex of a macaque monkey.

Testing the Ability to Decode Trajectory Information from Multichannel Local Field Potential Neural Input Signals

A recent set of experiments has shown that parietal cortex neurons tend to exhibit electrical activity predictive of arm or eye movement in a single preferred direction. Increases in γ-band (25–90 Hz) spectral activity of such tuned parietal neurons anticipate movements in the preferred directions of those neurons, so a potentially useful signal for decoding intended movement from neural activity is therefore an envelope curve describing the modulated amplitude of the power transmitted in the gamma band (Andersen, Musallam, & Pesaran, 2004; Musallam et al., 2004; Pesaran et al., 2002). As a preliminary demonstration of the ability of our convolutional decoder to interpret LFP-type neural input signals, we therefore generated simulated γ-band power envelopes in order to model the local field potentials recorded by a set of n neural recording electrodes. We modeled γ-band power envelopes using a set of sinusoids with randomized amplitudes and phases and a constant offset term, and stored the corresponding waveforms in the vector $\vec{N}(t)$, which was used as the input to the decoder. We then randomly generated an $m \times n$ matrix, $\mathbf{W}^*$, and used it to construct a vector of m motor control parameters, $\vec{M}(t)$. The decoder was permitted to observe $\vec{M}(t)$ during a learning period of variable length, over which it sought to optimize its $m \times n$-dimensional convolution kernel $\mathbf{W}(t)$. The parameter ε was set to 0.1 during these simulations, and both the $N_i(t)$ and the $M_i(t)$ were transformed using a hyperbolic-tangent normalization to constrain them to the interval [-1, 1]. We evaluated decoder performance using a scale-invariant and dimensionless conventional figure of merit, the normalized mean squared error, η, of the estimated trajectory, defined as

$$\eta \equiv \frac{1}{T}\int_{t_1=T}^{t_2=2T} dt \sum_{i=1}^{m} \left(\frac{M_i(t) - \hat{M}_i(t)}{L_i} \right)^2, \quad (1.16)$$

where L_i denotes the maximum extent of excursions permitted to $M_i(t)$ and the time T denotes the length of the training interval; $\eta^{(1)}$ is used to denote the average value of η for a single output dimension. It is possible to consider other figures of merit, including ones based on correlation rather than absolute error between $\vec{M}(t)$ and $\hat{\vec{M}}(t)$, but other authors have agreed that η-like figures of merit tend to reflect decoding system performance most reasonably (Wu et al., 2006). The results of these simulations are provided in the section entitled "Model Motor Trajectory Decoding from Simulated Multichannel Local Field Potential Inputs."

Testing the Decoding of Continuous Trajectories Using Neuronal Spike Recordings from the Thalamus of an Awake Behaving Rat

Head direction cells of the rat thalamus are neurons known to exhibit receptive fields tuned to specific orientations of the head relative to the environment (Taube, 1995). We explored the ability of our system to decode the temporal firing patterns of such cells in real time. The spike trains used as input signals to the decoder in this set of experiments were derived from tetrode recordings made in the thalamus of a laboratory rat that rat ran back and forth between two points on a circular maze for food reward over a 30-minute period. The position and head direction of the animal were continuously tracked using a pair of head-mounted light-emitting diode (LED) arrays imaged at a sampling frequency of 30 Hz using a 300 × 300-pixel charge-coupled device (CCD) array. Data from the imager were time-stamped in order to ensure synchronization with the neural recordings, and were used to generate a target output signal $\hat{\vec{M}}(t)$ for the decoder. In order to avoid learning the discontinuity associated with a mod-2π–based definition of the head direction angle $\theta(t)$, $\hat{\vec{M}}(t)$ was constructed as a two-dimensional vector having components $M_1(t) \equiv \cos\theta(t)$ and $M_2(t) \equiv \sin\theta(t)$. Spike-sorting analysis of the tetrode-derived waveforms isolated $n = 6$ single units, and the activity of each of these units was converted to a normalized spike rate $N_i(t)$, $i \in \{1, \ldots, n = 6\}$ so that $\vec{N}(t)$ could be used as an n-channel analog input to the decoder. As indicated in the section entitled "Input Signals for the Neural Decoder," the conversion of spike trains to analog input signals was achieved by treating each spike train as a train of pulses having uniform amplitude and pulse width, then passing the pulse trains through a third-order interpolation filter with transfer function

$$H_3(s) = \frac{1}{\left(1 + \tau_1 s\right)^3} \tag{1.17}$$

with $\tau_1 = 500$ ms. The filter output was then rescaled and recentered about a zero-offset in order to generate the normalized spike rates $N_i(t)$. The performance of the convolutional decoding algorithm in learning to map $\vec{N}(t)$ to $\vec{M}(t)$ was studied using a software implementation of the decoder, as well as a SPICE analog-circuit simulation of the convolutional decoder, the details of which are described in the section entitled "Functional Circuit Subunits of the Decoder Architecture." We discuss the results of these simulations in the section entitled "Continuous Real-Time Decoding of Head Direction from Neuronal Spike Activity in the Rat Thalamus."

Testing the Decoding of Discrete Decisions Using Neuronal Spike Recordings from the Posterior Parietal Cortex of a Macaque Monkey Engaged in an Arm-Reaching Task

Neurons in the posterior parietal cortex have been shown to encode intention to execute limb movements in both humans (Connolly, Andersen, & Goodale, 2003) and nonhuman primates (Snyder, Batista, & Andersen, 1997). The ability to decode signals from this region has provided proof of principle for neural prosthetic devices based on cognitive (as opposed to explicitly motor) control signals (Musallam et al., 2004). Using neural spike trains recorded during these proof-of-principle experiments, we investigated the performance of our system in the real-time decoding of discrete arm-reaching decisions.

The spike trains used as input signals to the decoder in this set of experiments were derived from recordings by a multielectrode array chronically implanted in the medial intraparietal area (within the 'parietal reach region') of a macaque monkey. The animal had previously been trained to perform a standard stimulus-response task involving center-out arm-reaching movements between visual targets. This task, which has been described in detail elsewhere (Musallam et al., 2004), was designed to isolate the neural correlates of motor intention from those of actual movement. The monkey initiated each iteration of the task by touching a central cue target and looking at a nearby visual fixation point at $t = -800$ ms (its gaze was monitored using an eye-tracking device, and cues were presented on a touch-sensitive screen). After a delay of 500 ms a peripheral cue target was flashed from $t = -300$ to $t = 0$ ms at one of four locations displaced up, right, down, or left from the starting point. The animal was rewarded if it touched the indicated target at the end of a memory period of 1500±300 ms. Neural activity as monitored by the implanted electrode array was recorded continuously during each trial. A spike-sorting algorithm isolated 54 units from the recorded signals, and spike trains from each unit were smoothed to spike rate waveforms using a filter of the form provided in Equation (1.17), with $\tau_1 = 50$ ms. Filter output was then rescaled and recentered about a zero-offset in order to generate the normalized spike rate input signals $N_i(t)$ for each of the isolated units indexed by $i \in \{1, \ldots, n - 1 = 54\}$; the $(n = 55)$-dimensional neural input signal $\vec{N}(t)$ contained an additional constant-offset component $N_n(t) = 1$.

The task of the decoder was to predict imminent arm movement on the basis of intention-related neuronal activity. Therefore, in order to ensure the absence from $\vec{N}(t)$ of residual neuronal activity corresponding to actual arm movement (such artifact signals are sometimes present at the beginning and end of a memory interval), only the segment of $\vec{N}(t)$ from $t \in [200, 1100]$ ms was fed into the decoder for each reach. The motor output $\vec{M}(t)$ was defined as a two-dimensional position vector corresponding to the target to which the monkey reached at the end of a corresponding memory period. Reach target positions were encoded as follows:

Analog outputs generated by the decoder were thresholded according to

$$M_i \to \operatorname{sgn} M_i, \tag{1.18}$$

so that positive and negative outputs were interpreted as +1 and –1, respectively.

We studied the performance of a software implementation of our convolutional decoding system in learning to use neural signals from the parietal reach region to predict the direction of subsequent reaching movements. We discuss the results of these simulations in the section entitled "Decoding Discrete Arm Reaches from Neuronal Spike Activity in the Macaque Monkey Posterior Parietal Cortex."

Table 2. Encoding vectors for reach targets

Direction	M_1	M_2
Up	+1	+1
Right	+1	–1
Down	–1	–1
Left	–1	+1

EVALUATING THE PERFORMANCE OF THE NEURAL DECODING SYSTEM

Model Motor Trajectory Decoding from Simulated Multichannel Local Field Potential Inputs

Parts (a) and (b) of Figure 9 respectively illustrate the training and post-training phases of decoder operation as the system learns to trace a three-dimensional trajectory in real time during a simulation of the kind described in the section entitled "Testing the Ability to Decode Trajectory Information from Multichannel Local Field Potential Neural Input Signals," with $(n, m) = (10, 3)$. The figure illustrates qualitatively that $\vec{M}(t)$ converges toward $\hat{\vec{M}}(t)$ reasonably quickly on the timescale set by full-scale variations in the trajectory.

Figure 10 presents the results of a set of computations of $\eta^{(1)}$ for the performance of the neural decoding system in simulations of the kind described in the section entitled "Testing the Ability to Decode Trajectory Information from Multichannel Local Field Potential Neural Input Signals." The system was trained for intervals of varying length up to one minute, $T \in [0, 60]$ s, and the value of $\eta^{(1)}$ was computed for each of 50 trials at each value of T. In a fraction f of trials at each value of T, the decoding performance as reflected by $\eta^{(1)}(T)$ was significantly worse than in the remaining fraction, $1-f$, of cases. In such cases markedly improved decoding, comparable

Figure 9. Trajectory decoding from simulated local field potential input signals. (a) The correct trajectory, $\hat{\vec{M}}(t)$, is plotted in light gray over the initial segment $t \in [0, 10]$ s of a 40-second training interval, while the decoded trajectory, $\vec{M}(t) \equiv \mathbf{W} \circ \vec{N}(t)$, is plotted as a darker line whose shade lightens as time progresses; $\vec{M}(t)$ converges toward $\hat{\vec{M}}(t)$. (b) For $t \in [40, 80]$ s following training, the correct trajectory is plotted in light gray while the decoded trajectory evolves with time from dark to lighter shades

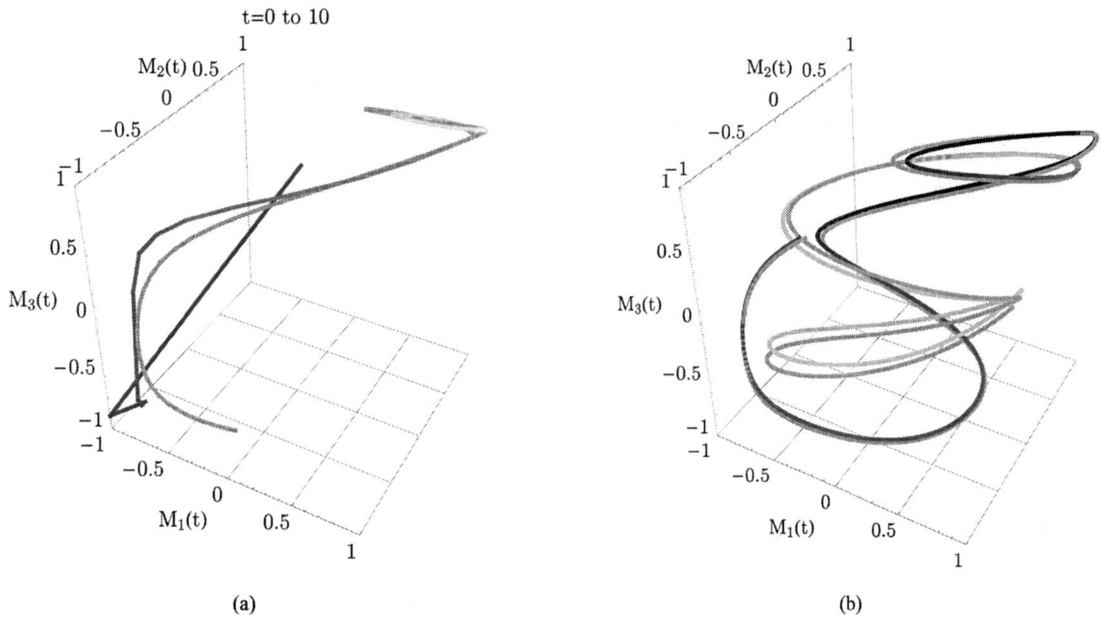

to that achieved in the (1–*f*)-majority of cases, could be achieved by randomly reinitializing the parameters $W_{ij}^{(k)}$ and decoding again. The data presented in Figure 10 were obtained by setting $f = 0.1$. Error in trajectory estimation by the decoder decreases rapidly as the training interval increases. At $T = 30$ s, for example, $\langle \eta^{(1)} \rangle \approx 0.008 \pm 0.008$, as compared with a baseline value of $\langle \eta^{(1)} \rangle \approx 0.118 \pm 0.106$ computed for an untrained system ($T = 0$) over 1000 trials.

Continuous Real-Time Decoding of Head Direction from Neuronal Spike Activity in the Rat Thalamus

Head direction was decoded from the activity of the $n = 6$ isolated thalamic neurons according to the method described in the section entitled "Testing the Decoding of Continuous Trajectories Using Neuronal Spike Recordings from the Thalamus of an Awake Behaving Rat." The adaptive filter parameters $\{W_{ij}^{(p)}\} = \{A_{ij}, \tau_{ij}\}$ were optimized through gradient descent over training intervals of length T during which the decoder error,

Figure 10. Mean squared trajectory prediction error as a function of training time for the convolutional decoding algorithm

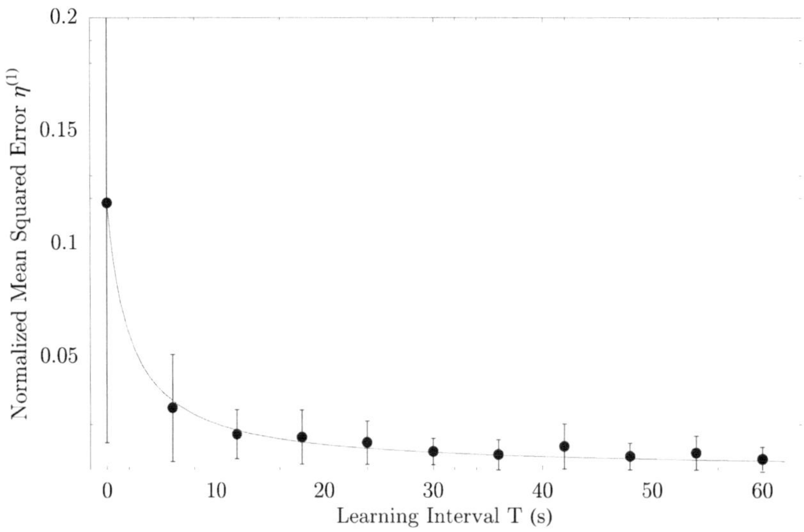

$$e_i(t) = M_i(t) - \hat{M}_i(t)$$
$$\vec{M}(t) = \left(\cos\theta(t), \sin\theta(t)\right), \quad (1.19)$$

(where θ denotes the head direction angle) was made available to the adaptive filter in the feedback configuration described in the section entitled "An Algorithm for Adaptive Convolutional Decoding of Neural Cell Ensemble Signals" for $t \in [0, T]$. Following these training intervals feedback was discontinued and the performance of the decoder was assessed by comparing the decoder output $\vec{M}(t)$ with $\hat{\vec{M}}(t)$ for $t>T$.

Figure 11(a) compares the output of the decoder to the measured head direction over a 240-s interval. The filter parameters were trained over the interval $t \in [0, T = 120]$ s. The figure shows $\vec{M}(t)$ (thick, light line) tracking $\hat{\vec{M}}(t)$ (thin, dark line) with increasing accuracy as training progresses, illustrating that while initial predictions are poor, they improve with feedback over the course of the training interval. Feedback is discontinued at $t = 120$ s. Qualitatively, the plots on the interval $t \in [120, 240]$ s illustrate that the output of the neural decoder reproduces the shape of the correct waveform, predicting head direction on the basis of neuronal spike rates. Figure 11(b) displays output over a brief interval from the neurons in the ensemble whose activity was decoded, showing individual action potentials as raster plots below the corresponding smoothened firing rate curve for each cell, as well as a plot of head direction over the same time interval; individual neurons evidently have distinct receptive fields in head-direction space, and their spatial selectivity makes decoding both possible and, in this case, intuitive.

The performance of the decoder in predicting head direction was assessed quantitatively using the normalized mean-squared error measure $\eta^{(1)}$ (in this context $L_i = 2$, $t_1 = T$, and $t_2 = T + 60$ s). In order to quantify the accuracy of head direction decoding as a function of training time T, $\eta^{(1)}$ was computed for a set of training and decoding trials with increasingly long training periods, averaging over randomized initial settings of the filter parameters and different choices of training interval.

Figure 11. (a) Continuous decoding of head direction from neuronal spiking activity. (b) Spiking activity in head direction cells and corresponding head direction plotted as functions of time. The paired plots illustrate neuronal receptive fields and the distribution of their peaks over the range of possible head direction angles

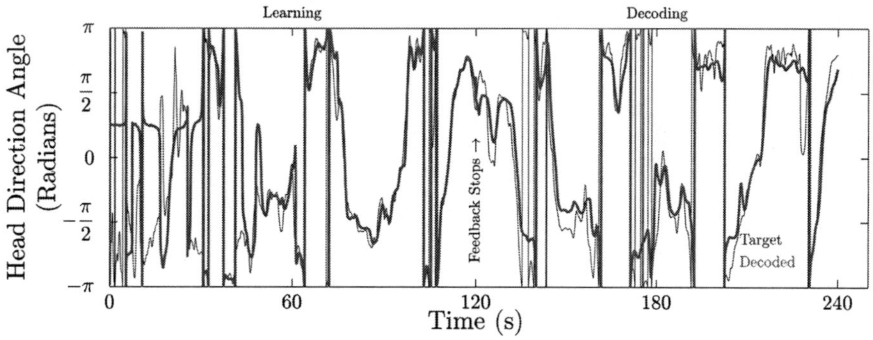

(a)

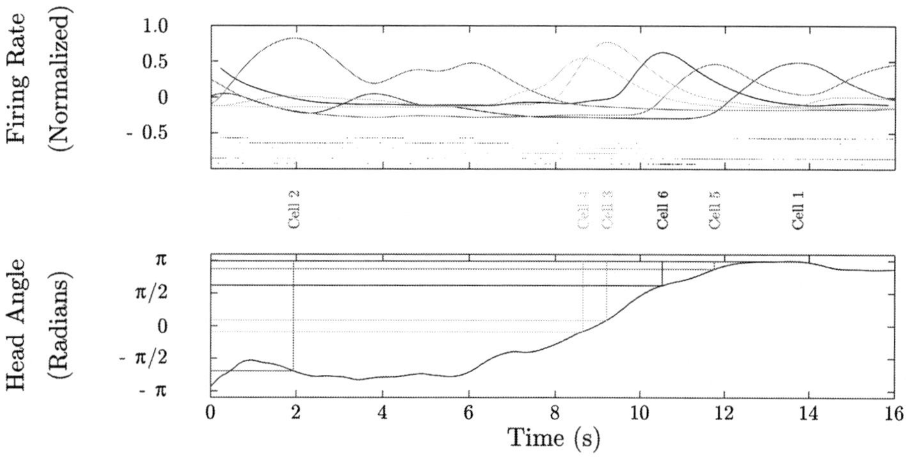

(b)

The results of this computation are displayed in Figure 12, which shows improving accuracy of head direction decoding with increased training.

Decoding Discrete Arm Reaches from Neuronal Spike Activity in the Macaque Monkey Posterior Parietal Cortex

The input signals to the neural decoder when decoding discrete reaches were piecewise-constant, as described in the section entitled "Testing the Decoding of Discrete Decisions Using Neuronal Spike Recordings from the Posterior Parietal Cortex of a Macaque Monkey Engaged in an Arm-Reaching Task." This form of input reflects a qualitative difference between the decoding problem in this experiment, which requires the decoder to make a series of decisions from among a finite set of options, and the decoding problems framed in the sections entitled "Testing the Ability to Decode Trajectory Information from Multichannel Local Field Potential Neural Input Signals" and "Testing the Decoding of Continuous

Figure 12. Performance improvements in head direction decoding with increasing training times

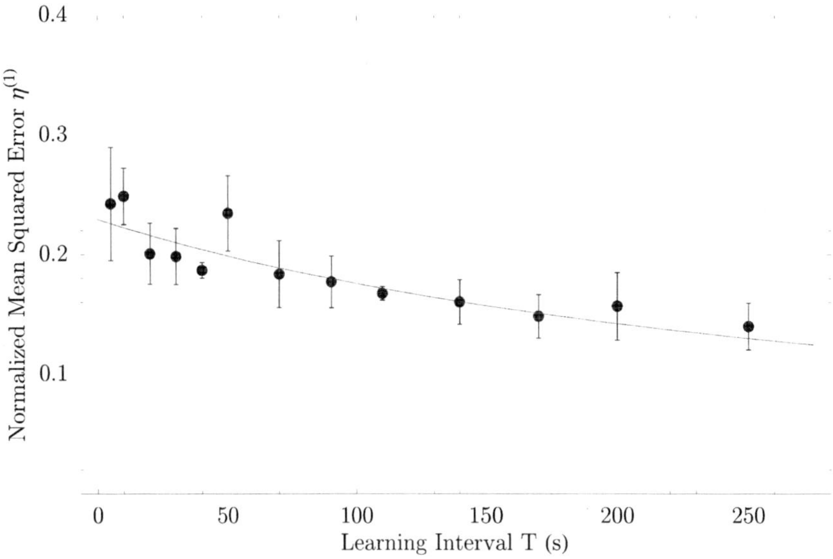

Trajectories Using Neuronal Spike Recordings from the Thalamus of an Awake Behaving Rat," and simulated in the sections entitled "Model Motor Trajectory Decoding from Simulated Multichannel Local Field Potential Inputs" and "Continuous Real-Time Decoding of Head Direction from Neuronal Spike Activity in the Rat Thalamus," which require the decoder to estimate smooth trajectories as functions of time. While the gradient-descent least-squares approach is applicable to both kinds of problem, the convolution kernel chosen to implement the neural decoder, $W_{ij} = \frac{A_{ij}}{\tau_{ij}} e^{-\frac{t}{\tau_{ij}}}$, is designed to exploit the predictive value of past input signals. The degree to which past inputs $\vec{N}(t' < t)$ have predictive value is reflected by the value of the time constant τ_{ij}, and as $\tau_{ij} \to 0$ the time interval over which $\vec{N}(t' < t)$ contributes significantly to the present-time output $\vec{M}(t)$ correspondingly vanishes. In this experiment the signal to be decoded corresponds to a time series of discrete decisions made every $\Delta t = w$; consecutive reach cues were guaranteed to be independent through experimental design. Consequently, $\vec{N}(t')$ is completely uncorrelated from $\vec{N}(t)$ and $\vec{M}(t)$ for $|t - t'| \geq w$. (In concrete terms, since successive reaches are independent, neural activity preceding one reach contains no predictive information concerning the direction of the next reach.) As a result, meaningful decoding requires $\tau_{ij} = 0$, which we enforce by taking τ_{ij} to be a small, unmodifiable constant. Therefore, our decoding scheme as applied to the reach-intention neural data reduces to an instantaneous linear decoder, analogous to a single-layer artificial neural network implemented in continuous time and trained with continuous-time feedback.

The neural data used in the experiments reported here were first obtained and analyzed in connection with a previously reported set of experiments (Musallam et al., 2004). The decoding method used in those experiments involved an analysis of variance to preselect a subset of neurons exhibiting the greatest directional tuning, followed by Bayesian inference on the mean firing rates and higher-order Haar wavelet coefficients of the signals obtained from the selected neurons. We consequently had the opportunity to compare the performance of the adaptive-filter decoder to that of the Bayesian decoder. The principal performance measure reported using the Bayesian decoder was a 64.4% success rate in predicting the correct one of four allowed reach directions (Musallam et al., 2004). Under corresponding training conditions the neural decoding system described in the present work generated accurate predictions in 65% ± 9% of trials (the uncertainty figure preceded by the ± symbol indicates the magnitude of one standard deviation). Improved decoding performances were demonstrated in (Musallam et al., 2004) by considering higher-order coefficients in the Haar wavelet decomposition of the neural input signals, but in the present study we considered only the zeroth-order coefficients, corresponding to mean firing rates.

The decoding scheme originally used to decode the data analyzed in this section was based in part on the known tendency of direction-sensitive neurons to 'tune' to preferred directions in the sense that only movement in certain preferred directions induces such neurons to modulate their firing rates away from a baseline (Cohen & Andersen, 2002). In preparing the Bayesian decoder, an off-line analysis of variance on the training set of spike trains (corresponding to arm reaches in each direction for each isolated neuron) was required to rank the isolated neurons by degree of directional sensitivity. The computational intensity of this decoding scheme was sufficiently high that inputs from only a subset of isolated neurons were used in decoding after the learning period ended, and this ranking provided a means of prioritizing neurons for use as decoder inputs. By contrast, the adaptive-filter decoder described here easily handles all 54 neuronal inputs in computer simulations of real-time decoding; in a certain sense the adaptive-filter decoder automatically learns which neural inputs are the most highly directionally tuned (Rapoport, 2007). Moreover, the analog-circuit–based implementation of the decoder described here processes all neuronal inputs in parallel, so the computational intensity of the decoding task does not constrain the number of neuronal inputs the system can handle. Consequently, the adaptive-filter approach to decoding scales favorably with the number of neuronal inputs to the system. This is an important virtue of adaptive-filter decoding, as decoding accuracy typically improves and more complex decoding tasks can be performed without sacrificing accuracy as more neuronal inputs are used (Chapin, 2004). Furthermore, improvements in multielectrode neural recording methodologies and technologies continue to facilitate recording from increasing numbers of neurons (Harrison et al., 2007; M. A. L. Nicolelis et al., 2003; Suner, Fellows, Vargas-Irwin, Nakata, & Donoghue, 2005; Wise, Anderson, Hetke, Kipke, & Najafi, 2004).

The ability of the adaptive-filter decoder to handle large numbers of neurons provides an opportunity to explore a decoding regime less amenable to the Bayesian analysis of (Musallam et al., 2004). Figure 13 plots decoder performance as a function of the number of neuronal inputs (the horizontal line across the plot indicates the 0.25 threshold corresponding to unbiased guessing). While the corresponding performance curves for the Bayesian decoding algorithm were originally analyzed for up to sixteen neurons (Musallam et al., 2004), the computational efficiency of the adaptive filter enables performance to be evaluated for considerably larger numbers of neuronal inputs; the computation illustrated in Figure 13 is limited only by the total number of neuronal inputs available. The computation was performed under the standard training condition of 30 trials, and the error bars indicate the magnitude of a standard deviation after averaging over sets of randomized initial conditions and training inputs. As expected, decoder performance increases from just above the 25% chance threshold to the maximum of approximately 65% reported earlier in this section. The lower curve corresponds to random selections of the input neurons, while the upper curve corresponds to preselection of neurons in order of decreasing variance in the mean firing rates over the four reach directions (higher variance indicates greater directional selectivity). The latter curve suggests that decoding input signals from the subset of neurons transmitting the greatest amount of directional information results in performance nearly equivalent to that obtained from using the full set of available signals.

The 65% success rate of the decoding system, while comparable to that of other decoding algorithms tested on the same data (Musallam et al., 2004), indicates that there is considerable room for improvement. An outstanding question in the field of neural prosthetics concerns the degree to which intelligent users can compensate for imperfect decoding through biofeedback. Marked improvements in performance along these lines have been observed over time in both monkeys and humans (Carmena et al., 2003; Hochberg et al., 2006; Musallam et al., 2004; Taylor et al., 2002), but such contributions from biological learning are evidently insufficient. The work of (Musallam et al., 2004) indicates that performance can be improved by considering the temporal structure of the input neural signals at higher than zeroth order, and this might be achieved through changing the form of the filter kernels W_{ij}.

EVALUATING DESIGN TRADEOFFS IN THE CONSTRUCTION OF AN IMPLANTABLE NEURAL DECODER

Power Efficiency

Simulations using the circuit designs presented in the section entitled "Implementation of the Decoding Algorithm in Analog Circuitry" indicate that a single decoding module (corresponding to an adaptive kernel W_{ij} and associated optimization circuitry, as diagrammed in Figure 3) should consume approximately 54 nW from a 1-V supply in 0.18 μm CMOS technology (and require less than 3000 μm^2 in area). This low power consumption is achieved through the use of subthreshold bias currents for transistors in the analog filters and other components. Analog preprocessing of raw neural input waveforms can be accomplished by dual thresholding to detect action potentials on each input channel and then smoothing the resulting spike trains to generate mean firing rate input signals. Simulations of the circuits presented in the section entitled "Spike–based decoding" indicate that each analog preprocessing module should consume approximately 241 nW from a 1-V supply in 0.18 μm CMOS technology. A full-scale system with $n = 100$ neuronal inputs comprising $\vec{N}(t)$ and $m = 3$ control parameters comprising $\vec{M}(t)$ would require $m \times n = 300$ decoding modules and consume less than 17 μW in the decoder and less than 25 μW in the preprocessing stages.

Savings in Telemetry Power

An advantage of our system is that its suitability for power- and area-efficient analog implementation can enable decoding in the implanted unit of a brain–machine interface, saving power by obviating the need for analog-to-digital conversion of neural signals before decoding, and by compressing data before wireless transmission. In this section we compare the power costs of internal analog decoding to those of external digital decoding. System power will depend on the bandwidth required to transmit digitized neural data to an external unit, so we consider three alternatives for digitization and telemetry, reflecting three approaches to trading algorithmic flexibility in decoding for total system power: (1) Transmission of digitized raw neural waveforms, preserving the greatest amount of neural information and requiring the greatest bandwidth; (2) Transmission of threshold-crossing events from neural waveforms,

Figure 13. Decoding performance as a function of neuron number for randomly selected neurons (dark) and neurons selected on the basis of directional selectivity (light)

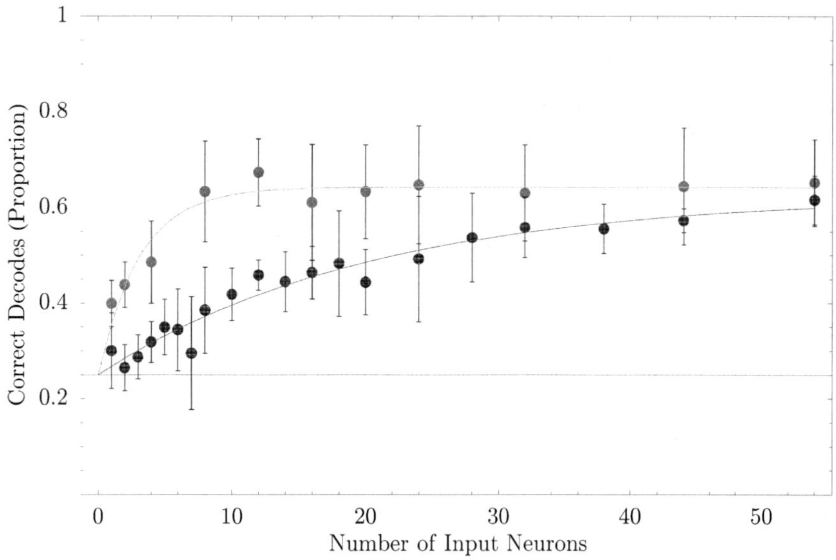

preserving only spike timing information and requiring intermediate bandwidth; (3) Transmission of control-parameter outputs from an implantable analog decoder, requiring minimal bandwidth and internal power consumption but sacrificing algorithmic flexibility.

In cases (1) and (2) initial 8-bit digitization of the input data at 30 kHz would require approximately 1 μW per channel (Yang & Sarpeshkar, 2006), contributing 100 μW in total. In these cases we consider implementing the external decoding system using a highly power-efficient digital signal processor (DSP) ("TMS320C55x Technical Overview (Literature Number SPRU393)," 2000) and analog-to-digital converters (A/Ds) (Yang & Sarpeshkar, 2006). (1) The first alternative requires transmitting all of the digitized data, corresponding to a bandwidth of 24 Mbs^{-1} for all n = 100 channels; at a rate of 1 mW per Mbs^{-1} (assuming typical link geometries and efficient topologies) (Mandal & Sarpeshkar, 2007, 2008) wireless data telemetry would consume 24 mW. (2) The second alternative requires dual thresholding for spike detection, followed by transmission of one bit per channel indicating the presence of a detected spike. Two comparison operations per period at 30 kHz across n = 100 input channels constitutes 6×10^6 operations per second. In practice (due to chip and board level parasitics) the most power-efficient DSPs operate at efficiencies of several hundred microwatts per MIPS (Millions of Instructions Per Second) (Verret, 2003); assuming an efficiency of 250 μW/MIPS, the power associated with these thresholding operations would be 1.5 mW. The bandwidth required to transmit the thresholded waveforms, assuming a maximal spike rate of 1 Hz per channel, would be 0.1 Mbs^{-1} for all n = 100 channels, corresponding to a transmission power of 0.1 mW. So the total power consumed by a system adopting this alternative for data digitization, compression and transmission would be approximately 1.7 mW.

In estimating the power consumed in cases (1) and (2) we have not included the overhead of a

DSP in excess of the power consumed in computations. In practice such overhead costs can be significant, contributing several milliwatts or more, depending on the processor used and its operating settings (Verret, 2003). However, it is important to note that all DSPs incur static power costs due to CMOS leakage currents, independent of device activity and operating frequency. Leakage power depends primarily on operating voltage and temperature, and the processing core of one highly power-efficient DSP dissipates approximately 180 μW at 1.6 V and room temperature (25°C); this leakage power increases to approximately 277 μW at body temperature (37°C) (Verret, 2003). Therefore, our power estimates for DSP-based processing represent lower bounds on what would be consumed in a practical implementation.

When our decoding algorithm is executed by a power-efficient DSP, the power expended in performing computations is negligible relative to the leakage power of the processor core. In a digital implementation of our decoder the adaptive filter kernels are transformed into discrete-time filters. A discrete-time implementation of the filter kernel $Ae^{-\frac{t}{\tau}}$ has a two-parameter z-transform, so each update cycle requires two multiplications. An update frequency of 10 Hz requires 20 multiplications per second, and scaling by $n \times m = 300$ yields the computational rate required to execute the algorithm, 0.006×10^6 multiplications per second. At an efficiency of 250 μW/MIPS, the power cost of the algorithm itself would therefore be only approximately 1.5 μW.

(3) As discussed in the section entitled "Power Efficiency," our simulations indicate that a low-power-analog implementation of our first-order adaptive kernel decoder with $(n, m) = (100, 3)$ could be built with a power budget of approximately 17 μW (54 nW per decoding module) and that an additional 25 μW is required for the preprocessing stages. Transmission of $m = 3$ decoded parameters for real-time control of an external device with 10-bit precision and an update frequency of 10 Hz requires a transmission rate of 300 bs^{-1} and an associated power of 300 nW. (Here we have assumed an impedance modulation telemetry scheme similar to the one reported in (Mandal & Sarpeshkar, 2007) and (Mandal & Sarpeshkar, 2008), which operates at an efficiency of <1 nJ per bit even for transmission rates greater than 1 Mbs^{-1}.) The total power consumption associated with internal decoding would therefore be approximately 43 μW.

So an implantable analog decoding system is capable of operating with 40- to 500-fold less power than would be required by digital preprocessing and telemetry in external decoding systems. Moreover, the 43 μW required by an implantable decoding system is 4–6 times less than even the leakage power of state-of-the-art power-efficient DSPs; this implies that when the implantable analog decoder is operating, it should consume at least 4 times less power than an external digital decoder that is doing nothing. The efficiency of our analog architecture arises from its exploitation of subthreshold currents (which are wasted as 'leakage' power in traditional digital implementations) to perform computations.

A further point of comparison concerns the sizes of the devices required to perform the decoding. In our simulations, a single decoder module implemented in 0.18 μm technology would require less than 3000 μm^2, so a system decoding 3 control parameters from 100 input channels would consume less than 1 mm^2 of chip area. By contrast, industry-standard low-power DSPs are typically 100 times larger, consuming approximately 1 cm^2 of board area ("TMS320C54x BGA Mechanical Data (Document MPBG021C)," 2002). Space limitations and skull curvature restrict the planar surface area of devices implanted within the cranial cavity to approximately 2×2 cm^2, so individual components that consume 1 cm^2 of area are likely impractical as elements of implantable units.

FUTURE RESEARCH DIRECTIONS

Neural Decoding in the Context of Implantable Brain–Machine Interfaces

In this section we describe five important emerging areas in the field of neural decoding for brain–machine interfaces: (1) *Biocompatibility and Stability:* Ideal neuroprosthetics must be capable of implantation in the brain for indefinite periods without damaging or eliciting unintended reactions from surrounding neural tissue, macro- and microanatomically optimized for the appropriate neural targets, and capable of stably recording neural signals of the selected types for indefinite periods of time; (2) *Biological versus Artificial Learning:* Achieving optimal long-term performance from brain–machine interfaces requires understanding the interplay between artificial and biological learning; (3) *Closed-Loop Neuroprosthetics:* Neuroprosthetics must be able to adapt in real time based on feedback from sensory input, neural populations, and other environmental variables; (4) *Integrated Electronic Systems:* General-purpose devices suitable for clinical intervention or neuroscientific research must have all functional subcomponents integrated within a single modularized package; (5) *Scalable Multi-Region Brain–Machine Interfaces:* Brain–machine interfaces should be capable of parallel or networked operation, in which multiple independent modules can operate either independently from neighboring or disparate neural populations without sacrificing performance quality, or while sharing information in a networked fashion in real time.

Biocompatibility and Stability

The difficulty of maintaining stable single-unit neural recordings for extended periods has long been acknowledged by electrophysiologists, and while some notable examples have been reported in the literature, such reports tend to be the exception rather than the rule. The field of brain–machine interfaces has responded to this problem in two principal ways, at once seeking to optimize electrode design and electrode-tissue interactions for stable long-term recording, while simultaneously exploring a range of neural signals, including local field potentials and unsorted multiunit activity as alternatives to single-unit action potentials. Biocompatibility as a concern for implantable brain–machine interface systems extends to multiple aspects of the implanted system, including the design and materials chosen for the packaging, but we restrict our comments here to neural electrodes.

Decoding neural signals presupposes the availability of such signals, and the quality of neural decoding depends not only on the particular algorithms used for the decoding, but also on the quality of the neural signals used as inputs to the neural decoder. An ideally biocompatible neural recording electrode must satisfy two sets of constraints, which respectively concern the static and dynamic properties of the tissue-electrode interface. Ideal static properties of the electrode include the following: (1) Suitability for insertion in a manner that does minimal damage to surrounding neural and vascular tissue; (2) Mechanical stiffness equal to that of the surrounding tissue, in order to avoid tissue-electrode shearing and electrode displacement during head acceleration; (3) Minimal electrode volume to minimize neural tissue displacement after insertion; (4) Shank and recording site geometry optimized for stereotactic placement relative to desired macro- and microanatomic targets; and (5) Tip or recording site geometry optimized for the neural signal of choice. Ideal dynamic properties of a neural recording electrode include the following: (1) Optimized electrode impedance given the local tissue properties and neural signals of interest; and (2) Ability to regulate the response of neural tissue to the presence of the electrode over time.

Almost all of these static and dynamic properties represent active areas of current research and potentially fruitful future work. In particular, microfabrication techniques (Kipke et al., 2008; Wise et al., 2004) and nontraditional materials (such as conducting polymers) (Abidian & Martin, 2008; Ludwig, Uram, Yang, Martin, & Kipke, 2006; Richardson-Burns, Hendricks, & Martin, 2007) present large parameter spaces within which to optimize electrode designs. Additionally, it is well known that the microanatomic environment of a recording electrode changes over time, generally in ways that degrade electrode performance, as neighboring neurons tend to die or recede from the electrode, for example, and astrocytes and microglia ensheath the electrode and change the impedance at the tissue-electrode interface. Consequently, understanding and controlling the dynamic response of neural and neurovascular tissue to neural recording electrodes is also an extremely important area for future research (Bjornsson et al., 2006; Shain et al., 2003).

Some differences of opinion exist as to the most appropriate signals to use as inputs for neural prosthetic devices. The difficulty of first reliably obtaining and subsequently maintaining stable single-unit recordings for indefinite periods has motivated the use of other forms of input signal, which in a number of studies have yielded equivalent decoding performance while exhibiting greater stability over time. Action potentials, multiunit activity, and local field potentials associated with movement, imagined movement, and motor planning have all been shown capable of affording neural control of external devices in conjunction with a variety of neural decoding techniques (Andersen, Burdick, Musallam, Pesaran, & Cham, 2004; Mehring et al., 2003; Pesaran et al., 2002; Shenoy et al., 2003; Stark & Abeles, 2007).

A related question concerns the ways in which the brain represents motor control information: Precisely what kinds of state space variables do neural populations encode, and how stable are the representations (Rokni, Richardson, Bizzi, & Seung, 2007)? In particular, in the context of neuromotor prosthetics, under what circumstances does neural activity reflect internal signals to muscles, external parameters such as those relating to limb kinematics or dynamics, or higher-level control signals such as those related to movement planning (Kakei, Hoffman, & Strick, 1999)? Questions such as these are particularly relevant to systems such as those in which functional electrical stimulation (FES) of muscles in a paralyzed limb is placed under real-time neural control to restore lost function (Moritz, Perlmutter, & Fetz, 2008).

Biological vs. Artificial Learning

A major question in the area of neural decoding to achieve neural control of prosthetic devices concerns the extent to which the brain can learn to decode processed neural data on its own. Given a particular prosthetic interface controlled by neural signals from a subject that receives feedback on decoder performance, what is the minimal decoder required to operate the device reliably? Under what circumstances, and with what degree of reliability, can biological learning compensate for deficiencies in an artificial neural decoder?

As indicated earlier in this chapter, experiments in both animals (Musallam et al., 2004; Taylor et al., 2002) and humans (Hochberg et al., 2006) have provided early evidence that users of neural prosthetic systems are capable of adapting to the particular rules governing the control of their brain–machine interfaces, demonstrating improved performance over time even after termination of the learning phases for their software-based decoders. Nevertheless, some of the same experiments have also demonstrated the apparent insufficiency of such contributions from biological learning, and so the degree to which a neural prosthetic system should rely on artificial or biological learning remains unclear. More recent work (Ganguly & Carmena, 2009) has helped clarify some of these issues by underscoring the importance of stable long-term neural recordings for reliable neural decoding and improvements through biological learning. In particular, it appears that the brain is capable not only of learning complex decoders, but also of correcting errors in corrupt decoders, provided the decoders are based on stable neural recordings. Much of the existing work on neural decoding has been limited by the inability to maintain stable recordings from multiple units over long time periods, and by the consequent need to retrain decoders at each training session. As biological learning can occur over longer timescales than those set by the instability of typical single- or multiunit neural recordings, optimal conditions for biological learning in the context of neural prosthesis control have rarely been achieved. Recent evidence suggests that a reliably high level of performance can be obtained as the brain forms motor memories in response to learning a decoder based on stable, long-term recordings. The implications of these findings for the design of neural decoders, neural electrodes, and neural prosthetic systems in general remain to be explored and will be an important area for future research.

Relatedly, decoder optimality is likely to be application dependent, as specific contexts will determine the constraints and performance criteria to be optimized by a particular neural decoder. Nevertheless, it may be important to ask under what circumstances is it possible to define and construct optimal neural decoders, and to understand how to make tradeoffs between biological and artificial learning that optimize system performance.

Closed-Loop Neuroprosthetics

Translating advances in neural decoding into clinical practice will require prosthetic devices, including robotic prosthetic limbs, that confer natural functionality (Aaron et al., 2006; Adee, 2009; Kuiken et al., 2009; Kuniholm, 2009). The form and quality of sensory and direct neural feedback signals are important in enabling devices to achieve such lifelike performances. Therefore, in the context of motor prosthetics, realistic sensory feedback from proprioceptive, haptic, and other modalities encoded by physiologic signals will improve motor prosthetic performance (Miguel A. L. Nicolelis, Chapin, & Wessberg, 2007). Implementation of such a system will require simultaneous neural recording and neural stimulation of somatosensory and motor brain regions.

An important class of future neural prosthetic systems will involve closed-loop neural decoding and neural stimulation, in which decoded neural firing patterns can be used to control neural stimulation in a feedback loop. This paradigm is applicable to deep brain stimulation (DBS) in which the stimuli delivered depend on sensory data and the state of local neural networks; current DBS systems use fixed, nonadaptive stimulation paradigms. Neural decoding for seizure detection, coupled with stimulation to preempt the seizure in a feedback fashion, represents another potential clinical application for closed-loop neural decoding and stimulation. The scope of clinical problems amenable to solutions of this kind is likely to expand over time.

Integrated Electronic Systems

We make reference in the Introduction to recent progress developing modular electronic components of implantable brain–machine interfaces, particularly in the areas of micropower neural amplification, low-power data telemetry, ultra-low-power analog-to-digital conversion, low-power and power-conserving schemes for neural stimulation, adaptive power biasing of multi-electrode arrays, and energy-efficient wireless recharging circuits (Sarpeshkar et al., 2008). Significant progress has also been made toward integrating and packaging these individual modules into functioning systems, in several cases together with neural recording electrodes (Harrison, 2008; Song et al., 2007; Wise et al., 2004). Work in this area is an important avenue for continuing research toward brain–machine interface systems that can be used in both clinical and experimental neuroscience.

Power efficiency and power management are extremely important concerns in small, biologically implantable systems. The development of high-performance biologically implantable power sources that are safe, compact, and easily rechargeable or schemes for scavenging energy from the biological environment could lift a variety of design constraints on the implantable electronics, as implantable batteries are typically the largest and most massive components of biologically implantable electronic devices.

Scalable Multi-Region Brain–Machine Interfaces

Scalability represents an important trend in contemporary neuroscience (Narasimhan, 2004). Neural computations underlying motor and other functions are distributed across a variety of brain regions, so it is likely that optimal control of neural prosthetic devices will be achieved using neural decoders that coordinate input signals from multiple brain regions (Andersen, Burdick et al., 2004; Chapin, 2004; M. A. L. Nicolelis et al., 2003). Coordinating signal processing over multiple input streams derived from distinct regions requires that brain–machine interface systems be designed in a modular fashion that permits individual modules not only to report data independently, but also to share information in a networked fashion in real time. Such scalable, networked systems represent an extremely interesting direction for future research, particularly in light of the observation that even rudimentary artificial networking of neural regions can induce long-term motor plasticity (Jackson et al., 2006). Systems of this kind might be used not only to establish functional connections among multiple regions within an individual brain, but also to connect individual brains to one another.

CONCLUSION

We have described a continuous-time, adaptive, biomimetic algorithm and a corresponding micropower analog circuit architecture for decoding neural signals (Figure 1 and Figure 2). The system is suitable for decoding both local field potentials and mean spike rates; in experimental trials it has successfully decoded both discrete decisions from the parietal cortex of a behaving primate (Figure 13) and continuous trajectories from the thalamus of a behaving rodent (Figure 11). The algorithm and architecture presented here offer a practical approach to computationally efficient neural signal decoding, independent of the hardware used for their implementation. While the system is suitable for analog or digital implementation, we discuss how a micropower analog implementation trades some algorithmic programmability for reductions in power consumption that could facilitate implantation of a neural decoder within the brain. In particular, circuit simulations of our analog architecture (comprised of standard building-block circuits described in the section entitled "Functional Circuit Subunits of the Decoder Architecture") indicate that a 100-channel, 3-motor-output neural decoder can be built with a total power budget of approximately 43 μW. Our work could also enable a 100,000-fold reduction in the bandwidth needed for wireless transmission of neural data, thereby reducing to nanowatt levels the power potentially required for wireless data telemetry from a brain implant.

Our work suggests that highly power-efficient and area-efficient analog neural decoders that operate in real time can be useful components of brain–implantable neural prostheses, with potential applications in neural rehabilitation and experimental neuroscience. Through front-end preprocessing to perform neural decoding and data compression, algorithms and architectures such as those presented here can complement digital signal processing and wireless data transmission systems (Figure 1), offering significant increases in power and area efficiency at little cost.

ACKNOWLEDGMENT

This work was supported in part by a grant from the National Institutes of Health, NS-056140, and in part by an MIT–CIMIT Medical Engineering Fellowship. Neural data were provided by Sam Musallam of the Andersen Laboratory at the California Institute of Technology, and by Hector Penagos of the Wilson Laboratory at the Massachusetts Institute of Technology.

REFERENCES

Aaron, R. K., Herr, H. M., Ciombor, D. M., Hochberg, L. R., Donoghue, J. P., & Briant, C. L. (2006). Horizons in Prosthesis Development for the Restoration of Limb Function. *The Journal of the American Academy of Orthopaedic Surgeons*, *14*(10), S198–S204.

Abidian, M. R., & Martin, D. C. (2008). Experimental and theoretical characterization of implantable neural microelectrodes modified with conducting polymer nanotubes. *Biomaterials*, *29*, 1273–1283. doi:10.1016/j.biomaterials.2007.11.022

Adee, S. (2009). The revolution will be prosthetized. *IEEE Spectrum*, *46*(1), 44–48. doi:10.1109/MSPEC.2009.4734314

Andersen, R. A., Burdick, J. W., Musallam, S., Pesaran, B., & Cham, J. G. (2004). Cognitive neural prosthetics. *Trends in Cognitive Sciences*, *8*(11), 486–493. doi:10.1016/j.tics.2004.09.009

Andersen, R. A., Musallam, S., & Pesaran, B. (2004). Selecting the signals for a brain-machine interface. *Current Opinion in Neurobiology*, *14*, 1–7. doi:10.1016/j.conb.2004.10.005

Arenz, A., Silver, R. A., Schaefer, A. T., & Margrie, T. W. (2008). The Contribution of Single Synapses to Sensory Representation in Vivo. *Science*, *321*, 977–980. doi:10.1126/science.1158391

Baker, M. W., & Sarpeshkar, R. (2007). Feedback Analysis and Design of RF Power Links for Low-Power Bionic Systems. *IEEE Transactions on Biomedical Circuits and Systems*, *1*(1), 28–38. doi:10.1109/TBCAS.2007.893180

Bjornsson, C. S., Oh, S. J., Al-Kofahi, Y. A., Lim, Y. J., Smith, K. L., & Turner, J. N. (2006). Effects of insertion conditions on tissue strain and vascular damage during neuroprosthetic device insertion. *Journal of Neural Engineering*, *3*, 196–207. doi:10.1088/1741-2560/3/3/002

Brockwell, A. E., Rojas, A. L., & Kass, R. E. (2004). Recursive Bayesian decoding of motor cortical signals by particle filtering. *Journal of Neurophysiology*, *91*, 1899–1907. doi:10.1152/jn.00438.2003

Carmena, J. M., Lebedev, M. A., Crist, R. E., O'Doherty, J. E., Santucci, D. M., & Dimitrov, D. F. (2003). Learning to Control a Brain-Machine Interface for Reaching and Grasping by Primates. *Public Library of Science Biology*, *1*(2), 1–16.

Chapin, J. K. (2004). Using multi-neuron population recordings for neural prosthetics. *Nature Neuroscience*, *7*(5), 452–455. doi:10.1038/nn1234

Chapin, J. K., Moxon, K. A., Markowitz, R. S., & Nicolelis, M. L. (1999). Real-time control of a robot arm using simultaneously recorded neurons in the motor cortex. *Nature Neuroscience*, *2*, 664–670. doi:10.1038/10223

Cohen, Y. E., & Andersen, R. A. (2002). A Common Reference Frame for Movement Plans in the Posterior Parietal Cortex. *Nature Reviews. Neuroscience*, *3*, 553–562. doi:10.1038/nrn873

Connolly, J. D., Andersen, R. A., & Goodale, M. A. (2003). fMRI evidence for a 'parietal reach region' in the human brain. *Experimental Brain Research*, *153*, 140–145. doi:10.1007/s00221-003-1587-1

Eden, U. T., Frank, L. M., Barbieri, R., Solo, V., & Brown, E. N. (2004). Dynamic analyses of neural encoding by point process adaptive filtering. *Neural Computation*, *16*(5), 971–998. doi:10.1162/089976604773135069

Eliasmith, C., & Anderson, C. H. (2003). *Neural Engineering*.

Ganguly, K., & Carmena, J. M. (2009). Emergence of a Stable Cortical Map for Neuroprosthetic Control. *Public Library of Science Biology, 7*(7).

Ghovanloo, M., & Atluri, S. (2007). A wideband power-efficieny inductive wireless link for implantable microelectronic devices using multiple carriers. *IEEE Transactions on Circuits and Systems. I, Fundamental Theory and Applications*, *54*(10), 71–77. doi:10.1109/TCSI.2007.905187

Harrison, R. R. (2008). The design of integrated circuits to observe brain activity. *Proceedings of the IEEE*, *96*, 1203–1216. doi:10.1109/JPROC.2008.922581

Harrison, R. R., Watkins, P. T., Kier, R. J., Lovejoy, R. O., Black, D. J., & Greger, B. (2007). A Low-Power Integrated Circuit for a Wireless 100-Electrode Neural Recording System. *IEEE Journal of Solid-state Circuits*, *42*(1), 123–133. doi:10.1109/JSSC.2006.886567

Haykin, S. (1999). *Neural Networks: A Comprehensive Foundation*. Upper Saddle River, New Jersey: Prentice Hall.

Hochberg, L. R., Serruya, M. D., Friehs, G. M., Mukand, J. A., Saleh, M., & Caplan, A. H. (2006). Neuronal ensemble control of prosthetic devices by a human with tetraplegia. *Nature*, *442*, 164–171. doi:10.1038/nature04970

Holleman, J., & Otis, B. (2007). 29th Annual International Conference of the IEEE Engineering in Medicine and Biology Society, *A sub-microwatt low-noise amplifier for neural recording* (pp. 3930-3933).

Jackson, A., Mavoori, J., & Fetz, E. E. (2006). Long-term motor cortex plasticity induced by an electronic neural implant. *Nature*, *444*, 55–60. doi:10.1038/nature05226

Kakei, S., Hoffman, D. S., & Strick, P. L. (1999). Muscle and Movement Representations in the Primary Motor Cortex. *Science*, *285*, 2136–2139. doi:10.1126/science.285.5436.2136

Kipke, D. R., Shain, W., Buzsáki, G., Fetz, E. E., Henderson, J. M., & Hetke, J. F. (2008). Advanced Neurotechnologies for Chronic Neural Interfaces: New Horizons and Clinical Opportunities. *The Journal of Neuroscience*, *28*(46), 11830–11838. doi:10.1523/JNEUROSCI.3879-08.2008

Kuiken, T. A., Li, G., Lock, B. A., Lipschultz, R. D., Miller, L. A., & Stubblefield, K. A. (2009). Targeted Muscle Reinnervation for Real-time Myoelectric Control of Multifunction Artificial Arms. *Journal of the American Medical Association*, *301*(6), 619–628. doi:10.1001/jama.2009.116

Kuniholm, J. (2009). Open Arms. *IEEE Spectrum*, *46*(3), 36–41. doi:10.1109/MSPEC.2009.4795454

Lazzaro, J., Wawrzynek, J., & Lippmann, R. P. (1997). A Micropower Analog Circuit Implementation of Hidden Markov Model State Decoding. *IEEE Journal of Solid-state Circuits*, *32*(8), 1200–1209. doi:10.1109/4.604076

Loeliger, H.-A., Tarköy, F., Lustenberger, F., & Helfenstein, M. (1999). Decoding in Analog VLSI. *IEEE Communications Magazine*, 99–101. doi:10.1109/35.755457

Ludwig, K. A., Uram, J. D., Yang, J., Martin, D. C., & Kipke, D. R. (2006). Chronic neural recordings using silicon microelectrode arrays electrochemically deposited with a poly(3,4-ethylenedioxythiophene) (PEDOT) film. *Journal of Neural Engineering*, *3*, 59–70. doi:10.1088/1741-2560/3/1/007

Mandal, S., & Sarpeshkar, R. (2007). A Bidirectional Wireless Link for Neural Prostheses that Minimizes Implanted Power Consumption. *Proceedings of the IEEE Biomedical Circuits and Systems Conference (BioCAS)*, 45-48.

Mandal, S., & Sarpeshkar, R. (2008). Power-Efficient Impedance-Modulation Wireless Data Links for Biomedical Implants. *IEEE Transactions on Biomedical Circuits and Systems*, *2*(4), 301–315. doi:10.1109/TBCAS.2008.2005295

Mead, C. (1989). *Analog VLSI and Neural Systems*. Addison Wesley.

Mehring, C., Rickert, J., Vaadia, E., de Oliveira, S. C., Aertsen, A., & Rotter, S. (2003). Inference of hand movements from local field potentials in monkey motor cortex. *Nature Neuroscience*, *6*(12), 1253–1254. doi:10.1038/nn1158

Mohseni, P., Najafi, K., Eliades, S. J., & Wang, X. (2005). Wireless Multichannel Biopotential Recording Using an Integrated FM Telemetry Circuit. *IEEE Transactions on Neural Systems and Rehabilitation Engineering*, *13*(3), 263–271. doi:10.1109/TNSRE.2005.853625

Moritz, C. T., Perlmutter, S. I., & Fetz, E. E. (2008). Direct control of paralysed muscles by cortical neurons. *Nature*, *456*, 639–642. doi:10.1038/nature07418

Musallam, S., Corneil, B. D., Greger, B., Scherberger, H., & Andersen, R. A. (2004). Cognitive Control Signals for Neural Prosthetics. *Science*, *305*, 258–262. doi:10.1126/science.1097938

Narasimhan, K. (2004). Scaling up neuroscience. *Nature Neuroscience*, *7*(5), 425. doi:10.1038/nn0504-425

Nicolelis, M. A. L., Chapin, J. K., & Wessberg, J. (2007). United States of America Patent No. Official Gazette of the United States Patent and Trademark Office Patents: U. S. P. a. T. Office.

Nicolelis, M. A. L., Dimitrov, D., Carmena, J. M., Crist, R., Lehew, G., & Kralik, J. D. (2003). Chronic, multisite, multielectrode recordings in macaque monkeys. *Proceedings of the National Academy of Sciences of the United States of America*, *200*(19), 11041–11046. doi:10.1073/pnas.1934665100

O'Halloran, M., & Sarpeshkar, R. (2004). A 10-nW 12-bit Accurate Analog Storage Cell with 10-aA Leakage. *IEEE Journal of Solid-state Circuits*, *39*(11), 557–560. doi:10.1109/JSSC.2004.835817

O'Halloran, M., & Sarpeshkar, R. (2006). An Analog Storage Cell with 5e$^-$/sec Leakage. *Proceedings of the IEEE International Symposium on Circuits and Systems (ISCAS)*, 557-560.

Olsson, R. H. III, & Wise, K. D. (2005). A Three-Dimensional Neural Recording Microsystem With Implantable Data Compression Circuitry. *IEEE Journal of Solid-state Circuits*, *40*(12), 2796–2804. doi:10.1109/JSSC.2005.858479

Pesaran, B., Pezaris, J. S., Sahani, M., Mitra, P. P., & Andersen, R. A. (2002). Temporal structure in neuronal activity during working memory in macaque parietal cortex. *Nature Neuroscience*, *5*(8), 805–811. doi:10.1038/nn890

Rapoport, B. I. (2007). *Neural Prosthetics for Paralysis: Algorithms and Low-Power Analog Architectures for Decoding Neural Signals*. Cambridge, Massachusetts: Massachusetts Institute of Technology.

Rapoport, B. I., Wattanapanitch, W., Penagos, H. L., Musallam, S., Andersen, R. A., & Sarpeshkar, R. (2009). *A Biomimetic Adaptive Algorithm and Low-Power Architecture for Implantable Neural Decoders*. Paper presented at the 31st Annual International Conference of the IEEE Engineering in Medicine and Biology Society (EMBC 2009).

Richardson-Burns, S. M., Hendricks, J. L., & Martin, D. C. (2007). Electrochemical polymerization of conducting polymers in living neural tissue. *Journal of Neural Engineering*, *4*, L6–L13. doi:10.1088/1741-2560/4/2/L02

Rokni, U., Richardson, A. G., Bizzi, E., & Seung, H. S. (2007). Motor Learning with Unstable Neural Representations. *Neuron*, *54*, 653–666. doi:10.1016/j.neuron.2007.04.030

Salthouse, C., & Sarpeshkar, R. (2003). A Practical Micropower Programmable Bandpass Filter for use in Bionic Ears. *IEEE Journal of Solid-state Circuits*, *38*(1), 63–70. doi:10.1109/JSSC.2002.806286

Sanchez, J. C., Erdogmus, D., Principe, J. C., Wessberg, J., & Nicolelis, M. A. L. (2005). Interpreting spatial and temporal neural activity through a recurrent neural network brain machine interface. *IEEE Transactions on Neural Systems and Rehabilitation Engineering*, *13*(2), 213–219. doi:10.1109/TNSRE.2005.847382

Santhanam, G., Ryu, S. I., Yu, B. M., Afshar, A., & Shenoy, K. V. (2006). A high-performance brain-computer interface. *Nature*, *442*, 195–198. doi:10.1038/nature04968

Sarpeshkar, R. (1998). Analog Versus Digital: Extrapolating from Electronics to Neurobiology. *Neural Computation*, *10*, 1601–1638. doi:10.1162/089976698300017052

Sarpeshkar, R. (2006). Brain Power: Borrowing from Biology Makes for Low-Power Computing. *IEEE Spectrum*, *43*(5), 24–29. doi:10.1109/MSPEC.2006.1628504

Sarpeshkar, R., Baker, M., Salthouse, C., Sit, J.-J., Turicchia, L., & Zhak, S. (2005). An Analog Bionic Ear Processor with Zero-Crossing Detection. *Proceedings of the IEEE International Solid State Circuits Conference (ISSCC)*, 78-79.

Sarpeshkar, R., Lyon, R. F., & Mead, C. (1997). A low-power wide-linear-range transconductance amplifier. *Analog Integrated Circuits and Signal Processing*, *13*(1-2), 123–151. doi:10.1023/A:1008292213687

Sarpeshkar, R., Salthouse, C., Sit, J.-J., Baker, M., Zhak, S., & Lu, T. (2005). An Ultra-Low-Power Programmable Analog Bionic Ear Processor. *IEEE Transactions on Bio-Medical Engineering*, *52*(4), 711–727. doi:10.1109/TBME.2005.844043

Sarpeshkar, R., Wattanapanitch, W., Arfin, S. K., Rapoport, B. I., Mandal, S., & Baker, M. W. (2008). Low-Power Circuits for Brain-Machine Interfaces. *IEEE Transactions on Biomedical Circuits and Systems*, *2*(3), 173–183. doi:10.1109/TBCAS.2008.2003198

Sarpeshkar, R., Wattanapanitch, W., Rapoport, B., Arfin, S. K., Baker, M. W., Mandal, S., et al. (2007). Low-Power Circuits for Brain-Machine Interfaces. *Proceedings of the IEEE Symposium on Circuits and Systems*, 2068-2071.

Serruya, M. D., Hatsopoulos, N. G., Fellows, M. R., Paninski, L., & Donoghue, J. P. (2003). Robustness of neuroprosthetic decoding algorithms. *Biological Cybernetics*, *88*(3), 219–228. doi:10.1007/s00422-002-0374-6

Shain, W., Spataro, L., Dilgen, J., Haverstick, K., Retterer, S., & Isaacson, M. (2003). Controlling cellular reactive responses around neural prosthetic devices using peripheral and local intervention strategies. *IEEE Transactions on Neural Systems and Rehabilitation Engineering*, *11*, 186–188. doi:10.1109/TNSRE.2003.814800

Shenoy, K. V., Meeker, D., Cao, S. Y., Kureshi, S. A., Pesaran, B., & Buneo, C. A. (2003). Neural prosthetic control signals from plan activity. *Neuroreport*, *14*(4), 591–596. doi:10.1097/00001756-200303240-00013

Snyder, L. H., Batista, A. P., & Andersen, R. A. (1997). Coding of intention in the posterior parietal cortex. *Nature*, *386*, 167–170. doi:10.1038/386167a0

Song, Y.-K., Patterson, W. R., Bull, C. W., Borton, D. A., Li, Y., Nurmikko, A. V., et al. (2007). *A Brain Implantable Microsystem with Hybrid RF/IR Telemetry for Advanced Neuroengineering Applications*. Paper presented at the 29th Annual International Conference of the IEEE Engineering in Medicine and Biology Society.

Srinivasan, L., Eden, U. T., Mitter, S. K., & Brown, E. N. (2007). General-purpose filter design for neural prosthetic devices. *Journal of Neurophysiology*, *98*, 2456–2475. doi:10.1152/jn.01118.2006

Stark, E., & Abeles, M. (2007). Predicting movement from multiunit activity. *The Journal of Neuroscience*, *27*(31), 8387–8394. doi:10.1523/JNEUROSCI.1321-07.2007

Suner, S., Fellows, M. R., Vargas-Irwin, C., Nakata, G. K., & Donoghue, J. P. (2005). Reliability of signals from a chronically implanted, silicon-based electrode array in non-human primate primary motor cortex. *IEEE Transactions on Neural Systems and Rehabilitation Engineering*, *13*(4), 524–541. doi:10.1109/TNSRE.2005.857687

Taube, J. S. (1995). Head Direction Cells Recorded in the Anterior Thalamic Nuclei of Freely Moving Rats. *The Journal of Neuroscience*, *15*(1), 70–86.

Taylor, D. M., Tillery, S. I. H., & Schwartz, A. B. (2002). Direct Cortical Control of 3D Neuroprosthetic Devices. *Science*, *296*, 1829–1832. doi:10.1126/science.1070291

Theogarajan, L., Wyatt, J., Rizzo, J., Drohan, B., Markova, M., Kelly, S., et al. (2004). *Low power neural stimulator for a retinal prosthesis*. Paper presented at the Annual Meeting of the Association for Research in Vision and Ophthalmology.

TMS320C54x BGA Mechanical Data (Document MPBG021C). (2002). Texas Instruments Incorporated.

TMS320C55x Technical Overview (Literature Number SPRU393). (2000). Texas Instruments Incorporated.

Velliste, M., Perel, S., Spalding, M. C., Whitford, A. S., & Schwartz, A. B. (2008). Cortical control of a prosthetic arm for self-feeding. *Nature*, *453*(7198), 1098–1101. doi:10.1038/nature06996

Verret, R. (2003). *TMS320VC5510 Power Consumption Summary (Application Report)*. Texas Instruments Incorporatedo. Document Number.

Warland, D., Reinagel, P., & Meister, M. (1997). Decoding visual information from a population of retinal ganglion cells. *Journal of Neurophysiology*, *78*(5), 2336–2350.

Wattanapanitch, W., Fee, M., & Sarpeshkar, R. (2007). An Energy-Efficient Micropower Neural Recording Amplifier. *IEEE Transactions on Biomedical Circuits and Systems*, *1*(2), 136–147. doi:10.1109/TBCAS.2007.907868

Wessberg, J., & Nicolelis, M. A. L. (2004). Optimizing a Linear Algorithm for Real-Time Robotic Control using Chronic Cortical Ensemble Recordings in Monkeys. *Journal of Cognitive Neuroscience*, *16*(6), 1022–1035. doi:10.1162/0898929041502652

Wessberg, J., Stambaugh, C. R., Kralik, J. D., Beck, P. D., Laubach, M., & Chapin, J. K. (2000). Real-time prediction of hand trajectory by ensembles of cortical neurons in primates. *Nature*, *408*, 361–365. doi:10.1038/35042582

Wise, K. D., Anderson, D. J., Hetke, J. F., Kipke, D. R., & Najafi, K. (2004). Wireless implantable microsystems: High-density electronic interfaces to the nervous system. *Proceedings of the IEEE*, *92*(1), 76–97. doi:10.1109/JPROC.2003.820544

Wu, W., Black, M. J., Mumford, D., Gao, Y., Bienenstock, E., & Donoghue, J. P. (2004). Modeling and decoding motor cortical activity using a switching Kalman filter. *IEEE Transactions on Bio-Medical Engineering, 51*(6), 933–942. doi:10.1109/TBME.2004.826666

Wu, W., Gao, Y., Bienenstock, E., Donoghue, J. P., & Black, M. J. (2006). Bayesian population decoding of motor cortical activity using a Kalman filter. *Neural Computation, 18*(1), 80–118. doi:10.1162/089976606774841585

Wu, W., & Hatsopoulos, N. G. (2008). Real-Time Decoding of Nonstationary Neural Activity in Motor Cortex. *IEEE Transactions on Neural Systems and Rehabilitation Engineering, 16*(3), 213–222. doi:10.1109/TNSRE.2008.922679

Wu, W., Shaikhouni, A., Donoghue, J. P., & Black, M. J. (2004). Closed-loop neural control of cursor motion using a Kalman filter. *Proceedings of the IEEE Engineering in Medicine and Biology Society*, 4126-4129.

Yang, H., & Sarpeshkar, R. (2006). A Bio-inspired Ultra-Energy-Efficient Analog-to-Digital Converter for Biomedical Applications. [Special Issue on Life Sciences and System Applications]. *IEEE Transactions on Circuits and Systems I, 53*(11), 2349–2356. doi:10.1109/TCSI.2006.884463

Zhak, S., Baker, M., & Sarpeshkar, R. (2003). A Low Power Wide Dynamic Range Envelope Detector. *IEEE Journal of Solid-state Circuits, 38*(10), 1750–1753. doi:10.1109/JSSC.2003.817599

ADDITIONAL READING

Brockwell, A. E., Rojas, A. L., & Kass, R. E. (2004). Recursive Bayesian Decoding of Motor Cortical Signals by Particle Filtering. *Journal of Neurophysiology, 91*, 1899–1907. doi:10.1152/jn.00438.2003

Brown, E. N. (2004). Theory of Point Processes for Neural Systems. In B. G. Carson Chow, David Hansel, Claude Meunier, Jean Dalibard (Ed.), *Methods and Models in Neurophysics, Session LXXX: Lecture Notes of the Les Houches Summer School 2003* (pp. 691-727): Elsevier.

Brown, E. N., Barbieri, R., Eden, U. T., & Frank, L. M. (2004). Likelihood Methods for Neural Spike Train Data Analysis. In Feng, J. (Ed.), *Computational Neuroscience: A Comprehensive Approach* (pp. 253–286). London: CRC Press.

Bullock, T. H. (1997). Signals and signs in the nervous system: The dynamic anatomy of electrical activity is probably information-rich. *Proceedings of the National Academy of Sciences of the United Sates of America, 94*(1-6), 1-6.

Buzsáki, G. (2004). Massively Parallel Recording of Unit and Local Field Potentials With Silicon-Based Electrodes. *Nature Neuroscience, 7*(5), 446–451.

Chorost, M. (2006). *Rebuilt: My Journey Back to the Hearing World*. Boston: Houghton Mifflin.

Csicsvari, J., Henze, D. A., Jamieson, B., Harris, K. D., Sirota, A., & Barthó, P. (2003). Massively Parallel Recording of Unit and Local Field Potentials With Silicon-Based Electrodes. *Journal of Neurophysiology, 90*, 1314–1323. doi:10.1152/jn.00116.2003

Eden, U. T. (2005). *Point Process Filters in the Analysis of Neural Spiking Models*. Cambridge: Unpublished Doctor of Philosophy, Harvard University.

Eliasmith, C., & Anderson, C. H. (2004). *Neural Engineering: Computation, Representation, and Dynamics in Neurobiological Systems*. Cambridge: MIT Press.

Georgopoulos, A. P., Kalaska, J. F., Caminiti, R., & Massey, J. T. (1982). On the Relations Between the Direction of Two-Dimensional Arm Movements and Cell Discharge in Primate Motor Cortex. *The Journal of Neuroscience*, *2*(11), 1527–1537.

Georgopoulos, A. P., Schwartz, A. B., & Kettner, R. E. (1986). Neural Population Coding of Movement Direction. *Science*, *233*, 1416–1419. doi:10.1126/science.3749885

Haykin, S. (2008). *Neural Networks and Learning Machines*. New York: Prentice Hall.

He, J., Ma, C., & Herman, R. (2008). Engineering Neural Interfaces for Rehabilitation of Lower Limb Function in Spinal Cord Injured. *Proceedings of the IEEE*, *96*(7), 1152–1166. doi:10.1109/JPROC.2008.922593

Kandel, E., Schwartz, J., & Jessell, T. (2000). *Principles of Neural Science* (4th ed.). New York: McGraw-Hill.

Lewicki, M. S. (1998). A review of methods for spike sorting: the detection and classification of neural action potentials. *Network (Bristol, England)*, *9*, R53–R78. doi:10.1088/0954-898X/9/4/001

MacKay, D. J. C. (2006). *Information Theory, Inference, and Learning Algorithms*. Cambridge: Cambridge University Press.

Martin, R. (2005). Mind Control. *Wired*, *13*(3).

Maynard, E. M., Nordhausen, C. T., & Normann, R. A. (1997). The Utah Intracortical Electrode Array: a recording structure for potential brain-computer interfaces. *Electroencephalography and Clinical Neurophysiology*, *102*, 228–239. doi:10.1016/S0013-4694(96)95176-0

Mead, C. (1989). *Analog VLSI and Neural Systems*. Reading: Addison-Wesley.

Mitra, P., & Bokil, H. (2007). *Observed Brain Dynamics*. Oxford University Press. doi:10.1093/acprof:oso/9780195178081.001.0001

Nicolelis, M. A. L. (Ed.). (1999). *Methods for Neural Ensemble Recordings*. New York: CRC Press.

Nordhausen, C. T., Rousche, P. J., & Normann, R. A. (1994). Optimizing recording capabilities of the Utah Intracortical Electrode Array. *Brain Research*, *637*, 27–36. doi:10.1016/0006-8993(94)91213-0

Paradiso, J., Borriello, G., & Bonato, P. (2008). Implantable Electronics. *IEEE Pervasive Computing / IEEE Computer Society [and] IEEE Communications Society*, *7*(1), 12–13. doi:10.1109/MPRV.2008.11

Ventura, V. (2008). Spike train decoding without spike sorting. *Neural Computation*, *20*(4), 923–963. doi:10.1162/neco.2008.02-07-478

Zhang, K., Ginzburg, I., McNaughton, B. L., & Sejnowski, T. J. (1998). Interpreting Neuronal Population Activity by Reconstruction: Unified Framework With Application to Hippocampal Place Cells. *Journal of Neurophysiology*, *79*(2), 1017–1044.

KEY TERMS AND DEFINITIONS

Adaptive Algorithm: In the present work we use the term "adaptive algorithm" to denote an optimization process in which a filter adjust its own transfer function. The associated filter is referred to as an "adaptive filter," and the adaptation process is referred to as "tuning." In other scientific literature, the term "adaptive algorithm" is sometimes used to refer to an algorithm that modifies its behavior in accordance with the computational resources available.

Biomimetic: Designed according to principles used by biological systems.

Brain–Machine Interface (BMI): A system enabling direct transfer of information between a brain and a machine; when the machine in question is a computer, such a system is sometimes called a "brain–computer interface" (BCI). The transfer of information is typically "direct" in one of two senses: Either information obtained from the brain remains encoded in physiologic signals (such as intracortical or electroencephalographic [EEG] voltage traces) that are recorded from the brain and transmitted to an external system for decoding, or information is sent to the brain by electrochemical stimulation of neural tissue. The present chapter focuses on brain-machine interfaces of the former kind, which decode information from electrophysiologically recorded neural signals.

Motor Control: "Motor" in the neurophysiologic sense refers to muscle activity and associated body movements coordinated by the nervous system; such neural coordination is referred to as "motor control."

Neural Cell Ensemble (Neuronal Ensemble): A group of neurons whose activity is considered simultaneously. The cells in the ensemble may or may not share functional or anatomic connections.

Neural Decoding: A process by which physiologic neural signals are translated into objectively defined state variables (which may correspond to parameters such as position, speed, or discrete values from a set of possibilities).

Neural Prosthetic (Neural Prosthesis): The term "prosthesis" refers to an artificial replacement for a body part, usually one whose function has been lost or impaired. The term "neural prosthesis" may refer literally to a system designed to replace or augment part of a brain or nervous system. The term may also refer to a prosthetic device, such as an artificial limb, that is controlled by a brain–machine interface.

Parietal Cortex: An anatomic region of the cerebral cortex whose functions relate primarily to spatial orientation and proprioception (the perception of body positioning), based on integration of information from multiple sensory information pathways. Experiments described in the present chapter involve neural data from the macaque monkey posterior parietal cortex, which computes transformations between eye-based and head-based coordinate systems, and which has been correspondingly implicated in the coordination of limb and eye movements for reaching and grasping.

Receptive Field: The "receptive field" of a neuron consists of all locations from which a stimulus is capable of altering the firing pattern of the neuron in question. When the cell of interest belongs to a sensory pathway, its receptive field may be spatial, corresponding to regions of the visual field for neurons of the visual system or to regions on the body surface for touch-sensitive neurons; the receptive field may also exist in a more abstract parameter space, corresponding, for example, to ranges in pitch for neurons of the auditory system. Functionally connected neurons may also be considered to comprise receptive fields for one another: One neuron whose firing constitutes a stimulus for a second neuron can be considered part of the receptive field of the second cell.

Thalamus: A structure in the brain whose functions include transmitting sensory information to the cerebral cortex, and relaying motor information from the cerebral cortex to the peripheral nervous system. The present chapter describes a set of experiments involving neural decoding from "head direction cells" of the rat thalamus, which are neurons within this region of the rat brain that are known to exhibit receptive fields tuned to specific orientations of the head relative to the environment.

Chapter 11
FPGA Coprocessor for Simulation of Neural Networks Using Compressed Matrix Storage

Jörg Bornschein
Goethe University Frankfurt am Main, Germany

ABSTRACT

An FPGA-based coprocessor has been implemented which simulates the dynamics of a large recurrent neural network composed of binary neurons. The design has been used for unsupervised learning of receptive fields. Since the number of neurons to be simulated (>10^4) exceeds the available FPGA logic capacity for direct implementation, a set of streaming processors has been designed. Given the state- and activity vectors of the neurons at time t and a sparse connectivity matrix, these streaming processors calculate the state- and activity vectors for time t + 1. The operation implemented by the streaming processors can be understood as a generalized form of a sparse matrix vector product (SpMxV). The largest dataset, the sparse connectivity matrix, is stored and processed in a compressed format to better utilize the available memory bandwidth.

INTRODUCTION

The connectionist model of information processing assumes that useful behavior is an emergent property of a huge number of relatively simple interacting units. A given connectionist model describes two things: On the one hand it describes the behavior of the individual units, the neurons; how they react to incoming stimuli and the output they generate. On the other hand it describes the connectivity between these units. Typically the exact structure of these connections varies over time; sometimes because of a learning process, sometimes, on smaller timescales, to facilitate dynamic plasticity.

For some models a mathematical abstraction can be found which allows the emergent macroscopic behavior to be understood without simulating the system at hand. In general, this is not the case and simulations are the predominant tool to understand the behavior of the modeled systems. Interesting systems often consist of more

DOI: 10.4018/978-1-60960-018-1.ch011

than 10,000 neurons with non-trivial connectivity between them. The human brain for example consists of about 10^{11} neurons with more than 10^{14} synapses between them. When considering strategies how to simulate connectionist systems, we can think of two extreme cases:

1. Sequentially simulate one neuron after another. For every neuron all input signals are collected and the neuron's output is computed.
2. Physically instantiate a simulation circuit for every neuron and make sure they all receive the input stimuli they need to compute a time step.

While in nature we find the second extreme realized, an arbitrary working point in between can be chosen. It is up to the software or hardware engineer to find a suitable trade-off, which makes best use of available hardware for a given system. In this work we assume that the number of neurons to be simulated exceeds the number of neurons that can be directly instantiated due to hardware resource limits. Given this assumption it is evident that, irrespective of the exact nature of the neuron simulator, be it software running on a CPU or a hardware implementation of a state-machine, some kind of multiplexing mechanism must exist to simulate a large number of neurons. The data needed to simulate a time step can be divided into three parts: A neural state vector $\vec{n}(t)$ which records the internal state of all neurons; an activity vector $\vec{a}(t)$, which can be directly derived from $\vec{n}(t)$ and stores if a neuron is firing or not, and a connection matrix $\mathbf{M}_{ij}$ which determines if and how a neuron *j* is connected to a neuron *i*. In this work we assume that the connection matrix **M** is best stored as a sparsely populated matrix, because only a small fraction of the matrix elements contain non-zero elements. We further assume, that the state and activity vectors $\vec{n}$ and $\vec{a}$ are stored as dense vectors.

It is crucial to understand that all currently available microprocessor architectures consist of processor elements with fast but relatively small local on-chip memory. External to these processor elements is larger, but much slower external DRAM (Wulf & McKee, 1995). Usually, at least for interesting systems, the data volume is larger than the size of the available internal on-chip memory. As a result the simulation performance is a function of memory bandwidth even with arbitrary fast processor elements.

Here we describe an architecture and the concrete implementation of an FPGA-based coprocessor which fully utilizes the available memory bandwidth to calculate $\vec{n}(t+1)$ given $\vec{n}(t), \vec{a}(t)$ and $\mathbf{M}$. Each of the three datasets is read sequentially, without random access, from external memory. The largest dataset, the connection matrix **M**, is stored in a compressed format using a variable-length entropy code to more efficiently use the available memory bandwidth.

This chapter is divided into 3 sections: In section 2 we introduce a model of the cortical macrocolumn, the artificial neural network we are going to simulate. This neural network has been successfully applied to unsupervised learning tasks and serves as an example for the types of networks the architecture can simulate.

Section 3 highlights the predominant operation when simulating cortical macrocolumns: The sparse matrix vector product (SpMxV). This operation is of general interest in engineering and computational science and we give a quick overview of the strategies deployed and the dataformats used when implementing SpMxV. In this section we also introduce a new storage format for sparse matrices, the *Compressed Incremental Row Storage* (CIRS) format. This format is designed to reduce bandwidth demand between the external memory and the processor elements performing SpMxV.

In section 4 we describe our implementation of an FPGA coprocessor which has been specifically designed to efficiently simulate neural networks similar to the one introduced in section 2. At its heart, this coprocessor implements the SpMxV operation for matrices stored in the compressed format introduced in section 3. We include benchmark results for (a) small scale implementation of the architecture running on a FPGA prototyping board and (b) scaling experiments that show what performance can be expected when this architecture is implemented on larger FPGAs and on platforms providing higher memory bandwidth.

UNSUPERVISED LEARNING USING BINARY NEURONS

In this section we describe a model of neural information processing as it was introduced by J. Lücke and C. von der Malsburg in "Rapid processing and unsupervised learning in a model of the cortical macrocolumn" in (Wulf & McKee, 1995). This model is on the one hand motivated by biological findings and on the other hand by its computational capabilities in unsupervised learning. This model of the macrocolumn consists of two principal elements: A layer of input neurons and a set of minicolums. Each minicolumn itself is composed of some hundred binary neurons.

Neural Dynamics of a Minicomlumn

We call a set of 100 to 200 neurons a cortical minicolumn. The neurons within a minicolumn maintain strong excitatory connections between each other. The individual neurons are modeled as McCulloch-Pitts neurons: Depending on the incoming stimuli, a given neuron takes one of two possible output states: 0 or 1. In addition, a refractory period of one time step is assumed:

$$\mathcal{H}(x) = \begin{cases} 0 & \text{if } x \leq 0 \\ 1 & \text{if } x > 0 \end{cases}$$

$$n_i(t+1) = \mathcal{H}\left(\sum_j \mathbf{T}_{ij} n_j(t) - \Theta\right) \underbrace{* \mathcal{H}(1 - n_i(t))}_{\text{refraction}},$$

where $n_i(t)$ denotes the activity of the i-th neuron at time step t, $\mathbf{T}$ denotes the recurrent connection matrix and Θ a common activity threshold. For the connection matrix $\mathbf{T}$ we assume that every neuron receives excitatory links from s random neurons of the same minicolumn. We set connection strength to

$$\mathbf{T}_{ij} = \begin{cases} 0 & \text{if not connected} \\ c & \text{if connected.} \end{cases}$$

Note that we allow for self excitatory links $T_{ii} = c$. For every c we can choose a Θ, so that the dynamics of the minicolumn does not change. Without loss of generality we can therefore choose $c = \frac{1}{s}$. We set the inhibition Θ to be a linear function of the average activity within the minicolumn:

$$\Theta(t) = \nu(t) \frac{1}{m} \sum_{i=1}^{m} n_i(t) + \Theta_0 + \mathcal{N}(0, \sigma_{noise}) \qquad \text{with} \qquad \Theta_0 = \frac{1}{s}$$

Here v is a time-dependent control parameter introduced in the next section. For the purpose of this model, we are primarily interested in the statistical properties of a minicolumn. To avoid repeating neural activity patterns, which are a direct consequence of the fixed recurrent connection matrix $\mathbf{T}$, we include sufficiently strong Gaussian threshold noise N(0, σ_{noise}) (e.g. $\sigma^2_{noise} = 0.1$). Another strategy to avoid these coherence effects would be to re-randomize the recurrent connection matrix $\mathbf{T}$ every timestep. Within this model, the state of the minicolumn is encoded by the activity vector of all the neurons $\vec{n}(t)$. Alternatively, we can express the state of the column by a single probabilistic scalar variable

$p(t)$, which can be interpreted as either the firing probability of a single neuron inside the minicolumn or as the mean activity within the minicolumn $p(t) = \frac{1}{m}\sum n_i(t)$. Without presenting the details of the stability analysis (Lücke & von Der Malsburg, 2004) we mention that the dynamical system described so far is bistable: If the average activity inside the minicolumn drops below a certain critical value, it will quickly drop to the inactive stable stationary point $p^- = 0$. Once the activity is above the critical value, it grows towards the ν-dependent active stable point $p^+ = \mathrm{P}_\nu$.

Neural Dynamics of a Macrocolumn

After having described the dynamics of a single minicolumn we now turn to macrocolumns. We define a macrocolumn to be a set of k minicolumns that interact via a common inhibition. A macrocolumn with k minicolumns can be written as a system of $k*m$ difference equations:

$$n_i^\alpha(t+1) = \mathcal{H}\left(\sum_j \mathbf{T}_{ij}^\alpha n_j^\alpha(t) - \Theta\right) * \mathcal{H}(1 - n_i^\alpha(t)) \qquad \text{with } 1 \leq \alpha \leq k$$

There are various ways to define the common inhibition Θ, but it has been demonstrated (Lücke & von Der Malsburg, 2004), that the system behaves favorably when the inhibition is defined to be proportional to the activity of the most active minicolum:

$$\Theta(t) = \nu \max_{\alpha=1,..,k}\{p_\alpha(t)\}.$$

Again we describe the macroscopic behaviour of this systems without going into the details of the stability analysis. Depending on the scalar parameter ν the system presented so far has a variable number of stable, stationary points. A detailed stability analysis shows, that there is a critical bifucation point ν_c:

- For $\nu < \nu_c$: Every minicolumn can be, independent of all other minicolumns, in one of two stationary stable points: $p_\alpha = 0$ or $p_\alpha = \mathrm{P}_\nu$. If we take the state of a macrocolumn to be defined as the vector of the states of its minicolumns, a macrocolumn can be in one of the 2^k possible stable states $\{0, \mathrm{P}_\nu\}^k$.
- For $\nu > \nu_c$: All stationary points with more than one active minicolumn loose their stability. The stable stationary points of the macrocolumn are now those $k + 1$ states with exactly one or no minicolumn active.

If the minicolumns inside a macrocolumn are initialized to be active at $t = 0$ and $\nu(t)$ is gradually increased from $\nu_{min} < \nu_c$ to $\nu_{max} > \nu_c$, it can be observerd that all minicolumns stay active until the bifurcation point ν_c is reached. Starting at $\nu(t) = \nu_c$ one minicolumn after the other deactivates until one single randomly choosen minicolumn remains active. We call this the "winning" minicolumn. In our experiments we set $\nu(t) = \nu_{reset} = 0.1$ for the period of two time steps to make sure that all minicolumns are activated. We then linearly increase $\nu(t)$ from $\nu_{min} = 0.4$ to $\nu_{max} = 1.1$ in 23 time steps. We call such a sequence of 25 time steps a ν-cycle. See Figure 1 for a graphical presentation of the macrocolumn dynamics. The critical value ν_c can be determined numerically and has been found to be $\nu_c \approx 0.69$ for $m = 100$, $s = 15$ and $\Theta_0 = \frac{1}{s}$.

Adding a Receptive Field

Close to the bifurcation point ν_c, the described system reacts very sensitively to external perturbations. A minor additional excitation of one minicolumn will give this minicolumn a significantly higher probability of winning the turn-off sequence. We exploit this behavior and use a macrocolumn as a decision unit. Let $n_j^E \in \{0,1\}$ with $1 \leq j \leq N$ be an additional set of binary neu-

Figure 1. Dynamic of a macrocolumn with 3 minicolumns over a period of 6 v-cycles (m = 100, s = 15)

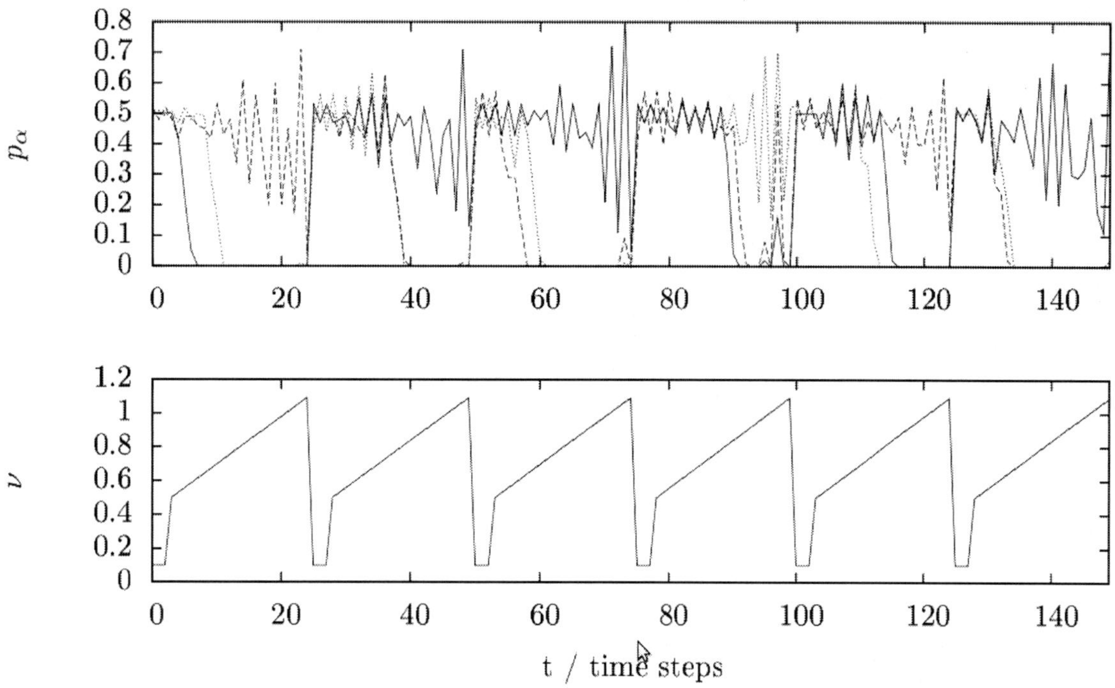

rons. These neurons represent some external input stimulus $\vec{I}$ with $1 \leq j \leq N$. For every time step, the probability of a given neuron $0 \leq I_j \leq 1$ being active is given by the corresponding input vector element:

$$P(n_j^E(t) = 1) = \frac{I_j(t)}{2}.$$

To connect the input layer neurons $\vec{n}^E$ with the macrocolumn, we add r incoming connections to every neuron n_i^α. In the beginning, these connections originate from random neurons of the receptive field. The afferent connection matrix representing these connections is named **R**:

$$n_i^\alpha(t+1) = \mathcal{H}\left(\sum_{j=1}^{m} \mathbf{T}_{ij}^\alpha n_j^\alpha(t) + \sum_{j=1}^{N} \mathbf{R}_{ij}^\alpha n_j^E(t) - \Theta\right) * \mathcal{H}(1 - n_i^\alpha(t))$$

See Figure 2 (a) for a sketch of the system. Instead of operating on individual matrices $\mathbf{T}^\alpha$ and $\mathbf{R}^\alpha$, we can consolidate these matrices into a single connectivity matrix **M** for the whole system. This aggregate matrix has $k*m$ rows and $k*m+r$ columns. A typical example of such an aggregate connection matrix is pictured in Figure 2 (b).

We now proceed by introducing learning into the system. Learning is implemented by adding Hebbian plasticity to the links between the receptive field neurons $\vec{n}^E$ and the neurons of all the minicolumns:

$\forall \alpha \in \{1..k\}, i \in \{1..m\}, j \in \{1..N\}$: If $A(t) < \chi$ and $n_i^\alpha(t) = n_j^E(t-1) = 1$ and $\mathbf{R}_{ij}^\alpha = 0$, with a probability of ò a random element $\mathbf{R}_{il}^\alpha = c$ ($l \neq j$) is set to zero and $\mathbf{R}_{ij}^\alpha$ is set to c.

Here $A(t)$ is the average activity within the macrocolumn: $A(t) = \frac{1}{k}\sum_\alpha p^\alpha(t)$. In the beginning of the v-cycle, when all minicolumns are

Figure 2. Connection structure in the model of the cortical macrocolumn. (a) Sketch of a k = 3, m = 8, s = 3, r = 2 system. Connections between the second and third minicolumn to the receptive field have been omitted for visual reasons. (b) Typical connection matrix for a k = 5, m = 100, s = 15 and r = 7 system. The block diagonal part of the matrix represents the recurrent connections; the section on the right incoming afferent connections from the receptive field

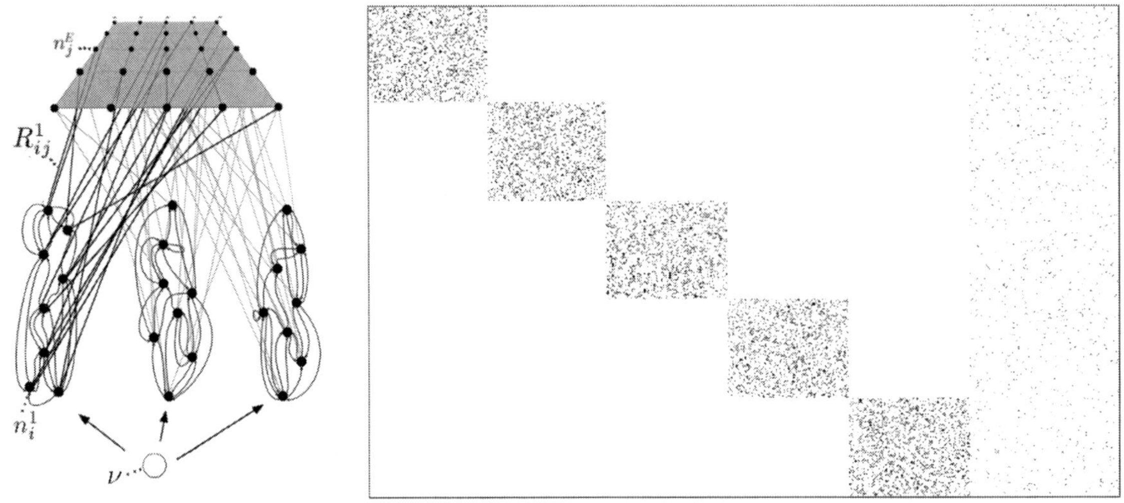

(a) (b)

active, the average activity $A(t)$ is larger than the learning threshold χ and no learning takes place. Later in the ν-cycle, when most minicolumns are inactive and only minicolumns whose receptive fields most closely matches the incoming stimulus are active, the average activity drops below χ and Hebbian learning further specializes the receptive field of the still active minicolumns. As a result the matrices R^{α} are reshaped according to the input patterns.

A typical training session consists of some hundred up to some thousand ν-cycles. In every ν-cycle, a different training pattern is presented to the system, which continuously adapts its receptive fields. Typically the receptive fields specialize for various classes into which the presented patterns can be clustered.

The parameters χ and ò can be used to fine-tune the learning characteristics. The parameter ò plays a role analogous to the learning rate in other machine learning algorithms. Threshold χ can be used to adjust the differentiation pressure between the receptive fields. In all of our experiments we set $\chi = 0.55$ and ò = 0.03.

Feature Extraction Problem: The Bars Test

Besides classification, the system can also be used for feature extraction. If, for instance, we have a system of k macrocolumns and present not only $\nu \leq k$ different basis patterns, but also all possible 2^{ν} superpositions (with $k < 2^{\nu}$) of these, the system is not able to store all combinations into specialized receptive fields. Instead, macrocolumns tend to learn the ν individual basis patterns. A standard problem of this kind is the bars test that was introduced by Földiak in (Földiak, 1990). The training patterns of the bars test consist of horizontal and vertical bars. A set of typical input patterns is shown in Figure 3 (a). In this case the set of basis patterns consist of four horizontal and

Figure 3. Bars test: (a) 20 example input patterns; (b) Afferent part of the connection matrix **M** *after 0, 250, 500 und 1000 v-cycles*

(a)

(b)

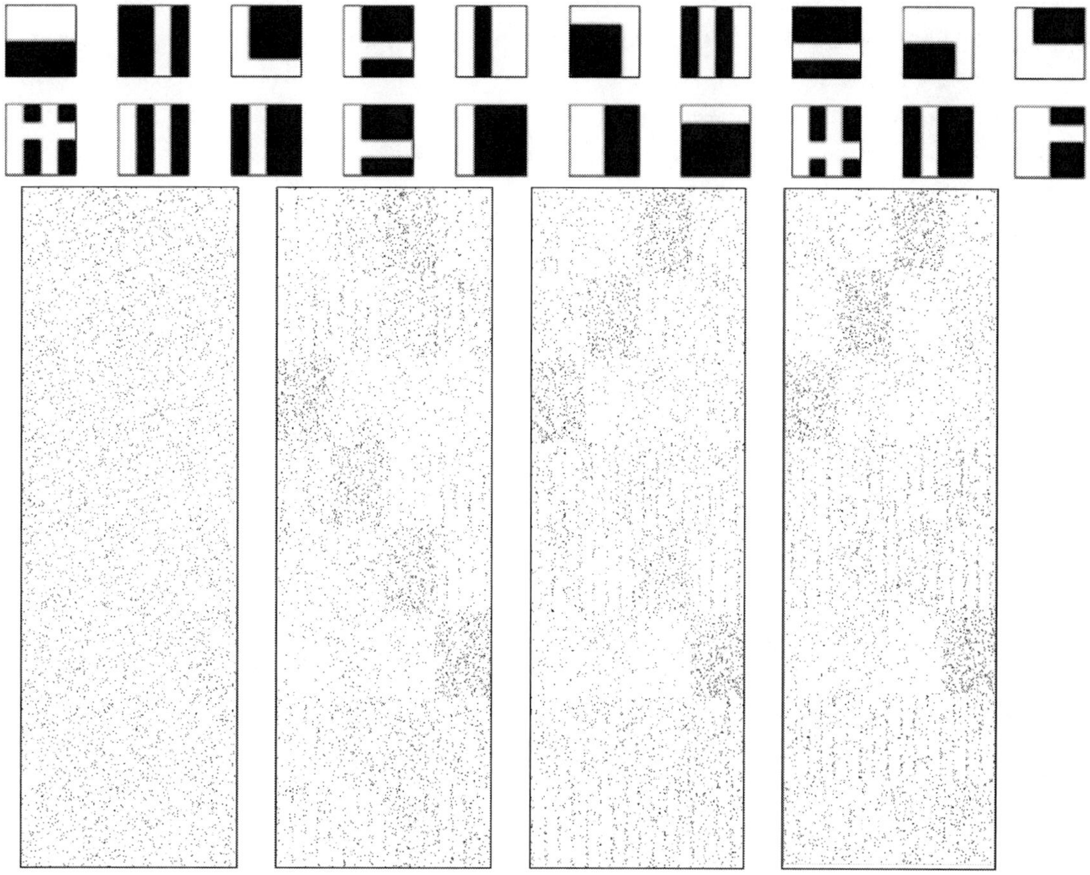

four vertical basis patterns ($v = 8$). Note that the superposition of a horizontal and a vertical white bar does not add up linearly, but overlapping white pixels result in a white pixel again.

We operate the system with the same set of parameters as we used in the clustering task. If $k > v$, the receptive fields of some minicolumns remain uncommitted, specialize for a bar already represented by another minicolum or specialize for a combination of two or more bars.

The original work (Lücke & von Der Malsburg, 2004) contains an in-depth discussion about the learning capabilities and properties of the system described here.

Larger System Containing Multiple Macrocolumns

Macrocolumns can be used as basic building block to construct larger systems, potentially containing many thousands of macrocolumns (Wolfrum, Wolff, Lücke, & von der Malsburg, 2008), (Jitsev & von der Malsburg, 2009), (Sato, Wolff, Wolfrum, & von der Malsburg, 2007). One instance of such a system demonstrated how to implement translation invariant pattern recognition in images using macrocolumns as decision units (Lücke, Keck, & von der Malsburg, 2008). The basic idea behind this correspondence finding system is, that at various points in the input image layer macrocolumns are placed. Each macrocolumn in the image domain has various minicolumns, each representing another potential correspondence match with a point in the model layer, where objects to be found are stored. Over the period of a system-wide *v*-cycle, every macrocolumn in the image domain decides for a single best correspondence match with a point in the model domain. As input to this decision process not only the similarity of the input image to various points in the model domain are taken into account, but also the current state of neighboring macrocolumns. Only minicolumns representing correspondence matches which are consistent with neighboring correspondence matches support each other: In terms of connection matrices this means, that the receptive field of one particular macrocolumn in the image domain consist of (a) a similarity measurement between the image domain and the various points in the model domain and (b) the current activity state of neighboring minicolumns. Note that for larger systems like this, in order to converge properly, the *v*-cycle has to be decelerated and more than 25 time steps have to be performed.

Again, analogously to the step where we joined the recurrent connection matrices $\mathbf{T}^{\alpha}$ and $\mathbf{R}^{\alpha}$ into an aggregate matrix **M** for a whole macrocolumn, we can join all matrices of all macrocolumns into one large aggregate matrix for the whole correspondence finding system. The size of such a aggregate matrix easily reaches the order of more than 10^5 rows with more than 10^6 non-zero elements.

Parallelism

In order to decide on what level to parallelize a concrete simulation algorithm, we consider the multiplicity of the nested loops:

For each *v*-cycle ($\geq$ 1000)
For each time step ($\geq$ 25)
For each neuron ($\geq$ 10000)
For each synapse ($\geq$ 10)

Given this structure it seems most promising to exploit parallelism at the neuron level. Not only has the neuron level the highest multiplicity, it also has low communication requirements. To update the state $n_i(t)$ of a given neuron to $n_i(t+1)$, only a single row of the matrix **M** and the activity vector $\vec{a}$ have to be accessed.

Sparse Matrix Vector Multiplication

The dominant operation for simulating the model of a cortical macrocolumn is the matrix-vector multiplication. Although the matrix is relatively large, every row has only $s + r$ non-zero matrix elements. Sparse matrices can be observed in various neural network models.

In contrast to storing the dense matrix, with most elements equal to zero, it is usually much more efficient to store, in conjunction with some index information, only the N_{nz} matrix elements that are non-zero. The optimal in-memory data representation first and foremost depends on the operation the matrix is primarily involved in. But even if we assume that the sparse matrix vector multiplication (SpMxV) is the predominant operation, the optimal storage format still depends on the spatial arrangement of the non-zero elements within the matrix and on the details of the processor architecture running the simulation.

Compressed Row Format

A basic data structure that is widely used especially in the context of SpMxV is the Compressed Row Storage format (CRS). Using this format, a sparse matrix is stored in three arrays: (1) a **val** array, that contains the values of all non zero elements starting in the upper left corner of the matrix; (2) a **colidx** array having the same number of entries as the **val** array, storing for every non-zero element the column-index and (3) a **rowptr** array storing for every row of the matrix a position in **val** and **colidx** where elements for this row can be found. To illustrate the CRS format we show the in-memory representation of a matrix $\mathbf{M}$ ($N_{nz}=7$):

$$\mathbf{M} = \begin{pmatrix} 11 & 12 & 0 & 0 \\ 21 & 0 & 23 & 0 \\ 0 & 0 & 33 & 34 \\ 0 & 0 & 0 & 44 \end{pmatrix}$$

Compressed Row Storage representation: (see Table 1 and Table 2)

A naive implementation of the SpMxV operation $\vec{y} = \mathbf{M}\vec{x}$ on a matrix stored in the CRS format looks like:

```
for i = 1 .. n:
    y(i) = 0
    for j = rowptr(i) ..
rowptr(i+1)-1
        y(i) = y(i) + val(j) *
x(colidx(j))
```

n denotes the number of rows in the matrix. SpMxV is a kernel of low computational density: for every non-zero element only a single multiplication and a single addition need to be performed.

Software Optimizations for SpMxV

Being of low computational density means that a software implementation on a modern superscalar[1] processor should be bound by the available memory bandwidth. But SpMxV is notorious for not reaching that level of performance. The reason why it is hard to come up with a generic, efficient implementation is the indirection via the field **colidx**. This indirection causes irregular memory access patterns to the source vector $\vec{x}$ with only limited spatial and temporal locality[2]. Missing memory access locality causes a low hit ratio in the CPUs cache subsystem and, in turn, causes the arithmetic units to often stall for the memory to deliver data. This situation gets worse as the gap between raw CPU performance and memory

Table 1.

val	11	12	21	23	33	34	44
colidx	1	2	1	3	3	4	4

Table 2.

rowptr	0	2	4	6

latency/bandwidth increases. The literature essentially describes four strategies to mitigate this problem:

- Prefetching, also known as software pipelining: Access to some needed vector element x_i can be issued one or multiple iterations before it is processed. In this way a superscalar CPU triggers a memory-load for some element x_i while at the same time executing the computation for some other element that has been fetched some iterations before (Wulf & McKee, 1995).
- Register blocking: Instead of storing individual non-zero elements in the **val** array, small fixed sized $r \times c$ dense matrices can be stored. As a result, the indirection via the **colidx**(i) array is done only once per block. This technique also allows for better register reuse: loaded elements from $\vec{x}$ are used r times for multiple rows. As an additional benefit, the operations on the dense matrix-blocks can make use of the SIMD (Single Instruction, Multiple Data) units present in modern processors. Note that this optimization only works if there is a sufficient probability for multiple non-zero elements per $r \times c$ block. Optimal block sizes strongly depend on the structure of the matrix and on the details of the proces-

sor architecture. Typical optimal block sizes are in the range from 2×4 to 4×8. The register-blocked version of the CRS storage format is called *Block Compressed Row Storage* (BCRS), (Geus & Röllin, 1999), (Vuduc et al., 2002).
- Cache blocking: The strategy behind cache blocking is to introduce temporal locality into the $\vec{x}$ element fetches by subdividing the sparse matrix into smaller sparse matrices of size $\tilde{r} \times \tilde{c}$. $\tilde{c}$ is chosen so that the fetches of $\vec{x}$ for a given sub-matrix are completely covered by the CPU cache (Im, Yelick, & Vuduc, 2004).
- Re-ordering: Re-ordering also aims at enhancing the temporal and spatial locality for $\vec{x}$ element lookups. Either by re-ordering rows and columns to create a more block-like structured matrix, or by re-ordering to a more band-matrix like structure (Pinar & Heath, 1999) (Catalyurek & Aykanat, 1999) (Temam & Jalby, 1992) (Vastenhouw & Bisseling, 2005).

Since many of these approaches depend on the structure of the matrix and on the details of the processor architecture, runtime optimization and auto-tuning techniques are commonly employed (Im, Yelick, & Vuduc, 2004) (Vuduc, Demmel, & Yelick, 2005). As a result of these efforts, a single thread of a Core 2 Duo processor for example typically processes between 50 and 300 M matrix elements per second, less than 30% of the theoretical peak performance.

Parallelized SpMxV on Multicore Architectures

Recently a detailed study on the SpMxV performance achievable on multicore systems has been presented (Williams et al., 2009). Although the authors point out that the per core performance sustains only a small fraction of the cores peak performance, the aggregate performance reaches the regime where the system is constrained by the available memory bandwidth. They mention that software optimizations that aim at bandwidth reduction might play an important role in the future. Their results also indicate that it is reasonable to deploy a higher number of "light-weight" in-order cores in order to saturate the available memory bandwidth—even at the cost of single core performance.

SpMxV on GPUs

GPUs typically consist of many parallelized SIMD execution units that provide a high theoretical peak performance. NVidia GT200 based GPUs like the GTX 280 for example provide nearly 1 TFlop/s single precision peak performance compared to about 0.1 TFlop/s peak performance for a Intel quad core Xeon 5400 generation CPU. GPUs also typically provide up to a factor 10 more memory bandwidth than general purpose CPUs. Recently there have been a number of publications on the implementation of SpMxV on GPUs (Bell & Garland, 2008) (Vazquez, Garzon, Martinez, & Fernandez, 2009) (Baskaran & Bordawekar, 2009). These implementations demonstrate an impressive performance of up to 10G matrix elements per second on a GeForce GTX 280 GPU. On the other hand these implementations again only reach a fraction of the theoretical peak performance which is, for the GTX 280 GPU, close to 1 TFlop/s.

Compressed Incremental Row Storage

In the attempt to find an optimal storage format for sparse matrices as they typically occur in simulations of macrocolumn systems, we aimed for two goals: Memory efficiency and streaming friendliness. Memory efficiency is important, because not only CPU-based architectures suffer from limited off-chip memory bandwidth and high latencies, but also FPGA architectures with external memory have to take this bottleneck into account. By looking at the matrices occurring in macrocolumn simulations, we identify two important characteristics:

1. The matrix elements are binary only: either two neurons are connected or they are not. As a result, the **val** array can be ignored without loss of information.
2. The matrices have a strong block-like structure. Non-zero matrix elements tend to be relatively close to each other. Close to the main diagonal, for example, $s*m$ non-zero matrix elements are populating $m \times m$ blocks.

The first observation allows the matrix to be represented by a single data-stream of column-indexes and *EndOfRow* control words. This allows for a compact implementation of a SpMxV streaming processor, as it will be presented later. The second observation allows us to deploy a simple but effective compression scheme. Instead of storing absolute column-indices, we transform the column-indexes into an array of incremental column-indices:

$$\text{incidx(l)}=\begin{cases}\text{colidx(l)} & \text{if colidx(l) first element in a row}\\ \text{colidx(l)-colidx(l-1)} & \text{else}\end{cases}$$

This format is similar to a format suggested by Bisseling (2004). From our point of view, this transformation not only allows to represent the matrix as a single stream of data, but also changes the distribution of values occurring in incidx. Because of the block-like structure, small increment values occur more often than large ones. This allows us to apply variable-length coding to the incremental-index vector: Similar to a general entropy coding, we encode elements that occur frequently in the incidx vector with short codewords, and rare elements with longer codewords. While a matrix-dependent optimal encoding can be constructed with the Huffman compression algorithm, we chose a static variable-length code.

The benefits of this static code are: (a) a small and efficient decoder can be build for the FPGA, (b) encoding matrix elements on a general purpose CPU is trivial and (c) the simple compression scheme shows reasonable good results. We identified the (2,4,8,16,24), (3,6,12,24) and (4,8,16,24)-codes to deliver the best compression results:

- (2,4,8,16,24)-coding

$$\begin{aligned}1 \le e \le 2, &\mapsto (0x)_2\\ 3 \le e \le 6, &\mapsto (10xx)_2\\ 7 \le e \le 38, &\mapsto (110xxxxx)_2\\ 39 \le e \le 4134, &\mapsto (1110xxxxxxxxxxxx)_2\\ 4135 \le e \le 528422, &\mapsto (11110xxxxxxxxxxxxxxxxxxx)_2\\ \text{control codes}\ , &\mapsto (111110xx)_2\end{aligned}$$

- (3,6,12,24)-coding

$$\begin{aligned}1 \le e \le 4, &\mapsto (0xx)_2\\ 5 \le e \le 20, &\mapsto (10xxxx)_2\\ 21 \le e \le 532, &\mapsto (110xxxxxxxxx)_2\\ 533 \le e \le 1049108, &\mapsto (1110xxxxxxxxxxxxxxxxxxxx)_2\\ \text{control codes}\ , &\mapsto (11110xx)_2\end{aligned}$$

- (4,8,16,24)-coding

$$\begin{aligned}1 \le e \le 8, &\mapsto (0xxx)_2\\ 9 \le e \le 72, &\mapsto (10xxxxxx)_2\\ 73 \le e \le 8265, &\mapsto (110xxxxxxxxxxxxx)_2\\ 8266 \le e \le 1056840, &\mapsto (1110xxxxxxxxxxxxxxxxxxxx)_2\\ \text{control codes}\ , &\mapsto (11110xx)_2\end{aligned}$$

where e is an element from the incidx-array. Beside *EndOfRow*, the control codes include symbols for *EndOfMinocolum*, *EndOfMacrocolumn* and *EndOfMatrix*. We call this format *Compressed Incremental Row Storage* (CIRS).

CIRS Applied to Connection Matrices

We applied the compression scheme to connection matrices as they typically occur in systems of cortical macrocolumns. The average storage requirements per non-zero element vary slightly depending on m, s and r and depending on the size and the structure of the receptive field. As-

Table 3.

Coding	Bits per non-zero element
(2,4,8,16,24)-coding	8.6
(3,6,12,24)-coding	7.3
(4,8,16,24)-coding	8.2

Table 4.

Coding	Median	Mean
(2,4,8,16,24)-coding	6.9	6.8 +/- 3.0
(3,6,8,12,24)-coding	6.6	6.7 +/- 2.3
(4,8,16,24)-coding	7.2	7.6 +/- 3.2

suming a macrocolumn with $k = 5$ minicolumns, our standard parameter-set $m = 100$, $s = 15$, $r = 7$ and a randomly structured receptive field of $N = 1000$ neurons, the storage requirements are: (see Table 3)

Figure 4 shows the development of the compression rate while a macrocolumn with $k = 8$ minicolumns is trained with bars patterns on 16×16 pixel sized input images ($N = 256$). In the beginning the system starts with a randomly structured receptive field. Over the course of some hundred v-cycles, the afferent part of the matrix gains structure (compare to Figure 3. (b)) and the storage requirements decrease. Note that the fact that the storage requirements do not decrease further after about 600 v-cycles, does not indicate that the training phase can be finished. Although not evident in the average storage size per non-zero element, the receptive fields still specialize further until about 2000 v-cycles.

CIRS Applied to Harwell-Boeing Matrices

Although the matrix compression scheme is tailored to connection matrices, it can also be applied to binary matrices originating from other disciplines. The Harwell-Boeing matrix collection (Duff, Grimes, & Lewis, 1992) provides a representative set of sparse matrices. We applied the compression schemes to all binary Harwell-Boeing matrices with more than 10^4 non-zero elements. 16 Harwell-Boeing matrices meet these conditions. Averaged over these 16 matrices, we measured the following storage requirements per non-zero element. (see Table 4)

Because of its generally good compression rate for the matrices that need to be processed, we chose the (3,6,12,24)-code for our coprocessor implementation.

FPGA COPROCESSOR ARCHITECTURE

We now describe the architecture of a coprocessor which has been designed to efficiently simulate neural systems similar to the one introduced earlier. Although our implementation simulates the relatively simple McCulloch-Pitts neurons, the architecture can be easily extended to simulate more elaborate neuron models.

Overall Structure

The logical structure of the parallel coprocessor is shown in Figure 5. The main components are:

- A set of streaming processors. Each streaming processors reads a continuous stream of neural-state vector elements and connection matrix elements from the external DRAM. It writes back a continuous stream of updated neural state elements.
- A crossbar switch which connects the streaming processors with a set of fast on-chip memory blocks. These are used to store the neural activity vector $\vec{a}(t)$.
- A 32-bit RISC CPU as control unit (Lattice Micro 32 (Lattice Semiconductor Corporation, 2007)). This component is responsible for general system orchestra-

Figure 4. Average storage size per non-zero element while training the bars pattern

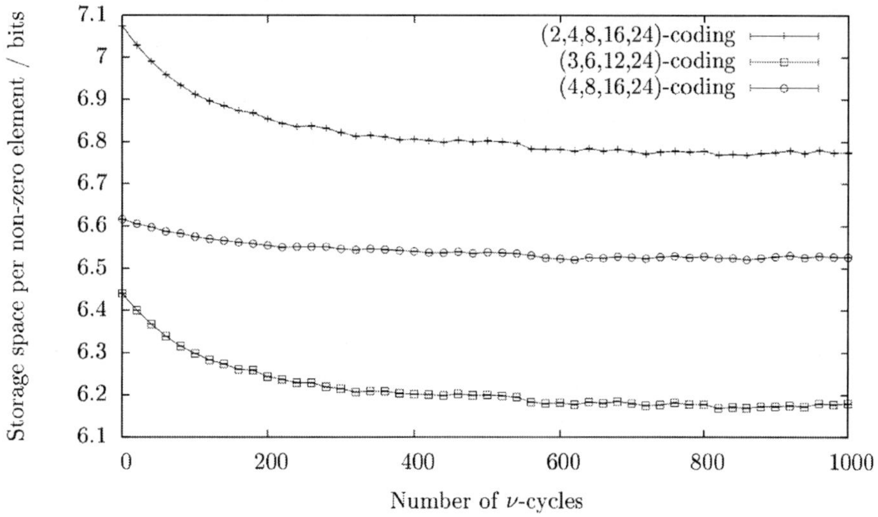

Figure 5. Overall structure of the coprocessor. ARAM refers to the activity memory blocks used to store elements of the neural activity vector $\vec{a}$

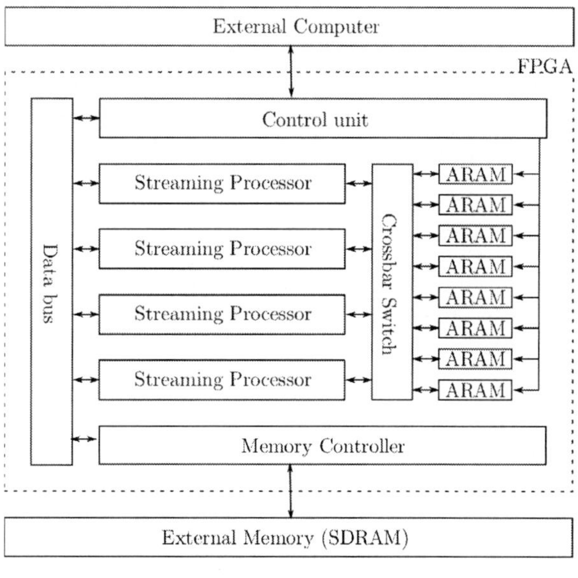

tion and handles the input/output with the external computer.

- An on-chip Wishbone bus (Peterson, 2002) to connect the control unit and the streaming processors to the memory controller.
- A memory controller optimized for maximal bandwidth to the external DRAM. The memory controller does not contain caches to speed up access to previously accessed memory locations.

We quantify the number of streaming processors with N_{PE}, the number of activity memory blocks with N_{ARAM} and the size of each activity memory block with S_{ARAM}. Note that S_{ARAM} is the number of activity vector elements a single memory block can store. For many neuron models, like McCulloch-Pitts, a single bit is sufficient to store the activity of a neuron. In this case S_{ARAM} is actually measured in bits.

The Streaming Processors

The actual computation is carried out by the streaming processors. Each streaming processor calculates a disjoint segment of the resulting vector $\vec{n}(t+1)$. It reads two data streams: The segment of the neural state vector $\vec{n}(t)$ and the relevant rows from the connection matrix **M**. It writes out a single data-stream, the updated segment of the neural state vector $\vec{n}(t+1)$. It is an important characteristic of these streaming processors that they never participate in random memory access to the external DRAM.

The design of the streaming processors is shown in Figure 6. Each streaming processor is fully pipelined and consists of two data paths: The first data path reads elements from the neural-state vector $\vec{n}(t)$ and updates them according to the rules implemented in the Neural-Finite-State-Machine (*NFSM*). Once all incoming stimuli for a neuron have been processed, the updated neuron state is written back to the external memory. The second data path reads compressed matrix elements from the external memory, decompresses them, fetches the activity $\vec{a}(t)$ via the crossbar switch from the on-chip memory blocks and finally feeds the resulting value into the *NFSM*. When simulating the model described in section 2, every neural state element loaded into the NFSM will receive $s+r$ matrix elements. An *EndOfRow* control word, which is part of the matrix element stream, indicates that there are no more stimuli to the currently loaded neural state element and that it can be written back to memory.

Every streaming processor contains three DMA[3] engines: Neural State Load (*NSL*), Matrix Element Load (*MEL*) and Neural State Store (*NSS*). Each DMA engine has its own independent address count register which always points to the next address to be loaded from external memory (or stored to, in case of the *NSS*). The DMA engines stop loading new data once the address counter equals a stop-address register, which is also configurable per DMA engine. In addition, each DMA engine contains its own FIFO buffer. The optimal size of these buffers depends on the number of streaming processors competing for external memory access and the number of bytes transferred in a single memory access burst. In our implementation, a FIFO buffer size of 64 bytes was sufficient to provide a close-to-continuous data stream.

Figure 6. Structure of a streaming processor: Neural-State-Load (NSL), Matrix-Element-Load (MEL), Neural-State-Save (NSS), Decompress (DC), Activity Lookup (AL) and Neural-Finite-State-Machine (NFSM)

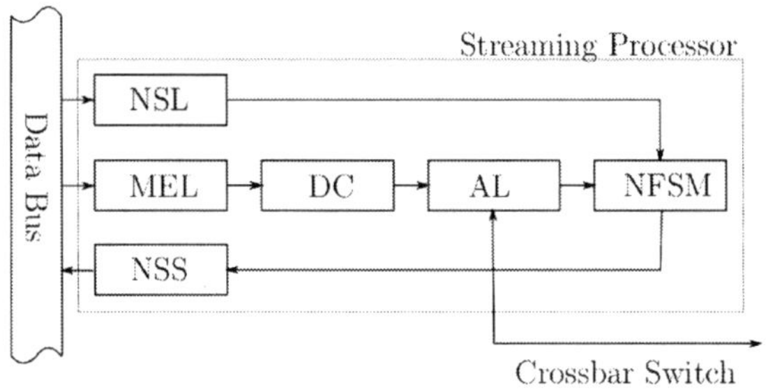

Crossbar Switch and On-Chip Memory

Critical to the streaming processor's performance is the activity lookup stage. In our implementation, we use N_{ARAM} on-chip memory blocks to store the activity vector. This design was chosen because fast on-chip memory is a scarce resource. We opted for a full cross-bar switch that connects the N_{PE} streaming processors with the N_{ARAM} memory blocks. The crossbar implementation closely follows the design of a Diagonal Propagation Arbiter with rotating priority (Hurt, May, Zhu, & Lin, 1999) and scales in terms of hardware resources $\mathcal{O}(N_{PE} * N_{ARAM})$.

In principle, the architecture allows every streaming processor to process one matrix element per clock cycle. But there are various reasons why a streaming processor might stall: The Neural State Load, the Matrix Element Load and the Neural State Save units access the external memory with short high bandwidth bursts. As long as there is sufficient average external memory bandwidth available, sufficient large FIFO buffers inside the DMA engines can hide these discontinuities. As mentioned earlier, in our case a FIFO buffer size of 64 byte is enough to provide a nearly uninterrupted data stream to the *NFSM*. Another important source of processor stalls is the activity lookup stage. Although the crossbar switch allows N_{PE} simultaneous requests to different memory blocks to be processed at the same time, wait-cycles will be introduced when multiple streaming processors access the same memory block. Assuming the activity elements looked up by the different streaming processors are uniformly distributed and independent from each other, the probability of at least one collision is given by the birthday paradox:

$$P_{coll} = 1 - \frac{N_{ARAM}!}{(N_{ARAM} - N_{PE})! \quad (N_{ARAM})^{N_{PE}}}$$

The collision probability is independent of the size of the individual memory blocks—each memory block stores a fraction $\frac{1}{N_{ARAM}}$ of the available activity elements. Unfortunately, when simulating macrocolumns, the access to the activity elements is not uniformly distributed and independent of each other. As a result, the probability of collision rises, causing processor stalls in the activity lookup stage and in effect decreasing the average processor performance.

We deploy the well known technique of interleaving to mitigate this effect: Instead of using the $log_2(S_{ARAM})$ lowest bits of the activity vectors element index to address within a memory block and the $log_2(N_{ARAM})$ highest bits to choose the memory block, we use the $log_2(S_{ARAM})$ highest bits to choose the memory block and the $log_2(N_{ARAM})$ lowest bits to address within a memory block. As a result, neighboring activity elements are stored in different memory blocks. Our measurements have shown that this simple change is enough to lower the observed collision rate to a value that is undistinguishable from the theoretical optimum given by the birthday paradox.

Arbitrary Network Sizes

Our implementation assumes that the complete activity vector can be loaded into the on-chip activity memory blocks ($N_{ARAM} * S_{ARAM} \geq k * (m + r)$). If this assumption does not hold, a relatively simple change to the implementation allows for arbitrary network sizes. These changes are analogous to the cache-blocking strategy used in software SpMxV implementations: The matrix **M** would be partitioned into smaller sparse sub-matrices, where each sub-matrix would span $\tilde{r} \times \tilde{c}$ elements, where $\tilde{c}$ needs to be chosen so that $\tilde{c} \leq N_{ARAM} * S_{ARAM}$. A side-effect of this multi-pass time step is that even for McCulloch-Pitts neurons the size of the neural state vector elements need to be enlarged: Instead of only storing the 1 bit activity state, each neural state element would store the (partial) excitation received so far. Note that this number can be clamped to Θ since once a neuron has received sufficient excitation to fire, additional excitation does not cause further state changes. Assuming our usual parameter $s = 15$, $r = 7$ this would require 4 bits of neural state per neuron ($\approx log_2(r + s)$).

Firmware and I/O with an External Computer

The various activities inside the coprocessor and especially the registers inside DMA engines are controlled by software running on the control CPU inside the FPGA. This firmware also handles memory management for the external DRAM connected to the FPGA. It provides the following slim set of operations that can be triggered by an external computer:

- *Upload*: Transfer either a compressed connection matrix **M** or a neuron state vector $\vec{n}$ from the computer to the coprocessor's external memory. The external computer has to ensure that the data is in the correct format to be later directly processed by the streaming processors. The firmware running on the FPGA allocates memory for this dataset and returns a device memory handle to the external computer for later usage. In general, device memory handles are used to refer to datasets uploaded or generated.
- *Download*: Given a device memory handle, the dataset referred to is transmitted to the external computer.
- *Delete*: Given a device memory handle, the dataset referred to is deleted and the memory freed.
- *LoadActivity*: This command takes a device memory handle of a neuron state vector $\vec{n}$. The elements of this vector are loaded into the on-chip activity memory. For McCulloch-Pitts neurons the neural state vector elements n_i, and the activity vector elements are exactly the same: Both contain 1 bit elements. For other, potentially more elaborate neuron models a more complicated translation function will have to be implemented. Since this function is a simple element-wise operation we don't expect a performance problem.

Table 5.

Component	Logic Resources / Slices	Percent
Wishbone Bus	216	5.1%
DDR Memory Controller	386	9.1%
ControlUnit (32 bit CPU)	1142	26.8%
CPU Periphery	245	5.8%
Activity Crossbar Switch	247	5.8%
4 Streaming Processors	2016	47.4%
Total	4253	100%

- *Step*: This command triggers the execution of a simulation step. The external computer has to provide three arguments: A device memory handle to a neural state vector $\vec{n}(t)$, a handle to a connection matrix **M** and the scalar parameter v. The firmware splits the datasets into N_{PE} equal sized strips and configures the DMA engines of the streaming processors accordingly. When the command finishes, it returns a device memory handle to a newly allocated neural state vector $\vec{n}(t+1)$.
- *ReadRegs*: This command reads the debug registers and sends their content to the external computer. Debug registers are used to count various events. For example the number of clock cycles needed to execute a simulation step, the number of collisions while accessing an activity memory block or the number of buffer-underruns inside the DMA engines that caused pipeline stalls.

Benchmarks and Scalability

We have implemented the architecture using the Verilog hardware description language. The same source code was used to (a) synthesize a running implementation for an FPGA prototyping board and (b) to run various simulations on how the architecture would scale when synthesized

Box 1.

$$throughput(N_{PE}) \approx \begin{cases} 0,53 * N_{PE} \text{ matrix elements per clock cycle} & \text{for } N_{ARAM} = 1 * N_{PE} \\ 0,68 * N_{PE} \text{ matrix elements per clock cycle} & \text{for } N_{ARAM} = 2 * N_{PE} \\ 0,76 * N_{PE} \text{ matrix elements per clock cycle} & \text{for } N_{ARAM} = 3 * N_{PE} \\ 0,81 * N_{PE} \text{ matrix elements per clock cycle} & \text{for } N_{ARAM} = 4 * N_{PE} \end{cases}$$

for larger FPGA platforms with more memory bandwidth available.

Running on a Spartan 3E-500 FPGA

We implemented a small scale version of the architecture on a Spartan-3E 500 FPGA evaluation board. This board features a Xilinx XC3S500E FPGA (Xilinx Inc., 2007) which provides 4656 slices logic capacity[4] and includes 20 on-chip memory blocks each providing 18 kbit storage. The evaluation board also features a 512 Mbit DDR SDRAM which is connected via 16 data lines to the FPGA. Although the memory can operate at a maximum frequency of 133 MHz, our memory controller is, due to technical constraints, only able to deliver about 220 MByte/s. We use a RS-232 serial connection operating at 1 Mbit/s to connect the FPGA board to an external computer. Both the available logic capacity of the FPGA but also the memory bandwidth of the single DDR SDRAM chip are relatively low. Off-the-shelf hardware with more than twenty times the logic capacity and more than forty times the memory bandwidth are available[5].

For our implementation running on the prototyping board we set the architecture parameter to $N_{PE}=4, N_{ARAM}=8$ and $S_{ARAM}=32k$. We synthesized and implemented the architecture using the Xilinx ISE 9.2 toolchain. The resulting design (Table 5) runs at a clock frequency of 80 MHz and allocates almost all available logic resources.

In terms of performance it processes on average 2.7 matrix elements per clock cycle, or about 217 M matrix elements per second. The gap between the observed throughput and the theoretical peak throughput of 4 matrix elements per clock cycle can be primarily attributed to the saturated external memory bandwidth.

Scaling to Larger FPGAs

To estimate the FPGA logic resources necessary to implement larger systems, we synthesized the design for various combinations of N_{PE} and N_{ARAM}. N_{PE} was varied in the range between 4 and 16; N_{ARAM} was varied in the range between 4 and 64. All numbers where obtained by using Xilinx ISE 9.2 with the target architecture set to Virtex-4 generation FPGAs. The necessary FPGA logic resources, excluding the size of the Control Unit and the Memory Controller can be estimated by:

$$S_{Logik} = \underbrace{14(\pm 2)\, N_{PE}\, N_{ARAM}}_{\text{crossbar switch}} + \underbrace{560(\pm 30)\, N_{PE}}_{\text{processor elements + Wishbone}} \text{ slices}$$

To evaluate the computational throughput to be expected from these large designs, we ran, for various combinations of N_{PE} and N_{ARAM}, a cycle-accurate simulation of the architecture. The results are shown in Figure 7. In all these simulations we assume that there is sufficient external memory bandwidth available and that the number of activity memory blocks is increased at a fixed ratio to the number of streaming processors. In the examined interval these results show a close-to linear scaling of the throughput with respect to the number of streaming processor elements: (see Box 1)

Figure 7. Performance: Matrix elements per clock cycle

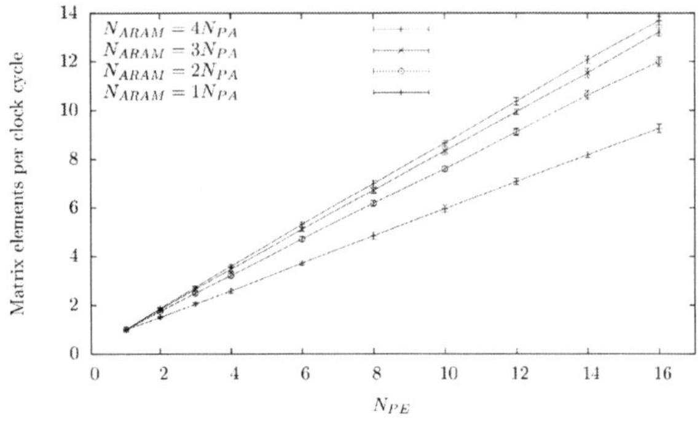

Note that for large systems the crossbar switch consumes most of the logic resources while at the same time provides sufficient interconnection resources to sustain a high computational throughput. Scaling the architecture to even larger FPGAs probably requires the replacement of the crossbar switch with an alternate, less resource consuming interconnect.

DISCUSSION AND FUTURE RESEARCH

The architecture we presented here was designed to efficiently simulate time steps in large connectionst systems. The design is based on a set of assumptions that we'd like to state here explicitly: (a) the number of neurons to be simulated exceeds the available hardware resources for a direct implementation; (b) the connection matrix is sparsely populated but nevertheless a large data set that does not fit into on-chip memory; and (c) the state- and the activity vectors are dense. It is likely that, whenever one ore more of these assumptions do not hold, another architectural approach is more promising.

Given that these assumptions hold true, and given the fact that SpMxV is an operation of low computational density, it is evident that any optimized implementation of a simulation step is bounded by the available memory bandwidth. The described coprocessor demonstrated, that a relatively simple FPGA design actually enters the regime of being memory-bound. In addition the architecture demonstrates that it is feasible to apply a compression scheme in order to reduce the size of an connection matrix and to increase the computational throughput. The proposed compression scheme based on a static variable-length code compressed the matrices typically occurring in macrocolumn simulations to about 7 bit per non-zero matrix element. Similar results were obtained when applying the same compression scheme to binary matrices from the Harwell-Boeing matrix set. Recent results for software SpMxV implementations on multicore architectures indicate that these implementations also become memory bandwidth-constrained. When the gap between CPU processing performance and memory bandwidth increases further, we expect that compression schemes gain importance for software implementations of SpMxV.

While our implementation demonstrated that an FPGA-based coprocessor can efficiently perform the SpMxV operation necessary to simulate a time step, it also highlighted the importance of a powerful general purpose processor. Controlling the *ν*-cycle, generating input stimuli and implementing Hebbian plasticity requires access to the neural state vector and to the connection matrix. From this point of view it seems most promising, to integrate FPGA-based streaming processors and general purpose processors into NUMA[6] shared memory systems. In such a system the FPGA-based streaming processors could simulate a time step for all neurons, while at the same time the general purpose processors could handle other important aspects of the connectionist system. For example to facilitate learning by changing the entries in the connection matrix.

REFERENCES

Baskaran, M. M., & Bordawekar, R. (2009). *Optimizing Sparse Matrix-Vector Multiplication on GPUs. RJ* (Vol. 24704, p. 11). Retrieved from http://domino.watson.ibm.com/library/CyberDig.nsf/1e4115aea78b6e7c85256b360066f0d4/1d32f6d23b99f7898525752200618339?OpenDocument.

Bell, N., & Garland, M. (2008). Efficient Sparse Matrix-Vector Multiplication on CUDA.

Bisseling, R. (2004). *Parallel Scientific Computation*. Oxford: Oxford Univ. Press. doi:10.1093/acprof:oso/9780198529392.001.0001

Duff, I. S., Grimes, R. G., & Lewis, J. G. (1992). *Users' Guide for the Harwell-Boeing Sparse Matrix Collection*. Release I.

Földiák, P. (1990). Forming sparse representations by local anti-Hebbian learning. *Biological Cybernetics, 64*(2), 165–170. doi:10.1007/BF02331346

Im, E., Yelick, K., & Vuduc, R. (2004). Sparsity: Optimization Framework for Sparse Matrix Kernels. *International Journal of High Performance Computing Applications, 18*(1), 135–158. doi:10.1177/1094342004041296

Jitsev, J., & von der Malsburg, C. (2009). Experience-driven formation of parts-based representations in a model of layered visual memory. *Frontiers in computational neuroscience, 3*(Special Issue on Complex systems science and brain dynamics), 15. Retrieved from http://www.ncbi.nlm.nih.gov/pubmed/19862345.

Lattice Semiconductor Corporation. (2007). *Lattice Mico 32 Processor Reference Manual*. Retrieved from http://www.latticesemi.com/.

Lücke, J., Keck, C., & von der Malsburg, C. (2008). Rapid convergence to feature layer correspondences. *Neural Computation, 20*(10), 2441–2463. doi:10.1162/neco.2008.06-07-539

Lücke, J., & von Der Malsburg, C. (2004). Rapid processing and unsupervised learning in a model of the cortical macrocolumn. *Neural Computation, 16*(3), 501–533. doi:10.1162/089976604772744893

Peterson, W. D. (2002). *WISHBONE system-on-chip (SoC) interconnection architecture for portable IP cores, revision: B.3*. Retrieved from http://www.opencores.org/.

Pinar, A., & Heath, M. T. (1999). Improving performance of sparse matrix-vector multiplication. *Proceedings of the 1999 ACM/IEEE conference on Supercomputing - Supercomputing '99*, 30-es. New York: ACM Press.

Sato, Y. D., Wolff, C., Wolfrum, P., & von der Malsburg, C. (2007). Dynamic Link Matching between Feature Columns for Different Scale and Orientation. *Lecture Notes In Computer Science*. Retrieved from http://portal.acm.org/citation.cfm?id=1423142.

Temam, O., & Jalby, W. (1992). Characterizing the behavior of sparse algorithms on caches. In *Proceedings of the 1992 ACM/IEEE conference on supercomputing* (pp. 578-587). Minneapolis: IEEE Computer Society Press.

Vastenhouw, B., & Bisseling, R. H. (2005). A Two-Dimensional Data Distribution Method for Parallel Sparse Matrix-Vector Multiplication. *SIAM Review, 47*(1), 67. .doi:10.1137/S0036144502409019

Vazquez, F., Garzon, E. M., Martinez, J. A., & Fernandez, J. J. (2009). The sparse matrix vector product on GPUs.

Vuduc, R., Demmel, J. W., & Yelick, K. A. (2005). A library of automatically tuned sparse matrix kernels. In *Institute of Physics Publishing*. OSKI.

Vuduc, R., Demmel, J. W., Yelick, K. A., Kamil, S., Nishtala, R., Lee, B., et al. (2002). Performance optimizations and bounds for sparse matrix-vector multiply. In *Supercomputing '02: Proceedings of the 2002 ACM/IEEE conference on Supercomputing* (pp. 1--35). {Baltimore, Maryland: IEEE Computer Society Press. Retrieved from http://portal.acm.org/citation.cfm?doid=762761.762822#.

Williams, S., Oliker, L., Vuduc, R., Shalf, J., Yelick, K., & Demmel, J. (2009). Optimization of sparse matrix–vector multiplication on emerging multicore platforms. *Parallel Computing, 35*(3), 178–194. doi:10.1016/j.parco.2008.12.006

Wolfrum, P., Wolff, C., Lücke, J., & von der Malsburg, C. (2008). A recurrent dynamic model for correspondence-based face recognition. *Journal of vision, 8*(7), 34.1-18.

Xilinx Inc. (2007). *Spartan 3 Generation User Guide*. San Jose.

Xilinx Inc. (2008). *Virtex-4 FPGA User Guide*. San Jose.

ENDNOTES

1 The term superscalar refers to the ability of a processor to execute multiple instructions per clock cycle to exploit instruction level parallelism. Modern CPUs typically issue multiple arithmetic and load-and-store memory operations at the same time.

2 Temporal locality means, that access to some memory location x_i implies a increased probability for a timely second access to the same location. Spatial locality refers to an increased probability of a memory access to some element x_i when a nearby memory element (e.g. x_{i-1}) has been accessed before.

3 Direct Memory Access

4 A slice can be understood as the basic unit of user-defined logic in Spartan-3 and Virtex-4 generation FPGAs. Conceptually, a slice in these FPGAs contains two 4bit to 1bit function generators, two clock synchronized 1bit storage elements (flip-flops) and some small multiplexers. The structure of these slices is highly optimized so that commonly used micro-architectural design-elements can be efficiently mapped onto slices. The details and the terminology varies between FPGA generations and between vendors.

5 For example: Xilinx Virtex-4 LX 200 with 89.088 Slice logic capacity and 336 internal RAM blocks. This chip can be connected to 300 MHz DDR2 SDRAM memory with 256 bit data-path (Xilinx Inc., 2008).

6 Non-Uniform Memory Architecture

APPENDIX A: TERMS, DEFINITIONS AND PARAMETERS USED

- $\vec{n}$: Neural state ($\vec{n}_i \in \{0,1\}$ for McCulloch-Pitts neurons)
- **T**, **R**, **M**: Connection matrices
- $m = 100$: Number of neurons within a minicolumn
- k: Number of minicolumns within a macrocolumn
- $\Theta(t)$: Time dependent neural threshold
- $\nu(t)$: Time dependent inhibition
- $\nu_{\text{reset}} = 0.1; \nu_{\text{min}} = 0.4; \nu_{\text{max}} = 1.1$: Parameters for ν-cycle
- $\varepsilon = 0.03$: Learning rate
- $\chi = 0.55$: Differentiation pressure
- N_{PE}: Number of processor elemens
- N_{ARAM}: Number of on-chip activity memory blocks
- S_{ARAM}: Number of neural activity elements an ARAM can store
- ARAM: On-chip neuron activity memory block
- CRS: Compressed Row Storage; data format for sparse matrices
- CIRS: Compressed Incremental Row Storage
- DMA: Direct Memory Access
- FPGA: Field Programmable Gate Array
- GPU: Graphics Processing Unit
- PE: Processor Element
- SpMxV: Sparse matrix vector multiplication

Chapter 12
Neural Network Circuits for Embedded Sensors Applications

N. Medrano
Universidad de Zaragoza, Spain

G. Zatorre
INCIDE S.A., Spain

M. T. Sanz
Instituto Nacional de Astrofísica, Óptica y Electrónica, México

B. Calvo
Universidad de Zaragoza, Spain

S. Celma
Universidad de Zaragoza, Spain

ABSTRACT

This chapter presents the suitability, development and implementation of programmable analogue artificial neural networks for sensor conditioning in embedded systems. Comments on the use of analogue instead of digital electronics due to the size and power constraints of these applications are included. Performance of an ad-hoc analogue architecture is evaluated, and its characteristics are analyzed. We will verify its low sensitivity to undesired effects, such as component mismatching, due to the capability of selecting and programming the proper weights for a given task. In addition, a brief discussion is offered on the selection of perturbative algorithms instead of classical error back-propagation techniques for weight tuning. At the end of the chapter, we will show the main characteristics of the proposed arithmetic cells implemented in a low-cost CMOS technology.

INTRODUCTION

Today's sensor market is advanced towards the so called smart sensors, that is, integrated sensor systems that contain on a single chip the sensing, interfacing, signal processing and intelligence (self-testing, self-identification and self-adaptation) functions (Meijer, 2008). Due to the capability of co-integration of sensors and sensor electronics, research challenges are focused on

DOI: 10.4018/978-1-60960-018-1.ch012

the implementation of low cost high performance CMOS smart sensors. Furthermore, if these smart sensors target the ever-increasing wireless sensor network (WSN) market, low-voltage low-power electronic circuits are required to maximize the lifetime of the battery operated systems.

To standardize the sensor output response, the transfer function from the sensor input to the electrical output should be the same for all sensors of the same type. However, due to process variations, properties vary from device to device and so do transfer characteristics. Therefore, calibration is mandatory to achieve a precise relationship between the electrical output and the physical signal being measured. Accurate sensors are usually more expensive than uncalibrated ones as the calibration process is individually carried out for each device, which pushes up production costs. Alternatively, automation of calibration is possible provided that the smart sensor contains a digitally programmable calibration function. This not only reduces costs and minimizes calibration time at the factory, but also allows the customer to perform recalibration if necessary (van der Horn, 1998).

Several methods are available for calibrating linearity errors in the sensor transfer characteristic, such as piecewise-linear interpolation, look-up table based linearization and electronic implementation of the inverse function of the sensor curve (Subramanian, 2005; Kolle, 2004; Pertijs, 2001). Another option is the use of artificial neural networks (ANNs), which, for linearization purposes, are made up of only a small number of programmable neurons or processing units. As a result, ANNs constitute a flexible solution at a low cost in terms of area, power consumption and computational complexity, thus being a valuable choice for adaptive sensor processing in embedded applications.

Recent technological advances allow a large number of battery-operated, inexpensive wireless networked sensor devices to be embedded in the physical environment. Wireless sensor networks allow for device mobility, fast and easy installation and relocation according to needs. Application fields cover natural habitat monitoring, structure health controlling, environmental pollutant detection, seismic structural damage monitoring, industrial process control and military target tracking, among others (Krishnamachari, 2005). The use of batteries to supply the system permits some of their main features, such as mobility or system ubiquity. In order to achieve long battery life (months or even years), power consumption must be carefully managed (Krishnamachari, 2005; Martinez, 2004).

A sensor unit can comprise smart sensors, with digital output and low power modes, and transducers that provide a raw analogue output. Interfacing between such sensors and the digital part of the system often requires conditioning electronics (Harb, 2004; Chao, 2004). An interface circuit consists of an analogue section to improve the sensor output by extending its linear range and reducing cross-sensitivity to other physical variables, and analogue-digital converters (ADC) to digitize the data to be processed by a microcontroller. Programmability allows a more versatile operation for the interface circuit, which can change its behavior according to the requirements. A classical programmable solution is a polynomial compensation (Khachab, 1991). This solution can be affected by mismatches, leading to reduced performance. Literature today shows more sophisticated solutions, (as in Cavalcanti, 2003), where a programmable analogue circuit is presented to amplify the signal supplied by a sensor, compensating the output offset. In this case, the system merely fits the output signal span to the input range of the ADC available in the microcontroller, but the sensor non-linearities are not corrected. In (Lopez-Martin, 2007), a versatile conditioning circuit for automotive applications is presented. In this case, the system consists of both analogue and digital elements, and power is provided by the car battery, so the adaptation to portable battery operated applications is difficult.

BACKGROUND

Adaptive circuits in sensor conditioning permit tuning the circuit operation to match changes in sensor response due to ageing, environmental effects or sensor replacement, providing optimum performance under any condition by means of a tuning/calibration process. We can consider these applications as function estimation problems, where the neural network input is the real sensor output and its output is the compensated, degradation-free output. Due to their flexibility and performance facing with these problems, ANNs based on multilayer perceptrons appear as a suitable choice for adaptive sensor conditioning applications.

Owing to the size and power consumption restrictions associated to portable sensor applications, mainly two possible implementation strategies exist for these adaptive systems: Digital implementation on low-cost microcontrollers and custom analogue circuits. Obviously, the use of software simulation on computers for implementing the conditioning system must be discarded.

Digital Implementation of Adaptive Sensor Conditioning

Today, embedded microcontrollers can be found everywhere: in industrial facilities, cars, kitchen appliances, mobile phones, mp3 players, watches, and even clothes. The generalization of microcontroller-based systems in industry has led to a fall in costs in parallel with a boosting of their computational power and, therefore, to the emergence of further unexpected applications. In the field of sensor systems, a microcontroller can use a part of its time in compensating for the non-idealities of the connected sensors. In this case, the sensor readings are formerly digitized, and the resulting values processed to cancel the effects of non-linearities and drifts in the sensor response. The compensation process is then programmed and run into the microcontroller. Literature offers some examples of this kind of solutions for adaptive sensor compensation systems based on neural networks (Medrano, 2001; Medrano, 2002). Due to the tough computational requirements of the classical learning algorithms for multilayer perceptrons (Haykin, 1999), and in order to reduce the memory size and resources required to implement the conditioning code in the microcontroller, weight fitting is usually done offline. The system operation is simulated on a computer; then the weight values are scaled from a 32 or 64 bits representation, which is usual in computers, to a 8 or 16 bits, usual in low-cost microcontrollers. In addition, to minimize the time required to compensate the output of a sensor, some arithmetic simplifications in the feed-forward algorithm have to be worked on: the most significant being fixed point instead of floating point numerical representation (Koren, 1993) and piecewise output functions for the hidden neurons.

Fixed point numerical representation is a condition that must be defined when the network weights are in the tuning (learning) phase. At this point, the weight precision must be determined by setting up the number of bits that will represent these numbers (8 or 16), and the value of the less significant bit (LSB) in the target microcontroller. For example, let 3.48556 be the value of a weight in a network implemented in an 8-bit microcontroller. If we set the value of the LSB at 2^{-5} (5 bits in the decimal part), the binary representation, including a sign bit in the most significant bit position, will be 01101011 (= 011.01111 including the decimal point), which represents exactly 3.46875. However, if we set the value of the LSB at 2^{-4}, the binary representation of 3.48556 will be 00110111 (= 0011.0111), which represents exactly 3.4375. In the first case the binary representation of the number is closer to the real value, but the highest positive number that can be encoded is 011.11111 (3.96875). On the other hand, the second case gives a lower resolution, but the highest positive number that can be encoded is 0111.1111 (7.9375). Thus, prior to training the ANN, the resolution of the binary representation must be determined, and then the maximum allowable decimal number in the network limited.

Piecewise output function representation is another important issue in the simplification of ANN algorithms. A typical transfer function for the processors in the hidden layer of a multilayer perceptron network (MLP) is the hyperbolic tangent:

$$\tanh(x) = \frac{e^x - e^{-x}}{e^x + e^{-x}} \tag{1}$$

This function could be calculated by the microcontroller using its Taylor series. However, this would consume too many computational resources. Instead of this approach, the use of a simplified piecewise version of this function gives similar results with far fewer computational requirements. A typical pseudo-code representation of a piecewise approximation of this function is given here:

```
function tanh(x)
   if (x>5.2)
      b=0; c=1.;
   elseif (x>3.42)
      b=0.05849; c=0.84101;
   elseif (x>2.38)
      b=0.20398; c=0.59284;
   elseif (x>1.62)
      b=0.42365; c=0.33143;
   elseif (x>0.72)
      b=0.72084; c=0.09071;
   elseif (x>-0.72)
      b=0.97281; c=0.;
   elseif (x>-1.62)
      b=0.72084; c=-0.09071;
   elseif (x>-2.38)
      b=0.42365; c=-0.33143;
   elseif (x>-3.42)
      b=0.20398; c=-0.59284;
   elseif (x>-5.2)
      b=0.05849; c=-0.84101;
   elseif (x<=-5.2)
      b=0; c=-1.;
   end
return(b*x+c);                                    (2)
```

Applying the previous modifications, it is possible to implement a reliable MLP network for sensor output conditioning into a low-cost microcontroller, giving response times lower than 1 ms for 5 MHz of clock frequency, as presented in (Medrano, 2002). Nevertheless, this option can have certain setbacks:

- In applications where several sensors must be compensated by the same microcontroller, as in WSN systems, the microcontroller must apply the same code for each sensor with the appropriate weight values. In this case, the conditioning time can increase dramatically and become the most time-consuming task, drastically reducing the system effectiveness.
- Low-cost microcontrollers usually include analogue-to-digital converters (ADC) with a resolution limited to 10 bits. For non-linear sensors, this resolution can not be high enough to differentiate between two significant sensor output values. The same binary value would be then assigned to several analogue inputs, consequently degrading the sensing process and affecting the system sensitivity. In such cases, the sensor output must be linearized before it is digitized.
- In some up-to-date battery-operated low-power applications, like WSN systems, the microcontroller program and data memories are mainly involved with wireless communication management and sensor data storage. These cover up to 90-95% of the memory resources, and drastically constrain the memory size available for the conditioning tasks. Furthermore, the use of the arithmetic unit of the microcontroller

in the conditioning process increases the microcontroller power consumption, and reduces battery life.

- The digital implementation of an adaptive algorithm for sensor output conditioning can, at times, become impractical. In these cases an analogue implementation is usually the best choice.

Analogue Implementation of Adaptive Sensor Conditioning

In low-power portable sensor network applications, an analogue electronic implementation of such adaptive conditioning circuits is a suitable choice due to its reduced size and power consumption, which allows it to be placed close to the sensor to be compensated. In addition, the use of digital register-based memories to store the programmable weights provides the system with more flexibility and greater reliability than when using analogue-based memories. Therefore, by combining analogue and digital electronics, it is possible to take advantage of both technologies, and so improve circuit performance.

An important issue regarding the use of digital weights encoding is the minimum resolution required. In (Lajusticia, 2003) it is shown that while 5-bit weights encoding is adequate for mixed-mode ANNs in realistic classification tasks, 8-bit weights are necessary in function estimation problems in order to achieve suitable results.

On the other hand, the analogue implementation of conditioning circuits has certain drawbacks, including, among others: component mismatching and changes in the system characteristics due to temperature drifts or offsets. However, adaptive circuits can compensate these errors in the system operation by properly selecting their weight values. As we will see in the next section, adaptive analogue systems resist well to component mismatching or loading effects by tuning its operation in order to give always the suitable transfer function.

The limited performance of error back-propagation-based learning algorithms applied to the tuning of non-ideal circuits, limits its use in analogue implementations (Dolenko, 1995). In this case, perturbative-based algorithms can be an appropriate choice (Jabri, 1992). These algorithms change the value of a set of weights $W = [w_{ij}]$ in the network with small random $[pert_{ij}]$ weight perturbations:

$$W' = W + \left[pert_{ij}\right] \tag{3}$$

Evaluating the root mean square error (RMSE) achieved in the system transfer function when the perturbation is added:

$$E(W') = rms(\sum_{k}\left(o_k - f\left(W'\right)\right) \tag{4}$$

where o_k are the target network outputs for each input pattern k, and $f(W')$ is the conditioning transfer function using the perturbed weights. If the resulting value $E(W')$ is smaller than the previous error $E(W)$, modified weights W' are kept; otherwise, weights W remain unchanged. This process is repeated until the system reaches the desired performance.

In contrast to a microcontroller-based neural network implementation, whose operation can be changed by reprogramming, analogue neural circuits must be designed to match the arithmetic operations required for a specific neural network model. Figure 1 shows the block diagram of an analogue implementation for a MLP for sensor output conditioning. The main blocks are the analogue-digital multiplier circuits (ADM), which multiply the neuron inputs with digital weights, and the activation function circuits (AF), which act upon the system non-linearities.

Figure 1. A typical analogue MLP architecture (top), processing unit architecture (bottom-left) and Analogue-Digital Multiplier diagram (bottom-right)

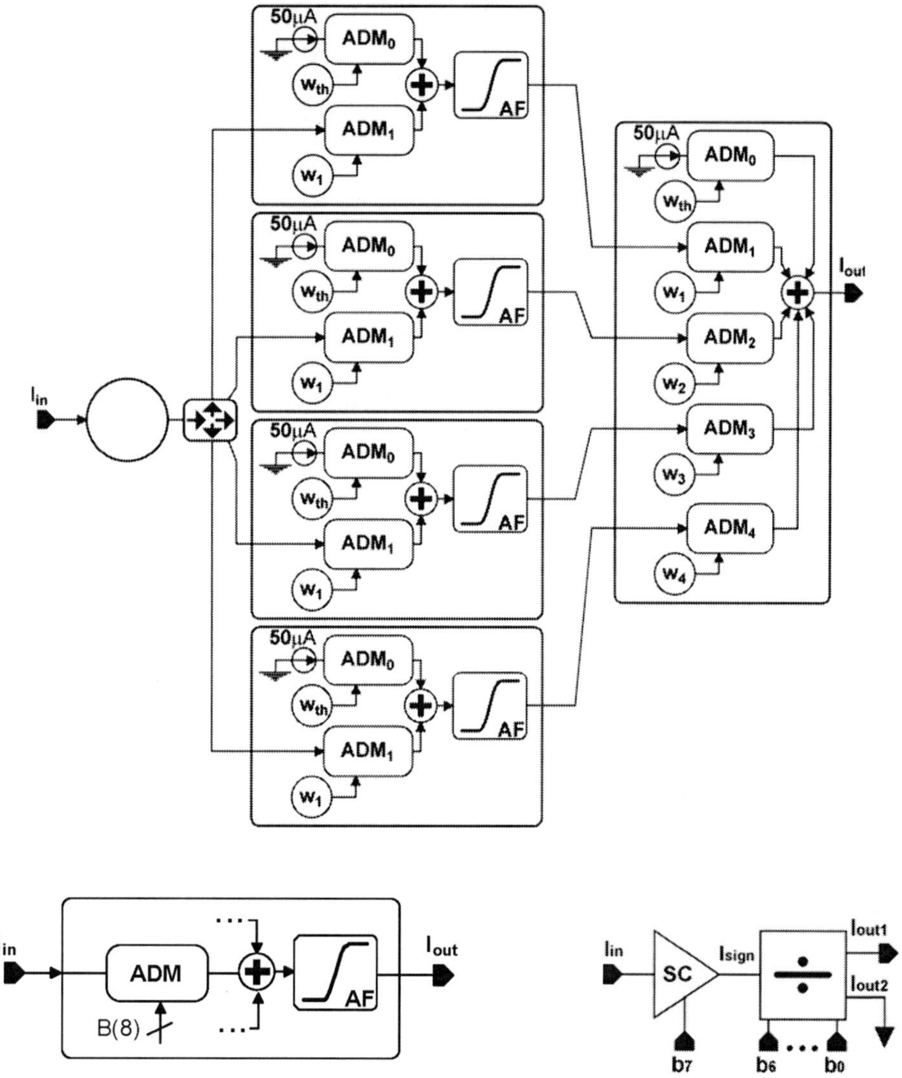

ANALOGUE NEURAL NETWORK CIRCUITS FOR LOW-POWER EMBEDDED SENSOR APPLICATIONS

The previous section stated how useful analogue neural circuits are for sensor compensation in low-power embedded applications. To design an adaptive analogue circuit, several points must be determined: the architecture of the arithmetic circuits, the algorithm to fit the weights to solve the proposed task and the network architecture. Both the arithmetic circuit architecture and the network algorithm are clearly related to the task to be resolved. Since sensor output compensation is a function estimation task, MLP is considered a worthy choice. Assuming this neural model, the arithmetic and circuits that have to be designed are those involved in the perceptron operation: the multiplier and the logistic function. Although voltage-mode is usually selected in analogue processing, current-mode circuits give better results at lower bias, which also reduces the power consumption (Tomazou, 1990). Therefore, due to the restrictions in bias voltage and power consumption related to portable embedded systems, the current-mode approach offers better characteristics for these applications.

Arithmetic Circuits

The design of a processing unit must favour the characteristics of the application. A portable application, as in the case of wireless sensor networks, is based on the use of batteries whose operating life must be as long as possible. Under these conditions, the analogue sensors connected to a wireless sensor unit provide low-level signals, which will input to the processing architecture. Thus, the processing circuits must be designed to condition the signals with no loss of information through impedance mismatching or other circuit non-idealities. A block diagram of a programmable current-mode four-quadrant multiplier is shown in Figure 1 (bottom-right). Basically, the multiplier consists of a sign circuit (SC) that selects the sign of the operation according to the direction of the input current and the sign bit of the digital weight, and a 7-bit programmable MOS-based R-2R (M-2M) current ladder (÷) that multiplies the current provided by the sign circuit by a factor equal or lower than 1.

Figure 2 (top) shows the sign circuit. Current mirrors are used to select the output either to I_{out} or nI_{out} according to the sign bit, while the non-selected output is set to high impedance. When b7 is '0', the input current flows through the right-side output of the circuit (I_{out}), keeping the same direction; when sign bit is '1', the current direction is reversed and it flows through the left-side output (nI_{out}). The sign circuit provides the output signal with a symmetrical path independently of the value of the sign bit. The output current from the sign circuit I_{sign} is driven to the next stage.

Figure 2 (middle) shows a 7-bit M-2M ladder. It is a classical circuit (Hammerschmied, 1998) which divides the input current into two branches depending on the value of a set of programmed bits. In our case, I_{out1} is the ladder output and I_{out2} is grounded. The input current is multiplied by a factor Δ that depends on the value of the first 7-bits of an 8-bit register, according to:

$$\Delta = \frac{1}{2^n}\left(\sum_{j=0}^{n-1} b_j 2^j\right) \quad \text{with n} = 7 \tag{5}$$

The complete operation is represented by:

$$I_{out1} = wI_{in} \quad \wedge \quad w = (-1)^{b_7}\frac{1}{2^7}\left(\sum_{j=0}^{6} b_j 2^j\right) \tag{6}$$

The transfer function of this circuit for 15 different digital weight values is shown in Figure 2 (bottom). The sign bit of the weight selects the slope sign: quadrants 2 and 4 in the graphic for positive values and quadrants 1 and 3 for negative, while the slope value is given by the 7 less significant bits: a higher weight value provides a higher slope value.

The logistic circuit shown in Figure 3 provides the non-linear output of the processing units. It consists of a current amplifier whose bias current has been set to I_{bias} = 25 μA (for I_{in} = 0). Current I_{Lim} (right side of the schematic) limits the maximum absolute value of the output current to a predetermined value of 50 μA, providing the non-linear operation.

Training Algorithms

The proposed analogue cells can be interconnected in order to build adaptive analogue processors. Figure 1 (bottom-left) shows the block diagram for an adaptive processing unit. The logistic circuit input is connected to several multiplier cells.

Figure 2. Four-quadrant multiplier: sign circuit (top), current ladder (middle) and operation (bottom)

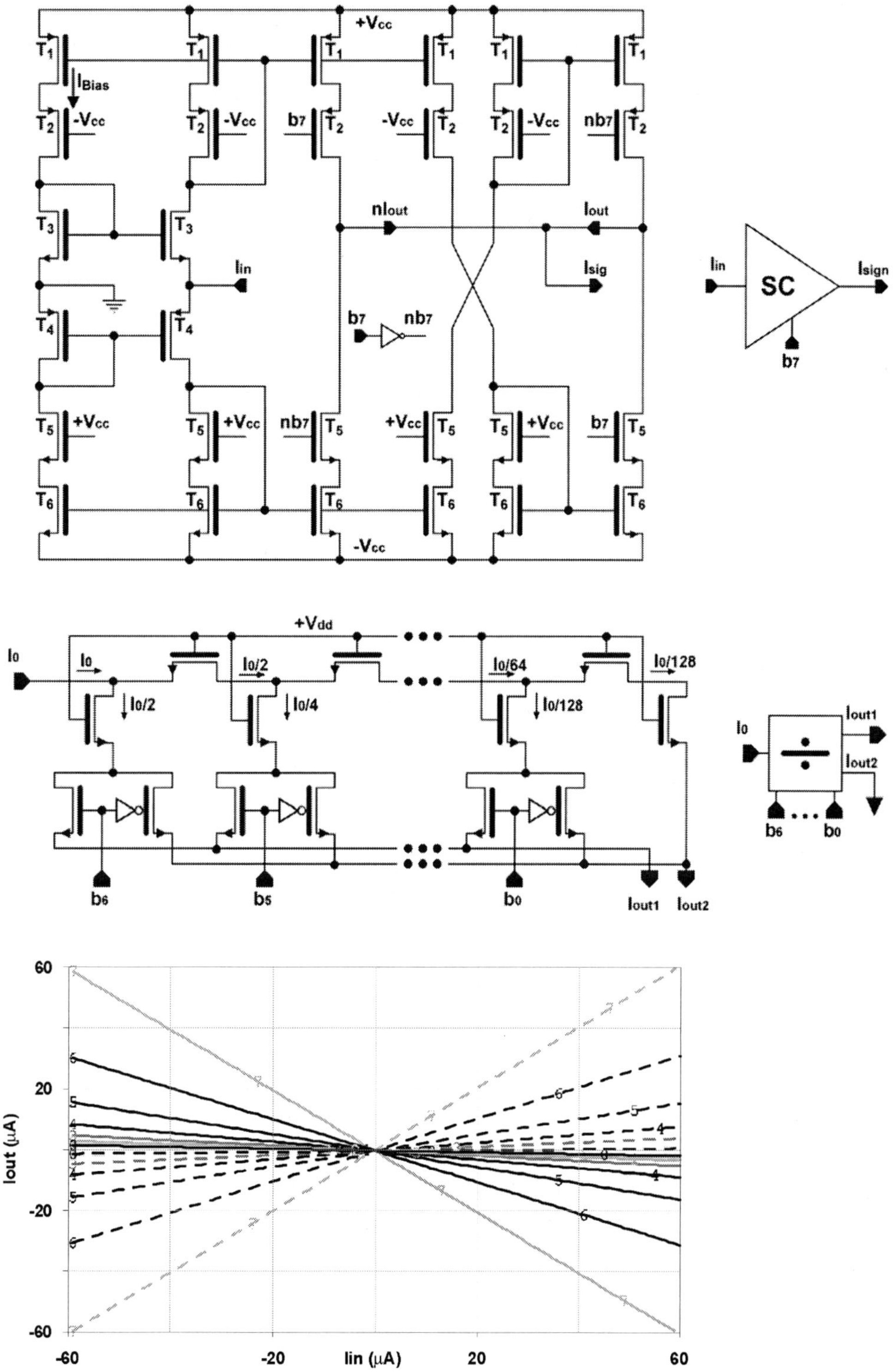

Figure 3. Non-linear circuit (top) and operation (bottom)

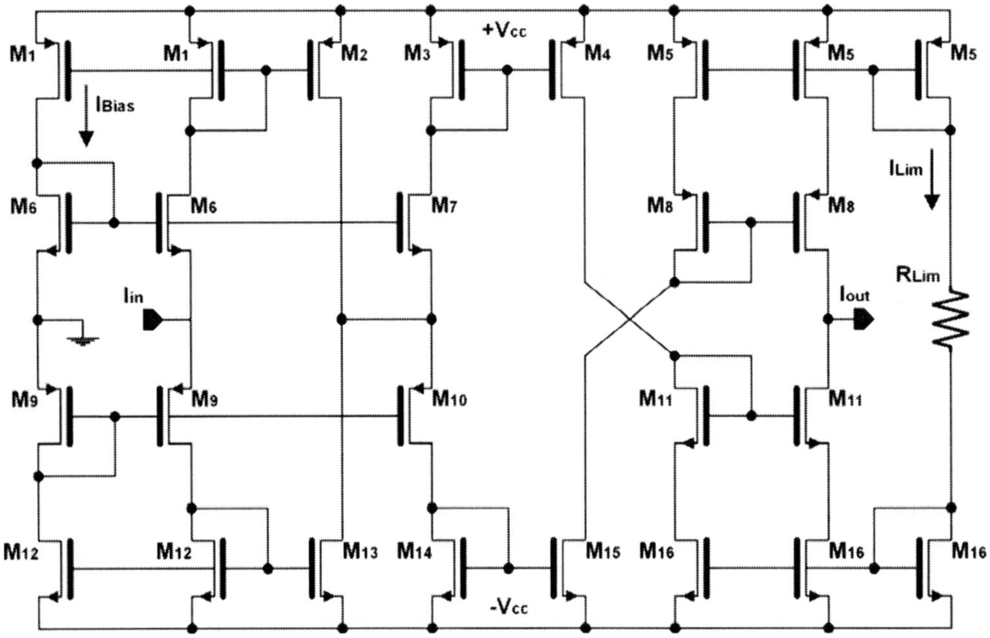

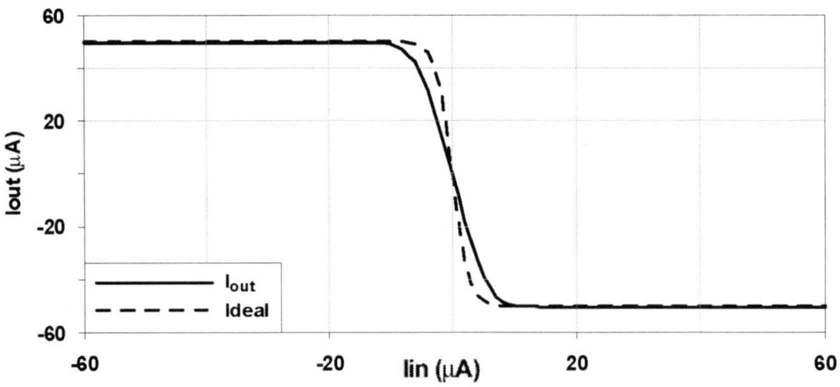

Depending on the number of multipliers connected to the non-linear circuit and the values B(7:0) stored in the corresponding weight registers, the current transfer to the logistic input changes, thus affecting the interface behavior. Post-layout simulations show that in the worst case (when multipliers present the minimum output impedance) the current transferred from a multiplier to a non-linear circuit decreases almost linearly with a mean value of about 3% per additional multiplier. Therefore, five multipliers connected to an output circuit, cause a mean error equal to or lower than 12.5% in the current transfer. Deviations of the system behavior must be compensated through the training algorithm by properly fitting the weight values in order to preserve the system performance.

An important issue in the field of adaptive systems is tuning the free parameters of the system, in our case the weights. As mentioned, when the arithmetic operations performed by the designed circuits match the ideal behavior, the best solution is an error back-propagation algorithm such as the Levenberg-Marquardt (Hagan, 1994). This is the case when the adaptive architecture is implemented using digital circuits. However, when the real operations performed by the processing architecture mismatch the ideal behavior, these algorithms become useless (Dolenko, 1995). Due to effects such as impedance mismatching, circuit simplifications, or faults in circuit manufacturing processes, arithmetic analogue implementations usually present considerable differences with the ideal operation. For the considered circuits, we can distinguish a negative output drift in the multiplier output (which can be seen in the zero-crossing of the curves, Figure 2), and a clear difference between the ideal and implemented hyperbolic tangent functions (Figure 3). In these cases, an algorithm independent of the arithmetic operations must be selected. A suitable training technique is perturbative learning. Perturbative algorithms give optimum results even for relative errors greater than 30% in the operation of the circuits, as we will see later.

In order to program the operation of a conditioning circuit, we have tested two different parameter perturbation strategies: multiple-parameter and single-parameter perturbation. In each tuning strategy, the number of perturbed bits per parameter is fixed (from 1 to 7) and the number of iterations (perturbations) is limited to 400. The problems proposed are to extend the linear range of four resistive sensors: two NTC thermistors and two giant magneto-resistive (GMR) sensors (Fraden, 2004). NTC thermistors are low-cost temperature sensors which are widely used in many applications, such as ambient control or room monitoring. GMR sensors are resistors whose resistive value varies depending on their position inside a magnetic field. These sensors are useful for instance in the automotive industry. In the NTC sensors, the maximum acceptable error is 1 °K, while in the GMR sensors the allowable error is 1 degree in the estimation of the angular position. Results are obtained by averaging 10 samples of training processes for each possible perturbation range and training strategy.

NTC patterns consist of 71 sensor readings from 253 °K to 323 °K. GMR patterns consist of 175 sensor output measurements collected in the 180°-355° range. Data are divided into two datasets: 10% of the patterns are used during the verification stage and the rest in the tuning or calibration process. Simulations are performed using the standard electric circuit models (with no mismatch effects), using a 1-4-1 architecture similar to that depicted in Figure 1.

In a Multiple-Parameter Perturbation (MPP), all the parameters of the conditioning circuit are modified in parallel and the RMSE of the output is calculated for the new parameter configuration. Only when the RMSE, calculated as the difference between the conditioned response and an ideal linear output decreases, are the new values kept; otherwise, they are discarded and old data are restored. Figure 4 (left) shows the final normalized RMSE as a function of the maximum number of bits that can be modified per parameter. We see that the minimum RMSE achieved after 400 iterations increases exponentially with the number of bits that can be modified, thus reducing the training performance.

In a Single-Parameter Perturbation (SPP), the RMSE of the output is calculated after perturbing only one parameter, using the same algorithm as in the MPP. Figure 4 (right) shows the final normalized RMSE in this case. As can be seen, the error is almost constant even for perturbations of six bits per parameter.

The linear range of the sensors can be extended according to the specifications by means of either a multiple-parameter or a single-parameter algorithm. In both cases, the conditioning system achieves the expected performance. However, the single-parameter algorithm is a better choice for hardware implementation, as only a 1-to-6 bits perturbation is calculated per iteration, in contrast with the set of N 1-to-3 bits perturbations per itera-

Figure 4. (left) RMSE vs. number of bits perturbed (multiple parameter algorithm); (right) RMSE vs. number of bits perturbed (single parameter algorithm)

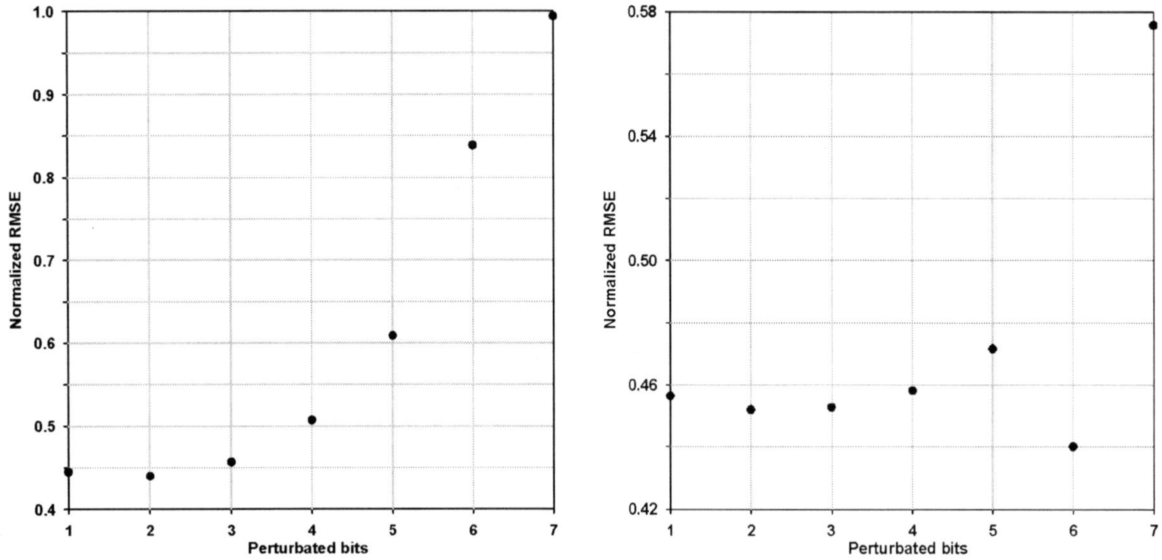

Table 1. Linear range extension (in %) for the four sensor samples

Sensor	Linear range	Extended range	%
NTC #1	274-308 °K	252-323 °K	108
NTC #2	274-308 °K	252-323 °K	108
GMR #1	252-305 deg	198-328 deg	145
GMR #2	234-292 deg	202-322 deg	107

tion required for the multiple parameter algorithm applied to an N-weight conditioning circuit.

Results of training the networks using a single parameter perturbation algorithm for the four sensor samples are shown in Table 1. The expected performance is well achieved in all cases.

Effects of Mismatch

As we have pointed out, component mismatching is one of the most important drawbacks in analogue circuit integration. To avoid these effects, special care must be taken in the layout design of the electronic components since mismatches can make the system ineffective. However, adaptability of neural network-based circuits could compensate for these errors in the operation of the system by properly tuning its weights. To study the effects of mismatch on an adaptive conditioning circuit, Monte-Carlo (MC) simulations were carried out. However, as these simulations are quite time-consuming and computationally intensive, they were first performed individually for each building block. Then, based on the obtained MC electrical simulation data, both the ADM and AF circuits were numerically modelled with Matlab at a system level. The activation and product functions provided in the Matlab Neural Network Toolbox models (MathWorks, 2009) were replaced by these more realistic electrical models. High level simulations were then carried out to study in a more efficient way mismatch effects on the whole processing architecture which was formerly described.

From Monte-Carlo simulation results, the 8-bit ADM operation can be modelled by:

$$I_{out1} = \alpha\, w I_{in} + \beta\, I_{in} + \gamma w + \delta \qquad (7)$$

where w is the programmable weight, I_{in} is the input current and the coefficients α, β, γ, and δ represent the mismatch effects, which will differ from one multiplier to another. Figure 5 (top) shows the mean error in the output current of 13 multiplier ADM cells (corresponding to the number of multipliers in the proposed architecture, see Figure 1) due to mismatches, considering 10 different mismatch-dependent case samples. Therefore, each multiplier in the processing architecture is affected differently by mismatches. Though the mean error is very high for some samples, this does not affect the correct processing of the sensor output, as will be shown in the following.

As for the AF sigmoid circuit, due to its complexity a polynomial approximation fails to fit the non-linear function properly. For this reason, the high-level circuit operation is modelled by means of a large look-up table. Figure 5 (bottom) shows the mean error in the output current of four AF circuits (see Figure 1) caused by mismatches, also considering 10 different mismatch-dependent case samples. Again, as shown in the figure, each AF circuit in the processing architecture is affected by mismatches in a different way.

Finally, these data were used to perform high level simulations of the whole adaptive conditioning circuit affected by mismatching, considering the previously studied practical case of extending the linear response of a GMR sensor. Table 2 shows the ranges where the error remains lower than 1° for the raw sensor output and the linearized span achieved for ten different mismatch case simulations for the complete processing circuit. Results show that the sensor compensated span is at least 100% higher than the raw output, even taking into account mismatch effects. Therefore, adaptive circuits based on mixed-mode perceptron processors work properly in sensor pre-processing electronics because of their adaptability and thus their ability to counteract mismatch effects.

Table 2. Linearization results for a GMR sensor using 10 different conditioning circuit models affected by mismatching

Simulation #	Angle (min)	Angle (max)	Improvement
Basic sensor	252	305	------------
Mismatch Case #1	215	331	119%
Mismatch Case #2	215	331	119%
Mismatch Case #3	216	323	102%
Mismatch Case #4	214	323	106%
Mismatch Case #5	214	329	117%
Mismatch Case #6	214	323	106%
Mismatch Case #7	211	323	111%
Mismatch Case #8	206	324	122%
Mismatch Case #9	214	323	106%
Mismatch Case #10	214	322	104%
Mean Results	216	322	100%

Hardware Implementation

The final step in the implementation of an electronic system is to fabricate its circuit components and verify their characteristics. Prototypes of multipliers and logistic circuits were integrated in the 3.3 V–0.35 μm standard CMOS technology from Austria Microsystems (AMS). This technology offers several advantages such as low-cost, a supply voltage compatible with the constraint of low-power and compatibility with digital systems. The corresponding layouts for these structures have been carefully realized taking into account the main design rules concerning transistor matching and symmetry between sections (Drennan, 2003). Figure 6 shows the microphotography of a part of the chip, in which the main processing blocks

Figure 5. Mean error for the mismatching-dependent multipliers (top) and non-linear circuits (bottom)

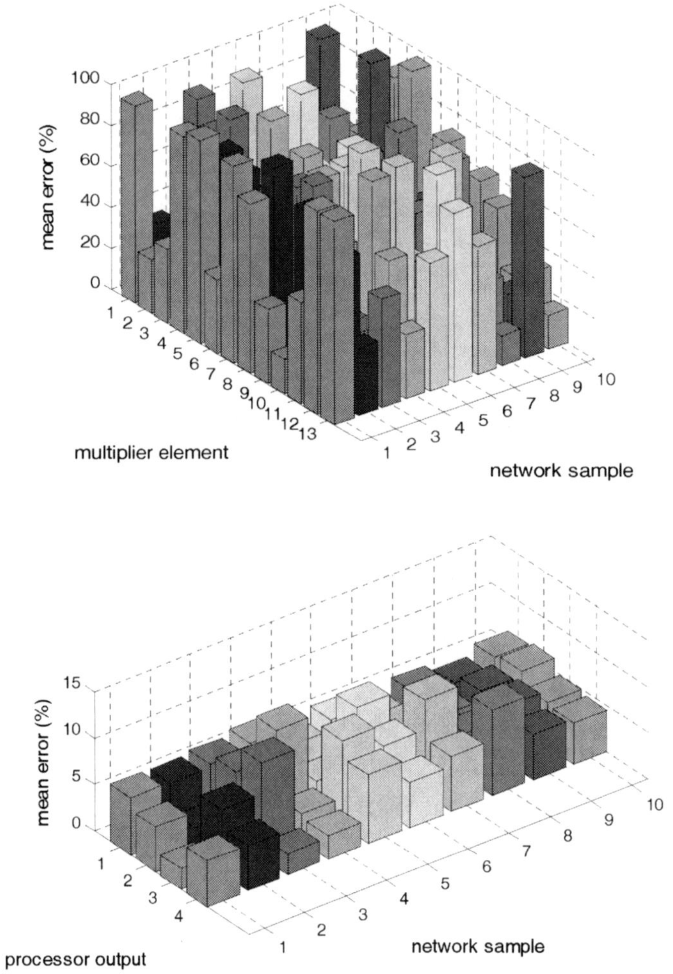

are highlighted: sign circuit, M-2M ladder and logistic circuit. Maximum current is limited by the sign and logistic circuits. Although the electronic components were designed to process low-level currents, limited to ±50μA, both circuits were oversized to provide more flexibility, so that they could be used in systems where higher currents are handled. The maximum output current of the logistic circuit can be increased or decreased by modifying the limiting resistor R_{Lim} (see Figure 3). Both Figure 2 and 3 show the experimental measurements of these circuits. Table 3 presents the main measured characteristics of the circuits. As seen, some values, such as active area or input/output impedances have been carefully adjusted to reduce signal loss in the processing path.

A processing architecture like the one proposed, built with these components has an active area of 0.25 mm^2, 10.8 mW of maximum operating power and a negligible quiescent power consumption (less than 105 nW), mainly due to the digital registers biasing. In embedded portable sensor applications, battery life can be extended by using intelligent power management, turning on (waking up) and off (sleeping) the corresponding electronics, keeping on only the power of the registers and turning off the analogue parts.

Figure 6. Chip microphotograph

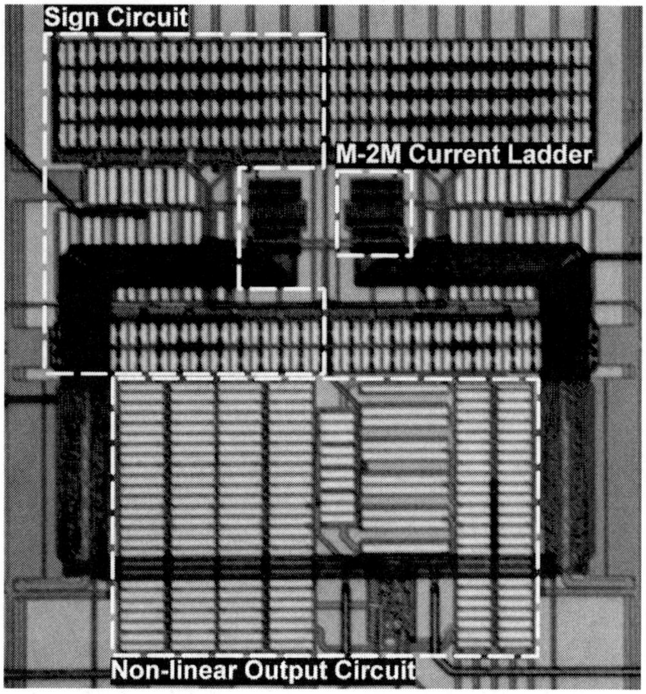

FUTURE RESEARCH DIRECTIONS

The growth of applications using portable embedded sensor systems is due to several facts: the increase of computing power and cost reduction in microcontrollers, the development of low-power electronics and battery technologies, and the use of low-cost sensors. These sensors present non-ideal characteristics that must be corrected for suitable information processing. To achieve the required accuracy, a conditioning operation must often be performed before digitizing the sensor readings. Analogue artificial neural networks offer adequate characteristics and properties for a suitable conditioning system to compensate these sensor non-linearities and drifts. However, sensor system design is evolving fast as the number of applications grows. The new ANNs designed for these applications should be adapted to the new requirements by reducing bias voltages, power and size, as well as increasing their flexibility by integrating not only programmable weights, but also programmable interconnections. This will allow for re-programming the ANN architecture on the fly, according to the changes in the characteristics of the task to be solved in each moment. The implementation of this feature requires developing suitable analogue switches, with low on and off switching times and ultra-low on resistance.

The design of a useful microelectronic analogue ANN must accomplish these considerations. In addition, the need to integrate analogue and digital electronics in the same silicon chip degrades the characteristics of the analogue circuit, making it necessary to improve the learning algorithms, in terms of adjusting the electronics operation and reducing the learning time. Integrating the learning algorithm into the system (or a part of it, leaving for instance the calculation of the RMSE to the microcontroller) will allow better weight tuning, due to the use of the real electronic components in the process, and not simply models.

Table 3. Characteristics of the real processor components

Sign Circuit	
Active area	13x10^{-3} mm^2
Max. input resistance	13 Ω
Mean input resistance	9 Ω
Min. output resistance	31 kΩ
Mean output resistance	149 kΩ
Maximum power	541 μW
Mean power	457 μW
$\pm V_{cc}$	±1.65 V
b_7, nb_7	±1.65 V
I_{Bias} (I_{in}=0)	30 μA
M-2M ladder	
Active area	165.4 μm^2
Input resistance	325 Ω
Min. output resistance	410 Ω
Mean output resistance	615 Ω
Quiescent power	79 pW
$+V_{dd}$	1.65 V
b_n	±1.65 V
Non-linear circuit	
Active area	4.73x10^{-3} mm^2
Max. input resistance	13 Ω
Mean input resistance	9 Ω
Min. output resistance	12 kΩ
Mean output resistance	15 kΩ
Maximum power	2.0 mW
Mean power	1.8 mW

CONCLUSION

Today, the trend towards embedding sensors in complex systems for the distributed measuring of relevant parameters has lead to the fast development of smart sensor systems. These systems are composed of low-cost sensors to measure physical variables (temperature, pressure, humidity, speed, gas concentration, etc.) that are processed and can eventually be transmitted to a remote monitoring center using low-power wireless communications. The needs to condition sensor output to make them compatible with the digital elements included in the sensing device and extend their characteristics make appropriate the use of adaptive sensor processing. Artificial neural networks have demonstrated their efficacy in sensor conditioning tasks. For these applications, ANNs can be implemented as software routines in the microcontroller that manages the measuring process in a sensor node. However, this is not the best solution in some applications, such as wireless sensor networks, where the microcontroller resources are mostly dedicated to the node management and wireless communications protocol and power consumption is an important restriction,. In these cases, the ANN implementation can be performed as an analogue or mixed application specific integrated circuit (ASIC)as proposed here.

In this chapter we have shown feasible current-mode analogue electronic cells to build a compact low-power easily programmable processor for adaptive systems based on a multilayer perceptron network. Digital programmability confers to the analogue circuitry the ability to compensate undesired effects such as sensor output drifts, non-idealities or circuit mismatches, while keeping the conditioning features. The blocks presented were implemented using a low-cost 0.35 μm standard digital CMOS technology, showing how they can be easily integrated in the analogue core of a sensor interface ASIC. Experimental results show accurate transfer functions, input and output impedances. In summary, the proposed processor is highly appropriate for implementing almost-analogue interfaces in integrated sensors being compact, robust and compatible with low bias voltage. For battery operated devices, operating life can be extended by using intelligent power management, switching the corresponding electronics on and off, and keeping on only the power of the registers and turning off the analogue parts.

An important issue in the development of analogue adaptive systems is the selection of a suitable training algorithm. It was shown that a single parameter perturbation algorithm provides a good performance vs. hardware complexity ratio. The use of perturbative learning compensates circuit non-idealities in multipliers and logistic circuits and current transfer loss, improving the full system operation. In sensor network applications, the tuning process can be controlled by the embedded low-cost processor that manages the node operation. Thus, updating time is mainly determined by the microprocessor operation and its clock frequency.

To provide a fully functional MLP-based sensor conditioning system, next important step is to provide a programmable connectivity that will allow for modifying the processing architecture according to the actual requirements.

The increasing use of low-power sensor networks in industry opens a new field of development for the design and implementation of analogue and mixed-mode artificial neural networks, the development of suitable training algorithms and configuration strategies which will make it possible to include an adaptive conditioning block embedded in these powerful and promising processing systems.

REFERENCES

Cavalcanti, S., Naviner, J. F., Deep, G., & Freire, R. (2003). Designing a Programmable Analog Signal Conditioning Circuit Without Loss of Measurement Range. *IEEE Transactions on Instrumentation and Measurement*, *52*, 1482–1487. doi:10.1109/TIM.2003.818556

Chao, G., & Meijer, G. (2004). A Universal Sensor Interface Chip Design in 0.5u CMOS Process. In *Proceedings 7th International Conference on Solid State and Integrated Circuits Technology Vol. 3* (pp. 1800-1803). Beijing: IEEE Press.

Dolenko, B. K., & Card, H. C. (1995). Tolerance to analog hardware of on-chip learning in backpropagation networks. *IEEE Transactions on Neural Networks*, *6*, 1045–1052. doi:10.1109/72.410349

Drennan, P. G., & McAndrew, C. C. (2003). Understanding MOSFET Mismatch for Analog Design. *IEEE Journal of Solid-state Circuits*, *38*(3), 450–456. doi:10.1109/JSSC.2002.808305

Fraden, J. (2004). *Handbook of Modern Sensors*. New York: Springer-Verlag.

Hagan, M., & Mohammad, B. (1994). Training feedforward networks with the Marquardt algorithm. *IEEE Transactions on Neural Networks*, *5*, 989–993. doi:10.1109/72.329697

Hammerschmied, C. M., & Huang, Q. (1994). Design and Implementation of an Untrimmed MOSFET-only 10-Bit A/D Converter with -79-db THD. *IEEE Journal of Solid-state Circuits*, *33*(8), 1148–1151. doi:10.1109/4.705353

Harb, A., Hu, Y., Sawan, M., Abdelkerim, A., & Elhilali, M. (2004). Low-Power CMOS Interface for Recording and Processing Very Low Amplitude Signals. *Analog Integrated Circuits and Signal Processing*, *39*, 39–54. doi:10.1023/B:ALOG.0000016642.76352.f8

Haykin, S. (1999). *Neural Networks, a Comprehensive Foundation*. Upper Saddle River, NJ: Prentice Hall.

Jabri, M., & Flower, B. (1992). Weight perturbation: An optimal architecture and learning technique for analog VLSI feedforward and recurrent multilayer networks. *IEEE Transactions on Neural Networks*, *3*, 154–157. doi:10.1109/72.105429

Khachab, N., & Ismail, M. (1991). Linearization Techniques for n th-Order Sensor Models in MOS VLSI Technology. *IEEE Transactions on Circuits and Systems*, *38*, 1439–1450. doi:10.1109/31.108498

Kolle, C., Scherr, W., Hammerschmidt, D., Pichler, G., Motz, M., Schaffer, B., et al. (2004). Ultra Low-Power Monolithically Integrated Capacitive Pressure Sensor for Tire Pressure Monitoring, In *Proceedings IEEE Sensors Conference 2004*, 244-247. Vienna: IEEE Press.

Koren, I. (1993). *Computer Arithmetic Algorithms*. Upper Saddle River, NJ: Prentice Hall.

Krishnamachari, B. (2005). *Networking Wireless Sensors*. New York: Cambridge University Press. doi:10.1017/CBO9780511541025

Lajusticia, C., Medrano, N., Zatorre, G., & Martin, B. (2003). Applying Non-Ideal Mixed Analog-Digital Multipliers in Electronic Processing Circuits Based on Neural-Networks. In *Proceedings of 2003 IEEE Conference on Emerging Technologies and Facttory Automation, ETFA 2003*, (pp. 362-367). Lisbon: IEEE Press.

Lopez-Martin, A., & Carlosena, A. (2007). Versatile Automotive Sensor Interface ASIC. In *Proceedings IEEE International Symposium on Industrial Electronics, ISIE 2007*, (pp. 1469-1472). Vigo: IEEE Press.

Martinez, K. K., Hart, J., & Ong, R. (2004). Sensor Network Applications. *Computer*, *8*, 50–56. doi:10.1109/MC.2004.91

MathWorks. The. (2009). *Neural Network Toolbox User's Guide*. Retrieved from http://www.mathworks.es/access/helpdesk/help/pdf_doc/nnet/nnet.pdf.

Medrano-Marqués, N. J., & Martín-del-Brío, B. (2001). Sensor linearization with neural networks. *IEEE Transactions on Industrial Electronics*, *48*, 1288–1290. doi:10.1109/41.969414

Medrano-Marques, N. J., & Martín-del-Brio, B. (2002). A Flexible Tool for Conditioning Sensor Signals based on Neural Networks. In *Proceedings IEEE Industrial Electronics Conference, IECON 2002*, (pp. 96-101). Sevilla: IEEE Press.

Meijer, G. (Ed.). (2008). *Smart Sensor Systems*. Wiltshire, UK: Wiley. doi:10.1002/9780470866931

Pertijs, M., Bakker, A., & Huijsing, J. H. (2001). A high-accuracy temperature sensor with second-order curvature correction and digital bus interface. In *Proceedings IEEE International Symposium on Circuits and Systems (ISCAS)* (pp. 368-371). Sydney: IEEE Press.

Subramanian, C. S., Pinelli, J. P., Lapilli, C. D., & Buist, L. (2005). A Wireless Multipoint Pressure Sensing System: Design and Operation. *IEEE Sensors Journal*, *5*(5), 1066–1074. doi:10.1109/JSEN.2005.854135

Toumazou, C., Lidgey, F. J., & Haigh, D. G. (1990). *Analogue IC Design: The Current-Mode Approach*. London: Peregrinus.

van der Horn, G., & Huijsing, J. L. (1998). *Integrated Smart Sensors, Design and Calibration*. Dordretch, The Netherlands: Kluwer Academic Publishers.

ADDITIONAL READING

Bae, H., Kim, S., Wang, B. H., Lee, M. H., & Harashima, F. (2006). Flame detection for the steam boiler using neural networks and image information in the Ulsan steam power generation plant. *IEEE Transactions on Industrial Electronics*, *53*, 338–348. doi:10.1109/TIE.2005.862209

Baker, J. (2008). *CMOS Circuit Design, Layout and Simulation*. New Jersey, USA: Wiley.

Boni, A., Pianegiani, F., & Petri, D. (2007). Low-Power and Low-Cost Implementation of SVMs for Smart Sensors. *IEEE Transactions on Instrumentation and Measurement*, *56*, 39–44. doi:10.1109/TIM.2006.887319

Bose, B. K. (2007). Neural Network Applications in Power Electronics and Motor Drives—An Introduction and Perspective. *IEEE Transactions on Industrial Electronics*, *54*, 14–33. doi:10.1109/TIE.2006.888683

Dündar, G., & Rose, K. (1995). The Effects of Quantization on Multilayer Neural Networks. *IEEE Transactions on Neural Networks*, *6*, 1446–1451. doi:10.1109/72.471364

King, D., Lyons, W., Flanagan, C., & Lewis, E. (2004). An Optical-Fiber Sensor for Use in Water Systems Utilizing Digital Signal Processing Techniques and Artificial Neural Network Pattern Recognition. *IEEE Sensors Journal*, *4*(1), 21–27. doi:10.1109/JSEN.2003.820344

Kinget, P. (2005). Device mismatch and tradeoffs in the design of analog circuits. *IEEE Journal of Solid-state Circuits*, *40*(6), 1212–1224. doi:10.1109/JSSC.2005.848021

Levenberg, K. (1944). A method for the solution of certain problems in least squares. *SIAM Journal on Numerical Analysis*, *16*, 588–604.

Linares-Barranco, B., Serrano-Gotarredona, T., & Serrano-Gotarredona, R. (2003). Compact Low-Power Calibration Mini-DACs for Neural Arrays With Programmable Weights. *IEEE Transactions on Neural Networks*, *14*, 1207–1216. doi:10.1109/TNN.2003.816370

Marquardt, D. (1963). An algorithm for least squares estimation of nonlinear parameters. *SIAM Journal on Applied Mathematics*, *11*, 431–441. doi:10.1137/0111030

Medrano, N., Zatorre, G., & Celma, S. (2008). A Tunable Analog Conditioning Circuit Applied to Magnetoresistive Sensors. *IEEE Transactions on Industrial Electronics*, *55*, 966–969. doi:10.1109/TIE.2007.896555

Milev, M., & Hristov, M. (2002). Analog Implementation of ANN with Inherent Quadratic Nonlinearity of the Synapses. *IEEE Transactions on Neural Networks*, *14*, 1187–1200. doi:10.1109/TNN.2003.816369

Omondi, A. (2004). *Computer Arithmetic Systems*. Cambridge, UK: Prentice Hall.

Razavi, B. (2001). *Design of Analog CMOS Integrated Circuits*. New York: McGraw Hill.

Saracoglu, Ö. G. (2008). An Artificial Neural Network Approach for the Prediction of Absorption Measurements of an Evanescent Field Fiber Sensor. *Sensors (Basel, Switzerland)*, *8*, 1585–1594. doi:10.3390/s8031585

Soloman, S. (1999). *Sensors Handbook*. New York: McGraw-Hill.

Stojmenovic, I. (Ed.). (2005). *Handbook of Sensor Networks*. New York: John Wiley & Sons. doi:10.1002/047174414X

Valle, M. (2002). Analog VLSI implementation of artificial neural networks with Supervised On-Chip Learning. *Analog Integrated Circuits and Signal Processing*, *33*, 263–287. doi:10.1023/A:1020717929709

van der Horn, G., & Huijsing, J. H. (1997). Integrated Smart Sensor Calibration. *Analog Integrated Circuits and Signal Processing*, *14*, 207–222. doi:10.1023/A:1008289918937

Wawryn, K., & Mazurek, A. (2001). Prototype Circuits for Programmable Neural Network. In *Proceedings European Conference on Circuits Theory and Design*, (pp. III/301-III/304). Espoo.

Webster, J. G. (Ed.). (1999). *The Measurement, Instrumentation and Sensors Handbook*. Washington, DC: IEEE Press.

Zatorre, G., Medrano, N., Aldea, C., Sanz, M. T., Digón, D., & Celma, S. (2008). A Tunable Mixed-Mode Interface Circuit for Sensor Conditioning. In *Proceedings IEEE International Symposium on Industrial Electronics, ISIE 2008* (pp. 980-985). Cambridge, UK: IEEE Press.

Zatorre, G., Medrano, N., & Celma, S. (2006). Analysis and Simulation of a Mixed-Mode Neuron Architecture for Sensor Conditioning. *IEEE Transactions on Neural Networks*, *17*, 1332–1335. doi:10.1109/TNN.2006.877535

Zatorre, G., Medrano, N., Sanz, M. T., Martinez, P., Celma, S., & Bolea, J. (2007). Robust Adaptive Electronics for Sensor Conditioning. In *Proceedings IEEE Sensors 2007 Conference* (pp. 1295-1298). Atlanta, GA: IEEE Press.

Zhuang, H., Low, K.-S., & Yau, W.-Y. (2007). A Pulsed Neural Network With On-Chip Learning and Its Practical Applications. *IEEE Transactions on Industrial Electronics*, *54*, 34–42. doi:10.1109/TIE.2006.888684

KEY TERMS AND DEFINITIONS

Adaptive Electronics: Electronic circuit which can change its operation according to modifications in the specifications of the problem to be solved. Usually these systems apply tuning algorithms that adjust the values of some variable or programmable parameters included in the circuit.

Embedded System: System designed to perform one or a few dedicated functions, embedded as part of a complete device.

Perturbative Algorithm: Adaptive system training technique based on the evolution of its performance when applying random perturbations to the programmable parameters of the system.

Circuit Mismatch: Process that causes variations between identically designed circuit components of an electronic system and that can lead to an incorrect system operation.

Current-Mode Circuit: Electronic circuit designed to process information as electric currents, instead of the more usual voltage codification. Current-mode operation can operate at lower voltage levels, thus allowing low-power operation, suitable for battery-based systems.

Mixed-Mode Circuit: Electronic circuit composed of analogue and digital components, combined to exploit the features of both technologies.

Resolution: Minimum variation of the value of a magnitude that can be detected by a device. In digital electronics, the number of bits that represents a numerical value: the greater number of bits, the higher resolution.

Multilayer Perceptron: Biologically-inspired processing system consisting of a set of artificial neurons arranged in layers. Each processor provides a non-linear output that is a function of the weighted sum of its inputs.

Sensor Conditioning: Processing techniques applied to the output of a sensor to improve its performance, extending the linear range and reducing offsets and drifts due to other physical magnitudes different from the principal.

Chapter 13
Parallel Hardware for Artificial Neural Networks Using Fixed Floating Point Representation

Nadia Nedjah
State University of Rio de Janeiro, Brazil

Rodrigo Martins da Silva
State University of Rio de Janeiro, Brazil

Luiza de Macedo Mourelle
State University of Rio de Janeiro, Brazil

ABSTRACT

Artificial Neural Networks (ANNs) is a well known bio-inspired model that simulates human brain capabilities such as learning and generalization. ANNs consist of a number of interconnected processing units, wherein each unit performs a weighted sum followed by the evaluation of a given activation function. The involved computation has a tremendous impact on the implementation efficiency. Existing hardware implementations of ANNs attempt to speed up the computational process. However, these implementations require a huge silicon area that makes it almost impossible to fit within the resources available on a state-of-the-art FPGAs. In this chapter, a hardware architecture for ANNs that takes advantage of the dedicated adder blocks, commonly called MACs, to compute both the weighted sum and the activation function is devised. The proposed architecture requires a reduced silicon area considering the fact that the MACs come for free as these are FPGA's built-in cores. Our system uses integer (fixed point) mathematics and operates with fractions to represent real numbers. Hence, floating point representation is not employed and any mathematical computation of the ANN hardware is based on combinational circuitry (performing only sums and multiplications). The hardware is fast because it is massively parallel. Besides, the proposed architecture can adjust itself on-the-fly to the user-defined configuration of the neural network, i.e., the number of layers and neurons per layer of the ANN can be settled with no extra hardware changes. This is a very nice characteristic in robot-like systems considering the possibility of the same hardware may be exploited in different tasks. The hardware also requires another system (a software) that controls the sequence of the hardware computation and provides inputs, weights and biases for the ANN in hardware. Thus, a co-design environment is necessary.

DOI: 10.4018/978-1-60960-018-1.ch013

INTRODUCTION

Artificial Neural Networks (ANNs) are useful for learning, generalization, classification and forecasting problems (Hassoun, 1995). They consist of a pool of relatively simple processing units, usually called artificial neurons, which communicates with one another through a large set of weighted connections. There are two main network topologies, which are feed-forward topology (Hassoun, 1995; Moerland & Fiesler, 1996), where the data flows from input to output neurons strictly forward and recurrent topology, where feedback connections are allowed. Artificial neural networks offer an attractive model that allows one to solve hard problems from examples or patterns. However, the computational process behind this model is complex. It consists of massively parallel non-linear calculations. Software implementations of artificial neural networks are useful but hardware implementations take advantage of the inherent parallelism of ANNs and so should answer faster.

Field Programmable Gate Arrays (FPGAs) (Xilinx, 2009) provide a re-programmable hardware that allows one to implement ANNs very rapidly and at very low-cost. However, FPGAs lack the necessary circuit density as each artificial neuron of the network needs to perform a large number of multiplications and additions, which consume a lot of silicon area if implemented using standard digital techniques, as floating-point operations.

The proposed hardware architecture described throughout this chapter is designed to process any fully connected feed-forward Multilayer Perceptrons (MLP) neural network. However, training is not included. It is now a common knowledge that the computation performed by the net is complex and consequently has a huge impact on the implementation efficiency and practicality. Existing hardware implementations of ANNs have attempted to speed up the computational process. However these designs require a considerable silicon area that makes them almost impossible to fit within the resources available on a state-of-the-art FPGAs (Bade & Hutchings, 1994; Brown & Card, 2001; Nedjah & Mourelle, 2007; Seul; & Sung, 2007, Tuffy *et. al.*, 2007; Harkin, *et. al.*, 2009). In this chapter, an original hardware architecture for ANNs that takes advantage of the dedicated adder blocks, commonly called MACs (short for Multiply, Add and Accumulate blocks) to compute both the weighted sum and the activation function is proposed.

Our system uses a specific number representation: Fractional Fixed Point (Saint-Jones & Gu, 2003). It means that a real number is treated (approximated) by a fraction. Fractional addition, subtraction and multiplication are inherently integer (fixed point) operations, which may be an attractive choice in decreasing silicon area, because integer mathematics can be done by combinational circuitry.

The weighted sum of a neuron is now a sum of fractional products. In this project, the activation function (for all neurons of the ANN) is the sigmoidal logistic function (*logsig*), whose mathematics is also reduced (approximated) to additions, subtractions and multiplications of fractions. The exponential term $\exp(\cdot)$ of the logsig function is approximated to 3 quadratic polynomials, using least-squares parabola method.

The proposed architecture requires a reduced silicon area considering the fact that the MACs come for free as these are FPGA's built-in cores. The hardware is fast because it is massively parallel. Besides, the proposed hardware can adjust itself on-the-fly to the user-defined configuration of the neural network, with no extra hardware changes, which is a very nice characteristic in robot-like systems considering the possibility of the same piece of hardware may be exploited in different tasks. This feature if the hardware is very used in bio-inspired learning application.

The remaining of this chapter is organized as follows: In Section 2, a brief introduction to the computational model behind artificial neural networks is given; In Section 3, it is shown how to approximate the sigmoid output function, so it can be implemented via the inherent computation using digital hardware; In Section 4, some hardware implementation issues about the proposed design, that makes it original, efficient and compact are explained; In Section 5, the detailed design of the proposed ANN hardware is presented; Last but no least important, In Section 6, some useful conclusions and new orientations for future work are drawn and pointed out respectively.

ANNS COMPUTATIONAL MODEL

In this section a brief introduction to the computational model used in neural networks is given. Generally, it is constituted of few layers, each of which includes several neurons. The number of neurons in distinct layers may be different and consequently the number of inputs and that of outputs may be different (Hassoun, 1995).

The model of one artificial neuron requires m inputs, say $x_1, x_2, \ldots, x_m$ and the synaptic weights associated with these inputs, say $w_1, w_2, \ldots, w_m$. The weighted sum v, also called activation of the neuron, is defined in (1). The model usually includes an output (activation) function $\varphi(\cdot)$ that is applied to the neuron activation before it is fed forwardly as input to the next layer neurons.

$$v = \sum_{i=0}^{m} x_i \cdot w_i \qquad (1)$$

where $x_0 = 1$ and $w_0 = b$ (a noise in v). The non-linearity of the neuron is often achieved by the output function, which may be the *hyperbolic tangent* (*tansig*) or *logistic sigmoid* (*logsig*) (Hassoun, 1995). In some cases, $\varphi(v)$ may be linear.

A typical ANN operates in two necessary stages: *learning* and *feed-forward computing*. The learning stage consists of supplying known patterns to the neural network so that the network can adjust the involved weights. Once the network has learned to recognize the provided patterns, the network is ready to operate, performing the feed-forward computing. In this stage, the network is supplied with an input data or pattern(s), which may or not be one of those given in learning stage, and verify how the network responds (in its output). This allows one to know whether the neural network could recognize the input data. The precision of the net in recognizing the new input patterns depends on the quality of its learning stage and on its generalization. As previously mentioned, here the only is with the implementation of the feed-forward computing stage of the MLP Neural Network.

It is now suitable to study the numeric representation used in this work: it is based on Fractional Fixed Point (FFP) (Saint-Jones & Gu, 2003). The idea of this technique is to represent a real number as a fraction of integers. The main objective is to escape from representation and mathematic operations (sum, subtraction and multiplication) of the IEEE floating Point, which require considerable silicon area, in hardware terms. When a real number is treated as a fraction, only basic-integer operations (performed by combinational circuitry) are used, so that a more simple hardware is required.

Given a real a, e.g., somehow it is converted to a fraction using one of know conversion algorithms. This conversion is not a responsibility of the ANN hardware. The latter gets directly a fraction in a binary representation of 33 bits: numerator (16 bits) and denominator (17 bits). Numerator is a non-negative integer, i.e., natural. The arithmetic sign of the fraction is chosen (arbitrarily) to be placed in the bit length of denominator. So, this one has 16 bits to allocate a non-zero-natural number and more 1 bit to express the sign of the fraction (see Figure 1). Thus, one can also say Denominator (17 bits) is a non-zero integer.

Figure 1. Binary representation of a fraction

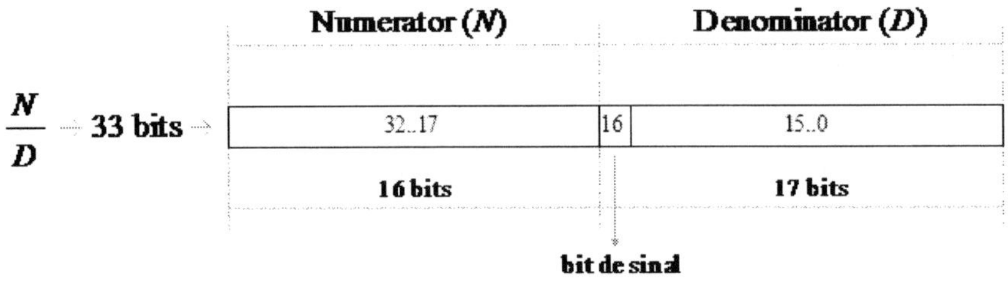

Conversion: $a \mapsto \frac{N_a}{D_a}$ or $a \mapsto frac(a)$

Example 1: $0.625 \mapsto \frac{5}{8}$

Example 2: $-0.0028 \mapsto \frac{7}{-2500}$

wherein a is a floating-point number, N_a is the numerator (natural) and D_a is the denominator (non-zero integer).

Any sum, subtraction and multiplication with fractions provide another fraction which may be put in the form of a natural numerator and a non-zero-integer denominator. Let a and b be two real numbers, the basic operations with fractions are presented below.

Sum: $a + b \mapsto \frac{N_a}{D_a} + \frac{N_b}{D_b} = \frac{N_a \times D_b + D_a \times N_b}{D_a \times D_b}$

$= \frac{\text{Natural}}{\text{Non} - \text{zero integer}}$

Subtraction:

$a - b \mapsto \frac{N_a}{D_a} - \frac{N_b}{D_b} = \frac{N_a \times D_b - D_a \times N_b}{D_a \times D_b}$

$= \frac{\text{Natural}}{\text{Non} - \text{zero integer}}$

Multiplication: $a \times b \mapsto \frac{N_a}{D_a} \times \frac{N_b}{D_b} = \frac{N_a \times N_b}{D_a \times D_b}$

$= \frac{\text{Natural}}{\text{Non} - \text{zero integer}}$

ANN hardware operates with a fraction in the binary representation of Figure 1. When a real number is converted into a fraction (considering a limited bit length for both numerator and denominator), there is a loss of accuracy involved. Therefore, it is quite important (in a conversion process) to search for a fraction that presents the minimum error regarding the given real number.

APPROXIMATION OF THE OUTPUT FUNCTION

Unlike the activation of a neuron (the weighted sum, v), which includes operations that can be easily and efficiently implemented in hardware, the output function requires a special care before the computation involved can be modeled in hardware. Without loss of generality, one can chose to use the logistic sigmoid, defined in (2), as the output function for all neurons in the ANN hardware.

$$Sigmoid(v) = \frac{1}{1 - \exp(-v)} \qquad (2)$$

To allow an efficient implementation of Eq. 2, in hardware, one can proceed with least-squares parabola method, using 3 quadratic polynomials in order to approximate the exponential decay: $\exp(-v)$. Initially, consider the case $v \geq 0$, as shown in Figures 2–5. The same method could be applied to the tangent hyperbolic function too.

Figure 2. exp(−v) in the interval [0,8]

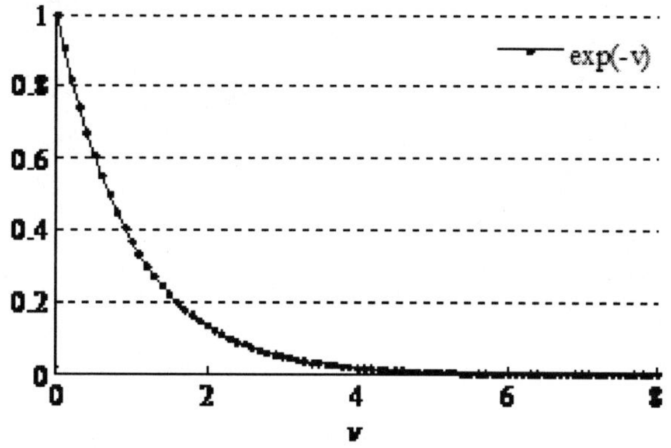

Figure 3. Second-degree curve fitting: 21 points of exp(−v), in [0,2]

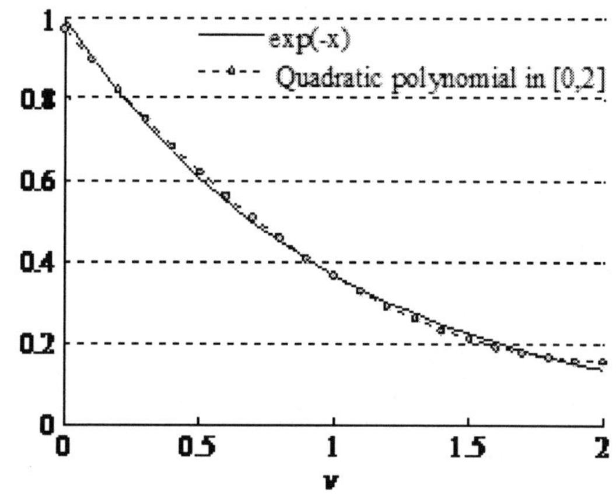

In Figure 3, for example, the approximation method generates the following quadratic polynomial, for $v \in [0, 2]$:

$$\exp(-v) \approx f_{[0,2]}(v) = 0.1987234 \cdot v^2 - 0.8072780 \cdot v + 0.9748092 \quad (3)$$

It is now known that the ANN hardware operates with fractions, which representation is depicted in Figure 1. So, it will be better to express the polynomial of Eq. (3) in the hardware parlance.

$$f_{[0,2]}(v) \approx \frac{12858}{64703} \cdot \left(\frac{N_v}{D_v}\right)^2 + \frac{11691}{-14482} \cdot \left(\frac{N_v}{D_v}\right) + \frac{56072}{57521} \quad (4)$$

In (4), there are 3 multiplications (2 represented by point and the one to compute the squaring) and 2 additions (represented by +) with fractions to be performed. As the computational time is also one of the concerns in this work, it is possible to save one operation (multiplication) using the identity $av^2+bv = v(av+b)$. Computation of the fraction polynomial in (4) leads to the fraction in (5), wherein $F_{[0,2]}(v)$ is a fractional function in $v \in [0, 2]$.

$$f_{[0,2]}(v) \approx F_{[0,2]}(v) = \frac{N_{F_{[0,2]}(v)}}{D_{F_{[0,2]}(v)}} \quad (5)$$

Figure 4. Second-degree curve fitting: 21 points of exp(−v), in [2,4]

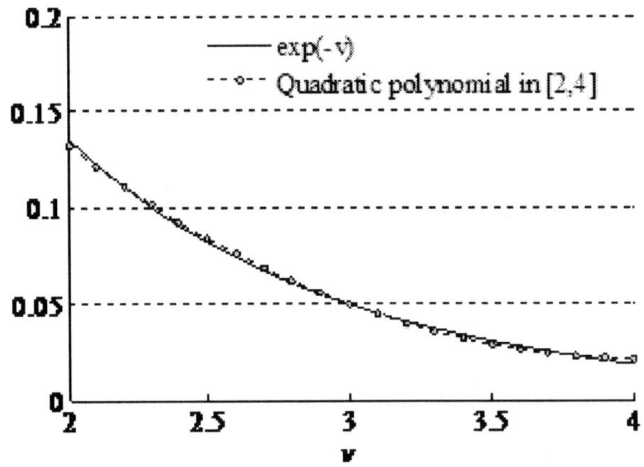

Figure 5. Second-degree curve fitting: 41 points of exp(−v), in [4,8]

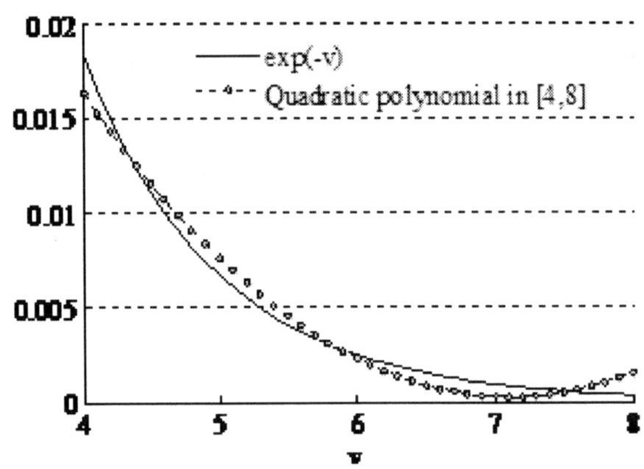

In general, for $v \geq 0$, one can say that $\exp(-v)$ is approximated by a fraction $F(v)$, so that $\exp(-v) \approx F(v)$, wherein $F(v)$ can be $F_{[0,2]}(v)$, $F_{[2,4]}(v)$, $F_{[4,8]}(v)$ or $frac(0)$. Therewith, the ANN hardware computes an approximate-quadratic polynomial in a fractional form, when $v \in [0, 8[$; and for $v \geq 0$, the hardware approximates $\exp(-v)$ to zero, i.e., to $frac(0)$. Thus, the fractional form of the logistic sigmoid, $\varphi(v)$, defined in (2), is obtained using the following considerations.

$$\exp(-v) \approx F(v) = \frac{N_{F(v)}}{D_{F(v)}} \Rightarrow \phi(v) = \frac{1}{1+\exp(-v)} \approx \frac{1}{1+F(v)} \quad (6)$$

So,

$$\phi(v) \approx \frac{1}{1+\dfrac{N_{F(v)}}{D_{F(v)}}} \Rightarrow \phi(v) \approx \frac{D_{F(v)}}{D_{F(v)}+N_{F(v)}},$$

wherein $v \geq 0$. (7)

Finally, the fractional form of $\varphi(v)$, for $v \geq 0$, is computed as follows:

Figure 6. Absolute Error: $|\varphi(v)-\varphi_q(v)|$

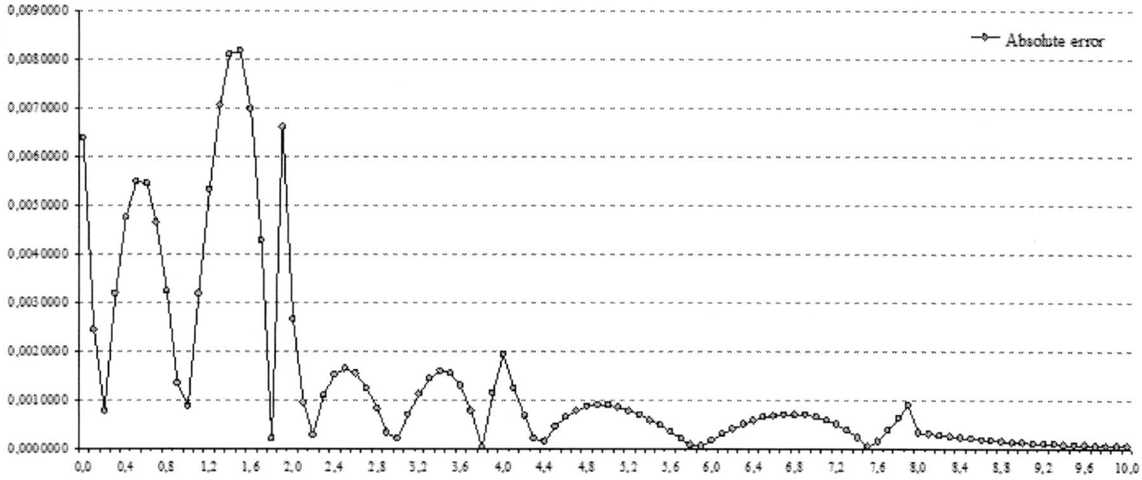

For $\frac{N_v}{D_v} < 0$, $frac(\phi(v)) = \frac{N_{\phi(v)}}{D_{\phi(v)}}$ is easily obtained from $\frac{D_{F(v)}}{D_{F(v)} + N_{F(v)}}$ (8)

When v is negative ($v<0$), one can take advantage of a logistic-sigmoid property: $\varphi(v)=1-\varphi(-v)$. Since $-v > 0$, there is no problem if (6) and (7) are used to determine $\varphi(-v)$, by replacing v to $-v$.

$$\phi(-v) \approx \frac{1}{1+\frac{N_{F(-v)}}{D_{F(-v)}}} \Rightarrow \phi(-v) \approx \frac{D_{F(-v)}}{D_{F(-v)} + N_{F(-v)}}$$

$-v \geq 0$ (9)

So,

$$\phi(v) \approx 1 - \frac{D_{F(-v)}}{D_{F(-v)} + N_{F(-v)}} \Rightarrow \phi(v) \approx \frac{N_{F(-v)}}{D_{F(-v)} + N_{F(-v)}}$$

$v \leq 0$ (8)

Finally, for $v < 0$, the fractional form of $\varphi(v)$ is computed as follows:

For $\frac{N_v}{D_v} < 0$, $frac(\phi(v)) = \frac{N_{\phi(v)}}{D_{\phi(v)}}$ is easily obtained from $\frac{N_{F(-v)}}{D_{F(-v)} + N_{F(-v)}}$ (9)

The intervals [0, 2], [2, 4] and [4, 8] were not chosen arbitrarily: the extremes 2, 4 and 8 are attractive for efficient evaluation if a fraction belongs to one of those intervals. For example, if $v \geq 0$, and so $frac(v) \geq 0$, the comparison in (10) is easily performed, in hardware, by left shifting and comparing (logical test). If, instead of 2 in (10), it were 4, hardware would shift twice, and so if it were 8, three times.

$$\frac{N_v}{D_v} < 2 \Leftrightarrow \frac{N_v}{2} < D_v \qquad (10)$$

Figure 6 shows the absolute error between $\varphi(v)$, calculated with no approximation, and $\varphi_q(v)$-obtained with an approximation of $\exp(-v)$ by one of the approximate-*q*uadratic polynomials (Figures 3, 4 and 5), for $v \in [0, 8[$; and if $v \geq 8$, $\exp(-v)$ is approximated to 0 (zero). The maximum error obtained is ≈ 0.0081757, in the interval $v \in [0, 2]$. One can conclude that the least-square-

Figure 7. Neural network with two inputs, three layers and one output Y

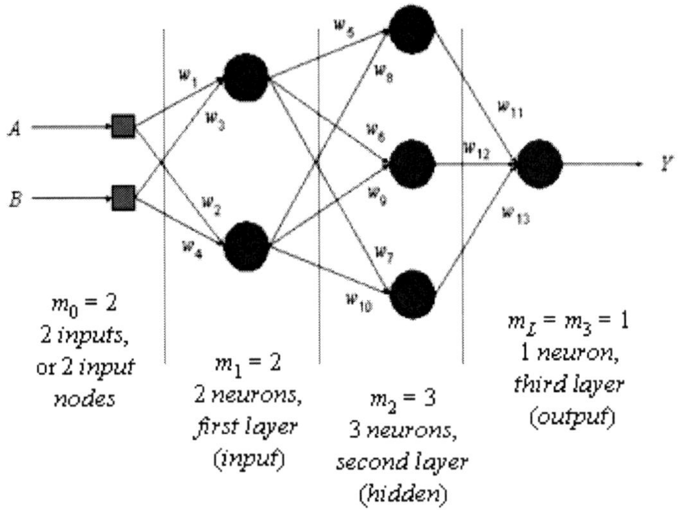

parabola approximation is better as curve-fitting in $v \in [2, 8[$

IMPLEMENTATION ISSUES

An Artificial Neural Network is a set of several interconnected neurons arranged in layers. Let L be the number of layers. Each layer has its own number of neurons. Let m_i be the number of neurons in layer i. The neurons are connected by the synaptic connections. Some neurons get the input data of the network, so they are called *input neurons* and thus compose the input layer ($i = 1$). Other neurons export their outputs to the outside world, so these are called output neurons ($i=L$) and thus compose the output layer. Neurons placed on the layer $i = 2$ up to layer $i = L-1$ are called the hidden neurons because they belong to the hidden layers. Figure 7 shows a simple example of an ANN. The output of each neuron, save output neurons, represents an input of all neurons placed in the next layer.

The computation corresponding to a given layer starts only when that of the corresponding previous layer has finished. Our ANN hardware has just one physical layer of neurons, which constitutes of n neurons, wherein n is maximum number of neurons per layer, considering all layers of the Neural Network to be computed. For instance, for the net of Figure 7, the parameter k is 3. This single real layer (or physical layer) is used to implement all layers of the network. As only one layer operates at a time, this allows us to minimize drastically the silicon area required without altering the response time of the net. Still considering Figure 7, the first stage of the computation would use only 2 neurons, then in the second stage all three physical neurons would be exploited and in the last stage, only one neuron would be useful. So instead of having 6 physically implemented neurons, our hardware requires only half that number to operate. ANN hardware treats each net layer of Figure 7 as virtual layers.

Besides reducing the number of neurons that are actually implemented in hardware, our design takes advantage of some built-in cores that come for free in now-a-days FPGAs. These blocks are called MACs (Multiply, add and Accumulate), which are usually used in DSPs (Digital Signal Processors) and their architecture is shown in Figure 8. The MACs blocks are perfect to perform

Figure 8. Built-in MAC blocks in FPGAs

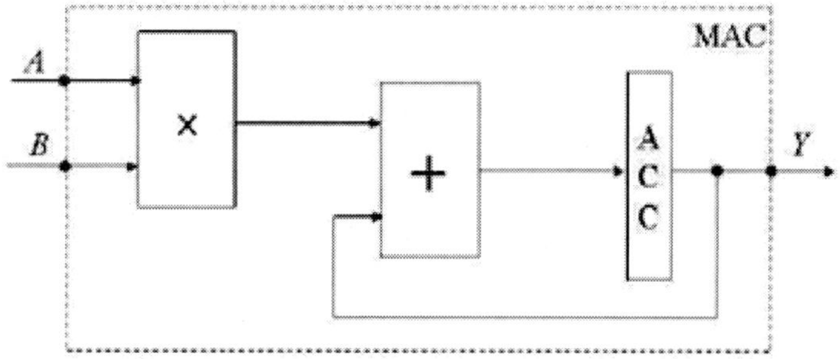

Figure 9. Interface of the ANN hardware

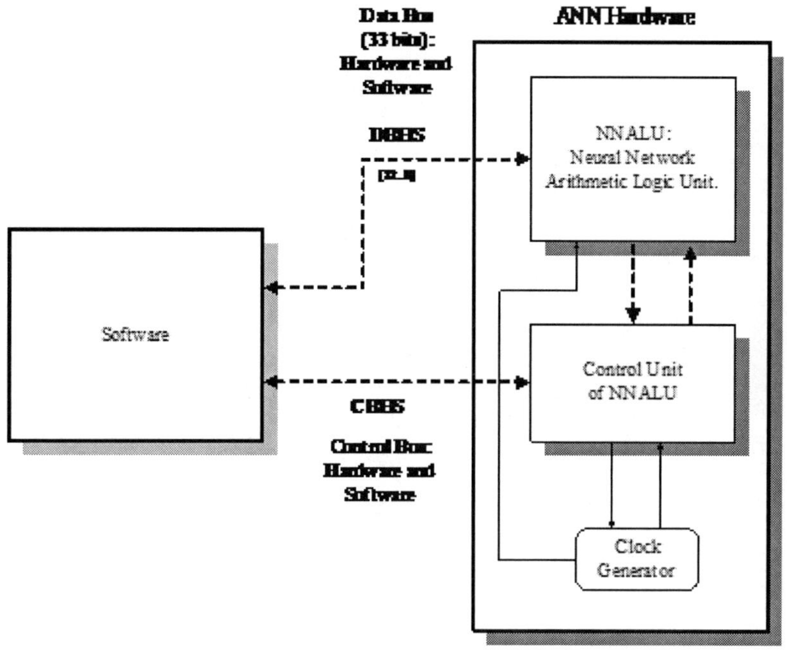

the weighted sum. Recall that the neuron output function, $\varphi(v)$, our ANN hardware will perform only additions and multiplications, as explained in Section 3. Observe that the computation involved in this function is sum of products, with fractions, from the approximate-quadratic polynomials of Figures 3, 4 and 5; so the MACs can be used in this purpose too. In this way, the block designed for computing the weighted sum is also used to compute the output function.

ANN HARDWARE ARCHITECTURE

The ANN hardware interface is illustrated in Figure 9, wherein three other components are included: NNALU, Control Unit of NNALU and Clock Generator. An external software is necessary to control ANN hardware computation. This software feeds the hardware (via DBHS) with the inputs, weights and biases which Neural Network needs. Software still defines (via CBHS) how

Figure 10. Details of the Arithmetic Logic Unit of the ANN hardware (NNALU)

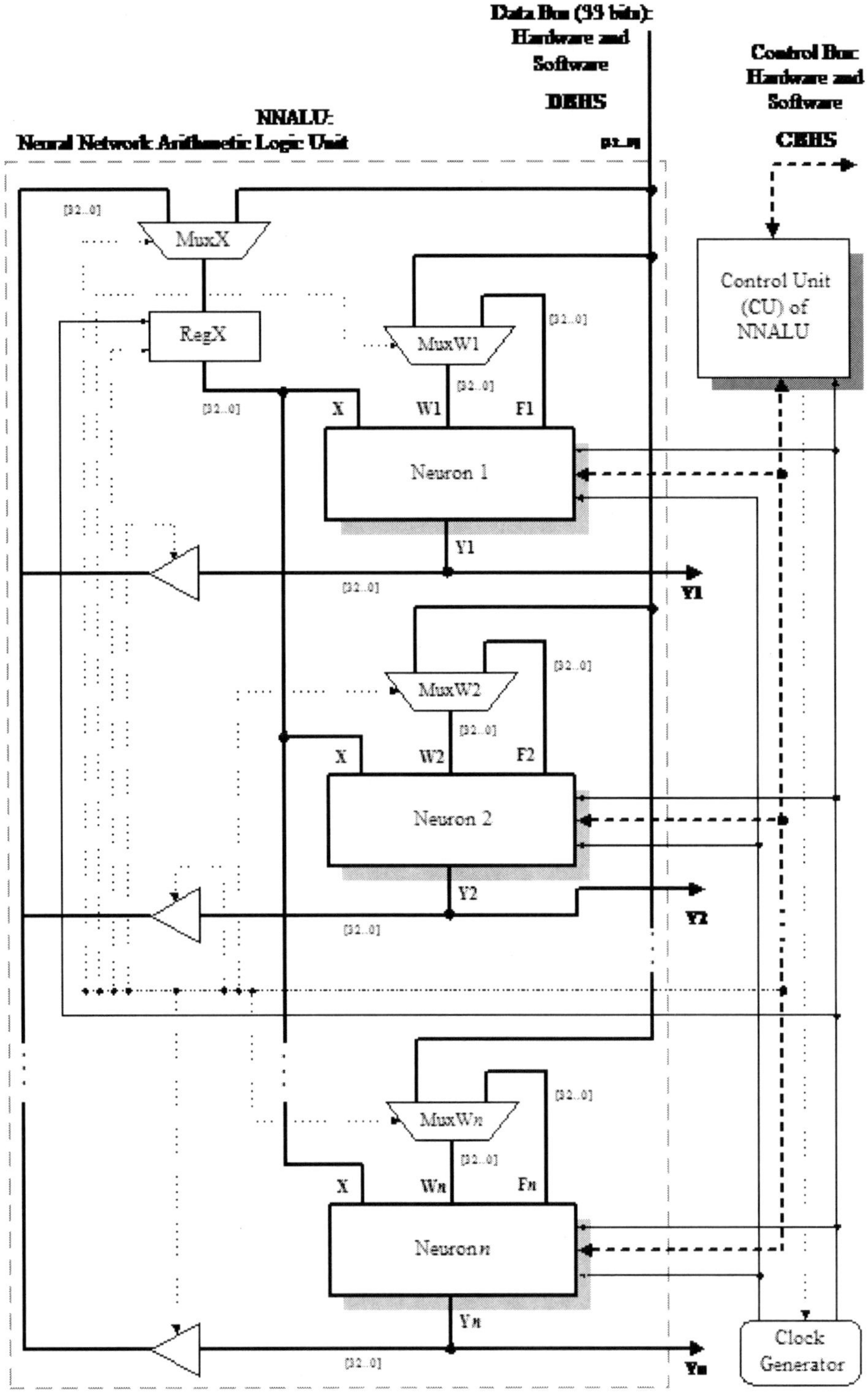

Figure 11. Details of the Neuron Architecture

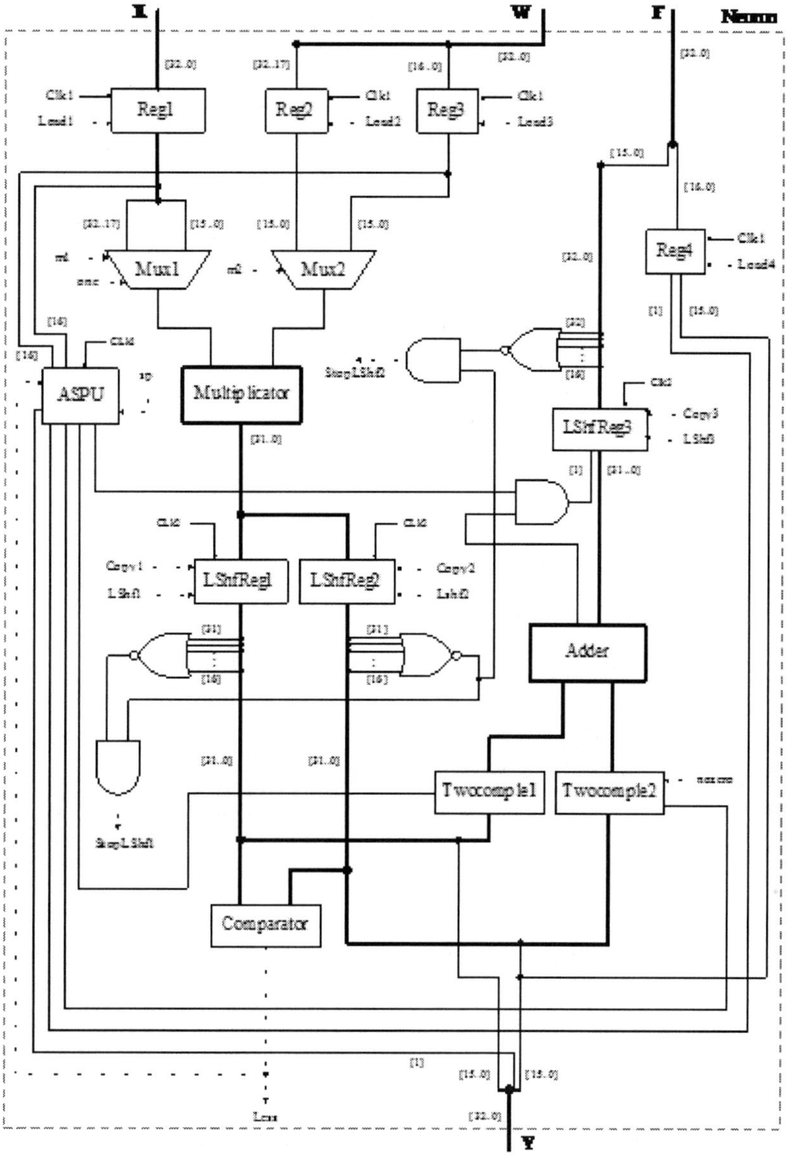

many neurons per layer hardware is going to work and all necessary steps for accomplishing the whole feed forward computing of the network.

Focusing on the ANN hardware, Control Unit of NNALU encompasses all control components for computing all neural network specific operations: sums, products and comparisons with fractions. The blocks that perform these operations are within NNALU-the Arithmetic Logic Unit of the ANN hardware. Clock Generator defines the time basis of the ANN hardware and synchronizes all operations in NNALU (which are commanded by the Control Unit).

Figure 10 shows details of NNALU. It is possible to see the physical layer with *n* Neurons. During the ANN hardware performance, the Neurons work in parallel, even though not necessarily all physical neurons are needed in the layer. Recall

Figure 12. Arithmetic Sign Processing Unit (fraction sign processing)

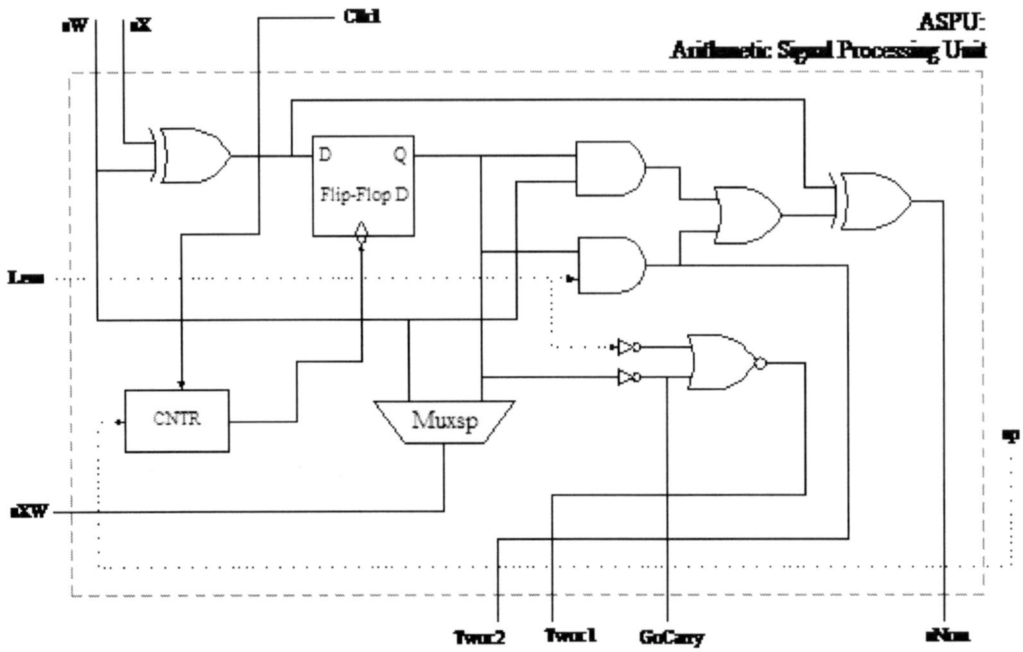

that some layers in the Neural Network may have fewer neurons than *n*.

One can see, the output of each hardware neuron (Y_i) goes out of the NNALU, to furnish the output of the network, when the whole computation is finished. Y_i also returns to the neurons by a buffer tri-state, a multiplexer MuxX and a register RegX. This Feedback action allows the reuse of one physical layer for computing all layers of the Neural Network (*virtual* layers). Multiplexer MuxX is also an interface of communication between software and NNALU, wherein the latter receives Inputs and Biases from software. MuxW*i*, on the other hand, allows the weights (from software) get into Neurons of the NALU.

All Neurons in Figure 10 have the same hardware architecture, which is depicted in Figure 11. The latter shows Multiplier and Adder, which are used for the operations between numerators and denominators of fractions (see Section 2). Still in Figure 11, the buses X, W, F and Y carry fractions in the model of Figure 1. Registers are useful to make data stable during multiplications, additions or any other operation. Mux1 allows the selection of an operand for the Multiplier: a numerator or a denominator of X. Mux2 do the similar task, regarding W. This way, it becomes feasible to perform X × Y (which are fractions).

The arithmetic signs of X and W (Figure 11) go to ASPU (Figure 12), where is given the sign of the fraction obtained by multiplying and adding two other fractions. ASPU also decides if an Adder operand will experiment the two's complement (Twocomple1 or Twocomple2, Figure 11). The Adder component is responsible to additions of the neuron's weighted sum. LShfReg3 and Reg4 are assigned to accumulate the weighted sum as a fraction: numerator in LShfReg3 and denominator in Reg4.

In Figure 11, Comparator performs the logical test in (10) of Section 3. Numerator is left-shifted by LShfReg1 and compared with the denominator, which comes from LShfReg2. Once the hardware computes the output function (*logsig*) using an approximate-quadratic polynomial, the same components used in the weighted sum are also taken advantage, because a polynomial involves sums and products. All Left Shifters (LShfReg1, LShfReg2 and LShfReg3) are responsible to keep numerator or denominator with 16 bits, each one, not considering the bit for arithmetic sign. For instance, if a multiplication is performed with two fractions, the result is a numerator and a denominator with 32 bits each one; then, left shifters are used to put them back with 16 bits, each one.

In Figure 12, component CNTR releases the negative transition of Clk1 to the Flip-Flop D, if *sp* = 1. ASPU works in parallel with multiplications and additions of fractions during weighted sum and output function computation.

Each Neuron, in Figure 10, works in parallel with another one. If one layer is in computation, the next one is being prepared to initialize. When all layers is completely ended, ANN hardware returns a sign to its Control Unit, informing that the output of the Neural Network is available. So, Control Unit returns to software that the whole computation is done.

CONCLUSION

In this chapter, a novel hardware architecture for processing an artificial neural network, whose configuration (number of neurons per layer and etc) can be changed on-the-fly without any extra effort, is designed. The design takes advantage of the built-in MACs block that come for free in modern FPGAs. The model was specified in VHDL (Navabi, 1998), simulated to validate its functionality. The main concern now is to work on the synthesis process to evaluate time and area requirements. The comparison of the performance result of our design will be then compared to both the binary-radix straight forward design and the stochastic computing based design.

ACKNOWLEDGMENT

The authors are grateful to FAPERJ (Fundação de Amparo à Pesquisa do Estado do Rio de Janeiro, http://www.faperj.br) and CNPq (Conselho Nacional de Desenvolvimento Científico e Tecnológico, http://www.cnpq.br) for their continuous financial support.

REFERENCES

Bade, S. L., & Hutchings, B. L. (1994). FPGA-Based Stochastic Neural Networks Implementation, *Proceedings of IEEE Workshop on FPGAs for Custom Computing Machines*, 189-198.

Brown, B. D., & Card, H. C. (2001). Stochastic Neural Computation II: Soft Competitive Learning. *IEEE Transactions on Computers*, *50*(9), 906–920. doi:10.1109/12.954506

Harkin, J., Morgan, F., McDaid, L., Hall, S., McGinley, B., & Cawley, S. (2009). A Reconfigurable and Biologically Inspired Paradigm for Computation using Networks-on-chip and Spiking Neural Networks. *International Journal of Reconfigurable Computing*, (908740): 1–13. doi:10.1155/2009/908740

Hassoun, M. H. (1995). *Fundamentals of Artificial Neural Networks*. Cambridge, MA: MIT Press.

Moerland, P., & Fiesler, E. (1996). Neural Network Adaptation to Hardware Implementations. In Fiesler, E., & Beale, R. (Eds.), *Handbook of Neural Computation*. New York: Oxford Press.

Navabi, Z. (1998). *Analysis and Modeling of Digital Systems* (2nd ed.). New York: McGraw Hill.

Nedjah, N., & Mourelle, L. M. (2007). Reconfigurable Hardware for Neural Networks: Binary radix vs. Stochastic. *Journal of Neural Computing and Applications*, *16*(3), 249–155. doi:10.1007/s00521-007-0086-x

Saint-Jones, P., & Gu, D. (2003). *Fractional Fixed Point Neural Network: an introduction*. Department of Computer Science, University of Essex.

Seul, J., & Sung, S. K. (2007). Hardware Implementation of a Real-Time Neural Network Controller With a DSP and an FPGA for Nonlinear Systems. *IEEE Transactions on Industrial Electronics*, *54*(1), 265–271. doi:10.1109/TIE.2006.888791

Tuffy, F., McDaid, L. J., Kwan, V. W., Alderman, J., McGinnity, T. M., & Santos, J. A. (2007). Inter-Neuron Communications Strategies for Spiking Neural Networks. *Neurocomputing*, *71*(1–3), 30–44. doi:10.1016/j.neucom.2006.11.027

Xilinx, Inc. (2009). *Foundation Series Software*. Retrieved from http://www.xilinx.com

Chapter 14
A Novel DCGA Optimization Technique for Guaranteed BIBO-Stable Frequency-Response Masking Digital Filters Incorporating Bilinear Lossless Discrete-Integrator IIR Interpolation Sub-Filters

Syed Bokhari
University of Alberta, Canada

Behrouz Nowrouzian
University of Alberta, Canada

ABSTRACT

This work is concerned with the development of a novel diversity-controlled (DC) genetic algorithm (GA) for the design and rapid optimization of frequency-response masking (FRM) digital filters incorporating bilinear lossless discrete-integrator (LDI) IIR interpolation sub-filters. The selection of FRM approach is inspired by the fact it lends itself to the design of practical sharp-transition band digital filters in terms of gradual-transition band FIR interpolation sub-filters. The proposed DCGA optimization is carried out over the canonical-signed-digit (CSD) multiplier coefficient space, resulting in FRM digital filters which are capable of direct implementation in digital hardware. A novel CSD look-up table (LUT) scheme is developed so that in every stage of DCGA optimization, the IIR interpolation sub-filters constituent in the intermediate and final FRM digital filters are guaranteed to be automatically BIBO stable. The proposed DCGA optimization permits simultaneous optimization of the magnitude-frequency as well of the group-delay frequency response of the desired FRM digital filters. An example is given to illustrate the application of the resulting DCGA optimization to the design of a lowpass FRM digital filter incorporating a fifth-order bilinear-LDI interpolation subfilter.

DOI: 10.4018/978-1-60960-018-1.ch014

INTRODUCTION

In many practical situations in the design and implementation of circuits and systems on hardware platforms, it is required for the resulting piece of hardware to be capable of adapting to changing environments. The main motivation behind this adaptability is to improve the performance characteristics of the resulting hardware implementation, and to prolong its operational lifetime. The notion of Evolvable Hardware (EH) has been developed to refer to a hardware piece that can change not only its performance parameters but also its configuration dynamically and autonomously by interacting with its environment. This is achieved through the use of reconfigurable hardware (e.g. programmable logic devices (PLDs) and field programmable gate arrays (FPGAs) on the one hand, and artificial intelligence computations (including evolutionary algorithms (EAs) and artificial neural networks (ANNs) on the other (Stoica, 2000).

The autonomous reconfigurabilty feature of EH makes it fundamentally different from conventional hardware, where the architecture and function of the hardware remain fixed past its implementation. Moreover, while programmable hardware devices like FPGAs allow for limited functional changes after implementation, such changes can only take place by human intervention. With the use of EAs and ANNs, however, EH is capable of autonomously changing its configuration and function, providing an attractive approach to making the hardware "soft" by adapting it to its environment dynamically (Higuchi, Liu, & Yao, 2006).

In principle, EH can be considered as a combination of hardware and its control subsystem, where the purpose of the control subsystem is to set the configuration and function of the hardware proper dynamically based on the environment. This is usually the case when the corresponding control subsystem has been developed and refined to the extent that it can co-exist with the hardware on the same platform for online operation. Otherwise, i.e. in offline applications, the control subsystem resides separately from the hardware proper, usually in the form of a computational engine. Of course, once the operation of the computational engine has been streamlined adequately, it can be incorporated as a part and parcel of the actual EH.

This work is concerned with the development of a control subsystem for a class of EH frequency-response masking (FRM) digital filters by employing an EA, where the EA is applied to the optimization of the values of the FRM digital multiplier coefficients based on given a set of target design specifications. Such an optimization turns out to have a multi-modal cost function, and requires built-in internal or external mechanisms for escaping from local optimal solutions during the course of optimization.

Genetic Algorithms (GAs), (Goldberg, 1989) are optimization techniques which simulate natural selection and reproduction to move towards an optimal solution, and closely resemble the concept of biological evolution. It is well known that GAs provide a promising approach to solve discrete and multimodal optimization problems due to the fact that they are capable of automatically finding near-optimal solutions while keeping the computational complexity of the optimization at moderate levels. Consequently, they have emerged as an attractive alternative for the optimization of FIR as well as IIR digital filters. These algorithms encode the digital filter design variables into a chromosome (usually as a binary string), and proceed towards an optimal solution through the evolution of a population of potential candidate chromosomes in an iterative manner from one generation to the next.

Unfortunately, the conventional GAs do not search the solution space robustly due to lack of mechanisms through which entrapment at local optimal solutions can be avoided. It was demonstrated by Shimodaira in (Shimodaira, 2001) that diversity control (DC) can be exploited to help to increase the convergence speed of conventional GAs. The main principle behind DCGA is to increase the diversity of the population pool through the incorporation of additional non-elite chromosomes based on a pair of external control parameters.

In principle, DCGA is capable of finding the global optimal solution provided that no bound is imposed on the constituent number of generations. However, in practical situations, DCGA is set to terminate once all of the design specifications have been satisfied. In such situations, the resulting solution may or may not represent the global optimal solution, but simply a solution that satisfies all of the given target design specifications.

The philosophy advocated to designing an EH FRM digital filter is to employ DCGA to generate a population of individual chromosomes, where each chromosome represents a candidate FRM digital filter. Subsequently, the candidate FRM digital filters can either be simulated in software or physically implemented on a reconfigurable device, and the performance characteristics of the resulting FRM digital filter can be assessed relative to the target design specifications. In the next iteration, a new population of candidate FRM digital filter chromosomes is generated from the best chromosomes from the preceding generation, resulting in increasingly better candidate FRM digital filters. If performed judiciously, over time, the DCGA controls the evolution of the EH FRM digital filter to exhibit near-optimal behavior.

This work focuses on the use of DCGA to optimize FRM digital filters lending themselves to direct implementation in hardware. In particular, it is demonstrated here how biologically inspired learning algorithms such as DCGA can be modified (for instance, by intelligently adjusting a pair of DC parameters) to satisfy application specific constraints, without recourse to extensive additional computational efforts. Of course, it may be possible to employ similar methods, e.g. other EAs or ANNs, instead, or in combination with DCGA, for this purpose.

It should be pointed out that as a software engine, DCGA tends to exhibit slow convergence especially for complex problems (see e.g., (Stoica, 2000)). Therefore, it may plausible to attempt to incorporate DCGA as an embedded hardware engine in a run-time reconfigurable (Sakr, & Groiza, 2005) FRM digital filter hardware. Such an attempt rests on the fact that a dedicated hardware DCGA engine offers a substantial reduction in evolution time, ultimately resulting in online EH FRM digital filters. However, run-time reconfigurable hardware is still awaiting corresponding adequate technological advances.

BACKGROUND

Digital filters play a central role in modern digital signal processing (DSP) systems. With the emerging DSP technologies and applications, there is an ever growing demand for computationally efficient digital filters. In practical applications, e.g. in audio signal processing or data compression, digital filters with sharp transition bands are required. However, narrow transition bandwidth digital filters become less economical if designed by using the conventional techniques.

Frequency-response masking (FRM) approach has been developed (Lim, 1986) for the design of practical sharp transition band digital filters in terms of a gradual transition band finite-impulse response (FIR) interpolation sub-filters. However, due to the fact that the lengths of the constituent FIR interpolation sub-filters are inversely proportional to their transition bandwidths, the FRM digital filter design approach may require FIR interpolation sub-filters with prohibitively high orders.

It is well known that infinite impulse-response (IIR) digital filters generally possess orders which are substantially lower than those of the corresponding FIR digital filters satisfying similar design specifications. Therefore, IIR digital filters prove to be attractive alternative candidates for interpolation sub-filters in the FRM digital filter design approach (Johansson, & Wanhammar, 1997). However, the resulting IIR interpolation digital sub-filters may suffer from BIBO stability problems, in addition to inevitably giving rise to group-delay distortions.

This work is concerned with the development of a novel technique for the rapid optimization of FRM digital filters employing hardware efficient IIR interpolation sub-filters. In this optimization, the corresponding design specifications include both the magnitude-frequency as well as the group-delay frequency response characteristics of the resulting FRM digital filters.

From a practical point of view, particularly in the hardware implementation of the FRM digital filters, there is every incentive to represent the constituent multiplier coefficients in computationally efficient number systems, e.g. in signed power- of-two (SPT) or canonical signed-digit (CSD) number systems, while still satisfying all the other design specifications. This is mainly due to the fact that such number systems permit the representation of the constituent multiplier coefficient values in terms of only a few non-zero digits within the coefficient wordlength, thereby reducing the corresponding multiplication operations to few shift-and-add operations.

In order to be compatible with a final digital hardware implementation in a direct manner (i.e. without any further transformations), the optimization of FRM digital filters must be carried out over the finite word-length multiplier coefficient space. The most widely used techniques for such optimizations include the simulated-annealing (SA) algorithms (Chen, & Lian, 2006) and GAs (Wu, & Nowrouzian, 2008). This work is concerned with the application of GAs.

(Wu, & Nowrouzian, 2008) applied GAs to the optimization of the magnitude frequency-response of an intermediate-frequency (IF) digital filters over the CSD multiplier coefficient space, where the IF digital filter chromosome was formed by the concatenation of the ternary representation of the constituent multiplier coefficient values. (Kilambi, & Nowrouzian, 2007) developed a nonlinear programming approach for the optimization of FRM digital filters incorporating FIR interpolation filters over the signed power-of-two (SPT) multiplier coefficient space. They also applied GAs to the same FRM digital filter optimization problem, leading to digital filters with superior magnitude frequency-response characteristics. In addition, they demonstrated the fact that the use of GAs overcomes the inherent drawback of the hitherto linear programming techniques which require the separate optimization of the constituent FIR interpolation digital sub-filters.

It is well known that GAs are likely to get trapped at local optimal solutions. DCGA resolves this problem by providing an external control over the population diversity throughout the course of optimization. In this way, DCGA leads to much faster optimization speeds arising from more intelligent exploration of the search space. The computational speed for DCGA is much more than those associated with using variable crossover and mutation rates reported by (Srinivas, & Patnaik, 1994), and of those of the SA technique reported by (Cen, & Lian, 2006). Seeker optimization algorithm (SOA), (Dai, Zhu, & Chen, 2007) uses empirical gradients and is therefore not very effective for highly irregular and non-linear systems. However, unfortunately, a direct application of DCGA to the optimization of the above FRM digital filters over the CSD multiplier coefficient space gives rise to two different problems:

- The first problem arises because of the fact that the operations of crossover and mutation in the course of DCGA optimization may lead to chromosomes that may no longer conform to the CSD number format.
- The second problem, on the other hand, stems from the fact that DCGA optimization may result in a solution chromosome that satisfies the given magnitude and group-delay frequency-response design specifications, but that the corresponding

IIR interpolation digital subfilter is not bounded-input bounded-output (BIBO) stable.

(Nowrouzian, Mercier, & Kilambi, 2007) resolved the first problem in the context of the DCGA optimization of FRM digital filters having FIR interpolation digital sub-filters. This was facilitated by generating an indexed LUT of permissible CSD multiplier coefficient values (with pre-specified word-lengths and pre-specified maximum number of nonzero digits), and by employing the indices of the resulting multiplier coefficient values (as opposed to their values) to represent FRM digital filter chromosomes. The key point in generating the CSD LUT is to ensure that the constituent indices form a closed set under the operations of crossover and mutation (or other similar operations) in the course of the underlying DCGA optimization so as to preserve adherence to the CSD number format.

In this work, the latter problem mentioned above is resolved by resorting to use of a set of CSD look-up tables (LUTs). These LUTs are constructed to consist of such CSD multiplier coefficient values which automatically lead to FRM digital filter chromosomes whose IIR interpolation sub-filters remain BIBO stable under the operations of crossover and mutation throughout the course of DCGA optimization. In this way, the resulting FRM digital filter chromosomes not only conform to the CSD number system, but also lead to BIBO stable interpolation sub-filters (without ever making recourse to the process of gene repair).

The proposed DCGA optimization starts from a seed FRM digital filter consisting of infinite-precision multiplier coefficient values. The corresponding infinite-precision IIR interpolation sub-filter is realized in terms of bilinear lossless discrete-integrator (bilinear-LDI) all-pass digital networks (Nowrouzian, 1989). The main advantage of the bilinear-LDI design approach is that it leads to digital filters which exhibits exceptionally low pass-band sensitivity to their multiplier coefficient values (permitting reduced multiplier coefficient word-lengths), while being minimal in the number of digital multipliers and digital unit-delays (and practically minimal in the number of digital adders as well).

The infinite-precision multiplier coefficient values are subsequently quantized to their closest CSD counterparts (to within the pre-specified word-length and the pre-specified maximum number of non-zero digits), in order to obtain a corresponding FRM digital filter consisting of finite-precision multiplier coefficient values. The resulting CSD seed FRM digital filter is subsequently used to form an initial population pool of CSD FRM digital filter chromosomes for DCGA optimization.

FRM APPROACH

The block diagram in Figure 1 shows a conventional FRM digital filter, where $H_a(z)$ represents a FIR interpolation low-pass digital sub-filter, and where $H_b(z)$ represents a power complementary counterpart of $H_a(z)$ in accordance with

$$|H_a(e^{j\omega})|^2 + |H_b(e^{j\omega})|^2 = 1 \qquad (1)$$

Here, z represent the discrete-time complex frequency, and ω represents the corresponding (normalized) real frequency-variable. Moreover, $F_0(z)$ and $F_1(z)$ represent FIR masking digital sub-filters. In addition, $H_a(z^M)$ and $H_b(z^M)$ represent M-fold interpolated versions of $H_a(z)$ and $H_b(z)$, respectively.

The FRM digital filter in Figure 1 has an overall transfer function

$$H(z) = H_a(z^M)F_0(z) + H_b(z^M)F_1(z) \qquad (2)$$

Figure 1. Block diagram representation of frequency-response masking

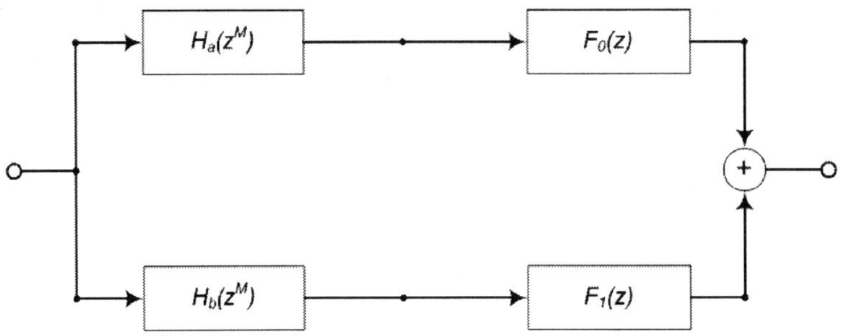

The masking digital sub-filters $F_0(z)$ and $F_1(z)$ are employed to suppress the unwanted image bands produced by the interpolated digital sub-filters $H_a(z^M)$ and $H_b(z^M)$. The interpolated digital sub-filters $H_a(z^M)$ and $H_b(z^M)$ can realize transition bands which are a factor of M sharper than those of $H_a(z)$ and $H_b(z)$, without increasing the number of required non-zero digital multipliers.

This work is concerned with the DCGA optimization of FRM digital filters over the CSD multiplier coefficient space, where the constituent interpolation digital sub-filter $H_a(z)$ and its power complementary counterpart $H_b(z)$ are realized in terms of bilinear-LDI digital all-pass networks.

Bilinear-LDI IIR Interpolation Sub-Filters

The bilinear-LDI digital filter design technique employs the bilinear frequency transformation

$$s = \frac{2}{T}\frac{(z-1)}{(z+1)} \tag{3}$$

for mapping the transfer function of a prototype reference filter from the analog to the digital domain, while using the LDI frequency transformation

$$s = \frac{1}{T}\left(z^{1/2} - z^{-1/2}\right) \tag{4}$$

for mapping the hardware realization of the prototype reference filter from the analog to digital domain, where s represents the continuous-time analog complex frequency-variable. In this work, a class of symmetrical digital filters referred to as the "elliptic filters with minimum Q-factor" (EMQF) (Rabrenovic and Lutovac, 1994) is selected for the bilinear-LDI realization of the digital sub-filters $H_a(z)$ and $H_b(z)$.

It is expedient to assume $H_a(z)$ and $H_b(z)$ are a pair of odd-ordered power complementary symmetrical low-pass (LP) and high-pass (HP) digital filters. Such digital filters can be represented as the sum and the difference of two all-pass digital networks (Willson, & Orchard, 1995) $G_0(z)$ and $G_1(z)$ in accordance with

$$\begin{aligned} H_a(z) &= \frac{G_0(z) + G_1(z)}{2} \\ H_b(z) &= \frac{G_0(z) - G_1(z)}{2} \end{aligned} \tag{5}$$

where $G_0(z)$ is odd-ordered and $G_1(z)$ is even ordered.

The bilinear-LDI digital all-pass network design technique can now be used to realize the all-pass digital networks $G_0(z)$ and $G_1(z)$. Let us represent the corresponding prototype reference analog all-pass networks $G_0(s)$ or $G_1(s)$ in the general form

$$G_{0 \text{ or } 1}(s) = \frac{P_{0 \text{ or } 1}(-s)}{P_{0 \text{ or } 1}(s)} \quad (6)$$

where $P_{0 \text{ or } 1}(s)$ is a Hurwitz polynomial of, say, order $\tilde{n}$. Then, the bilinear-LDI realization of the analog all-pass network $G_{0 \text{ or } 1}(s)$ is achieved through the following three steps:

Step 1: The transfer function $G_{0 \text{ or } 1}(s)$ is decomposed in the form

$$G_{0 \text{ or } 1}(s) = 1 - 2g_{LP \text{ or } HP}(s) \quad (7)$$

where

$$g_{LP \text{ or } HP}(s) = \frac{Z_{0 \text{ or } 1}(s)}{1 + Z_{0 \text{ or } 1}(s)} \quad (8)$$

represents a low-pass or high-pass analog filter, and where $Z_{0 \text{ or } 1}(s)$ represents a realizable reactance (consisting of capacitors and inductors only). In this way, the $Z_{0 \text{ or } 1}(s)$ can be decomposed into its Foster II canonical form in accordance with

$$Z_{0 \text{ or } 1}(s) = sC_{1,0 \text{ or } 1} + \frac{1}{sL_{1,0 \text{ or } 1}} + \sum_{i=2}^{m} \frac{sC_{i,0 \text{ or } 1}}{1 + s^2 C_{i,0 \text{ or } 1} L_{i,0 \text{ or } 1}} \quad (9)$$

where $C_{p,0 \text{ or } 1}$ (for $p = 1, 2, \ldots m$) represent capacitances, and where $L_{p,0 \text{ or } 1}$ represent inductances. In the following, in order to simplify notations, the subscripts "*LP* or *HP*" and "0 or 1" are omitted from explicit mention whenever possible.

Step 2: The pre-compensation technique in (Green, & Turner, 1990) is applied to the analog low-pass or high-pass filter $g(s)$, resulting, among others, the following capacitance and inductance modifications

$$L'_1 = L_1$$

$$C'_1 = C_1 + \frac{T}{2} + \frac{T^2}{4L_1} + \sum_{i=2}^{m} \frac{C_i \frac{T^2}{4L_i}}{C_i + \frac{T^2}{4L_i}} \quad (10)$$

and

$$L'_i = L_i \left[\frac{C_i + \frac{T^2}{4L_i}}{C_i} \right]^2$$

$$C'_i = \frac{C_i^2}{C_i + \frac{T^2}{4L_i}} \quad (11)$$

for $i = 2, 3, \ldots m$, with $m = \tilde{n} / 2$ for even $\tilde{n}$, and with $m = (\tilde{n} + 1) / 2$ for odd $\tilde{n}$.

Step3: $G(z)$ is realized as bilinear-LDI digital all-pass network as shown in Figure 2, where

$$m_{Lp} = \frac{T}{L'_p}$$

$$m_{Cp} = \frac{T}{C'_p} \quad (12)$$

where m_{Lp} and m_{Lp} represent infinite-precision multiplier coefficient values.

Finally, the interpolated digital sub-filters $H_a(z^M)$ and $H_b(z^M)$ are simply derived via an M-fold interpolation of the all-pass digital networks $G_0(z)$ and $G_1(z)$ (by replacing z by z^M throughout).

DCGA Optimization

Broadly speaking, there are two main approaches available for the optimization of digital filters. One approach is based on the conventional continuous optimization techniques, while the other is based on heuristic discrete evolutionary optimization

Figure 2. Realization of bilinear-LDI Allpass digital network G(z)

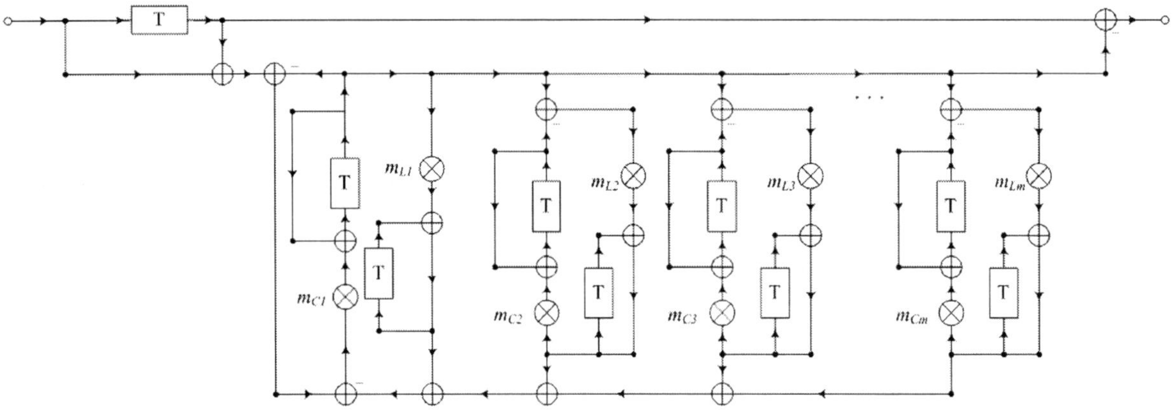

techniques. Continuous optimization techniques are usually greedy (i.e. they make use of gradient information). These techniques are used to optimize applications with continuous (infinite-precision) design variables, and they utilize the gradient information of the objective function for guiding the direction of search. Examples of continuous optimization techniques include the classical Newton's method and Parks-McClellan filter design approach, (Lee, & Oppenheim, 1997). While continuous optimization schemes usually have a well defined search direction and are capable of converging rapidly to an optimal solution, they also tend to lack mechanisms that allow them to escape local minima, in the case of design problems having multimodal cost-functions. Also, continuous optimization techniques are not directly applicable to finite-precision realizations and hardware implementations unless one uses such techniques as branch-and-bound (computationally extensive).

Discrete optimization techniques, on the other hand, may or may not require gradient information. These techniques can be successfully employed over discrete domain (i.e. when the optimization parameters are discrete variables). The most commonly used discrete optimization techniques are the GA and simulated annealing (SA).

In GAs, the method of selection is such that if there is a dominant chromosome (one that shows a comparatively high fitness value) in the population pool, then it is likely that it will produce several offspring. On the other hand, other chromosomes with lower fitness values contribute less or even no offspring at all. Consequently, in such cases, as the GA progresses from one generation to the next, the population pool experiences a rapid decline in diversity and all its chromosomes start looking very similar to or are exact replicas of the dominant chromosome.

The solution to avoiding this entrapment at local optima is to ensure that the population pool remains diverse. However, care must be taken that the GA is not made to be so diverse that the convergence rate starts to look like that of a completely random search. Consequently, an appropriate level of diversity must be constantly maintained in the population pool at all times. DCGA is a promising method developed to achieve this goal of maintaining an optimal diversity threshold within the population.

In DCGA, the members of a current population pool $P(t)$ of size N are combined together with their offspring chromosomes to form an enlarged population pool $\hat{P}(t)$ of $2N$ chromosomes, where t represents the generation number ($t = 0$ initially). This is followed by ranking the chromosomes in the enlarged population pool $\hat{P}(t)$) by evaluating their fitness values. Then, the chromosome in $\hat{P}(t)$ with the best fitness value is selected as a member of the next-generation population pool $P(t + 1)$. The remaining $N - 1$ chromosomes in the population pool $P(t + 1)$ are selected from $\hat{P}(t)$ probabilistically based on the relationship:

$$p_s = [(1 - c)\,h/L + c]^{\alpha} \tag{13}$$

where h represents the hamming distance (i.e. the number of bit locations at which a given chromosome is different from another chromosome) between a candidate chromosome and the best chromosome in $\hat{P}(t)$, where L represents the total bit-length of the individual (binary) chromosomes, and where c and α denote, respectively, the shape coefficient and the exponent parameter. In this way, the selected chromosome with hamming distance h is chosen as a candidate for the next generation population pool if $p_s s$ is greater than a locally generated uniform random number between 0 and 1. This selection process is referred to as the cross-generational probability survival selection (CPSS) scheme.

The CPSS scheme is repeated until N chromosomes are selected for the next generation population pool $P(t + 1)$. However, in situations when CPSS leads to less than N chromosomes, the remaining chromosomes are formed by randomly complementing bits in the chromosome with the highest fitness value. By choosing the values of c and α appropriately, CPSS facilitates the desired external control over the diversity of the population pool permitting a rapid convergence to an optimal solution. In the absence of analytical solutions, the values of the shape coefficient c and the exponent parameter α are usually selected through an empirical investigation. This investigation is conducted over suitable range of values for c and α.

In accordance with Equation (13), chromosomes with large hamming distances from the chromosome with the highest fitness value in the population pool have a high chance of survival. The selection of such chromosomes increases the diversity of the population pool, giving rise to a substantial increase in the convergence speeds. In particular, if the fitness function has a few local optima only, then by using a high value of c and/or small value of α, one can achieve a rapid convergence to an optimal solution. On the other hand, when the fitness function is multimodal, lower values of c and/or higher values of α can be chosen to increase the probability of selecting chromosomes that are different from the chromosome with the highest fitness value.

CONSTRAINTS FOR GAURANTEED BIBO STABILITY

Let us consider a FRM digital filter consisting of CSD multiplier coefficients $\hat{m}_{FRM} \in CSD(W, w)$, where $CSD(W, w)$ represents the set of all possible CSD numbers having a word-length of W digits and a maximum number of w nonzero digits. In this way, the CSD multiplier coefficients $\hat{m}_{FRM}$ can be expressed in the general form

$$\hat{m}_{FRM} = \sum_{n=1}^{W} D_n \times 2^{(R-n)} \tag{14}$$

and satisfying the constraints

$$\begin{aligned} & D_n \in \{-1 \quad 0 \quad 1\} \\ & D_n \times D_{n+1} = 0 \\ & \sum_{n=1}^{W} \left| D_n \right| \le w \end{aligned} \tag{15}$$

with R representing a fixed value radix-point in the range $0 < R < W$.

In order for the FRM digital filter consisting of CSD multiplier coefficients $\hat{m}_{FRM}$ to be BIBO stable, it is both necessary and sufficient that the bilinear-LDI IIR interpolation sub-filters $H_0(z)$ and $H_1(z)$ be BIBO stable. Similarly, in order for the interpolation sub-filters $H_0(z)$ and $H_1(z)$ to be BIBO stable, it is both necessary and sufficient that the bilinear-LDI all-pass digital networks $G_0(z)$ and $G_1(z)$ be BIBO stable. In this way, it is required that the bilinear-LDI digital all-pass networks $G_0(z)$ and $G_1(z)$ remain BIBO stable throughout the course of the DCGA optimization over the CSD multiplier coefficient space $CSD(W, w)$.

In the course of DCGA optimization, the infinite-precision multiplier coefficients m_{Lp} and m_{Cp} can only take quantized values $\hat{m}_{Lp} \in CSD(W, w)$ and $\hat{m}_{Cp} \in (W, w)$. In this way, by taking into account the mapping properties of the bilinear analog-to-digital frequency transformation, in order for the bilinear-LDI digital all-pass networks $G_0(z)$ and $G_1(z)$ to remain BIBO stable, it required that the values of the corresponding reactive elements $\hat{L}_p$ and $\hat{C}_p$ remain positive (Valkenburg, 1965). To this end, in accordance with Equation (12), one has

$$\begin{aligned} \hat{L}'_p &= \frac{T}{\hat{m}_{Lp}} \\ \hat{C}'_p &= \frac{T}{\hat{m}_{Cp}} \end{aligned} \tag{16}$$

Moreover, in accordance with Equations (10)-(11), one has

$$\begin{aligned} \hat{L}'_1 &= \hat{L}_1 \\ \hat{C}'_1 &= \hat{C}_1 + \frac{T}{2} + \frac{T^2}{4\hat{L}_1} + \sum_{i=2}^{m} \frac{\hat{C}_i \dfrac{T^2}{4\hat{L}_i}}{\hat{C}_i + \dfrac{T^2}{4\hat{L}_i}} \end{aligned} \tag{17}$$

and

$$\begin{aligned} \hat{L}'_i &= \hat{L}_i \left[\frac{\hat{C}_i + \dfrac{T^2}{4\hat{L}_i}}{\hat{C}_i} \right]^2 \\ \hat{C}'_i &= \frac{\hat{C}_i^2}{\hat{C}_i + \dfrac{T^2}{4\hat{L}_i}} \end{aligned} \tag{18}$$

where $\hat{L}_1 = \infty$ for odd-ordered all-pass network $G(z)G(z)$. By substituting Equation (16) into Equations (17)-(18), and by solving the resulting equations for the reactive elements $\hat{L}_p$ and $\hat{C}_p$, one can obtain

$$\begin{aligned} \hat{L}_1 &= \frac{T}{\hat{m}_{L1}} \\ \hat{C}_1 &= \frac{-T\left\{2\hat{m}_{C1} + \hat{m}_{C1}\hat{m}_{L1} + 4\hat{m}_{C1}\left(\sum_{i=2}^{m} \dfrac{-\hat{m}_{Li}}{\hat{m}_{Li}\hat{m}_{Ci} - 4}\right) - 4\right\}}{4\hat{m}_{C1}} \end{aligned} \tag{19}$$

and

$$\begin{aligned} \hat{L}_i &= \frac{T\left(\hat{m}_{Li}\hat{m}_{Ci} - 4\right)^2}{16\hat{m}_{Li}} \\ \hat{C}_i &= \frac{-4T}{\hat{m}_{Ci}\left(\hat{m}_{Li}\hat{m}_{Ci} - 4\right)} \end{aligned} \tag{20}$$

From (19)-(20), $\hat{L}_p > 0$ and $\hat{C}_p > 0$ provided that

$$\begin{aligned} \hat{m}_{L1} &> 0 \\ \hat{m}_{Li} &> 0 \end{aligned} \tag{21}$$

and

$$\hat{m}_{Ci} < \frac{4}{\hat{m}_{Li}}$$

$$\hat{m}_{C1} < \frac{4}{\left\{2 + \hat{m}_{L1} + 4\left(\sum_{i=2}^{m} \frac{-\hat{m}_{Li}}{\hat{m}_{Li}\hat{m}_{Ci} - 4}\right)\right\}} \tag{22}$$

Then, in order to make the CSD FRM digital filter section BIBO stable, it is necessary and sufficient to choose the values of the multiplier coefficients $\hat{m}_{FRM} \in CSD(W, w)$ such that the inequality constraints (21)-(22) are satisfied

GENERATION OF CSD LUTS

The proposed approach for DCGA optimization of BIBO stable FRM digital filters over the multiplier coefficient space *CSD(W, w)* is based on a set of indexed CSD LUTs. These LUTs are constructed as follows:

- One LUT is constructed to include all permissible CSD values for the multiplier coefficient $\hat{m}_{L1}$ in inequality constraint $\hat{m}_{L1} > 0$, and $2(m - 1)$ for the multiplier coefficients $\hat{m}_{Li}$ and $\hat{m}_{Ci}$ in the inequality constraints in (22).
- Unlike the inequality second constraints in (21) along with the first in (22), the inequality constraint, which is the second in (22) for the multiplier coefficient $\hat{m}_{C1}$ involves more than one other multiplier coefficient. To circumvent this problem, let us replace the second inequality constraint in (22) by a corresponding equality constraint in accordance with

$$\hat{m}_{C1} = \frac{4}{\left\{2 + \hat{m}_{L1} + 4\left(\sum_{i=2}^{m} \frac{-\hat{m}_{Li}}{\hat{m}_{Li}\hat{m}_{Ci} - 4}\right)\right\}} - \varepsilon \tag{23}$$

where ε is a positive infinite-precision slack variable. Then the problem under consideration amounts to a judicious selection of ε>0. In this way, one can bypass any direct reference to the value of the multiplier coefficient $\hat{m}_{C1}$. Instead, one can incorporate the value of the slack variable ε as a gene in the construction of the FRM digital filter chromosome. This is best facilitated by replacing the slack variable ε by a corresponding finite-precision counterpart $\hat{\varepsilon}$, and by representing $\hat{\varepsilon}$ by a binary number having a suitable word-length. Then, the equality constraint in (23) is replaced by the best approximation

$$\hat{m}_{C1} \in CSD(W, w) \approx \frac{4}{\left\{2 + \hat{m}_{L1} + 4\left(\sum_{i=2}^{m} \frac{-\hat{m}_{Li}}{\hat{m}_{Li}\hat{m}_{Ci} - 4}\right)\right\}} - \hat{\varepsilon} \tag{24}$$

- Finally, one LUT is constructed for all permissible CSD values for the multiplier coefficients of the masking digital sub-filter $F_0(z)$ and $F_1(z)$.

If necessary, the above LUTs are increased in size in such a manner that the number of CSD values in each LUT is a power-of-two. Then, the indices into the CSD LUT in each LUT can be represented by a finite word-length binary number, and the resulting index sets become automatically closed under the operations of crossover and mutations throughout the course of the underlying DCGA optimization.

Design Methodology

The design methodology for the proposed DCGA optimization of BIBO stable FRM digital filters over the CSD multiplier coefficient space can be summarized as follows:

1. *Generation of seed FRM digital filter chromosome*: The seed FRM digital filter chromosome is formed in an ordered manner by concatenating
   - A block of B_{IIR} bits serving as the binary index into the corresponding CSD LUT for each multiplier coefficient in the bilinear-LDI interpolation digital subfilters $H_0(z)$ and $H_1(z)$ (except for the multiplier coefficient $\hat{m}_{C1}$).
   - A block of $B_{\hat{\varepsilon}}$ bits serving as the binary value of the slack variable $\hat{\varepsilon}$.
   - A block of B_{FIR} bits serving as the binary index into the corresponding CSD LUT for each multiplier coefficient in the FIR masking digital subfilters $F_0(z)$ and $F_1(z)$.

In this way, each of the above blocks of bits forms a gene in FRM digital filter chromosome.

2. *Generation of Initial Population Pool*: An initial population pool of N chromosomes is formed by scanning the FRM digital filter seed chromosome successively one gene at a time, and by randomly flipping the bits in the p-th bit in a given gene in accordance with the probabilistic relationship $p_F \times 0.5^{B_p+1-b_p}$ (with $1 \leq b_p \leq B_p$ representing the current bit position within the gene, and with B_p representing the word-length of the gene), where p_F is a fixed probability factor.
3. *Formation of the Next Generation Population Pool*: The current population pool $P(t)$ of size N is replaced by an enlarged population pool $P(t)$ of size N by using the following genetic operations:
   - *Crossover Operations*: Chromosomes in the population pool $P(t)$ are randomly paired as parents in such a manner that each chromosome is chosen only once as a parent. The resulting parent chromosome pairs undergo two-point crossover operations, reproducing two offspring for each parent pair. The resulting offspring are then combined with the initial population pool $P(t)$ to form the enlarged population pool $\hat{P}(t)$.
   - *Mutation Operations*: A few chromosomes (determined by a small mutation probability) in the enlarged population pool $\hat{P}(t)$ undergo mutation operation by randomly flipping their bits to enhance diversity.

Any resulting duplicate chromosomes are eliminated so as to maintain diversity, and the chromosomes in the enlarged population pool $\hat{P}(t)$ are ranked by evaluating their fitness values. The next generation population pool of $P(t+1)$ is then formed by using the CPSS scheme.

Fitness Evaluation: The fitness of each of the resulting FRM digital filter chromosomes in the enlarged population pool $\hat{P}(t)$ is evaluated in accordance with

$$\begin{aligned} fitness_{\text{magnitude response}} &= -20\log[\max(\varepsilon_p, \varepsilon_s)] \\ fitness_{\text{group-delay response}} &= \varepsilon_{gd} \\ fitness = fitness_{\text{magnitude response}} &- fitness_{\text{group-delay response}} \end{aligned} \tag{25}$$

where

$$\begin{aligned} \varepsilon_p &= \underbrace{\max}_{\omega=\omega_p}\left[W_p \left|H(e^{j\omega}) - 1\right|\right] \\ \varepsilon_s &= \underbrace{\max}_{\omega=\omega_s}\left[W_s \left|H(e^{j\omega})\right|\right] \\ \varepsilon_{gd} &= \underbrace{\max}_{\omega=\omega_p}\left[W_{gd} \left|\tau(\omega) - \mu_\tau\right|\right] \end{aligned} \tag{26}$$

with ω_p representing the pass-band frequency region, with ω_s representing the stop-band frequency region, and with $\tau(\omega)$ representing the group-delay frequency response of the FRM digital filter. Here, W_p, W_s, and W_{gd} represent the pass-band, stop-band, and group-delay weighting factors, and μ_τ represent the average group-delay over the pass-band region.

The group-delay of $H(e^{j\omega})$ is given by

$$\tau(\omega) = -\operatorname{Im}\left\{\frac{1}{H(e^{j\omega})}\frac{\partial H(e^{j\omega})}{\partial \omega}\right\} \quad (27)$$

The pass-band and stop-band weighting factors are W_p and W_s, are easily determined from user specifications. The group-delay weighting factor is formulate as

$$W_{gd} = \frac{\xi \times fitness_{\text{magnitude response}}}{fitness_{\text{group-delya response}}} \quad (28)$$

where ξ is a fixed constant such that $0 < \xi < 1$, and where $fitness_{\text{magnitude response}}$ and $fitness_{\text{group-delya response}}$ are determined from the seed FRM digital filter chromosome. The importance of group-delay in the optimization increases as $\xi \rightarrow 1$.

Application Example

This section is concerned with the design of a low-pass FRM digital filter with the following design specifications:

- Maximum Passband Ripple $A_p = 0.05$[dB]
- Minimum Stopband Los $A_a = 38$[dB]
- Passband-Edge Normalized Frequency $\omega_p = 0.20\pi$[Rad]
- Stopband-Edge Normalized Frequency $\omega_a = 0.20\pi$[Rad]
- Normalized Sampling Period $T = 1$[s]
- Interpolation Factor $M = 7$

The remaining DCGA optimization parameters are given by

Table 1. Analog components & corresponding digital multiplier

Variable	Value
$C_{1,0}$; $C'_{1,0}$; $m_{C1,0}$	0.3828 [F]; 1.0123 [F]; 0.9878
$C_{2,0}$; $C'_{2,0}$; $m_{C2,0}$	0.3173 [F]; 0.1878 [F]; 5.3253
$L_{2,0}$; $L'_{2,0}$; $m_{L2,0}$	1.1423 [H]; 3.2615 [H]; 0.3066
$C_{1,1}$; $C'_{1,1}$; $m_{C1,1}$	0.4081 [F]; 1.2888 [F]; 0.7759
$L_{1,1}$; $L'_{1,1}$; $m_{L1,1}$	0.6567 [H]; 0.6567 [H]; 1.5227

- $c = 0.8$; $\alpha = 0.3$
- $p_F = 0.5$
- $\xi = 0.4$

The above specifications entail $\tilde{n} = 5$. Then, the values of the inductances and capacitances $L_{p,0 \text{ or } 1}$ and $C_{p,0 \text{ or } 1}$, the values of the precomensated inductances $L'_{p,0 \text{ or } 1}$ and capacitances $C'_{p,0 \text{ or } 1}$, and the values of the multiplier coefficients $m_{Lp,0 \text{ or } 1}$ and $m_{Cp,0 \text{ or } 1}$ can be obtained as summarized in Table 1.

In this example, a set of five CSD LUTs are required, four LUTs with entries belonging to $CSD(11, 3)$ (with 7-bit fractional part) for the multiplier coefficients $m_{C2,0}$, $m_{L2,0}$, $m_{C1,1}$, and $m_{L1,1}$ constituent in the interpolation digital sub-filters $H_0(z)$ and $H_1(z)$, and one LUT with entries belonging to $CSD(11,3)$ (with 10-bit fractional part) for all the multiplier coefficients constituent in the masking digital sub-filters $F_0(z)$ and $F_1(z)$. The analysis of the resulting seed FRM digital filter revealed that before the DCGA optimization,

- Maximum Passband Ripple A_p = 0.1286[dB]
- Minimum Stopband Los $A_a = 31.7879$[dB]
- Maximum Group-Delay $\tau = 48.7$

An initial population size of N=500 was chosen for the ensuing DCGA optimization. The DCGA optimization converged in around 300 generations to a desired FRM digital filter with the following frequency response characteristics:

Figure 3. Magnitude and Group-Delay Response of FRM Digital Filter, Before (dotted), and After (Solid) DCGA Optimization

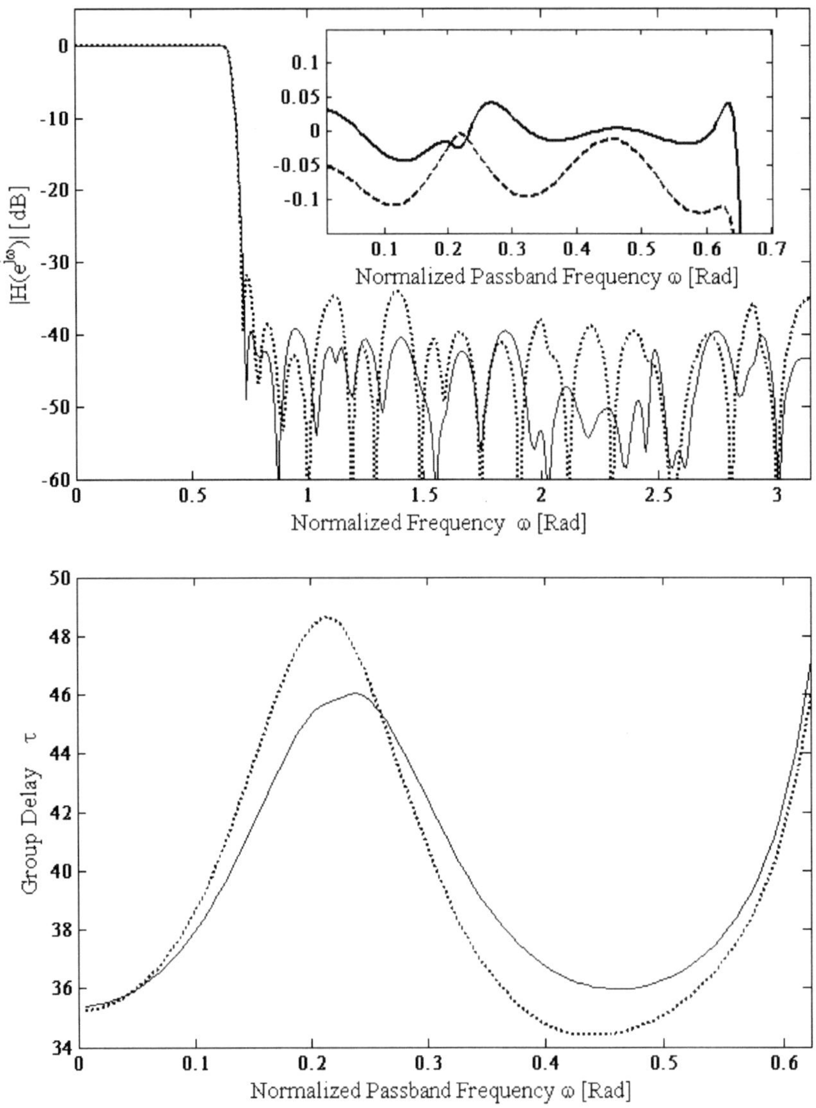

- Maximum Pass-band Ripple A_p = 0.0440[dB]
- Minimum Stop-band Los A_a = 38.9540[dB]
- Maximum Group-Delay τ = 46.0

The magnitude and group-delay frequency-responses of the FRM digital filter before and after the DCGA optimization are obtained as shown in Figure 3.

FUTURE WORK

Although the constituent CPSS removes similar chromosomes from the population pool, it does not produce suitable substitutes in their place. The substitutes can be produced by adaptively changing the probability of mutation, and adaptively changing the number of bits flipped by each application of the mutation operation.

The performance of DCGA may similarly be improved through the development of novel adaptive mechanisms for the shape coefficient c and the exponent parameter α.

CONCLUSION

This work has presented a novel technique for the design of FRM digital filters incorporating bilinear-LDI IIR interpolation sub-filters through a rapid DCGA optimization over the CSD multiplier coefficient space. The resulting DCGA design technique permits simultaneous optimization of the magnitude-frequency as well of the group-delay frequency response of the desired FRM digital filters. A novel CSD look-up table (LUT) scheme has been developed so that the IIR interpolation sub-filters in the intermediate and the final FRM digital filters are guaranteed to be automatically BIBO stable throughout the course of DCGA optimization. The usefulness of the proposed DCGA optimization has been demonstrated through its application to the design of a low-pass FRM digital filter satisfying stringent specifications.

REFERENCES

Cen, L., & Lian, Y. (2006). Hybrid Genetic Algorithm for the Design of Modified Frequency-Response Masking Filters in a Discrete Space. *Journal of Circuits, Systems, and Signal Processing*, *25*, 153–174. doi:10.1007/s00034-005-2502-8

Dai, C., Zhu, Y., & Chen, W. (2006). Seeker Optimization Algorithm. *Proceedings of International Conference on Computational Intelligence and Security*, (CIS), *1*, 225-229.

Goldberg, D. E. (1989). *Genetic Algorithms in Search, Optimization, and Machine Learning*. USA: Addison-Wesley.

Green, B., & Turner, L. E. (1990). Digital LDI Ladder Filters Using Lattice Equivalents and Wave Concepts. *IEEE Transactions on Circuits and Systems*, *37*(1), 133–135. doi:10.1109/31.45701

Higuchi, T., Liu, Y., & Yao, X. (Eds.). (2006). *Evolvable Hardware, VIII*. New York: Springer. doi:10.1007/0-387-31238-2

Johansson, H., & Wanhammar, L. (1997). High-Seed Recursive Filtering Using the Frequency-Response Masking Approach. In *Proceedings of the IEEE International Symposium on Circuits and Systems*, (ISCAS), 2208-2211.

Kilambi, S., & Nowrouzian, B. (2007). A Diversity Controlled Genetic Algorithm for Optimization of FRM Digital Filters over DBNS Multiplier Coefficient Space. *Proceedings of IEEE International Symposium on Circuits and Systems*, (ISCAS), 2331-2334.

Lee, L., & Oppenheim, A. (1997). Properties of Approximate Parks-McClellan Filters. *Proceedings of IEEE International Conference on Acoustics, Speech, and Signal Processing*, (ICASSP), *3*, 2165.

Lim, Y. (1986). Frequency-Response Masking Approach for the Synthesis of Sharp Linear Phase Digital Filters. *IEEE Transactions on Circuits and Systems*, *33*(4), 357–364. doi:10.1109/TCS.1986.1085930

Lim, Y. (1986). A Digital Filter Bank for Digital Audio Systems. *IEEE Transactions on Circuits and Systems*, *33*(8), 848–849. doi:10.1109/TCS.1986.1085988

Lutovac, M., & Milid, L. (1999). Design of Multiplierless Elliptic IIR Filters with a Small Quantization Error. *IEEE Transactions on Signal Processing*, *47*(2), 469–479. doi:10.1109/78.740130

Nowrouzian, B. (1989). Minimal Multiplier Realization of Bilinear-LDI Digital All-Pass Networks. *IEE Proceedings on Devices and Systems*, *G-136*, 114–117. doi:10.1049/ip-g-2.1989.0018

Nowrouzian, B., Mercier, P., & Kilambi, S. M. (2007). Optimization of FRM FIR Digital Filters over CSD and CDBNS Multiplier Coefficient Spaces Employing a Novel Genetic Algorithm. *Journal of Computers*, *2*(7), 20–31.

Rabrenovic, D., & Lutovac, M. (1994). Elliptic Filters with Minimal Q-factors. *IEE Electronics Letters*, *30*(3), 206–207. doi:10.1049/el:19940180

Sakr, N., & Groza, V. (2005). Run-time Reconfigurable Hardware Blocks for Multimedia Applications. *Proceedings of Canadian Conference on Electrical and Computer Engineering*: *(1996-1999)*.

Shimodaira, H. (2001). A Diversity-Control-Oriented Genetic Algorithm (DCGA): Performance in Function Optimization. Proceedings of 2001 Congress on Evolutionary Computation, 1, *44-51*.

Srinivas, M., & Patnaik, L. M. (1994). Adaptive Probabilities of Crossover and Mutation in Genetic Algorithms. *IEEE Transactions on Systems, Man, and Cybernetics*, *24*, 656–667. doi:10.1109/21.286385

Stoica, A. (2000). Evolvable Hardware: From On-Chip Circuit Synthesis to Evolvable Space Systems. In *Proceedings of IEEE 30th International Symposium on Multiple-Valued Logic*, (ISMVL), 161.

Valkenburg, V. (1965). *Introduction to Modern Network Synthesis*. New York: John Wiley and Sons.

Willson, A., & Orchard, H. (1995). Insights into Digital Filters Made as the Sum of Two All-Pass Functions. *IEEE Transactions on Circuits and Systems*, *42*, 129–137. doi:10.1109/81.376877

Wu, Y., & Nowrouzian, B. (2008). A Novel Technique for the Design and DCGA Optimization of Bilinear-LDI Lattice-Based Digital IF Filters. Proceedings of IEEE International Symposium on Circuits and Systems, (ISCAS), 1184-1187.

ADDITIONAL READING

Antoniou, A. (1993). *Digital Filters: Analysis, Design, and Applications*. New York: Mc-Graw Hill.

Lee, L. (1998). *Design Techniques for Bilinear-LDI Digital All-pass Networks*. M.Sc. Thesis. Canada: Department of Electrical and Computer Engineering, University of Calgary, Calgary, Alberta.

Lutovac, M., & Milid, L. (1997). Design of Computationally Efficient Elliptic IIR Filters with a Reduced Number of Shift-and-Add Operations in Multipliers. *IEEE Transactions on Signal Processing*, *45*(7), 2422–2430. doi:10.1109/78.640708

Lutovac, M., & Milid, L. (2001). IIR Filters Based on Frequency-Response Masking Approach. *Proceedings of Telecommunications in Modern Satellite, Cable and Broadcasting Service, (*TELSIKS), *1*, 163-170.

Nowrouzian, B. (1990). A Novel Approach to the Exact Design of LDI Symmetrical Digital and Switched-Capacitor Filters. *Proceedings of 33rd Midwest Symposium on Circuits and Systems, 2*, 967-972).

Temes, G. C. (1970). Exact Computation of Group-Delay and its Sensitivities Using Adjoint-Network Concept. *IEE Electronics Letters*, *6*, 483–485. doi:10.1049/el:19700338

KEY TERMS AND DEFINITIONS

Diversity Controlled Genetic Algorithms: A class of genetic algorithms incorporating external control over the population diversity in genetic algorithms.

Frequency Response Masking: A cascade digital filter structure using (easily realizable) subfilters with gradual transition bands to realize an overall digital filter with very sharp transition bands.

Bilinear-LDI Digital Filters: A class of digital filters incorporating bilinear analog-to-digital frequency transformation in their transfer functions and the LDI analog-to-digital transformation in their realizations.

FIR and IIR Digital Filters: Finite impulse-response and infinite impulse-response digital filters.

CSD Number System: A number system for the representation of finite wordlength numbers in canonical signed-digit format.

BIBO Stability: A stability criterion implying a bounded-output signal for a bounded-input signal.

Chapter 15
Neuromodeling and Natural Optimization of Nonlinear Devices and Circuits

Paulo H. da F. Silva
Federal Institute of Education, Science and Technology of Paraiba, Brazil

Rossana M. S. Cruz
Federal Institute of Education, Science and Technology of Paraiba, Brazil

Adaildo G. D'Assunção
Federal University of Rio Grande do Norte, Brazil

ABSTRACT

This chapter describes some/new artificial neural network (ANN) neuromodeling techniques and natural optimization algorithms for electromagnetic modeling and optimization of nonlinear devices and circuits. Neuromodeling techniques presented are based on single hidden layer feedforward neural network configurations, which are trained by the resilient back-propagation algorithm to solve the modeling learning tasks associated with device or circuit under analysis. Modular configurations of these feedforward networks and optimal neural networks are also presented considering new activation functions for artificial neurons. In addition, some natural optimization algorithms are described, such as continuous genetic algorithm (GA), a proposed improved-GA and particle swarm optimization (PSO). These natural optimization algorithms are blended with multilayer perceptrons (MLP) artificial neural network models for fast and accurate resolution of optimization problems. Some examples of applications are presented and include nonlinear RF/microwave devices and circuits, such as transistors, filters and antennas.

INTRODUCTION

Versatility, efficient computation, reduced memory occupation, stability of learning algorithms and generalization from representative data are some characteristics that have motivated the use of neural networks in many areas of microwave engineering (Patnaik & Mishra, 2000; Zhang & Gupta, 2000). In circuit simulation, neuromodeling applications reported in literature to improve

DOI: 10.4018/978-1-60960-018-1.ch015

the harmonic balance method have been used as nonlinear device models for microwave circuit steady-state analysis (Santos, Romariz, & Carvalho, 1997). On the order hand, neuromodeling technique is evaluated in time-domain, in order to improve nonlinear GaAs MESFET logic gate circuit transient and sensitivity analysis (Silva, Melo, & Neto, 2001; Silva, Melo, & Neto, 2002).

Circuit simulators like SPICE (with integrated circuit emphasis) are formed around semiconductor devices like diodes, BJTs, MOSFETs, MESFETs etc. (Raghuram, 1989). In general, the quality of simulation is decided by the accuracy of device models. On the other hand, a very detailed model would naturally slow down the program. A compromise between accuracy and speed of computation has to be struck. Using neural networks enables to overcome this problem.

Generally, the use of circuit simulation packages presents difficulties to the designer in implementing their own nonlinear model applied to a new device (Raghuram, 1989). Numerical simplifications are required. Then, the use of empirical models increases the computational efficiency of numerical simulations. In this context, artificial neural networks trained by accurate electromagnetic (EM) data, are very suitable for developing computer aided design (CAD) tools. Neural models combine the accuracy of EM-simulators with the computational efficiency of empirical models (Silva, 2002). For this reason, ANN models for nonlinear RF/microwave devices and circuits have been widely used (Zhang & Gupta, 2000). Various hybrid neuromodeling techniques incorporate previously EM knowledge to ANN in order to obtain more consistent training, reliability and accuracy for the resulting ANN models. Versatility, stability of learning algorithms and generalization abilities permit us to employ neural models for complex ill-defined input-output mappings in new (not well-known) devices (Santos et al., 1997).

Neuromodeling methodology can be described by two steps: i) neural network model development - that includes selection of representative training data, network configuration and training algorithms; ii) neural model validation - the neural network model is tested and validated according to its interpolation and generalization capacities in a given region of interest.

Natural optimization algorithms, which are stochastic population-based global search methods inspired by nature, such as simulated annealing (SA), genetic algorithm (GA) and particle swarm optimization (PSO) are effective for optimization problems with a large number of design variables and inexpensive cost function evaluation (Haupt & Werner, 2007; Kennedy & Eberhart, 1995). However, the main computational drawback for optimization of nonlinear devices and circuits relies on the repetitive evaluation of numerically expensive cost (or fitness) functions. Finding a way to shorten the optimization cycle is highly desirable. In the case of GA, for example, several schemes are available in order to improve its performance, such as: the use of fast full-wave methods, micro-genetic algorithm, which aims to reduce the population size, and parallel GA associated with parallel computation (R. Haupt & S. Haupt, 2004).

In this chapter, we present neuromodeling techniques based on single hidden layer feedforward neural network configurations – trained by the efficient resilient back-propagation (RPROP) algorithm (Ridmiller & Braun, 1993) - to solve modeling learning tasks associated with device or circuit under analysis. In particular, we focus on the use of new hidden neuron activation functions in order to improve learning, reliability and generalization of neural models. Some optimal neural network activation functions are described. Modular configurations of these feedforward networks, as well as mathematical formulation and implementation details are presented. An overview of the applications of proposed neuromodeling techniques based on previous developed researches are shown.

Figure 1. (a) Nonlinear model of an artificial neuron; (b) FNN configuration with two hidden layers

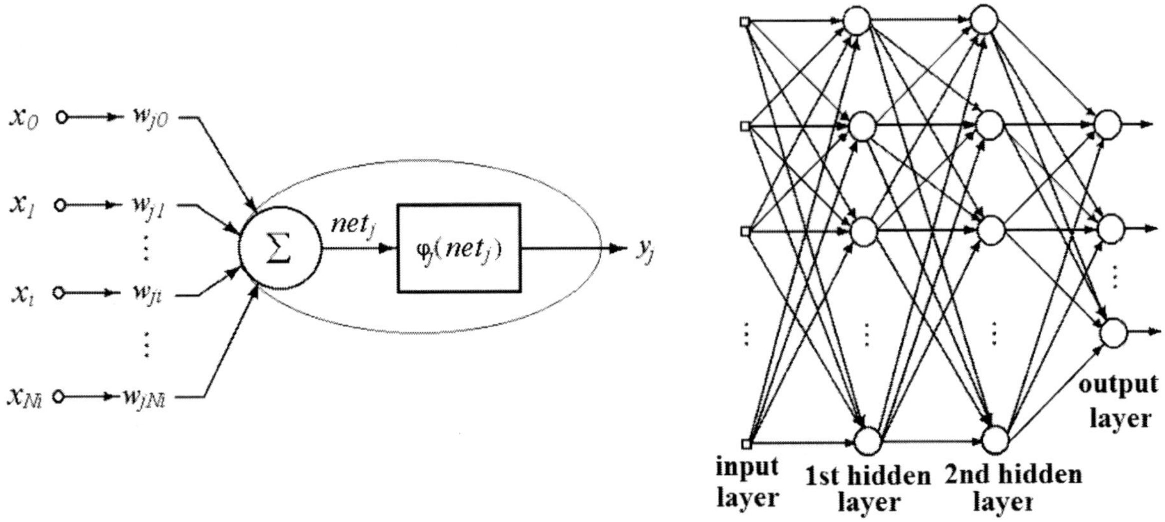

(a) (b)

In addition, this chapter also describes the mathematical formulation and implementation of some natural optimization algorithms and hybrid EM-optimization methods, using improved versions of continuous-GA and PSO algorithms, blended with multilayer perceptrons (MLP) artificial neural network models. Such methods are applied to design spatial mesh filters, such as frequency selective surfaces (FSSs). MLP models are used for fast and accurate evaluation of cost function into continuous-GA and PSO simulations, in order to overcome the computational requirements associated with full-wave numerical simulations.

ARTIFICIAL NEURAL NETWORKS

Fundamentals

Rosenblatt (1958) perceptron is the most used artificial neuron in neural network configurations and is based on the nonlinear model proposed by McCulloch and Pitts (1943). In this model, neurons are signal processing units composed by a set of input connections (weights), an adder (for summing the input signals, weighted by the respective synapses of a neuron, constituting a linear combiner) and an activation function, that can be linear or nonlinear, as shown in Figure 1(a). The input signals are defined as x_i, $i = 0,1,\cdots,N_i$, whose result corresponds to the level of internal activity of a neuron net_j, as defined in (1), where $x_0 = +1$ is the polarization potential (or bias) of the neurons. The output signal y_j is the activation function response $\phi(\cdot)$ to the activation potential net_j, as shown in (2).

$$net_j = \sum_{i=0}^{Ni} w_{ji} \cdot x_i \quad (1)$$

$$y_j = \phi(net_j) \quad (2)$$

For a feedforward neural network (FNN), the artificial neurons are set into layers. Each neuron of a layer is connected to those of the previous

Figure 2. (a) Block diagram of supervised learning; (b) neural network "black box" model

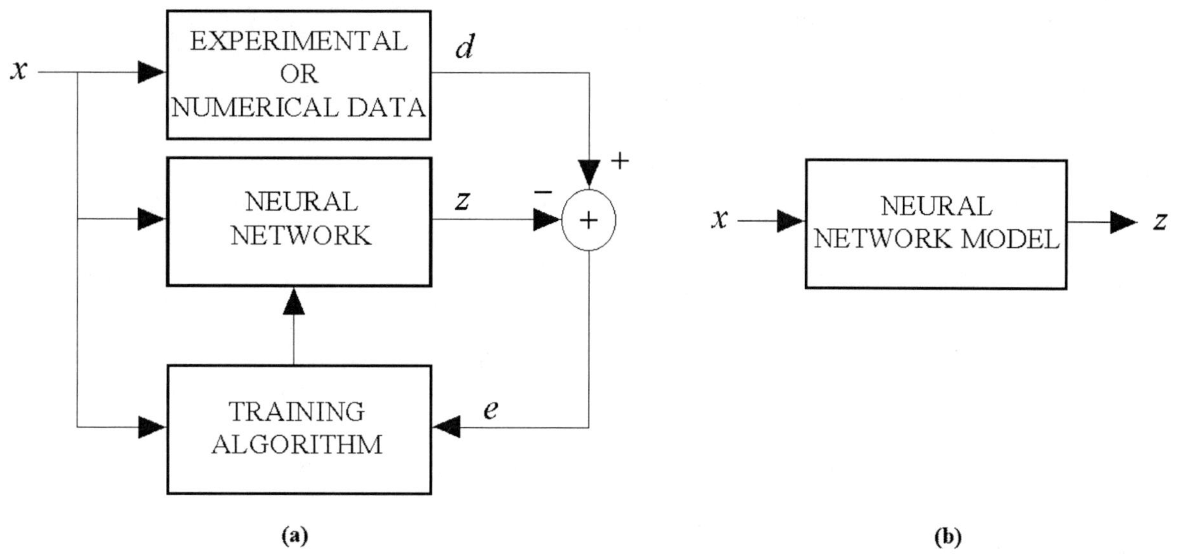

layer, as illustrated in Figure 1(b). Signal propagation occurs from input to output layers, passing through the hidden layers of the FNN. Hidden neurons represent the input characteristics, while output neurons generate the neural network responses (Haykin, 1999).

Methodology

Generally, the design of a neural network is composed by three main steps: configuration − how layers are organized and connected; learning − how information is stored; generalization − how neural network produces reasonable outputs for inputs not found in the training (Haykin, 1999). In this work, we use feedforward neural networks and supervised learning to develop neural network models.

In the computational simulation of supervised learning process, a training algorithm is used for the adaptation of neural network synaptic weights. The instantaneous error $e(n)$, as defined in (3), represents the difference between the desired response, $d(n)$, and the neural network output, $z(n)$, at the iteration n, corresponding to the presentation of the nth training pattern $\left(x(n);d(n)\right)$.

$$e(n) = z(n) - d(n) \quad (3)$$

Supervised learning can be illustrated through the block diagram of Figure 2(a) and has as objective the minimization of the mean square error $E(t)$, given in (4), where the index t represents the number of training epochs (one complete presentation of all training examples, $n = 1, 2, \ldots, N$, where N is the total number of examples, is called an epoch).

$$E(t) = \frac{1}{N}\sum_{n=1}^{N}\frac{1}{2}e(n)^2 \quad (4)$$

Currently, there are several algorithms for the training of neural networks that use different optimization techniques. The most popular training algorithms are those derived from backpropagation algorithm (Rumelhart, Hinton, & Williams, 1986). Among the family of backpropagation algorithms, the RPROP shows to be very efficient in solving complex electromagnetic problems. In this work, the stop criteria are defined in terms of the maximum number of epochs and/or the minimum error.

After training, the neural network is submitted to a test, in order to verify its capability of generalizing to new values that do not belong to the training dataset, for example, parts of the region of interest where there is not enough knowledge about the modeled device/circuit. Therefore, the neural network operates like a "black box" model that is illustrated in Figure 2(b).

Resilient back-propagation algorithm is a first-order local adaptive learning scheme. The basic principle of RPROP is to eliminate the harmful influence of the partial derivative size in the weight update. Only the sign of the derivative is considered to indicate the direction of the weight update, Δw_{hp}, as given in (5).

$$\Delta w_{hp}(t) = \begin{cases} -\Delta_{hp}(t), \; if \; \dfrac{\partial E}{\partial w_{hp}}(t) > 0 \\ +\Delta_{hp}(t), \; if \; \dfrac{\partial E}{\partial w_{hp}}(t) < 0 \\ 0, \; elsewhere \end{cases} \tag{5}$$

The second step of RPROP algorithm is to determine the new update-values $\Delta_{hp}(t)$. This is based on a sign-dependent adaptation process, similar to the learning-rate adaptation shown by Jacobs (1988). The changes in the weight size are exclusively determined by a weight 'update-value', Δ_{hp}, as given in (6).

$$\Delta_{hp}(t) = \begin{cases} \eta^{+} \cdot \Delta_{hp}(t-1), & \dfrac{\partial E}{\partial w_{hp}}(t-1) \cdot \dfrac{\partial E}{\partial w_{hp}}(t) > 0 \\ \eta^{-} \cdot \Delta_{hp}(t-1), & \dfrac{\partial E}{\partial w_{hp}}(t-1) \cdot \dfrac{\partial E}{\partial w_{hp}}(t) < 0 \\ \Delta_{hp}(t-1), & elsewhere \end{cases} \tag{6}$$

Here, the following RPROP parameters were employed: $\eta^{+} = 1.2$ and $\eta^{-} = 0.5$. The update-values were restricted to the range $10^{-6} \leq \Delta_{hp} \leq 50$.

NATURAL OPTIMIZATION ALGORITHMS

Natural optimization algorithms are stochastic population-based global search methods that start with an initial population of candidate individuals for an optimal solution. Assuming an optimization problem with N_{var} input variables and N_{pop} individuals, the population at the kth iteration is a matrix $P(k)_{Npop \times Nvar}$ of floating-point elements, denoted by $p^{k}_{m,n}$, with each row corresponding to an individual. Under GA and PSO jargons, for example, individuals are named *chromosomes* and *particles* (or agents), respectively. The implementation details of these algorithms are described.

Continuous Genetic Algorithm

Continuous genetic algorithm is very similar to the binary-GA but works with floating-point variables. Continuous-GA chromosomes are defined by (7), where each one corresponds to a vector with N_{var} floating-point optimization variables. Each chromosome is evaluated by means of its associated cost, which is computed through the cost function E given in (8).

$$chromosome(k,m) = \left[p^{k}_{m,1}, \quad p^{k}_{m,2}, \quad \ldots, \quad p^{k}_{m,N\,\mathrm{var}} \right], \\ m = 1, 2, \ldots, Npop \tag{7}$$

$$\cos t(k,m) = E\left(chromosome(k,m) \right) \tag{8}$$

Based on the cost associated with each chromosome, the population evolves through generations

Figure 3. Flow charts of the natural optimization algorithms: (a) continuous-GA; (b) PSO

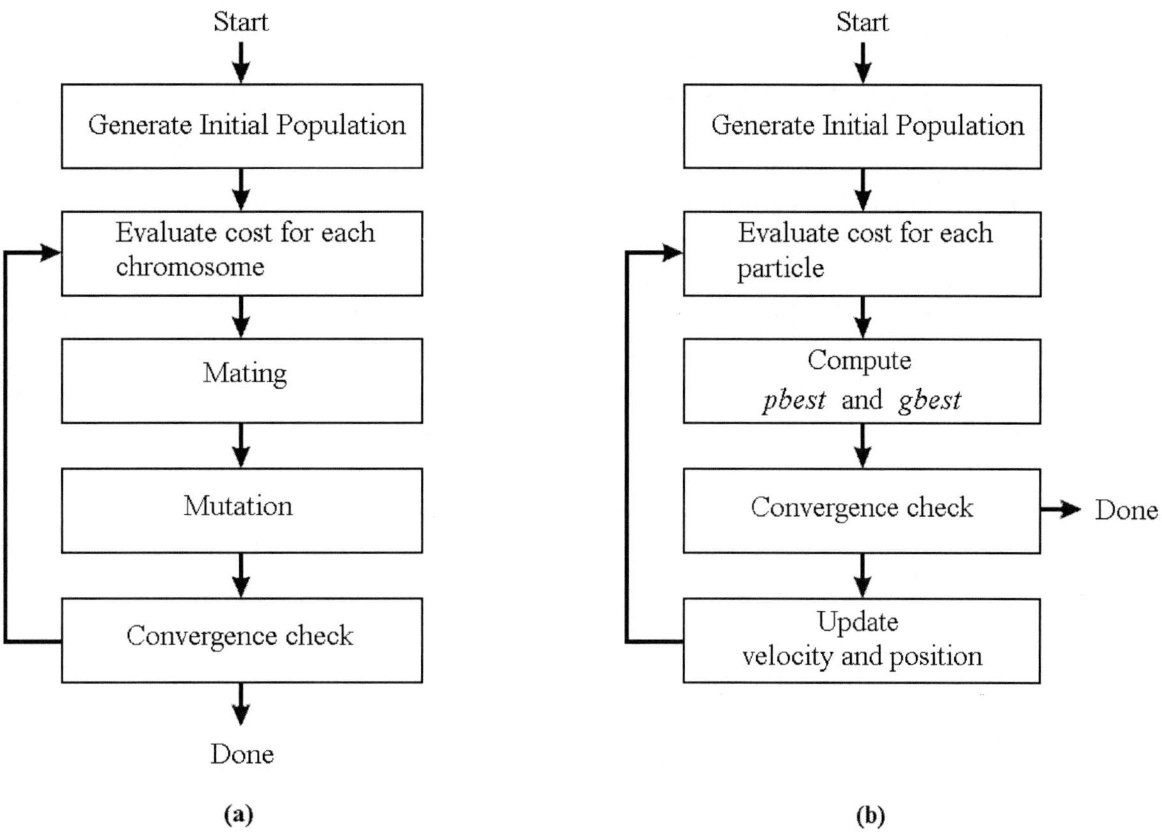

with the application of genetic operators, such as: selection, crossover and mutation. Figure 3(a) gives a "big picture" overview of continuous-GA. Mating step includes roulette wheel selection presented in (Haupt & Werner, 2007; R. Haupt & S. Haupt, 2004). Population selection is performed after the N_{pop} chromosomes are ranked from lowest to highest costs. Then, the N_{keep} most-fit chromosomes are selected to form the mating pool and the rest are discarded to make room for the new offspring. Mothers and fathers pair in a random fashion through the blending crossover method (R. Haupt & S. Haupt, 2004). Each pair produces two offspring that contain traits from each parent. In addition, the parents survive to be part of the next generation. After mating, a fraction of chromosomes in the population will suffer mutation. Then, the chromosome variable selected for real-value mutation is added to a normally distributed random number.

Improved Genetic Algorithm

Most users of continuous-GA add a normally distributed random number to the variable selected for mutation with a constant standard deviation (R. Haupt & S. Haupt, 2004). In particular, we propose a new real-value mutation operator for continuous-GA as given in (9), where p_{max} and p_{min} are constant values defined according to the limits of the region of interest composed by input parameters. Function *randn*() returns a normal distribution with mean equal to zero and standard deviation equal to one. This mutation operator was inspired by simulating annealing cooling schedules (R. Haupt & S. Haupt, 2004) and is used to improve continuous-GA convergence at the neighborhood of global minimum. The quotient function Q given in (10) is crescent when the number of iterations increases and the global cost decreases. Thus, similar to the decrease of temperature in a simulating annealing algorithm, the standard deviation is decreased when the number of continuous-GA iterations is increased. The parameter A is a constant value and B is a value of cost function neighbor to the global minimum. The continuous-GA using the real-value mutation definition given in (9) and (10) is denominated improved genetic algorithm.

$$p_{m,n}^{k+1} = p_{m,n}^{k} + randn() \cdot \frac{\left(p_{\max} - p_{\min}\right)}{Q\left(k, global\cos t(k)\right)} \quad (9)$$

$$Q\left(k, global\cos t(k)\right) = \begin{cases} A, & global\cos t \geq B \\ A + k \cdot \left[\log\left(global\cos t(k)\right)\right]^2, & global\cos t < B \end{cases} \quad (10)$$

Particle Swarm Optimization

Particle swarm optimization algorithm was first formulated by Kennedy and Eberhart (1995). The thought process behind the algorithm was inspired by the social behavior of animals, such as bird flocking or fish schooling. PSO algorithm is similar to continuous-GA since it begins with a random population matrix. Unlike GA, PSO has no evolution operators such as crossover and mutation. Each particle moves along the cost surface with an individual velocity. A flow chart of the PSO algorithm is shown in Figure 3(b). The implemented PSO algorithm updates the velocities and positions of the particles based on the best local and global solutions according to (11) and (12), respectively.

$$v_{m,n}^{k+1} = C\left[r_0 v_{m,n}^{k} + \Gamma_1 \cdot r_1 \cdot \left(p_{m,n}^{local\,bes(k)} - p_{m,n}^{k}\right) + \Gamma_2 \cdot r_2 \cdot \left(p_{m,n}^{global\,best(k)} - p_{m,n}^{k}\right)\right] \quad (11)$$

$$p_{m,n}^{k+1} = p_{m,n}^{k} + v_{m,n}^{k+1} \quad (12)$$

Here, $v_{m,n}$ is the particle velocity, $p_{m,n}$ is the particle variables, r_0, r_1 and r_2 are independent uniform random numbers; Γ_1 and Γ_2 are is the cognitive and social parameters, respectively, $p_{m,n}^{localbest(k)}$ **and** $p_{m,n}^{globalbest(k)}$ are the best local and global solutions, respectively; C is the constriction parameter (Kennedy & Eberhart, 1995). If the best local solution has a cost less than the best cost of the current global solution, then the best local solution replaces the best global solution. PSO is a very simple natural optimization algorithm, easy to implement and with few parameters to adjust.

APPLICATIONS

Neural Network Models for GaAs MESFET Nonlinear Circuits

Since the commercial development of GaAs MESFET integrated circuit technology, its models proposed for SPICE simulators are rising. For example, in Schichman-Hodges analytical model (Schichman & Hodges, 1968), used in SPICE2 program, the drain current is defined by (13) considering V_{DS}>0, where V_T is the threshold voltage, β and λ are constants.

$$I_{DS}\left(V_{GS}, V_{DS}\right) = \begin{cases} 0, V_{GS} + V_T < 0 \\ \beta\left(V_{GS} + V_T\right)^2\left(1 + \lambda V_{DS}\right), 0 \leq V_{GS} + V_T \leq V_{DS} \\ \beta V_{DS}\left[2\left(V_{GS} + V_T\right) - V_{DS}\right]\left(1 + \lambda V_{DS}\right), 0 \leq V_{DS} \leq V_{GS} + V_T \end{cases} \quad (13)$$

Figure 4. (a) GaAs MESFET equivalent circuit; (b) Characteristic curves of the GaAs MESFET microwave transistor models

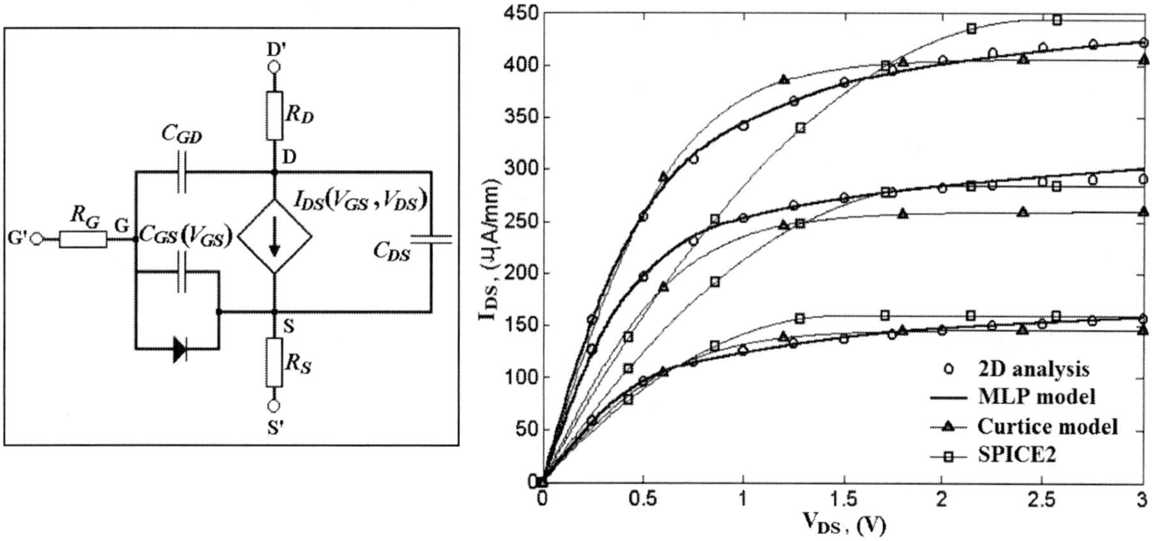

(a) (b)

This expression seems to fit experimental devices quite well in the region of current saturation. However, the fit is quite poor below current saturation. Curtice model (Curtice, 1980) using hyperbolic tangent function is derived of Schichman and Hodges (1968) JFET model, modified to provide a proper knee voltage for the *I-V* characteristic curves. This model used for the n-channel GaAs MESFET is given by (14) and (15), where V_{BI} is the built-in voltage. The transit time under the gate, τ, is also a model parameter, although the dependence upon τ is not stated explicitly in (14).

$$I_{DS}\left(V_{GS}, V_{DS}\right) = \beta\left(V_{GS} + V_T\right)\cdot\left(1 + \lambda V_{DS}\right) \cdot \tanh\left(\alpha V_{DS}\right) \qquad (14)$$

$$C_{GS}\left(V_{GS}\right) = C_{GS}\left(0\right) / \left(1 - V_{GS} / V_{BI}\right)^{1/2} \qquad (15)$$

The model developed by Curtice (1980) has been implemented into a source code of the SPICE simulator, (Sussman-Fort, Narasimhan, & Mayaram, 1984), with thirteen parameters. Figure 4(a) shows the respective equivalent circuit for GaAs MESFET. Other models try improving these aproximations (Parker & Skellern, 1997). MESFET devices are extremely complex internally and simple external models cannot accurately describe their behavior under all conditions.

In the design of the neural network model to describe the GaAs MESFET characteristic, we chose a configuration to the MLP network with one hidden layer that was trained with different algorithms (Silva, 2002). MLP networks perform global approximations to nonlinear input-output mapping with good generalization capacity, but sometimes with slow learning. The proposed neural modeling technique is evaluated in time-domain, in order to improve nonlinear circuit transient and sensitivity analysis (Silva, Melo, & Neto, 2001; Silva, Melo, & Neto, 2002). The design of MLP network model considered logistic activation functions, as shown in (16) for the hidden layer, while output layer is linear.

$$\phi(net) = 1/\left[1+\exp(-net)\right] \quad (16)$$

The forward computation for MLP network is defined by (17)-(20), where $x^T = [x_0, x_1, \ldots, x_{Ni}]$ is the input vector; $y^T = [y_0, y_1, \ldots, y_{Nh}]$ is the vector of hidden neuron outputs; $z^T = [z_1, z_2, \ldots, z_{Nq}]$ is the network output vector; W and V are weight matrix network; net_h and net_q are activation potentials; $\varphi(\cdot)$ denotes the logistic function.

$$net_h = \sum_{i=0}^{Ni} w_{hi} x_i, \quad h = 1, 2, \ldots, Nh \quad (17)$$

$$y_h = \phi(net_h) \quad (18)$$

$$net_q = \sum_{h=0}^{Nh} v_{qh} y_h, \quad q = 1, 2, \ldots, Nq \quad (19)$$

$$z_q = net_q \quad (20)$$

The 2-D numerical results for GaAs MESFET given by Curtice (1980) were utilized to train the MLP model. In this way, we adopt a MLP network with two inputs (V_{GS}, V_{DS}); thirty hidden units and one output, which represents the drain current. Because of the slow convergence of back-propagation training algorithm, other local learning schemes were implemented (Jacobs, 1988; Silva, 2002). In particular, RPROP algorithm was chosen for MLP training, since it presents the best convergence properties, in comparison to other training algorithms implemented. In addition, RPROP is robust in value attributions to the algorithm's parameters.

A comparison of the implemented model responses for the MESFET transistor is shown in Figure 4(b). It is observed that the MLP model is more accurate than the empirical ones, because it shows a better approximation to accurate results of the 2-D numerical analysis.

Optimal Neural Network Models

In this application example, an optimal neural network is used to develop fast and accurate analitical models, defined through basis function expansions (activation function φ), for the interpolation of special functions. In this method, a neural network is trained for each basis function chosen for the model. Some problems such as the choice of number and type of basis functions and their parameter optimization are included at the training step. After a trial and error investigation, it is possible to find an optimal neural network that fits the desired specifications for the model.

For example, a model used to describe the directivity of a circular loop antenna was considered to elaborate an optimal neural network model. The integral expressions for the radiation resistance, $R_r(\alpha)$, and directivity, $D(\alpha)$, according to the radius, a, of the loop antenna can be found in Balanis (2005). For convenience, these expressions are placed here:

$$R_r(\alpha) = 60(\pi\alpha)^2 T(\alpha) \quad (21)$$

$$D(\alpha) = F_m(\alpha)/T(\alpha). \quad (22)$$

For the current uniform and co-sinusoidal distributions, the auxiliary functions $F_m(\alpha)$ and $T(\alpha)$ are given by (23) and (24), respectively.

$$F_m(\alpha) = \begin{cases} \begin{cases} 2J_1^2(1.840) = 0.677, & \alpha > 1.840 \\ 2J_1^2(\alpha) & \alpha < 1.840 \end{cases}, & I_\phi = I_0 \\ 1, & I_\phi(\phi) = I_0\cos(\phi) \end{cases} \quad (23)$$

$$T(\alpha) = \begin{cases} Q_{11}^{(1)}(\alpha), & I_\phi = I_0 \\ \frac{1}{2}\left[Q_{00}^{(1)}(\alpha)\text{-}2Q_{11}^{(1)}(\alpha)/\alpha^2 + Q_{22}^{(1)}(\alpha)\right], & I_\phi(\phi) = I_0\cos(\phi) \end{cases} \quad (24)$$

The objective is to find a neural network to model the Q integrals shown in (24). The Q integrals representation was given by Savov (2006) and is shown in (25), using the Bessel functions notation, where $\alpha = ka$, $k = 2\pi / \lambda$, and $J_m(\cdot)$ is the Bessel function of first type and *m*th order.

$$Q_{mn}^{(p)}(\alpha) = \int_0^{\pi/2} J_m[\alpha \sin(\theta)] J_n[\alpha \sin(\theta)] \sin^{(p)}(\theta)\, d, \quad (25)$$

The computational solution of Q integrals is a difficult numerical problem, mainly with respect to large loop antennas, due to the fast oscilations shown by the integral operator, which represents an exaustive and inneficient numerical procedure. However, according to Mahony (2003), for $n = m$ **and** $p = 1$, it is possible to overcome this problem, by rewriting (25) as a function of a simplified integral, shown in (26).

$$Q_{nn}^{(1)}(\alpha) = \frac{1}{2\alpha} \int_0^{2\alpha} J_{2n}(t)dt \quad (26)$$

In addition, an analitical approximation through Bessel function series can be done and is given in (27).

$$Q_{nn}^{(1)}(\alpha) = \frac{1}{\alpha} \sum_{k=n}^{\infty} J_{2k+1}(2\alpha) \quad (27)$$

A neural network configuration similar to that of Figure 1(b) was used with only one input node and one hidden layer to model the expression defined in (26). After several tests to choose the appropriate basis function, among sigmoid, exponential, polynomial and sinusoidal functions, the basis function defined in (28) was chosen, where $\mathbf{w}_j = [k_j \;\; \xi_j \;\; \tau_j \;\; \omega_j \;\; \varphi_j]^{\mathrm{T}}$ is the weight vector of the *j*th hidden neuron and $0 \le \bar{\alpha} \le 1$ is the normalized input of the neural network. The activation function proposed in (28) has five independent parameters and for this reason is very flexible, presenting a variety of formulations, depending on the value of each parameter.

$$q_j(\mathbf{w}_j, \bar{\alpha}) = \frac{k_j}{\sqrt{|1-\xi_j^2|}} \exp\left(-\xi_j \tau_j \bar{\alpha}\right) \cdot \sin\left(\omega_j \bar{\alpha} + \varphi_j\right) \quad (28)$$

The resulting neural network is called DSFNN – *Damped-Sinusoid Functions Neural Network* and is very efficient at the solution of Q integrals (Silva, Passos, D'Assunção, 2007; Silva, Passos, & Fernandes, 2007). DSFNN works according to the forward computation defined in (29) and approximates the Q integrals using (30).

$$q_{nn} = \left| 1 - \sum_{j=0}^{N_h - 1} q_j(\mathbf{w}_j, \bar{\alpha}) \right| \quad (29)$$

$$Q_{nn}^{(1)}(\alpha) \approx \frac{1}{\alpha} q_{nn} \quad (30)$$

The radiation resistance and directivity of the circular loop antenna were obtained using four approximations: numerical integration, empirical expressions, series of Bessel functions (30 terms) and the DSFNN model (which used 10 basis functions). The numerical integration of (26) using Lobatto quadrature returned accurate values and verified the precision of the other approximations.

Some of the obtained results are shown in Figure 5. Figure 5(a) shows the excellent approximation obtained through the DSFNN model, considering $n = 0, 1, 2$. In this case, a number of 1000 points were used for testing the DSFNN model, at the range of $0.1 \le \alpha \le 16$. Figure 5(b) shows the results obtained for the antenna directivity, considering the uniform and co-sinusoidal current distributions at the range of $0.1 \le \alpha \le 10$.

Figure 5. (a) DSFNN model approximation for Q integrals; (b) simulated results for the directivity of the circular loop antenna through Lobatto quadrature, approximated expressions and DSFNN model

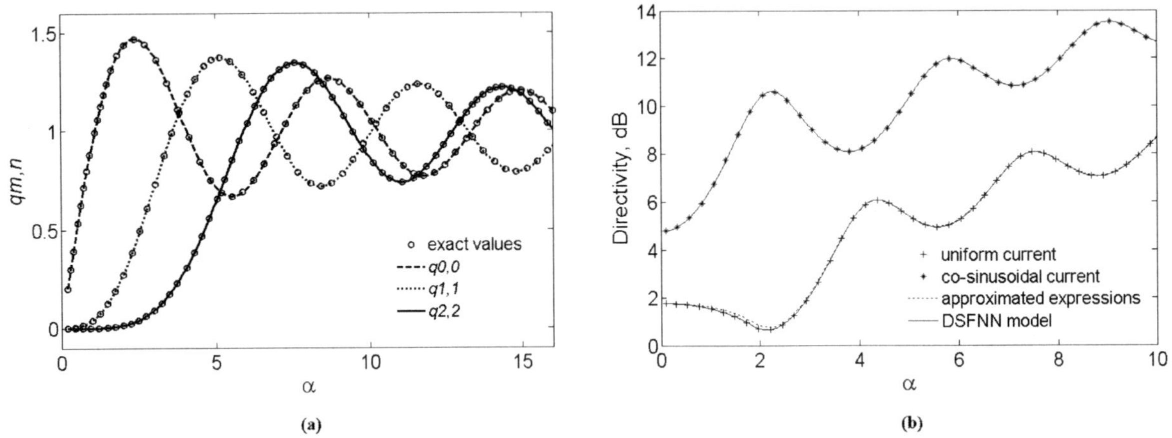

It is worth to say that while the approximated expressions return a maximum error of 0.2 dB, the DSFNN model returns a maximum error of 0.00006 dB, validating the accuracy of the proposed model.

On the other hand, the computational efficiency is almost the same for both numerical expressions and the DSFNN model, except for the fact that the DSFNN model showed to be ten times faster than the series of Bessel functions.

Modular Neural Networks

In recent years, some techniques have been proposed that exploit the microwave knowledge by incorporating empirical models to single neural network models. Some advantages by the use of prior information in neural networks trainings include: a better neural model accuracy, a good generalization ability, a model reliability improvement and a decrease in the number of training examples. These interesting characteristics contribute to reduce the neural network complexity. Some examples of these techniques are: hybrid EM-ANN (Watson & Gupta, 1996), Prior Knowledge Input - PKI (Watson, Gupta, & Mahajan, 1998), Knowledge Based ANN - KBNN (Wang & Zhang, 1997), and space mapping ANN (Rayas-Sanchez, 2001).

However, the larger is the training dataset (which represents a high complex mapping) the more complex is the single neural network configuration. The addition of more hidden units naturally results in a slow learning, which may contribute to a poor generalization. On the other hand, for an insufficient number of hidden units, the overload of the single neural network occurs. In this case, custom methods are not able to give good responses in the mapping regions that have high oscillatory and complex nonlinear behavior. To overcome these difficulties, we can use a modular configuration of neural networks.

The idea of using a modular neural network associated to complex input-output mapping functions was discussed as far as the middle of 1990s (Jacobs, Jordan, Nowlan, & Hinton, 1991). The most popular modular architectures are the mixture of experts (ME) and the hierarchical mixture of experts (HME) (Jordan & Jacobs, 1994). These models attempt to solve problems using the '*divide and conquer*' principle. In this context, expert networks share the complex nonlinear modeling task. The gating network computes the output of modular structure from weighting the outputs of expert networks.

This section presents a new class of modular neural networks based on Prior Knowledge Input - PKI technique and that has been used to model nonlinear devices in microwave/optical bands. The proposed modular configuration employs three or more feedforward neural networks each one with one hidden layer of activation functions. Furthermore, the proposed modular configuration is able to generalize for new values of input parameters, validating it as a good estimator into the mapping regions where no previous numerical or experimental information is available.

The simplest modular configuration with two expert networks is illustrated in Figure 6(a). The expert networks share the entire mapping, reducing the complexity of the learning task. The technique uses training datasets for initial and final input parameter values that are presented to the expert networks. For three or more experts, the obtained training data from intermediate input parameter values can be used to train additional experts. The entire training set is then used for the output network training.

The first definition of the proposed modular network paradigm is that all the individual neural networks have the same configuration: the Sample Function Neural Network – SFNN (Silva, 2002). The configuration of the SFNN is similar to the configuration of a RBF (Radial Basis Function) neural network. The activation function of the hidden neurons is defined with a set of modified sample functions, given by (13), where x is the input vector; c and σ are the centers (translations) and the widths (dilatations) of sample functions, respectively; ε is an exponent that manages the amplitude of main (central) and side lobes of sample functions. The range of variation of these parameters are given by: $c = x + \gamma$, where γ is a random variable, $0.1 \leq \sigma \leq 2.0$, and $0.1 \leq \varepsilon \leq 2.0$.

$$\phi(\mathbf{x}) = \frac{\sin\left(\left\|\mathbf{x} - \mathbf{c}\right\|^{2}\right)}{\tilde{\mathbf{A}} \cdot \left\|\mathbf{x} - \mathbf{c}\right\|^{2\mu}} \qquad (31)$$

The choice of a sample function is based on signal processing theory. The computation of (31) involves only one elementary sine function. From this simple definition, it is obtained a more efficient training algorithm. For instance, sigmoid (MLP) and Gaussian (RBF) activation functions need more complex gradient calculations, naturally slowing down the training algorithm. Training SFNN networks involves the adjustment of the free parameters, $w = [c\,\sigma\,\varepsilon\,v]$. The efficient RPROP algorithm was used to adjust the free parameters of the SFNN.

Here, a modular configuration of SFNNs is applied for modeling a parallel plate waveguide on electromagnetic band gap (EBG) structure. The EBG and PBG (photonic band gap) structures are composed by periodic lattices of metallic, dielectric or composite elements, which exhibit filter characteristics in their frequency responses. These structures have been extensively investigated for their versatility in controlling the propagation of electromagnetic waves (Joannopoulus, Jonhson, Winn, & Meade, 2008). Usually, the EBG devices are analyzed by full-wave techniques, like integral equation or Finite-Difference Time-Domain (FDTD) methods (Radisic, Qian, Coccioli, & Itoh, 1998). These methods have been extensively studied and accomplished good results. However, they require a well-established electromagnetic theory and intensive computational efforts.

The SFNN configuration is composed by two expert networks and one output network, each one with 10 neurons in the hidden layer. Besides, two input nodes are used for the parameters: a hole diameter d and an operation frequency f. The output layer has one node that represents the transmission parameter S_{21}. In the training process was employed a set of 60 results, available in (Dawn, Ohashi, & Shimura, 2002), that were obtained by electromagnetic simulation with the commercial software Ansoft HFSS. The parallel plate waveguide on EBG structure parameters are shown in Figure 6(b), which assume the following values: a shielding plate with circular hole diameters d

Figure 6. (a) The proposed modular neural network configuration; (b) parallel plate waveguide on EBG structure; (c) generalization of SFNN modular model for EBG structure

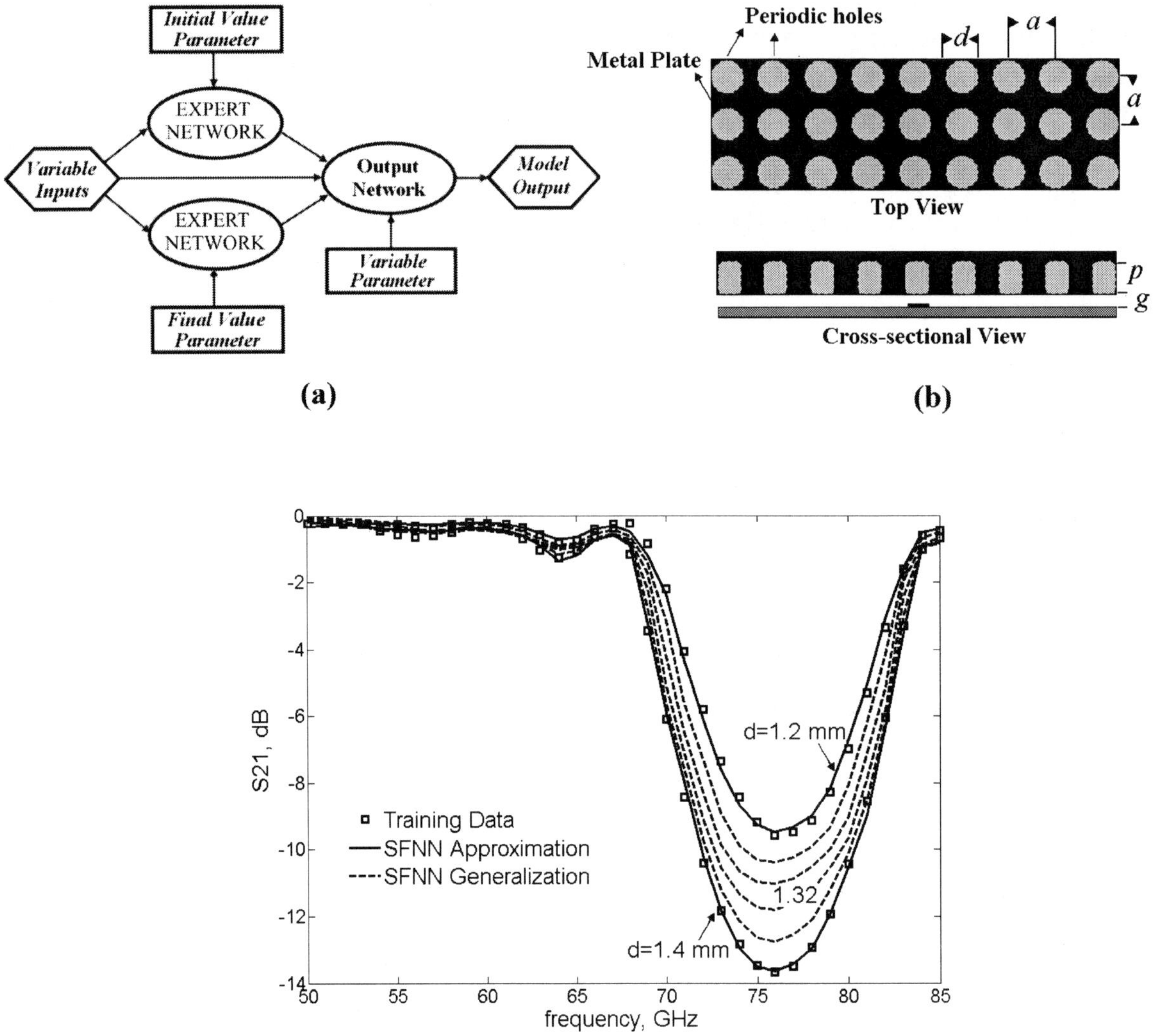

(c)

= 1.2 mm and d = 1.4 mm, a = 1.62 mm, p = 1.2 mm, and g = 0.5 mm.

Some of the simulated results are shown in Figure 6(c). A good agreement was observed between the simulations and the SFNN model response. Some of reported SFNN neuromodeling applications for microwave devices with EBG/PBG structures include: microstrip filters on PBG structure, UC-EBG rectangular waveguide and parallel plate waveguide on EBG structure, and can be found in (Fernandes, 2004).

Other applications of the proposed modular network configuration include fast and accurate modeling of frequency selective surfaces using a modular neural network configuration of multilayer perceptrons (Silva & Campos, 2008), as well as using a RBF/MLP modular configuration for device modeling in microwave and optical bands (Passos, Silva, & Fernandes, 2007).

HYBRID EM-OPTIMIZATION METHOD FOR OPTIMAL DESIGN OF FSS

Frequency selective surface (FSS) is a two-dimensional periodic array of elements (patches or apertures) in a conducting screen, which could be either freestanding or supported by dielectric substrates, as shown in Figure 7(a). FSSs are used for a variety of applications, such as: hybrid radomes, polarizers and dichroic reflectors, waveguide filters, artificial magnetic conductors, microwave absorbers etc. To provide high-performance filtering properties at microwave bands, electromagnetic engineers have investigated various types of FSS devices: reconfigurable FSS screens, fractal self-similar geometries, pixelized FSS screens, multilayered FSS structures, as well as FSSs on anisotropic substrates (Silva, Lacouth, Fontgalland, Campos, & D'Assunção, 2007; Campos, D'Assunção, & Melo, 2001).

There is no closed form solution directly from a given desired frequency response to the corresponding FSS (Hwang, Chan, & Marks, 1990). The analysis of scattering characteristics from FSS devices requires the application of rigorous full-wave techniques. Besides that, due to the computational complexity of using a full-wave simulator to evaluate the FSS scattering variables, many electromagnetic engineers still use a trial-and-error process until to achieve a given design criterion. Obviously this procedure is very laborious and human dependent. Therefore, optimization techniques are required to design practical FSSs with desired filter specifications. Some authors have employed neural networks, PSO and GA for FSS design and optimization.

The FSS design methodology, which blends MLP models, GA and PSO algorithms, is applied for thin dipole FSS synthesis considering electromagnetic parameters such as resonant frequency (f_r) and –3dB bandwidth (BW) as a function of the substrate thickness (h) and the periodicity of elements ($\tau = t_x = t_y$) corresponding to a square unit cell. The width and length of the thin dipole were kept constant: $W = 1.27$ mm and $L = 12.7$ mm, respectively. The region of interest (or search space) defined by desired input variables is a rectangle: $0.1 \leq h \leq 2.0$ mm and $15.24 \leq \tau \leq 19.05$ mm. The FSS optimization problem consists of obtaining an optimal solution ($h^*; \tau^*$) in the search space that results in a minimal thickness FSS with the desired specifications for resonant frequency and bandwidth.

After the definition of the FSS filter-type, design input variables and search space, a parametric analysis is performed in order to observe the FSS EM-behavior. At this step, the FSS transmission coefficients at 6.0−14.0 GHz band were obtained by means of Method of Moments (MoM) simulations considering substrate anisotropy (Campos et al., 2001). Representative EM-datasets must be obtained from the parametric analysis for supervised learning of FSS analysis and synthesis MLP models.

At the second step, a modular MLP/MLP model for FSS analysis is developed to approach the transmission coefficient $S_{21}(f, h, \tau)$. The MLP/MLP model estimates the EM-relations $f_r(h, \tau)$ and $BW(h, \tau)$ for FSS resonant frequency and bandwidth, respectively (Silva & Campos, 2008). Then, f_r and BW mappings are modeled by the synthesis MLP network using the conventional neuromodeling technique (Zhang & Gupta, 2000). The third step just consists of implementing the natural optimization algorithms for FSS optimal synthesis. In particular, the continuous-GA and PSO algorithms were used.

Through the FSS neuromodeling, we avoid the very intensive application of the CPU for MoM analysis in GA and PSO simulations. Two ANN models were developed for FSS analysis and synthesis using one hidden layer MLP configurations. The MLP learning processes were carried out using the RPROP training algorithm, with

Figure 7. (a) Frequency selective surface structure; (b) synthesis MLP configuration; (c) modular MLP/MLP configuration

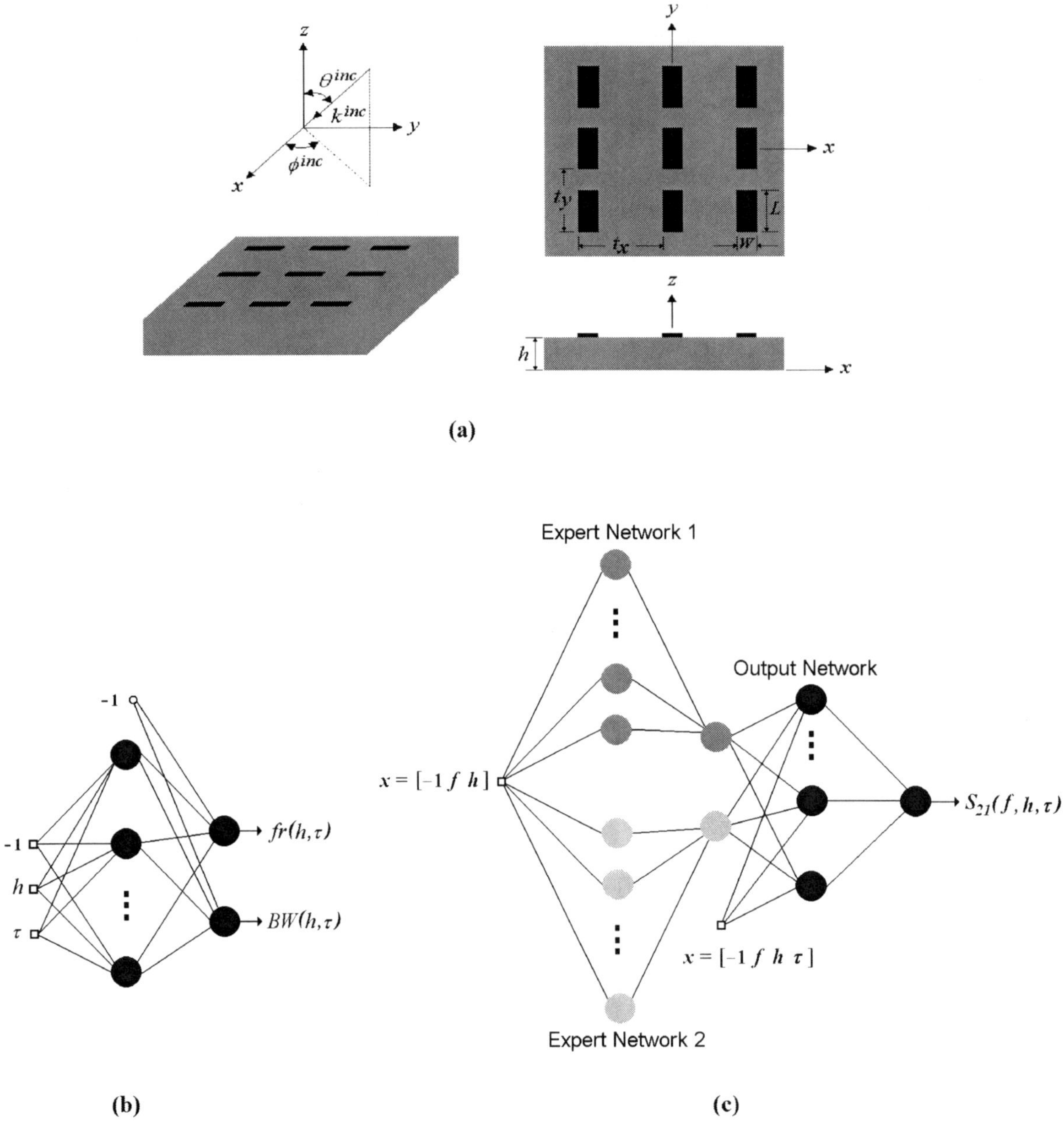

standard parameters (Ridmiller & Braun, 1993), in order to minimize the mean square error as defined in (4). In this case, the RPROP training is performed until the mean square error reaches a minimum pre-established value.

The synthesis MLP network configuration (composed by three inputs, ten hidden neurons and two outputs) simultaneously approaches both the mappings $f_r(h, \tau)$ and $BW(h, \tau)$. The MLP configuration with one hidden layer is illustrated in Figure 7(b). To generate the synthesis training

Table 1. GA and PSO parameters used in the simulations

Continuous-GA	Improved-GA	PSO
crossover probability = 0.5	crossover probability = 0.5	constriction parameter, $C = 0.8$
mutation rate = 0.5	mutation rate = 0.5	
$A = 30$	$A = 30$ and $B = 10^{-9}$	cognitive parameter, $\Gamma_1 = 2$
		social parameter, $\Gamma_2 = 2$

dataset were assumed the vectors given in (32) for the design input variables h and τ, adding up 72 training examples.

$$\begin{cases} \mathbf{h} = \begin{bmatrix} 0.1 & 0.3 & 0.5 & 0.7 & 0.9 & 1.0 & 1.2 & 1.4 & 1.5 & 1.6 & 1.8 & 2.0 \end{bmatrix} \text{ mm} \\ \text{Ä} = \mathbf{tx} = \mathbf{ty} = \begin{bmatrix} 15.24 & 15.87 & 16.51 & 17.14 & 18.41 & 19.05 \end{bmatrix} \text{ mm} \end{cases} \quad (32)$$

The ANN model for FSS analysis approximates the EM relation $S_{21}(f, h, \tau)$ from 6.0 GHz up to 14.0 GHz with increments of $\Delta f = 100$ MHz, totalizing 81 samples. Considering the design input variable vectors according to (32), the entire analysis training dataset comprises 5,832 examples. To accomplish this complex modeling learning task, the '*divide-and-conquer*' principle was applied to develop a modular MLP/MLP configuration of MLP networks (two experts and one output) as illustrated in Figure 7(c). The hidden layer of each expert MLP was assumed with 30 neurons. The output MLP network was configured with 40 hidden neurons. The modular MLP/MLP model development and the EM dataset subdivision scheme can be found in (Silva & Campos, 2008).

GA and PSO algorithms were implemented in Matlab® for optimal FSS synthesis. The assumed design input variables (substrate thickness and periodicity) were symbolized by h_m^k and τ_m^k to take into account the m-th individual at the k-th iteration. Given a desired FSS filter specification, $(fr_{desired}, BW_{desired})$, the aim is the minimization of the quadratic cost function as defined in (33) in terms of absolute percent errors.

$$\cos t(k,m) = \left(\frac{\left| fr_{desired} - fr\left(h_m^k, \tau_m^k\right) \right|}{f_{desired}} + \frac{\left| BW_{desired} - BW\left(h_m^k, \tau_m^k\right) \right|}{BW_{desired}} \right)^2, \quad m = 1, 2, \ldots, Npop \quad (33)$$

To evaluate the cost function (33) the synthesis MLP approach the EM relations $f_r\left(h_m^k, \tau_m^k\right)$ and $BW\left(h_m^k, \tau_m^k\right)$. When the population evolves, each individual is constrained to the region of interest using (34), where the dummy variable ξ can be replaced by h or τ.

$$\xi_m^k = \min\left(\max\left(\xi_m^k, \xi_{\min}\right), \xi_{\max}\right) \quad (34)$$

The parameters used for continuous-GA, improved-GA, and PSO simulations are shown in Table 1.

Here, an example that uses the hybrid EM-optimization technique for the optimal synthesis of FSSs is shown. It was considered a previously known design solution provided by MoM simulation, which was used in the training of the synthesis MLP network, corresponding to input/output data: $(h^*; \tau^*) = (0.10; 16.51)$ mm and $(f_r; BW) = (11.1; 2.2)$ GHz.

The algorithms start with the same initial population far from the optimum known solution and composed by one hundred of individuals

Figure 8. FSS optimization example: (a) continuous-GA simulation; (b) improved-GA and PSO simulations; (c) continuous-GA, improved-GA and PSO cost functions

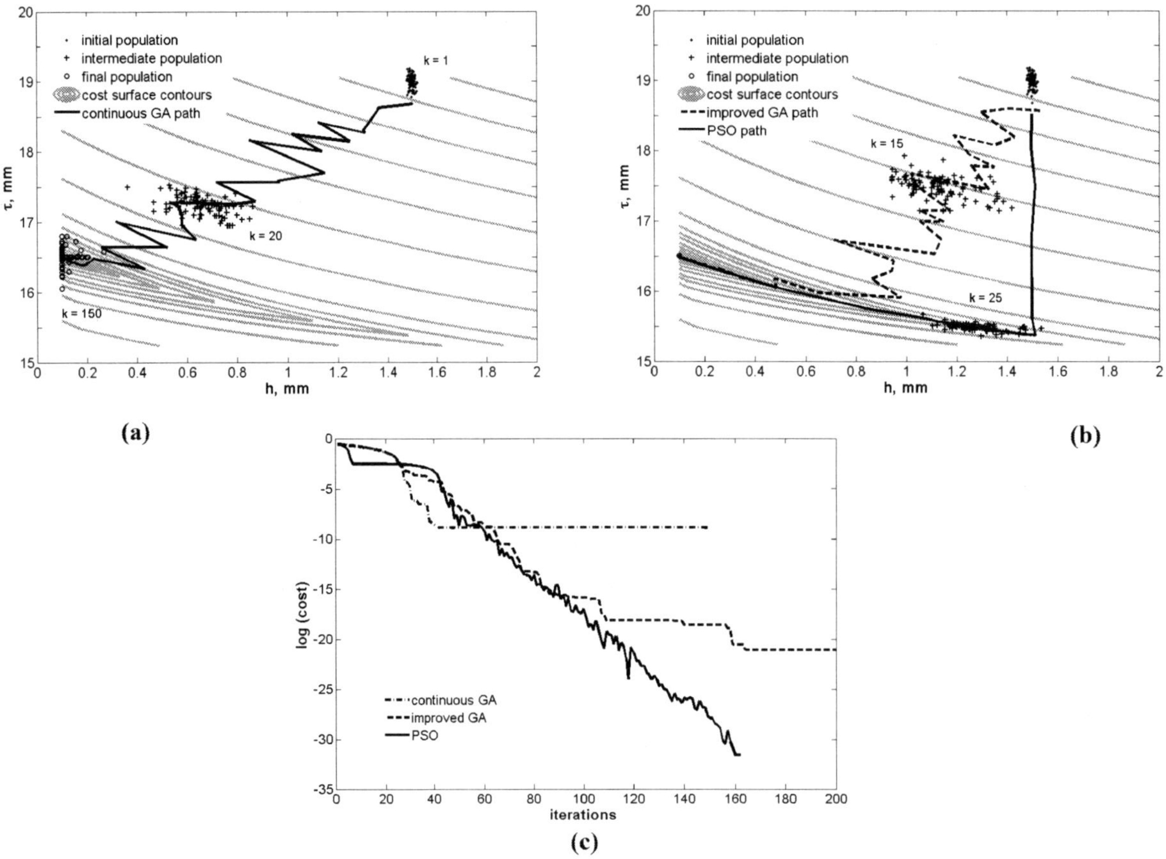

(N_{pop}=100) distributed according to (35) and subject to the restriction given in (34). The *randn*() function on the right side of (35) returns normally distributed random numbers, chosen from a normal distribution with mean equal to zero, variance and standard deviation equal to one.

$$\left(h_i;\tau_i\right) = \left(1.5 + randn() \,/\, 1000;\ 19 + randn() \,/\, 100\right), \quad i = 1, 2, \cdots, 100 \tag{35}$$

Figures 8(a) and 8(b) show the cost surface contours, the initial, intermediate, and final populations, as well as the best path obtained from the algorithm simulations. The zigzag paths at flat regions of cost surface contribute to slow down the convergence of genetic algorithms. The final population of continuous-GA algorithm oscillates around the global minimum of cost function, according to Figure 8(a), while the improved-GA final population is closely to the global minimum, which can be observed in Figure 8(b). On the other hand, PSO algorithm path is quite linear and, for the global minimum neighborhoods, its direction is normal to the contours of the cost surface, also seen in Figure 8(b).

Figure 8(c) shows the evolution of the global cost for each algorithm simulation. It is observed that improved-GA converges closely to global minimum while continuous-GA final cost is relatively very high. The best-fit individual of the PSO final population converges to the global minimum of the cost function (36) and the algorithm is limited in precision to the round off error of the computer.

CONCLUSION

This chapter described some of the neuromodeling methodology applications, where the artificial neural networks showed to be a powerful tool to be used in Engineering, in particular, to model RF/microwave circuit/devices. Some original contributions were shown, such as the optimal neural network DSFNN and the hybrid EM-optimization (which blends MLP/MLP modular neural network), genetic algorithms and particle swarm optimization, used in the design of frequency selective surfaces. The choice of the activation function of a FNN strongly influences the neural model performance. However, there is not an universal activation function that can be used to solve any kind of nonlinear modeling problem. Using additional information from the hybrid neural models, as well as sharing the training process with modular neural networks, increased the efficiency and therefore the generalization ability and model reliability of the resulting neural models. The MLP model developed to map MESFET's parameters was successful employed in association to time-domain method for MESFET logic gate circuit transient analysis. The fast and accurate obtained results demonstrated the improvements with the utilization of this model, and proved that the MLP network global approximation is able to generalize. The efficient computation and accuracy of the GaAs MESFET MLP model developed lead to further utilization in time-domain simulation programs, like SPICE. On the other hand, the proposed SFNN modular network and DSFNN optimal neural network also presented a great capacity of approximation and generalization. Some advantages include computational efficiency and reduced use of memory. In addition, the idea of blending natural optimization algorithms and ANNs for EM-optimization shows to be very interesting. The characteristics of ANN models (precision, CPU-efficiency and flexibility) can be blended with natural optimization algorithms to develop powerful EM-optimization soft computing tools. For example, one thousand of continuous-GA or PSO cycles iterations can be carried out below 30 seconds to the FSS optimal design when the MLP/MLP modular neural network was used for cost function evaluation of developed natural algorithms.

REFERENCES

Balanis, C. A. (2005). *Antenna theory: Analysis and design* (3rd ed.). New York: John Wiley & Sons.

Campos, A. L. P. S., D'Assunção, A. G., & Melo, M. A. B. (2001). Investigation of scattering parameters for frequency selective surfaces using thin dipoles on anisotropic layers. *Proceedings of the SBMO/IEEE MTT-S International Microwave and Optoelectronics Conference, 1,* 413-416.

Curtice, W. R. (1980). A MESFET model for use in design of GaAs integrated circuits. *IEEE Transactions on Microwave Theory and Techniques, 28*(5), 448–456. doi:10.1109/TMTT.1980.1130099

Dawn, K., Ohashi, Y., & Shimura, T. (2002). A novel electromagnetic band gap metal plate for parallel plate mode suppression in shielded structures. *IEEE Microwave and Wireless Components Letters, 12*(5), 166–168. doi:10.1109/7260.1000191

Fernandes, E. N. R. Q. (2004). *Modelagem Neurocomputacional de Dispositivos de Microondas com Estruturas EBG.* (Doctoral dissertation, Federal University of Campina Grande, 2004).

Haupt, R. L., & Haupt, S. E. (2004). *Practical genetic algorithms* (2nd ed.). Hoboken, NJ: John Wiley & Sons.

Haupt, R. L., & Werner, D. H. (2007). *Genetic algorithms in electromagnetics*. Hoboken, NJ: John Willey & Sons. doi:10.1002/047010628X

Haykin, S. (1999). *Neural networks: a comprehensive foundation* (2nd ed.). Upper Saddle River, NJ: Prentice-Hall.

Hwang, J. N., Chan, C. H., & Marks, R. J. (1990). Frequency selective surface design based on iterative inversion of neural networks. *Proceedings of the International Joint Conference on Neural Networks, 1*, 39–44. doi:10.1109/IJCNN.1990.137541

Jacobs, R. A. (1988). Increase rate of convergence through learning rate adaptation. *Neural Networks, 1*(4), 295–307. doi:10.1016/0893-6080(88)90003-2

Jacobs, R. A., Jordan, M. I., Nowlan, S. J., & Hinton, G. E. (1991). Adaptive mixture of local experts. [Cambridge, MA: MIT Press.]. *Neural Computation, 3*, 79–87. doi:10.1162/neco.1991.3.1.79

Joannopoulus, J. D., Jonhson, S. G., Winn, J. N., & Meade, R. D. (2008). *Photonic crystal molding the flow of light* (2nd ed.). New Jersey: Princenton University Press. Retrieved February 06, 2010, from http://ab-initio.mit.edu/book/photonic-crystals-book.pdf.

Jordan, M. I., & Jacobs, R. A. (1994). Hierarchical mixtures of experts and the EM algorithm. [MIT Press.]. *Neural Computation, 6*, 181–214. doi:10.1162/neco.1994.6.2.181

Kennedy, L., & Eberhart, R. C. (1995). Particle swarm optimization. *Proceedings of the IV IEEE Conference on Neural Networks, 4*, 1942–1948.

Mahony, J. D. A. (2003). Comment on Q-type integrals and their use in expressions for radiated power. *IEEE Antennas and Propagation Magazine, 45*(3), 127–128. doi:10.1109/MAP.2003.1232169

McCculloch, W. S., & Pitts, W. (1943). A logical calculus of the ideas immanent in nervous activity. *The Bulletin of Mathematical Biophysics, 5*, 115–133. doi:10.1007/BF02478259

Parker, A. E., & Skellern, D. J. (1997). A realistic large-signal MESFET model for SPICE. *IEEE Transactions on Microwave Theory and Techniques, 45*(9), 1563–1571. doi:10.1109/22.622923

Passos, M. G., Silva, P. H. da F., & Fernandes, H. C. C. (2007). Applications of modular RBF/MLP neural networks in the modeling of microstrip photonic band gap structures. *Proceedings of Progress In Electromagnetics Research Symposium, 2*(5), 695–700.

Patnaik, A., & Mishra, R. K. (2000). ANN techniques in microwave engineering. *IEEE Microwave Magazine, 1*(1), 55–60. doi:10.1109/6668.823828

Radisic, V., Qian, Y., Coccioli, R., & Itoh, T. (1998). Novel 2-D photonic band-gap structures for microstrip lines. *IEEE Microwave Guided Wave Letters, 8*(2), 69–71. doi:10.1109/75.658644

Raghuram, R. (1989). *Computer simulation of electronic circuits*. New Delhi: Wiley Eastern Limited.

Rayas-Sanchez, J. E. (2001). *Neural space mapping methods for modeling and design of microwave circuits*. (Doctoral dissertation, McMaster University, 2001).

Ridmiller, M., & Braun, H. (1993). *A direct adaptive method for faster backpropagation learning: The RPROP algorithm*. Paper presented at the IEEE International Conference on Neural Networks, San Francisco, EUA.

Rosenblatt, F. (1958) The Perceptron: A probabilistic model for information storage and organization in the brain. *Psychological Review, 65*(6), p. 386-408. Retrieved February 06, 2010, from http://www.ling.upenn.edu/courses/Fall_2007/cogs501/Rosenblatt1958.pdf.

Rumelhart, D. E., Hinton, G. E., & Williams, R. J. (1986). Learning internal representations by error propagation. In D. E. Rumelhart & J. L. McClelland (Ed.), *Parallel Distributed Processing: Explorations in the microstructure of cognition, Vol. 1: Foundations* (pp. 318-362). Cambridge, MA: MIT Press.

Santos, A. L., Romariz, A. R. S., & Carvalho, P. H. P. (1997). Neural model of electrical devices for circuit simulation. *Proceedings of the SBMO/IEEE MTT-S International Microwave and Optoelectronics Conference, Vol. 1,* 253-258.

Savov, S. V. (2002). An efficient solution of a class of integrals arising in antenna theory. *IEEE Antennas and Propagation Magazine, 44*(5), 98–101. doi:10.1109/MAP.2002.1077781

Schichman, H., & Hodges, D. A. (1968). Modeling and simulation of insulated-gate field-effect transistor switching circuits. *IEEE Journal of Solid-state Circuits, 3*(3), 285–289. doi:10.1109/JSSC.1968.1049902

Silva, P. H. da F. (2002). *Modelos através de redes neurais artificiais sem realimentação para dispositivos e circuitos de RF/Microondas.* (Doctoral dissertation, Federal University of Campina Grande, 2002).

Silva, P. H. da F., & Campos, A. L. P. S. (2008). Fast and accurate modeling of frequency selective surfaces using a new modular neural network configuration of multilayer perceptrons. *IET Microwaves. Antennas & Propagation, 2*(5), 503–511.

Silva, P. H. da F., Lacouth, P., Fontgalland, G., Campos, A. L. P. S., & D'Assunção, A. G. (2007), Design of frequency selective surfaces using a novel MoM-ANN-GA technique. *Proceedings of the SBMO/IEEE MTT-S International Microwave and Optoelectronics Conference, Vol. 1,* 275-279.

Silva, P. H. da F., Melo, M. A. B., & Neto, A. D. D. (2001). Fast and accurate neural network GaAs MESFET model for time-domain circuit simulation. *Proceedings of the SBMO/IEEE MTT-S International Microwave and Optoelectronics Conference, Vol. 1,* 53-56.

Silva, P. H. da F., Melo, M. A. B., & Neto, A. D. D. (2002). Using neural network models for efficient GaAs MESFET time-domain nonlinear circuit analysis. *Proceedings of the International Joint Conference on Neural Networks, 3,* 2282–2287.

Silva, P. H. da F., Passos, M. G., & D'Assunção, A. G. (2007). Fast and accurate analysis for the directivity of circular-shape antennas using optimal neural networks. *Microwave and Optical Technology Letters, 49*(11), 2721–2726. doi:10.1002/mop.22839

Silva, P. H. da F., Passos, M. G., & Fernandes, H. C. C. (2007). Novel neural network models of Q-type integrals and their use for circular-loop antenna analysis. *Proceedings of Progress In Electromagnetics Research Symposium, 1,* 2137–2141.

Sussman-Fort, S. E., Narasimhan, S., & Mayaram, K. (1984). A complete GaAs MESFET computer model for SPICE. *IEEE Transactions on Microwave Theory and Techniques, 32*(4), 471–473. doi:10.1109/TMTT.1984.1132707

Wang, F., & Zhang, Q. J. (1997). Knowledge based neural models for microwave design. *IEEE Transactions on Microwave Theory and Techniques, 45*(12), 2333–2343. doi:10.1109/22.643839

Watson, P. M., & Gupta, K. C. (1996). EM-ANN models for microstrip vias and interconnects in datasets circuits. *IEEE Transactions on Microwave Theory and Techniques, 44*(12), 2495–2503. doi:10.1109/22.554584

Watson, P. M., Gupta, K. C., & Mahajan, R. L. (1998). *Development of knowledge based artificial neural networks models for microwave components*. Paper presented at the IEEE MTT-S International Microwave Symposium, Baltimore.

Zhang, Q. J., & Gupta, C. (2000). *Neural networks for RF and microwaves design*. Norwood, MA: Artech House.

ADDITIONAL READING

Balanis, C. A. (1989). *Advanced engineering electromagnetics*. New York: John Wiley & Sons.

Bonabeau, E., Dorigo, M., & Theraulaz, G. (1999). *Swarm intelligence: From natural to artificial system*. New York: Oxford University Press.

Christodoulou, C., & Georgiopoulos, M. (2001). *Applications of neural networks in electromagnetics*. Boston, MA: Artech House.

Cruz, R. M. S., D'Assunção, A. G., & Silva, P. H. da F. (2009). Synthesis of crossed dipole frequency selective surfaces using genetic algorithms and artificial neural networks. *Proceedings of the International Joint Conference on Neural Networks, Vol. 1*, 627- 633.

Cruz, R. M. S., Silva, P. H. da F., & D'Assunção, A. G. (2009). Neuromodeling stop-band properties of Koch island patch elements for FSS filter design. *Microwave and Optical Technology Letters, 15*(12), 3014–3019. doi:10.1002/mop.24795

Cruz, R. M. S., Silva, P. H. da F., & D'Assunção, A. G. (2009, November). *Blending PSO and ANN for optimal design of FSS filters with Koch island patch elements.* Paper presented at the Conference on the Computation of Electromagnetic Fields, Florianópolis, Brasil.

Duch, W., & Jankowski, N. (2001, April). *Optimal transfer function neural networks*. Paper presented at the European Symposium on Artificial Neural Networks, Bruges, Belgium. Retrieved February 06, 2010, from http://www.fizyka.umk.pl/ftp/papers/kmk/01Esann-ND.pdf.

Fernandes, E. N. R. Q., Silva, P. H. da F., Melo, M. A. B., & D'Assunção, A. G. (2002, September). *A new neural network model for accurate analysis of microstrip lines on PBG filters*. Paper presented at the 32nd European *Microwave Conference*, Milano, Italy.

Fernandes, E. N. R. Q., Silva, P. H. da F., Melo, M. A. B., & D'Assunção, A. G. (2003, June). *A neural network modeling of microwave circuits on PBG structures*. Paper presented at the *IEEE MTT-S International Microwave Symposium*, Philadelphia.

Fernandes, E. N. R. Q., Silva, P. H. da F., Melo, M. A. B., & D'Assunção, A. G. (2005, June). *Modular configuration RPROP/SF-ANN for microwave waveguide on EBG structures modeling*. Paper presented at the *IEEE MTT-S International Microwave Symposium*, Long Beach, USA.

Hashem, S., & Schmeiser, B. (1995). Improving model accuracy using optimal linear combinations of trained neural networks. *IEEE Transactions on Neural Networks, 6*(3), 792–794. doi:10.1109/72.377990

Haupt, R. L. (1995). An introduction to genetic algorithms for electromagnetics. *IEEE Antennas Propagation Magazine, 37*(2), 7–15. doi:10.1109/74.382334

Haykin, S. (2008). *Neural networks and learning machines* (3rd ed.). Upper Saddle River, NJ: Prentice-Hall.

Johnson, J. M., & Rahmat-Samii, Y. (1997). Genetic algorithm in engineering electromagnetics. *IEEE Antennas Propagation Magazine, 39*(4), 7–21. doi:10.1109/74.632992

Lendaris, G. G., Rest, A., & Misley, T. R. (1997, June). *Improving ANN generalization using a priori knowledge to pre-structure ANNs*. Paper presented at the IEEE International Conference on Neural Networks, Houston.

Maas, S. A. (2003). *Nonlinear microwave and RF circuits* (2nd ed.). Norwood, MA: Artech House.

Munk, B. A. (2000). *Frequency-selective surfaces: Theory and design*. New York: John Wiley & Sons. doi:10.1002/0471723770

Passos, M. G., Silva, P. H. da F., & Fernandes, H. C. C. (2006). A RBF/MLP modular neural network for microwave device modeling. *International Journal of Computer Science and Network Security, 6*(5A), 81-86. Retrieved February 06, 2010, from http://paper.ijcsns.org/07_book/200605/200605A12.pdf.

Passos, M. G., Silva, P. H. da F., & Fernandes, H. C. C. (2006, September). *A new RBF/MLP modular neural network for device modeling in microwave/optical bands*. Paper presented at the XXVII Iberian Latin American Congress On Computational Methods In Engineering, Belém, Brazil.

Rahmat-Samii, Y., & Michielssen, E. (Eds.). (1999). *Eletromagnetic Optimization by Genetic Algorithms*. John Wiley and Sons.

Silva, P. H. da F., Cruz, R. M. S., & D'Assunção, A. G. (2009, November). *An improved continuous genetic algorithm for electromagnetic optimization*. Paper presented at the Conference on the Computation of Electromagnetic Fields, Florianópolis, Brasil.

Silva, P. H. da F., Fernandes, E. N. R. Q., & Neto, A. D. D. (2002). A feedforward neural network with resolution properties for function approximation and modeling. *Proceedings of the 7th Brazilian Symposium on Neural Networks, Vol. 1*, 55-60.

Tretyakov, S. (2003). *Analytical modeling in applied electromagnetics*. Norwood, MA: Artech House.

Wiak, S., Dolezel, I., & Krawczyk, A. (2008). *Intelligent computer techniques in applied electromagnetics*. Berlin, Germany: Springer.

KEY TERMS AND DEFINITIONS

Continuous Genetic Algorithm: A genetic algorithm that works with floating-point variables and presents some advantages in relation to the binary-GA, such as: precision in representation, less memory storage and CPU requirements.

Feedforward Neural Network: A layered neural network fully connected (every neuron in each layer of the network is connected to every other neuron in the adjacent forward layer) with no feedback connections between layers. Thus, neurons in each layer of the network have as their inputs the output signals of the preceding layer only.

Knowledge-Based Neural Networks (KBNN): A neuromodeling technique where the existing device or circuit knowledge in the form of empirical functions or analytical approximations is embedded into the neural network internal structure to improve the performance of the resultant neural network models.

Improved Genetic Algorithm: A proposed continuous genetic algorithm that uses a special real function for mutation operator that improves GA-convergence on the neighborhood of global minimum of cost function.

Modular Neural Network: In the present work, a modular neural network is composed by one hidden layer feedforward neural networks that are distributed on two or more expert networks and one output neural network.

Natural Optimization: The term natural optimization is used here to describe a class of optimization algorithms inspired by nature, such as genetic algorithms, particle swarm optimization, ant colony optimization, simulated annealing, etc.

Neuromodeling: In this work, the term 'neuromodeling' is used for the method through feedforward neural networks that is applied to model the nonlinear behavior of devices and circuits in a given region of interest previously established.

Optimal Neural Network: A feedforward neural network that uses special activation or transfer functions to compute responses of nonlinear neurons and are used in complex learning task problems where common neural networks like MLP and RBF fail.

Particle Swarm Optimization (PSO): A stochastic, population-based evolutionary computer algorithm for problem solving that is based on social-psychological principles. PSO is a kind of swarm intelligence motivated by the social behavior of organisms, such as bird flocking and fish schooling.

Prior Knowledge Input (PKI): A neuromodeling technique where empirical model outputs are used as inputs to the neural network model, in addition to the original problem inputs.

Compilation of References

Aaron, R. K., Herr, H. M., Ciombor, D. M., Hochberg, L. R., Donoghue, J. P., & Briant, C. L. (2006). Horizons in Prosthesis Development for the Restoration of Limb Function. *The Journal of the American Academy of Orthopaedic Surgeons*, *14*(10), S198–S204.

Abidian, M. R., & Martin, D. C. (2008). Experimental and theoretical characterization of implantable neural microelectrodes modified with conducting polymer nanotubes. *Biomaterials*, *29*, 1273–1283. doi:10.1016/j.biomaterials.2007.11.022

Adee, S. (2009). The revolution will be prosthetized. *IEEE Spectrum*, *46*(1), 44–48. doi:10.1109/MSPEC.2009.4734314

Ahissar, M., & Hochstein, S. (2004). The reverse hierarchy theory of visual perceptual learning. *Trends in Cognitive Sciences*, *8*, 457–464. doi:10.1016/j.tics.2004.08.011

Alberini, C. M., Milekic, M. H., & Tronel, S. (2006). Mechanisms of Memory Stabilization and Destabilization. *Cellular and Molecular Life Sciences*, *63*(9), 999–100. doi:10.1007/s00018-006-6025-7

Amsel, A., & Rashotte, M. E. (1984). *Mechanisms of adaptive behavior: Clark Hull's theoretical papers, with commentary*. New York: Columbia University Press.

Andersen, R. A., Burdick, J. W., Musallam, S., Pesaran, B., & Cham, J. G. (2004). Cognitive neural prosthetics. *Trends in Cognitive Sciences*, *8*(11), 486–493. doi:10.1016/j.tics.2004.09.009

Andersen, R. A., Musallam, S., & Pesaran, B. (2004). Selecting the signals for a brain-machine interface. *Current Opinion in Neurobiology*, *14*, 1–7. doi:10.1016/j.conb.2004.10.005

Anderson, J. R. (1983). *The architecture of cognition*. Cambridge, MA: Harvard University Press.

Anderson, J. R. (2000). *Learning and memory* (2nd ed.). New York: Wiley.

Anderson, J. A. (1972). A Simple Neural Network Generating an Interactive Memory. *Mathematical Biosciences*, *14*, 197–220. doi:10.1016/0025-5564(72)90075-2

Angelov, P. P., & Filev, D. (2004). An approach to online identification of Takagi-Sugeno fuzzy models, *IEEE Trans. on Systems, Man and Cybernetics*, part B, *34*(1), 484-498.

Angulo, J. R., Acevedo, G. D., Carvajal, R. G., & Martin, A. L. (2005). Low-voltage High-performance Current-mode WTA Circuits Based on Flipped-voltage Followers. *IEEE Transactions on Circuits and Wystems. II, Express Briefs*, *52*(7), 420–423. doi:10.1109/TCSII.2005.850433

Arbib, M. A. (1987). *Brains, Machines, and Mathematics* (2nd ed.). Berlin: Springer-Verlag.

Arenz, A., Silver, R. A., Schaefer, A. T., & Margrie, T. W. (2008). The Contribution of Single Synapses to Sensory Representation in Vivo. *Science*, *321*, 977–980. doi:10.1126/science.1158391

Arik, S. (2000). Global asymptotic stability of a class of dynamic neural networks. *IEEE Transactions on Circuits and Systems I*, *47*(4), 568–571. doi:10.1109/81.841858

Ariniello, L., & McComb, M. (2002). *Brain Facts: A Primer on the Brain and Nervous System*. Washington: The Society for Neuroscience.

Asada, M., Mac Dorman, K. F., Ishiguro, H., & Kuniyoshi, Y. (2000). Cognitive developmental robotics as a new paradigm for the design of humanoid robots. In *Proc. Of the 1st IEEE-RAS Int. Conf. on Humanoid Robotics*, Cambridge, MA: MIT Press.

Asloni, M., Khoei, A., & Hadidi, K. (2006). Design of Analog Current-mode Looser-take-all Circuit. *IEICE Transactions on Electronics . E (Norwalk, Conn.)*, *89-C*(6), 819–822.

Astrom, K. J., & Wittenmark, B. (1995). *Adaptive Control* (2nd ed.). Reading, MA: Addison-Wesley.

Azeem, M. F., & Baig, A. (2007). Design and Fabrication of Basic Building Blocks for Analog Implementation of Programmable Fuzzy Logic Controller. *Proceedings of IEEE Information Reuse and Integration*, 563-569.

Baars, B. J. (2006). Conscious cognition and blackboard architectures. *The Behavioral and Brain Sciences*, *22*, 70–71.

Baars, B. J., & Franklin, S. (2003). How conscious experience and working memory interact. *Trends in Cognitive Sciences*, *7*, 166–172. doi:10.1016/S1364-6613(03)00056-1

Bade, S. L., & Hutchings, B. L. (1994). FPGA-Based Stochastic Neural Networks Implementation, *Proceedings of IEEE Workshop on FPGAs for Custom Computing Machines*, 189-198.

Baker, R. J., Li, H. W., & Boyce, D. E. (1998). *CMOS Circuit Design, Layout, and Simulation*. New York: IEEE Press.

Baker, M. W., & Sarpeshkar, R. (2007). Feedback Analysis and Design of RF Power Links for Low-Power Bionic Systems. *IEEE Transactions on Biomedical Circuits and Systems*, *1*(1), 28–38. doi:10.1109/TBCAS.2007.893180

Balanis, C. A. (2005). *Antenna theory: Analysis and design* (3rd ed.). New York: John Wiley & Sons.

Balkenius, J., & Moren, A. (1988). Computational Model Of Emotional Conditioning In The Brain. In *Proceeding of the workshop on Grounding Emotions in Adaptive* Systems, Zurich.

Baron-Cohen, S. (1995). The eye direction detector (EDD) and the shared attention mechanism (SAM): Two cases for evolutionary psychology . In Moore, C., & Dunham, P. (Eds.), *Joint attention: Its origins and role in development* (pp. 41–59). Hillsdale, NJ: Erlbaum.

Barsalou, L. W. (1999). Perceptual symbol systems. *The Behavioral and Brain Sciences*, *22*, 577–660.

Basar, T., & Bernhard, P. (1995). *Optimal Control and Related Minimax Design Problems: A Dynamic Game Approach* (2nd ed.). Boston: Birkhauser. doi:10.1007/978-0-8176-4757-5

Baskaran, M. M., & Bordawekar, R. (2009). *Optimizing Sparse Matrix-Vector Multiplication on GPUs. RJ* (Vol. 24704, p. 11). Retrieved from http://domino.watson.ibm.com/library/CyberDig.nsf/1e4115aea78b6e7c8525 6b360066f0d4/1d32f6d23b99f7898525752200618339?OpenDocument.

Bateson (1980) *Mind and Nature - A Necessary Unity*. New York: Bantam Books.

Baturone, I., Huertas, J. L., Barriga, A., & Solano, S.-S. (1994). Current-Mode Multiple-input MAX Circuit, *IEE . Electronics Letters*, *30*(9), 678–680. doi:10.1049/el:19940510

Baturone, I., Solano, S. S., & Huertas, J. L. (1994). Current-mode Singleton Fuzzy Controller. In *Proceedings of the 3rd International Conference on Fuzzy Logic, Neural Networks and Soft Computing*, IIZUKA, 647-648.

Bell, N., & Garland, M. (2008). Efficient Sparse Matrix-Vector Multiplication on CUDA.

Berthouze, H., Kozima, D., Bullock, G., & Stojanov, C. (Eds.). (2003) *Balkenius*. In *Proceedings of the Third International Workshop on Epigenetic Robotics: Modeling Cognitive Development in Robotic Systems*. Lund, Sweden: Lund University Cognitive Studies Volume 101.

Berthouze, L., & Prince, C. G. (2003) Introduction *The Third International Workshop on Epigenetic Robotics.*

Bezdek, J. C., Keller, J., Krisnapuram, R., & Pal, N. R. (2005). *Fuzzy Models and Algorithms for Pattern Recognition and Image Processing*. New York: Springer.

Billard, A., Dautenhahn, K., & Hayes, G. (1998). *Experiments on human robot communication with robots: an imitative learning and communicating doll robot*. (Technical Report CPM-98-38), Centre for Policy Modelling

Birattari, M., Bontempi, G., & Bersini, H. (1999). *Lazy learning meets the recursive least-squares algorithm, Advances in Neural Information Processing Systems 11* (Kearns, M. S., Solla, S. A., & Cohn, D. A., Eds.). Cambridge: MIT Press.

Bishop, C. M. (2004). *Neural Networks for Pattern Recognition* (3rd ed.). Oxford: Oxford University Press.

Bisseling, R. (2004). *Parallel Scientific Computation*. Oxford: Oxford Univ. Press. doi:10.1093/acprof:oso/9780198529392.001.0001

Bjornsson, C. S., Oh, S. J., Al-Kofahi, Y. A., Lim, Y. J., Smith, K. L., & Turner, J. N. (2006). Effects of insertion conditions on tissue strain and vascular damage during neuroprosthetic device insertion. *Journal of Neural Engineering*, *3*, 196–207. doi:10.1088/1741-2560/3/3/002

Bloom, P. (2000). *How children learn the meanings of words*. Cambridge, MA: MIT Press.

Boring, E. G. (1950). *A history of experimental psychology* (2nd ed.). New York: Appleton-Century-Crofts.

Boukabou, W. R., & Bouridane, A. (2007). An Improved LDA Approach with DFB Preprocessing for Face Recognition. In *Proceedings of IEEE International Symposium on Bio-inspired Learning, and Intelligent Systems for Security*, 106-110.

Bradbury, J. (2004). Taste perception: Cracking the code. *PLOS BIOL.*, *2*(3). Retrieved September 20, 2008 from http://biology.plosjournals.org

Breazeal, C. (2000, May). *Social Machines: Expressive Social Exchange Between Humans and Robots*. (PhD Thesis), Cambridge, MA: Massachusetts Institute of Technology.

Brockwell, A. E., Rojas, A. L., & Kass, R. E. (2004). Recursive Bayesian decoding of motor cortical signals by particle filtering. *Journal of Neurophysiology*, *91*, 1899–1907. doi:10.1152/jn.00438.2003

Brown, M., Di Gello, E., Milewsky, M., Wilson, M., & Kozak, M. (2000). Spatial pattern learning in rats: conditional control by two patterns. *Animal Learning & Behavior*, *28*(3), 278–287.

Brown, B. D., & Card, H. C. (2001). Stochastic Neural Computation II: Soft Competitive Learning . *IEEE Transactions on Computers*, *50*(9), 906–920. doi:10.1109/12.954506

Bubic, A., von Cramon, D. Y., & Schubotz, R. I. (2010), Prediction, cognition and the brain, *Frontiersin Journal, 4, 12 pages*

Buchel, C., Coull, J. T., & Friston, K. J. (1999). The predictive value of changes in effective connectivity for human learning. *Science*, *283*, 1538–1541. doi:10.1126/science.283.5407.1538

Buckley, J. J., & Hayashi. (1994). Fuzzy Neural Networks: A survey. *Fuzzy Sets and Systems*, *66*, 1–13. doi:10.1016/0165-0114(94)90297-6

Budik, D., & Elhanany, I. (2006, August). TRTRL: A localized resource efficient learning algorithm for recurrent neural networks. In *Proc. IEEE Midwest Symp. Circuits Syst.*, (pp. 371–374).

Bult, K., & Geelen, G. J. G. M. (1990). A Fast-Settling CMOS Operational Amplifier for SC Circuits with 90-dB DC Gain. *IEEE Journal of Solid-state Circuits*, *25*(6), 1379–1384. doi:10.1109/4.62165

Bult, K., & Wallinga, H. (1987). A Class of Analog CMOS Circuits Based on the Square-law Characteristic of an MOS Transistor in Saturation. *IEEE Journal of Solid-state Circuits*, *SC-22*(3), 357–365. doi:10.1109/JSSC.1987.1052733

Burgsteiner, H. (2006). Imitation learning with spiking neural networks and real-world devices. *Engineering Applications of Artificial Intelligence, 1*, 741–752. doi:10.1016/j.engappai.2006.05.007

Campos, A. L. P. S., D'Assunção, A. G., & Melo, M. A. B. (2001). Investigation of scattering parameters for frequency selective surfaces using thin dipoles on anisotropic layers. *Proceedings of the SBMO/IEEE MTT-S International Microwave and Optoelectronics Conference, 1,* 413-416.

Carmena, J. M., Lebedev, M. A., Crist, R. E., O'Doherty, J. E., Santucci, D. M., & Dimitrov, D. F. (2003). Learning to Control a Brain-Machine Interface for Reaching and Grasping by Primates. *Public Library of Science Biology, 1*(2), 1–16.

Carvajal, R., Angulo, J. R., & Tombs, J. (2000). High-Speed High-Precision Voltage-mode MIN/MAX Circuits in CMOS Technology. In . *Proceedings of IEEE International Symposium on Circuits and Systems, V*, 13–16.

Carvajal, R. G., Angulo, J. R., & Martin, A. J. L. (2005). The Flipped-voltage Follower: A Useful Cell for Low-voltage Low-power Circuit Design. *IEEE Transactions on Circuits and Systems II, 52*(7), 1276–1291. doi:10.1109/TCSI.2005.851387

Caticha, N., Pelado, J. E. P., Lancet, D., & Domany, E. (2002). Computational Capacity of an Odorant Discriminator: The Linear Separability of Curves. *Neural Computation, 14*(9), 2201–2220. doi:10.1162/08997660232026405l

Caton, R. (1875). The electric currents of the brain. *British Medical Journal, 2*, 278.

Cavalcanti, S., Naviner, J. F., Deep, G., & Freire, R. (2003). Designing a Programmable Analog Signal Conditioning Circuit Without Loss of Measurement Range. *IEEE Transactions on Instrumentation and Measurement, 52*, 1482–1487. doi:10.1109/TIM.2003.818556

Cen, L., & Lian, Y. (2006). Hybrid Genetic Algorithm for the Design of Modified Frequency-Response Masking Filters in a Discrete Space. *Journal of Circuits, Systems, and Signal Processing, 25*, 153–174. doi:10.1007/s00034-005-2502-8

Chandrashekar, J., Hoon, M. A., Ryba, N. J., & Zuker, C. S. (2006). The receptors and cells for mammalian taste. *Nature, 444*, 288–294. doi:10.1038/nature05401

Chao, G., & Meijer, G. (2004). A Universal Sensor Interface Chip Design in 0.5u CMOS Process. In *Proceedings 7th International Conference on Solid State and Integrated Circuits Technology Vol. 3* (pp. 1800-1803). Beijing: IEEE Press.

Chapin, J. K. (2004). Using multi-neuron population recordings for neural prosthetics. *Nature Neuroscience, 7*(5), 452–455. doi:10.1038/nn1234

Chapin, J. K., Moxon, K. A., Markowitz, R. S., & Nicolelis, M. L. (1999). Real-time control of a robot arm using simultaneously recorded neurons in the motor cortex. *Nature Neuroscience, 2*, 664–670. doi:10.1038/10223

Chen, W., Shan, C., & de Haan, G. (2009). Optimal Regularization Parameter Estimation for Spectral Regression Discriminant Analysis. *IEEE Transactions on Circuits and Systems for Video Technology, 19*(12), 1921–1926. doi:10.1109/TCSVT.2009.2026953

Chen, G., & Pham, T. T. (2001). *Introduction to Fuzzy Sets, Fuzzy Logic, and Fuzzy Control Systems*. Boca Raton, FL: CRC Press.

Chen, J. -J., Chen, Chen, C. -C., & Tsao, H. -W. (1992). Tunable Membership Function Circuit for Fuzzy Control Systems Using CMOS Technology. *IEE Electronics Letters, 28*(22), 2101-2103.

Cho, J. –W., park. C., -W., & Park, M. (2002). An Indirect Model Reference Adaptive Fuzzy Control for SISO Takagi–Sugeno Model. *Fuzzy Sets and Systems, 131*, 197–215. doi:10.1016/S0165-0114(02)00105-7

Cohen, L. B., & Amsel, G. (1998). Precursors to infants' perception of causality. *Infant Behavior and Development, 21*(4), 713–732. doi:10.1016/S0163-6383(98)90040-6

Cohen, L. B., & Younger, B. A. (1984). Infant perception of angular relations. *Infant Behavior and Development*, *7*, 37–47.doi:10.1016/S0163-6383(84)80021-1

Cohen, Y. E., & Andersen, R. A. (2002). A Common Reference Frame for Movement Plans in the Posterior Parietal Cortex. *Nature Reviews. Neuroscience*, *3*, 553–562. doi:10.1038/nrn873

Cohen (1970). *Il linguaggio del bambino*, La nuova Italia Editrice, Bologna.

Cohen, L. B., Amsel, G., Redford, M. A., & Casasola, M. (1998). The development of infant causal perception. Chapter . In Slator, A. (Ed.), *Perceptual Development: Visual, auditory and speech perception in infancy*. London: UCL Press and Taylor and Francis.

Cohen, L. B., & Cashon, C. H. (2003). Infant object segregation implies information integration In R. Lerner, A. Easterbrooks, and J. Mistry (Eds.), *Comprehensive handbook of psychology. Volume 6, Developmental Psychology*. II. Infancy.(pp 65-89) New York: Wiley and Sons.

Cohen, P. R., Atkin, M., Oates, T., & Beal, C. R. (1997). Neo: Learning conceptual knowledge by sensorimotor interaction with an environment. In *Proceedings of the First International Conference on Autonomous Agents*. 170-177.

Connolly, J. D., Andersen, R. A., & Goodale, M. A. (2003). fMRI evidence for a 'parietal reach region' in the human brain. *Experimental Brain Research*, *153*, 140–145. doi:10.1007/s00221-003-1587-1

Cortina, M., Duran, A., Alegret, S., & del Valle, M. (2006). A sequential injection electronic tongue employing the transient response from potentiometric sensors for anion multidetermination. *Analytical and Bioanalytical Chemistry*, *358*(7), 1186–1194. doi:10.1007/s00216-006-0530-2

Cox, D. D., Meier, P., Oertelt, N., & DiCarlo, J. J. (2005). 'Breaking' position invariant object recognition. *Nature Neuroscience*, *8*, 1145–1147. doi:10.1038/nn1519

Coyle, D. (2009). Neural network based auto association and time-series prediction for biosignal processing in brain-computer interfaces . *IEEE Computational Intelligence Magazine*, *4*(4), 47–59. doi:10.1109/MCI.2009.934560

Coyle, D., Prasad, G., & McGinnity, T. M. (2009). Faster self-organizing fuzzy neural network training and a hyperparameter analysis for a brain-computer interface [Part B]. *IEEE Transactions on Systems, Man, and Cybernetics*, *39*(6), 1458–1471. doi:10.1109/TSMCB.2009.2018469

Coyle, D. (2006). *Intelligent Preprocessing and Feature Extraction Techniques for a Brain Computer Interface*, Unpublished Doctoral Dissertation, University of Ulster, UK.

Coyle, D., Prasad, G., & McGinnity (2006). Enhancing autonomy and computational efficiency of the self-organizing fuzzy neural network for a brain-computer interface, *FUZZ-IEEE, World Congress on Computational Intelligence*, pp. 10485-10492. Coyle et al., 2006

Curtice, W. R. (1980). A MESFET model for use in design of GaAs integrated circuits. *IEEE Transactions on Microwave Theory and Techniques*, *28*(5), 448–456. doi:10.1109/TMTT.1980.1130099

Dai, C., Zhu, Y., & Chen, W. (2006). Seeker Optimization Algorithm. *Proceedings of International Conference on Computational Intelligence and Security*, (CIS), *1*, 225-229.

Das, S., & Olurotimi, O. (1998). Noisy recurrent neural networks: the continuous-time case. *IEEE Transactions on Neural Networks*, *9*(5), 913–936. doi:10.1109/72.712164

Dawn, K., Ohashi, Y., & Shimura, T. (2002). A novel electromagnetic band gap metal plate for parallel plate mode suppression in shielded structures. *IEEE Microwave and Wireless Components Letters*, *12*(5), 166–168. doi:10.1109/7260.1000191

Dawson, M. E. (1970). Cognition and conditioning: Effects of masking the CS-UCS contingency on human GSR classical conditioning. *Journal of Experimental Psychology*, *85*, 389–396. doi:10.1037/h0029715

Dawson, M. E., & Biferno, M. A. (1973). Concurrent measurement of awareness and electrodermal classical conditioning. *Journal of Experimental Psychology, 101*, 55–62. doi:10.1037/h0035524

Dayan, P., & Abbot, L. F. (2001). *Theoretical Neuroscience: Computational and Mathematical Modeling of Neural Systems*. Cambridge, MA: MIT Press.

De Houwer, J., & Beckers, T. (2003). Secondary task difficulty modulates forward blocking in human contingency learning. *Quarterly Journal of Experimental Psychology, 56B*, 345–357.

de Sousa, H. C., Carvalho, A. C. P. L. F., Riul, A., Jr., & Mattoso, L. H. C. (2002). Using MLP networks to classify red wines and water readings of an artificial tongue. *The VII Brazilian Symposium on Neural Networks SBRN'02*, 13-18.

Deák, G. O., Flom, R., & Pick, A. D. (2000). Perceptual and motivational factor affecting joint visual attention in 12- and 18-month-olds. *Developmental Psychology, 36*, 511–523.

Delorme, A., Gautrais, J., van Rullen, R., & Thorpe, S. (1999). SpikeNET: A simulator for modelling large networks of integrate and fire neurons. *Neurocomputing, 26-27*, 989–996. doi:10.1016/S0925-2312(99)00095-8

Di Lorenzo, P. M., & Victor, J. D. (2003). Taste response variability and temporal coding in the nucleus of the solitary tract of the rat. *Journal of Neurophysiology, 90*, 1418–1431. doi:10.1152/jn.00177.2003

Diedrich, F. J., Roberts, B., Diller, D. E., MacMillan, J., & Deutsch, S. (2002). Hybrid Team Training Testbed for AWACS Aircraft Controllers. In *Proceedings of the Human Factors and Ergonomics Society 46th Annual Meeting*, Baltimore, MD.

Dolan, R. J., Fink, G. R., Rolls, E., Booth, M., Holmes, A., Frackowiak, R. S., & Friston, K. J. (1997). How the brain learns to see objects and faces in an impoverished context. *Nature, 389*, 596–599. doi:10.1038/39309

Dolenko, B. K., & Card, H. C. (1995). Tolerance to analog hardware of on-chip learning in backpropagation networks. *IEEE Transactions on Neural Networks, 6*, 1045–1052. doi:10.1109/72.410349

Donckers, N., Dualibe, C., & Verleysen, M. (2000). A Current-mode CMOS Loser-take-all with Minimum Function for Neural Computations. In . *Proceedings of IEEE International Symposium on Circuits and Systems, I*, 415–418.

Drennan, P. G., & McAndrew, C. C. (2003). Understanding MOSFET Mismatch for Analog Design. *IEEE Journal of Solid-state Circuits, 38*(3), 450–456. doi:10.1109/JSSC.2002.808305

Drescher, G. L. (1991). *Made-Up Minds: A Constructivist Approach to Artificial Intelligence*. Cambridge, MA: MIT Press.

Driankov, D., Hellendoorn, H., & Reinfrank, M. (1993). *An Introduction to Fuzzy Control*. Berlin Heidelberg, Germany: Springer-Verlag.

Dualibe, C., Jespers, P., & Verleysen, M. (2001). Embedded Fuzzy Control for Automatic Channel Equalization After Digital Transmissions. In . *Proceedings of IEEE International Symposium on Circuits and Systems, III*, 73–176.

Dualibe, C., Verleysen, M., & Jespers, P. G. A. (2003). *Design of Analog Fuzzy Logic Controllers in CMOS Technologies: Implementation, Test and Application.* Dordrecht: Springer.

Duff, I. S., Grimes, R. G., & Lewis, J. G. (1992). *Users' Guide for the Harwell-Boeing Sparse Matrix Collection.* Release I.

Dulac, C. (2000). The physiology of taste, vintage 2000. *Cell, 100*, 607–610. doi:10.1016/S0092-8674(00)80697-2

Eden, U. T., Frank, L. M., Barbieri, R., Solo, V., & Brown, E. N. (2004). Dynamic analyses of neural encoding by point process adaptive filtering. *Neural Computation, 16*(5), 971–998. doi:10.1162/089976604773135069

Efron, B., & Tibshirani, R. (1997). Improvements on Cross-validation: The. 632 + Bootstrap Method. *Journal of the American Statistical Association, 92*(438), 548–560. doi:10.2307/2965703

Eliasmith, C., & Anderson, C. H. (2003). *Neural Engineering*.

Elman, J. L. (1995). Language as a dynamical system . In *R. F. Port and T. Van Gelder. Mind as motion. Explorations in the dynamics of cognition* (pp. 195–226). Cambridge, MA: Bradford Book/MIT Press.

Elman, J. L. (1991). Distributed representations, simple recurrent networks, and grammatical structure. *Machine Learning, 7*, 195–225. doi:10.1007/BF00114844

Ensari, T., & Arik, S. (2005). Global stability analysis of neural networks with multiple time varying delays. *IEEE Transactions on Automatic Control, 50*(11), 1781–1785. doi:10.1109/TAC.2005.858634

Ensari, T., & Arik, S. (2005). Global stability analysis of neural networks with multiple time varying delays. *IEEE Transactions on Automatic Control, 50*, 1781–1785. doi:10.1109/TAC.2005.858634

Er, M. J., & Wu, S. (2002). A fast learning algorithm for parsimonious fuzzy neural systems. *Fuzzy Sets and Systems, 126*, 337–351. doi:10.1016/S0165-0114(01)00034-3

Ezal, K., Pan, Z., & Kokotovic, V. P. (2000). Locally optimal and robust backstepping design. *IEEE Transactions on Automatic Control, 45*, 260–271. doi:10.1109/9.839948

Fahle, M. (2004). Perceptual learning: a case for early selection. *Journal of Vision (Charlottesville, Va.), 4*, 879–890. doi:10.1167/4.10.4

Favorov, O., & Ryder, D. (2004). SINBAD: a neocortical mechanism for discovering environmental variables and regularities hidden in sensory input. *Biological Cybernetics, 90*, 191–202. doi:10.1007/s00422-004-0464-8

Felleman, D. J., & van Essen, D. C. (1991). Distributed hierarchical processing in the primate cerebral cortex. *Cerebral Cortex, 1*, 1–47. doi:10.1093/cercor/1.1.1-a

Fernandes, E. N. R. Q. (2004). *Modelagem Neurocomputacional de Dispositivos de Microondas com Estruturas EBG*. (Doctoral dissertation, Federal University of Campina Grande, 2004).

Fine, I., & Jacobs, R. A. (2002). Comparing perceptual learning tasks: a review. *Journal of Vision (Charlottesville, Va.), 2*, 190–203. doi:10.1167/2.2.5

Finke, R. A., & Ward, T. B. Smith S. M (1992). *Creative cognition: theory, research and application*. Cambridge MA: MIT Press.

Fisch, B. J. (1999). *Fisch & Spellmann's EEG Primer: Basic principles of digital and analog EEG*. New York: Elsevier.

Fisher, R. A. (1936). The Use of Multiple Measurements in Taxonomic Problems. *Annals of Eugenics, 7*, 179–188.

Fletcher, R., & Reeves, C. M. (1964). Function Minimization by Conjugate Gradients. *The Computer Journal, 7*, 149–154. doi:10.1093/comjnl/7.2.149

Florchinger, P. (1995). Lyapunov-like techniques for stochastic stability. *SIAM Journal on Control and Optimization, 33*(4), 1151–1169. doi:10.1137/S0363012993252309

Fodor, J. A. (2000). *The mind doesn't work that way*. Cambridge, MA: MIT Press.

Fodor, J. A., & Pylyshyn, Z. W. (1988). Connectionism and cognitive architecture: A critical analysis . In Pinker, S., & Mehler, J. (Eds.), *Connections and symbols* (pp. 3–71). Cambridge, MA: MIT Press.

Földiák, P. (1990). Forming sparse representations by local anti-Hebbian learning. *Biological Cybernetics, 64*(2), 165–170. doi:10.1007/BF02331346

Fraden, J. (2004). *Handbook of Modern Sensors*. New York: Springer-Verlag.

Freedman, D. J., Riesenhuber, M., Poggio, T., & Miller, E. K. (2003). A comparison of primate prefrontal and inferior temporal cortices during visual categorization. *The Journal of Neuroscience, 23*, 5235–5246.

Freedman, D. J., Riesenhuber, M., Poggio, T., & Miller, E. K. (2006). Experience dependent sharpening of visual shape selectivity in inferior temporal cortex. *Cerebral Cortex*, *16*, 1631–1644. doi:10.1093/cercor/bhj100

Freeman, J. A., & Skapura, D. M. (1991). *Neural Networks: Algorithms, Applications, and Programming Techniques*. Reading, MA: Addison-Wesley.

Freeman, R., & Kokotovic, V. P. (1996). Inverse optimality in robust stabilization. *SIAM Journal on Control and Optimization*, *34*(4), 1365–1391. doi:10.1137/S0363012993258732

Freitas, D. A., & Current, K. W. (1983). CMOS Current Comparator Circuit. *IEE Electronics Letters*, *19*(17), 695–697. doi:10.1049/el:19830474

Furber, S., & Temple, S. (2007). Neural Systems Engineering. *Journal of the Royal Society, Interface*, *4*, 193–206. doi:10.1098/rsif.2006.0177

Furmanski, C. S., Schluppeck, D., & Engel, S. A. (2004). Learning strengthens the response of primary visual cortex to simple patterns. *Current Biology*, *14*, 573–578. doi:10.1016/j.cub.2004.03.032

Gallardo, J., Alegret, S., Muñoz, R., De-Román, M., Leija, L., Hernández, P. R., & del Valle, M. (2003). An electronic tongue using potentiometric all-solid-state PVC-membrane sensors for the simultaneous quantification of ammonium and potassium ions in water. *Analytical and Bioanalytical Chemistry*, *377*(2), 248–256. doi:10.1007/s00216-003-2042-7

Ganguly, K., & Carmena, J. M. (2009). Emergence of a Stable Cortical Map for Neuroprosthetic Control. *Public Library of Science Biology*, *7*(7).

Ghose, G. M., Yang, T., & Maunsell, J. H. (2002). Physiological correlates of perceptual learning in monkey V1 and V2. *Journal of Neurophysiology*, *87*, 1867–1888.

Ghovanloo, M., & Atluri, S. (2007). A wideband power-efficieny inductive wireless link for implantable microelectronic devices using multiple carriers. *IEEE Transactions on Circuits and Systems. I, Fundamental Theory and Applications*, *54*(10), 71–77. doi:10.1109/TCSI.2007.905187

Glendinning, J. I., Davis, A., & Rai, M. (2006). Temporal coding mediates discrimination of "bitter" taste stimuli by an insect. *The Journal of Neuroscience*, *26*(35), 8900–8908. doi:10.1523/JNEUROSCI.2351-06.2006

Goldberg, D. E. (1989). *Genetic Algorithms in Search, Optimization, and Machine Learning*. USA: Addison-Wesley.

Gong, G. (1986). Cross-validation, the Jackknife, and the Bootstrap: Excess Error Estimation in Forward Logistic Regression. *Journal of the American Statistical Association*, *81*(393), 108–113. doi:10.2307/2287975

Gonzalez, J., Rojas, I., Pomares, H., Ortega, J., & Prieto, A. (2002). A new clustering technique for function approximation. *IEEE Transactions on Neural Networks*, *13*, 132–142. doi:10.1109/72.977289

Gopalan, A., & Titus, A. H. (2003). A New Wide Range Euclidean Distance Circuit for Neural Network Hardware Implementations. *IEEE Transactions on Neural Networks*, *14*(5), 1176–1186. doi:10.1109/TNN.2003.816034

Gottarredona, S., & Barranco, B.-L. (2006). A Low-Power Current Mode Fuzzy-ART Cell. *IEEE Transactions on Neural Networks*, *17*(6), 1666–1673. doi:10.1109/TNN.2006.883725

Green, B., & Turner, L. E. (1990). Digital LDI Ladder Filters Using Lattice Equivalents and Wave Concepts. *IEEE Transactions on Circuits and Systems*, *37*(1), 133–135. doi:10.1109/31.45701

Greene, J., Sommerville, R. B., Nystorm, L. E., Darley, J. M., & Cohen, J. D. (2001). An FMRI Investigation of Emotional Engagement in Moral Judgment. *Science*, *293*, 2105–2108. doi:10.1126/science.1062872

Gregory, R. L. (1974). A look at biological and machine perception . In Meltzer, B., & Michie, D. (Eds.), *Machine intelligence 7*. Edinburgh, UK: Edinburgh University Press.

Grill-Spector, K., & Malach, R. (2004). The human visual cortex. *Annual Review of Neuroscience*, *27*, 649–677. doi:10.1146/annurev.neuro.27.070203.144220

Griva, I., Nash, S. G., & Sofer, A. (2009). *Linear and Nonlinear Optimization* (2 nd ed.).

Guastello, J. (1995). *Chaos catastrophe and human affairs*. Upper Saddle River, NJ: Lawrence Erlbaum Ass.

Guger, C. (1999). *Real-time Data Processing Under Windows for an EEG-based Brain-Computer Interface*, Unpublished Doctoral Dissertation, Technical University Graz, Austria

Gulz, A. (1991). *The planning of action as a cognitive and biological phenomenon*. Lund University Cognitive Studies 2.

Gutés, A., Ibáñez, A. B., Céspedes, F., Alegret, S., & del Valle, M. (2005). Simultaneous determination of phenolic compounds by means of an automated voltammetric electronic tongue. *Analytical and Bioanalytical Chemistry*, *382*, 471–476. doi:10.1007/s00216-005-3201-9

Gutiérrez, M., Gutiérrez, J. M., Alegret, S., Leija, L., Hernández, P. R., & Favari, L. (2008). Remote environmental monitoring employing a potentiometric electronic tongue. *International Journal of Environmental Analytical Chemistry*, *88*, 103–117. doi:10.1080/03067310701441005

Guyon, I., & Elisseeff, A. (2003). An Introduction to Variable and Feature Selection. *Journal of Machine Learning Research*, *3*, 1157–1182. doi:10.1162/153244303322753616

Hadley, R. F. (2008). The problem of rapid variable creation. *Neural Computation*, *20*, 1–23.

Hagan, M., & Mohammad, B. (1994). Training feedforward networks with the Marquardt algorithm. *IEEE Transactions on Neural Networks*, *5*, 989–993. doi:10.1109/72.329697

Hammerschmied, C. M., & Huang, Q. (1994). Design and Implementation of an Untrimmed MOSFET-only 10-Bit A/D Converter with -79-db THD . *IEEE Journal of Solid-state Circuits*, *33*(8), 1148–1151. doi:10.1109/4.705353

Hansmann, U., Merk, L., Nicklous, M. S., & Stober, T. (2003). *Pervasive computing* (2nd ed.). Springer.

Harb, A., Hu, Y., Sawan, M., Abdelkerim, A., & Elhilali, M. (2004). Low-Power CMOS Interface for Recording and Processing Very Low Amplitude Signals. *Analog Integrated Circuits and Signal Processing*, *39*, 39–54. doi:10.1023/B:ALOG.0000016642.76352.f8

Härdle, W., & Simar, L. (2003). *Applied Multivariate Statistical Analysis*. Berln, Germany: Springer-Verlag.

Hardy, G., Littlewood, J., & Polya, G. (1989). *Inequalities* (2nd ed.). London: Cambridge University Press.

Harkin, J., Morgan, F., McDaid, L., Hall, S., McGinley, B., & Cawley, S. (2009). A Reconfigurable and Biologically Inspired Paradigm for Computation using Networks-on-chip and Spiking Neural Networks . *International Journal of Reconfigurable Computing*, (908740): 1–13. doi:10.1155/2009/908740

Harnad, S. (1991). The symbol grounding problem . In Forrest, S. (Ed.), *Emergent computation: Self-organizing, collective, and cooperative phenomena in natural and artificial computing networks*. Cambridge, MA: MIT Press.

Harrison, R. R. (2008). The design of integrated circuits to observe brain activity. *Proceedings of the IEEE*, *96*, 1203–1216. doi:10.1109/JPROC.2008.922581

Harrison, R. R., Watkins, P. T., Kier, R. J., Lovejoy, R. O., Black, D. J., & Greger, B. (2007). A Low-Power Integrated Circuit for a Wireless 100-Electrode Neural Recording System. *IEEE Journal of Solid-state Circuits*, *42*(1), 123–133. doi:10.1109/JSSC.2006.886567

Hartman, K., Keeler, J. D., & Kowalski, J. M. (1990). Layered Neural Networks with Gaussian Hidden Units as Universal Approximations. *Neural Computation, 2*, 210–215. doi:10.1162/neco.1990.2.2.210

Hassibi, B., & Stork, D. G. (1993). Second order derivatives for network pruning: Optimal brain surgeon . *Advances in Neural Information Processing Systems, 4*, 164–171.

Hassoun, M. H. (1995). *Fundamentals of Artificial Neural Networks*. Cambridge, MA: MIT Press.

Haupt, R. L., & Haupt, S. E. (2004). *Practical genetic algorithms* (2nd ed.). Hoboken, NJ: John Wiley & Sons.

Haupt, R. L., & Werner, D. H. (2007). *Genetic algorithms in electromagnetics*. Hoboken, NJ: John Willey & Sons. doi:10.1002/047010628X

Hauser, M. D. (1994). How monkeys feel about how they see the world. *Language & Communication, 14*, 31–36. doi:10.1016/0271-5309(94)90018-3

Haykin, S. (2003). *Neural Networks: A Comprehensive Foundation* (4th ed.). Upper Saddle River, New Jersey: Prentice Hall.

Haykin, S. (1999). *Neural Networks: A Comprehensive Foundation*. Upper Saddle River, New Jersey: Prentice Hall.

Hebb, D. O. (1949). *The Organization of Behavior: A Neuropsychological Theory*. New York: John Wiley & Sons.

Higuchi, T., Liu, Y., & Yao, X. (Eds.). (2006). *Evolvable Hardware, VIII*. New York: Springer. doi:10.1007/0-387-31238-2

Himavathi, S., Anitha, D., & Muthuramalingam, A. (2007). Feedforward neural network implementation in FPGA using layer multiplexing for effective resource utilization. *IEEE Transactions on Neural Networks, 18*(3), 880–888. doi:10.1109/TNN.2007.891626

Hochberg, L. R., Serruya, M. D., Friehs, G. M., Mukand, J. A., Saleh, M., & Caplan, A. H. (2006). Neuronal ensemble control of prosthetic devices by a human with tetraplegia. *Nature, 442*, 164–171. doi:10.1038/nature04970

Hodgkin, A. L., & Huxley, A. F. (1952). A Quantitative Description of Membrane Current and its Application to Conduction and Excitation in Nerve . *The Journal of Physiology, 117*, 500–544.

Holleman, J., & Otis, B. (2007). 29th Annual International Conference of the IEEE Engineering in Medicine and Biology Society, *A sub-microwatt low-noise amplifier for neural recording* (pp. 3930-3933).

Hopfield, J. J. (1984). Neurons with graded response have collective computational properties like those of two-state neurons. *Proceedings of the National Academy of Sciences of the United States of America, 81*(10), 3088–3092. doi:10.1073/pnas.81.10.3088

Hu, S., & Wang, J. (2002). Global asymptotic stability and global exponential stability of continuous-time recurrent neural networks. *IEEE Transactions on Automatic Control, 47*(5), 802–807. doi:10.1109/TAC.2002.1000277

Huang, Y. J., Maruyama, Y., Lu, K. S., Pereira, E., & Roper, S. D. (2005). Mouse taste buds release serotonin in response to taste stimuli. *Chemical Senses, 30*(Supplement 1), i39–i40. doi:10.1093/chemse/bjh102

Huang, C. Y., Wang, C. J., & Liu, B. D. (1996). Modular Current-mode Multiple Input Minimum Circuit for Fuzzy Logic Controllers' . *IEE Electronics Letters, 32*(12), 1067–1069. doi:10.1049/el:19960728

Huang, C.-Y, & Liu, B.-D. (1994). Current-mode Multiple Input Maximum Circuit for Fuzzy Logic

Huang, G. B., Saratchandran, P., & Sundararajan, N. (n.d.). An efficient sequential learning algorithm for growing and pruning RBFNs, *IEEE Transactions on Systems, Man and Cybernetics, Part B, 34*(6).

Hull, C. L. (1930). Knowledge and purpose as habit mechanisms. *Psychological Review, 37*, 511–525. doi:10.1037/h0072212

Hull, C. L. (1935). The mechanism of the assembly of behavior segments in novel combinations suitable for problem solution. [Reprinted in Amsel, A. & Rashotte, M. E., 1984.]. *Psychological Review, 42*, 219–245. doi:10.1037/h0063473

Hwang, J. N., Chan, C. H., & Marks, R. J. (1990). Frequency selective surface design based on iterative inversion of neural networks. *Proceedings of the International Joint Conference on Neural Networks*, *1*, 39–44. doi:10.1109/IJCNN.1990.137541

Im, E., Yelick, K., & Vuduc, R. (2004). Sparsity: Optimization Framework for Sparse Matrix Kernels. *International Journal of High Performance Computing Applications*, *18*(1), 135–158. doi:10.1177/1094342004041296

Inoue, T., Ueno, F., Motomura, R. M., & Setoguchi, O. (1991). Analysis and Design of Analog CMOS Building Blocks For Integrated Fuzzy Inference Circuits. *Proceedings of IEEE International Symposium on Circuits and Systems*, *4*, 2024–2027.

Ivarsson, P., Kikkawa, Y., Winquist, F., Krantz-Rülcker, C., Höjer, N.-E., & Hayashi, K. (2001). Comparison of a voltmetric electronic tongue and a lipid membrane taste sensors. *Analytica Chimica Acta*, *449*, 59–68. doi:10.1016/S0003-2670(01)01349-6

Jabri, M., & Flower, B. (1992). Weight perturbation: An optimal architecture and learning technique for analog VLSI feedforward and recurrent multilayer networks. *IEEE Transactions on Neural Networks*, *3*, 154–157. doi:10.1109/72.105429

Jackson, A., Mavoori, J., & Fetz, E. E. (2006). Long-term motor cortex plasticity induced by an electronic neural implant. *Nature*, *444*, 55–60. doi:10.1038/nature05226

Jacobs, R. A. (1988). Increase rate of convergence through learning rate adaptation. *Neural Networks*, *1*(4), 295–307. doi:10.1016/0893-6080(88)90003-2

Jacobs, R. A., Jordan, M. I., Nowlan, S. J., & Hinton, G. E. (1991). Adaptive mixture of local experts. [Cambridge, MA: MIT Press.]. *Neural Computation*, *3*, 79–87. doi:10.1162/neco.1991.3.1.79

Jain, A. K., Bolton, R. J., & Abd-El-Barr, M. (1993). CMOS Multiple-valued Logic Design, Part I and II. *IEEE Transactions on Circuits and Systems-Fundamental Theory and Applications*, *40*(8), 503–522. doi:10.1109/81.242320

Jang, J.-S. R. (1993). ANFIS: Adaptive-network-based fuzzy inference system . *IEEE Transactions on Systems, Man, and Cybernetics*, *23*, 665–685. doi:10.1109/21.256541

Jang, J.-S. R., Sun, C.-T., & Mizutani, E. (1997). *Neuro-Fuzzy & Soft Computing*. Upper-Saddle River, NJ: Prentice Hall.

Jang, R. (1992). Self-Learning Fuzzy Controllers Based on Temporal Back Propagation. *IEEE Transactions on Neural Networks*, *3*(5), 714–723. doi:10.1109/72.159060

Jean, P. (1952). *The Origins of Intelligence in Children*. New York: Norton.

Jitsev, J., & von der Malsburg, C. (2009). Experience-driven formation of parts-based representations in a model of layered visual memory. *Frontiers in computational neuroscience, 3*(Special Issue on Complex systems science and brain dynamics), 15. Retrieved from http://www.ncbi.nlm.nih.gov/pubmed/19862345.

Joannopoulus, J. D., Jonhson, S. G., Winn, J. N., & Meade, R. D. (2008). *Photonic crystal molding the flow of light* (2nd ed.). New Jersey: Princenton University Press. Retrieved February 06, 2010, from http://ab-initio.mit.edu/book/photonic-crystals-book.pdf.

Johansson, H., & Wanhammar, L. (1997). High-Seed Recursive Filtering Using the Frequency-Response Masking Approach. In *Proceedings of the IEEE International Symposium on Circuits and Systems*, (ISCAS), 2208-2211.

Johnson, S., Slaughter, V., & Carey, S. (1998). Whose gaze will infants follow? The elicitation of gaze-following in 12-month-olds. *Developmental Science*, *1*, 233–238. doi:10.1111/1467-7687.00036

Jordan, M. I., & Jacobs, R. A. (1994). Hierarchical mixtures of experts and the EM algorithm. [MIT Press.]. *Neural Computation*, *6*, 181–214. doi:10.1162/neco.1994.6.2.181

Juang, C. F. (2002). A TSK-type recurrent fuzzy network for dynamic systems processing by neural network and genetic algorithms . *IEEE Transactions on Fuzzy Systems*, *10*(2), 155–170. doi:10.1109/91.995118

Juang, C. F., & Lin, C. T. (1999). A recurrent self-organising neural fuzzy inference network . *IEEE Transactions on Neural Networks*, *10*(4), 829–845.

Juang, C. F., & Hsieh, C. D, (In Press). A locally recurrent fuzzy neural network with support vector regression for dynamic system modelling, *IEEE Transactions on Fuzzy Systems*.

Kasabov, N. K. (2001). Evolving Fuzzy Neural Networks for Supervised/Unsupervised Online Knowledge-Based Learning, *IEEE Transactions on Systems, Man, and Cybernetics, 31*(6), 902-918.

Kakei, S., Hoffman, D. S., & Strick, P. L. (1999). Muscle and Movement Representations in the Primary Motor Cortex. *Science*, *285*, 2136–2139. doi:10.1126/science.285.5436.2136

Kamin, L. J. (1969). Predictability, surprise attention and conditioning. In B. A.Campbell & R. M. Church (Eds.), *Punishment and aversive behavior* (pp. 279-296). NewYork: Appleton-Century – Crofts.

Kasabov, N. (2007). *Evolving connectionist systems. The knowledge engineering approach*. London: Springer-Verlag London Limited.

Kasabov, N. (2009). Integrative Connectionist Learning Systems Inspired by Nature: Current Models, Future Trends and Challenges. *Natural Computing*, *8*(2), 199–210. doi:10.1007/s11047-008-9066-z

Kasabov, N. (2010). To spike or not to spike: A probabilistic spiking neural model . *Neural Networks*, *23*(1), 16–19. doi:10.1016/j.neunet.2009.08.010

Kasabov, N. K. (2003). *Evolving connectionist systems: methods and applications in bioinformatics*. New York: Springer.

Kasabov, N. K., & Song, Q. (2002). DENFIS: Dynamic evolving neural-fuzzy inference system and its application for time-series prediction . *IEEE Transactions on Fuzzy Systems*, *10*(2), 144–154. doi:10.1109/91.995117

Kasabov, N. K. (1998). *Foundations of Neural Networks, Fuzzy Systems, and Knowledge Engineering*, (2nd ed.). Cambridge, MA: MIT Press. Philapdelphia: SIAM.

Kashtiban, M. M-., Khoei, A., & Hadidi, K. (2007). A Current-mode, First-order Takagi-Sugeno-Kang Fuzzy Logic Controller, Supporting Rational-powered Membership Functions. *IEICE Transactions on Electronics . E (Norwalk, Conn.)*, *90-C*(6), 1258–1266.

Katz, D. B., Nicolelis, M. A. L., & Simon, S. A. (2002). Gustatory processing is dynamic and distributed. *Current Opinion in Neurobiology*, *12*, 448–454. doi:10.1016/S0959-4388(02)00341-0

Kellman, P. J., & Arterberry, M. E. (1998). *The Cradle of Knowledge*. Cambridge, MA: MIT Press. A Bradford Book.

Kennedy, L., & Eberhart, R. C. (1995). Particle swarm optimization. *Proceedings of the IV IEEE Conference on Neural Networks*, *4*, 1942–1948.

Kettner, T., Heite, C., & Schumacher, K. (1993). Analog CMOS Realization of Fuzzy Logic Membership Functions . *IEEE Journal of Solid-state Circuits*, *28*(7), 857–861. doi:10.1109/4.222189

Khachab, N., & Ismail, M. (1991). Linearization Techniques for n th-Order Sensor Models in MOS VLSI Technology. *IEEE Transactions on Circuits and Systems*, *38*, 1439–1450. doi:10.1109/31.108498

Khalil, H. (1996). *Nonlinear Systems* (2nd ed.). Upper Saddle River, NJ: Prentice Hall.

Kilambi, S., & Nowrouzian, B. (2007). A Diversity Controlled Genetic Algorithm for Optimization of FRM Digital Filters over DBNS Multiplier Coefficient Space. *Proceedings of IEEE International Symposium on Circuits and Systems,* (ISCAS), 2331-2334.

Kipke, D. R., Shain, W., Buzsáki, G., Fetz, E. E., Henderson, J. M., & Hetke, J. F. (2008). Advanced Neurotechnologies for Chronic Neural Interfaces: New Horizons and Clinical Opportunities. *The Journal of Neuroscience*, *28*(46), 11830–11838. doi:10.1523/JNEUROSCI.3879-08.2008

Klawonn, F., & Keller, A. (1998). Grid clustering for generating fuzzy rules. *European Congress on Intelligent Techniques and Soft Computing*, 1365-1369.

Kneer, S., Personnaz, L., & Dreyfus, G. (1992). Handwritten Digit Recognition by Neural Networks with Single-Layer Training. *IEEE Transactions on Neural Networks*, *3*(6), 962–968. doi:10.1109/72.165597

Kobatake, E., Wang, G., & Tanaka, K. (1998). Effects of shape-discrimination training on the selectivity of inferotemporal cells in adult monkeys. *Journal of Neurophysiology*, *87*, 324–330.

Kohler, W. (1969). *The task of Gestalt psychology*. Princeton, NJ: Princeton University Press.

Kohonen, T. (1982). Self-organized Formation of Topographically Correct Feature Maps. *Biological Cybernetics*, *43*, 59–69. doi:10.1007/BF00337288

Kohonen, T. (1990). Improved Versions of Learning Vector Quantizations. *Proceedings of International Joint Conference on Neural Networks*, *1*, 545–550. doi:10.1109/IJCNN.1990.137622

Kohonen, T. (1990). The Self-organizing Map. *Proceedings of the IEEE*, *78*(9), 1464–1480. doi:10.1109/5.58325

Kohonen, T. (1993). Physiological Interpretation of the Self-organising Map Algorithm. *Neural Networks*, *6*, 895–905.

Kolb, B., & Whishaw, I. Q. (2008). *Fundamentals of Human Neuropsychology. Hampshire*. Macmillan.

Kolle, C., Scherr, W., Hammerschmidt, D., Pichler, G., Motz, M., Schaffer, B., et al. (2004). Ultra Low-Power Monolithically Integrated Capacitive Pressure Sensor for Tire Pressure Monitoring, In *Proceedings IEEE Sensors Conference 2004*, 244-247. Vienna: IEEE Press.

Kolman, E., & Margaliot, M. (2005). Are artificial neural networks white boxes? *IEEE Transactions on Neural Networks*, *16*(4), 844–852. doi:10.1109/TNN.2005.849843

Koren, I. (1993). *Computer Arithmetic Algorithms*. Upper Saddle River, NJ: Prentice Hall.

Kosko, K. (1992). *Neural Networks and Fuzzy Systems*. Upper Saddle River, NJ: Prentice-Hall.

Krantz-Rülcker, C., Stenberg, M., Winquist, F., & Lundström, I. (2001). Electronic tongues for environmental monitoring based on sensor arrays and pattern recognition: a review. *Analytica Chimica Acta*, *426*, 217–226. doi:10.1016/S0003-2670(00)00873-4

Kreiman, G. (2004). Neural Coding: Computational and Biophysical Perspectives. *Physics of Life Reviews*, *1*(2), 71–102. doi:10.1016/j.plrev.2004.06.001

Krishnamachari, B. (2005). *Networking Wireless Sensors*. New York: Cambridge University Press. doi:10.1017/CBO9780511541025

Krstic, M., & Deng, H. (1998). *Stabilization of Nonlinear Uncertain Systems*. New York, NY: Springer-Verlag.

Krstic, M., Kanellakopoulos, I., & Kokotovic, P. V. (1995). *Nonlinear and Adaptive Control Design*. New York: John Wiley & Sons.

Kuiken, T. A., Li, G., Lock, B. A., Lipschultz, R. D., Miller, L. A., & Stubblefield, K. A. (2009). Targeted Muscle Reinnervation for Real-time Myoelectric Control of Multifunction Artificial Arms. *Journal of the American Medical Association*, *301*(6), 619–628. doi:10.1001/jama.2009.116

Kulawski, G. J., & Brdys, M. A. (2000). Stable adaptive control with recurrent networks. *Automatica*, *36*(1), 5–22. doi:10.1016/S0005-1098(99)00092-8

Kuniholm, J. (2009). Open Arms. *IEEE Spectrum*, *46*(3), 36–41. doi:10.1109/MSPEC.2009.4795454

Kuniyoshi, Y., & Berthouze, L. (1998). Neural learning of embodied interaction dynamics. *Neural Networks*, *11*, 1259–1276. doi:10.1016/S0893-6080(98)00085-9

Kursun, O., & Favorov, O. (2004). SINBAD automation scientific discovery: From factor analysis to theory synthesis. *Natural Computing*, *3*(2), 207–233. doi:10.1023/B:NACO.0000027756.50327.26

Lajusticia, C., Medrano, N., Zatorre, G., & Martin, B. (2003). Applying Non-Ideal Mixed Analog-Digital Multipliers in Electronic Processing Circuits Based on Neural-Networks. In *Proceedings of 2003 IEEE Conference on Emerging Technologies and Facttory Automation, ETFA 2003*, (pp. 362-367). Lisbon: IEEE Press.

Lakoff, G., & Johnson, M. (1980). *Metaphors We Live By*. Chicago, IL: The University of Chicago Press.

Landolt, O., Vittoz, E., & Heim, P. (1992). CMOS Self-biased Euclidean Distance Computing Circuit with High Dynamic Range, *IEE. Electronics Letters*, *28*(4), 352–354. doi:10.1049/el:19920220

Lattice Semiconductor Corporation. (2007). *Lattice Mico 32 Processor Reference Manual*. Retrieved from http://www.latticesemi.com/.

Lazzaro, J., Wawrzynek, J., & Lippmann, R. P. (1997). A Micropower Analog Circuit Implementation of Hidden Markov Model State Decoding. *IEEE Journal of Solid-state Circuits*, *32*(8), 1200–1209. doi:10.1109/4.604076

Lazzaro, J., Rykebusch, R., Mahowald, A., & Mead, C. (1989). Winner-take-all Networks of O(n) Complexity . In Touretzky, D. (Ed.), *Advances in Neural Information Processing Systems 1* (pp. 703–711). San Francisco: Morgan Kaufmann.

Lee, C. C. (1990). Fuzzy logic in control systems: Fuzzy logic controller – Part I and II. *IEEE Transactions on Systems, Man, and Cybernetics*, *20*, 404–435. doi:10.1109/21.52551

Lee, L., & Oppenheim, A. (1997). Properties of Approximate Parks-McClellan Filters. *Proceedings of IEEE International Conference on Acoustics, Speech, and Signal Processing*, (ICASSP), *3*, 2165.

Lee, Y., & Ko, S.-B. (2006). FPGA implementation of a face detector using neural networks. *IEEE Conference on Electrical and Computer Engineering CCECE/CCGEI*, 1914-1917.

Lee, Y., Oh, S. H., Song, H. K., & Kim, M. W. (1982). Design Rules of Multilayer Perceptron. *Proceedings of SPIE, Science of Artificial Neural Networks,* 1710, 329–339.

Leng, G., Prasad, G., & McGinnity, T. M. (2004). An on-line algorithm for creating self-organising fuzzy neural networks . *Neural Networks*, *17*(10), 1477–1493. doi:10.1016/j.neunet.2004.07.009

Leng, G. (2003). *Algorithmic Developments for Self-Organizing Fuzzy Neural Networks*, (Unpublished doctoral dissertation), University of Ulster, UK.

Leung, C. S., Wong, K. W., Sum, P. F., & Chan, L. W. (2001). A pruning method for the recursive least squared algorithm. *Neural Networks*, *14*, 147–174. doi:10.1016/S0893-6080(00)00093-9

Li, P., Abarbanell, L., & Shusterman, A. (2003). *Spatial Reference, Laboratory of Development at the Cambridge*. MA: Harvard.

Liberati, C., Howe, J. A., & Bozdogan, H. (2009). Data Adaptive Simultaneous Parameter and Kernel Selection in Kernel Discriminant Analysis Using Information Complexity. *Journal of Pattern Recognition*, *4*(1), 119–132.

Lim, Y. (1986). Frequency-Response Masking Approach for the Synthesis of Sharp Linear Phase Digital Filters. *IEEE Transactions on Circuits and Systems*, *33*(4), 357–364. doi:10.1109/TCS.1986.1085930

Lin, G., & Shi, B. (1999). A Multi-input Current-mode Fuzzy Integrated Circuit for Pattern Recognition. In *Proceedings of IEEE 2nd International Conference on Intelligent Processing and Manufacturing of Materials,* 1, 687-693.

Liu, Z., Torres, R., Patel, N., & Wang, Q. (2008). Further development of input-to-state stabilizing control for dynamic neural network systems. *IEEE Transactions on Systems, Man, and Cybernetics A*, *38*, 1425–1433. doi:10.1109/TSMCA.2008.2003464

Liu, Z., Wang, Q., & Schurz, H. (2009). Inverse optimal noise-to-state stabilization of stochastic recurrent neural networks driven by noise of unknown covariance. *Optimal Control Applications and Methods*, *30*(2), 163–178. doi:10.1002/oca.851

Liu, Z., Shih, S., & Wang, Q. (2009). Global robust stabilizing control for a dynamic neural network system. *IEEE Transactions on Systems, Man, and Cybernetics A*, *39*, 426–436. doi:10.1109/TSMCA.2008.2010749

Liu, Z., & Wang, Q. (2007). Further result on input-to-state stabilization of dynamic neural network systems. *Proceedings of American Control Conference,* 4798-4803.

Loeliger, H.-A., Tarköy, F., Lustenberger, F., & Helfenstein, M. (1999). Decoding in Analog VLSI. *IEEE Communications Magazine*, 99–101. doi:10.1109/35.755457

Logothetis, N. K., Pauls, J., & Poggio, T. (1995). Shape representation in the inferior temporal cortex of monkeys. *Current Biology*, *5*, 552–563. doi:10.1016/S0960-9822(95)00108-4

Lopez-Martin, A., & Carlosena, A. (2007). Versatile Automotive Sensor Interface ASIC. In *Proceedings IEEE International Symposium on Industrial Electronics, ISIE 2007*, (pp. 1469-1472). Vigo: IEEE Press.

Lorenz, K. (1977). *Behind the mirror*. London: Methuen and co Ltd. Oxford University Press

Lovibond, P. F. (2003). Causal beliefs and conditioned responses: Retrospective revaluation induced by experience and by instruction. *Journal of Experimental Psychology. Learning, Memory, and Cognition*, *29*, 97–106. doi:10.1037/0278-7393.29.1.97

Lücke, J., Keck, C., & von der Malsburg, C. (2008). Rapid convergence to feature layer correspondences. *Neural Computation*, *20*(10), 2441–2463. doi:10.1162/neco.2008.06-07-539

Lücke, J., & von Der Malsburg, C. (2004). Rapid processing and unsupervised learning in a model of the cortical macrocolumn. *Neural Computation*, *16*(3), 501–533. doi:10.1162/089976604772744893

Ludwig, K. A., Uram, J. D., Yang, J., Martin, D. C., & Kipke, D. R. (2006). Chronic neural recordings using silicon microelectrode arrays electrochemically deposited with a poly(3,4-ethylenedioxythiophene) (PEDOT) film. *Journal of Neural Engineering*, *3*, 59–70. doi:10.1088/1741-2560/3/1/007

Lughofer, E., & Klement, E. P. (2005). FLEXFIS: A Variant for Incremental Learning of Takagi-Sugeno Fuzzy Systems. In . *Proceedings of FUZZ-IEEE, 2005*, 915–920.

Lungarella, M., Pfeifer, R., & Iida, F. (2007). Self-Organization, Embodiment, and Biologically Inspired Robotics. *Science*, *318*, 1088–1093. doi:10.1126/science.1145803

Lungarella, M., & Metta, G. (2003). Beyond Gazing, Pointing, and Reaching: A Survey of Developmental Robotics. In *Proceedings of the 3rd International Workshop on Epigenetic Robotics*. (pp.81-89). Boston

Lutovac, M., & Milid, L. (1999). Design of Multiplierless Elliptic IIR Filters with a Small Quantization Error. *IEEE Transactions on Signal Processing*, *47*(2), 469–479. doi:10.1109/78.740130

Maass, W. (1999). Computing with spiking neurons . In Maass, W., & Bishop, C. H. (Eds.), *Pulsed Neural Networks*. WA: Bratford Book.

MacLahlan, G. J. (1992). *Discriminant Analysis and Statistical Pattern Recognition*. New York: Wiley & Sons.

Maguire, L. P., McGinnity, T. M., Glackin, B., Ghani, A., Belatreche, A., & Harkin, J. (2007). Challenges for large-scale implementations of spiking neural networks on FPGAs. *Neurocomputing*, *71*(1-3), 13–29. doi:10.1016/j.neucom.2006.11.029

Mahony, J. D. A. (2003). Comment on Q-type integrals and their use in expressions for radiated power. *IEEE Antennas and Propagation Magazine*, *45*(3), 127–128. doi:10.1109/MAP.2003.1232169

Mak, T. S., Rachmuth, G., Lam, K. P., & Poon, C.-S. (2005). Field programmable gate array implementation of neuronal ion channel dynamics. *The 2th International IEEE EMBS Conference on Neural Engineering*, v-ix.

Malisoff, M., Rifford, L., & Sontag, E. D. (2004). Global asymptotic controllability implies input-to-state stabilization. *SIAM Journal on Control and Optimization*, *42*, 2221–2238. doi:10.1137/S0363012903422333

Maltzman, I. (1955). Thinking: From a behaviorist point of view. *Psychological Review*, *62*, 275–286. doi:10.1037/h0041818

Mamdani, E. H. (1977). Application of Fuzzy Logic to Approximate Reasoning Using Linguistic Synthesis. *IEEE Transactions on Computers*, *C-26*(12), 1182–1191. doi:10.1109/TC.1977.1674779

Mamdani, E. H., & S. Assilian. (2008). An experiment in linguistic synthesis with a fuzzy logic controller. *International Journal of Man-Machine Studies, 7*(1), 1:13

Mandal, S., & Sarpeshkar, R. (2008). Power-Efficient Impedance-Modulation Wireless Data Links for Biomedical Implants. *IEEE Transactions on Biomedical Circuits and Systems*, *2*(4), 301–315. doi:10.1109/TBCAS.2008.2005295

Mandal, S., & Sarpeshkar, R. (2007). A Bidirectional Wireless Link for Neural Prostheses that Minimizes Implanted Power Consumption. *Proceedings of the IEEE Biomedical Circuits and Systems Conference (BioCAS)*, 45-48.

Marco, M., Forti, M., & Tesi, A. (2004). On absolute stability of convergence for nonlinear neural network models. In W. Kang et al. (Eds.), *New Trends in Nonlinear Dynamics and Control and their Applications, Lecture Notes in Control and Information Sciences,* 209-220, Berlin: Springer.

Marcus, G. F. (2001). *The algebraic mind.* Cambridge, MA: MIT Press.

Margolskee, R. F. (1993). The molecular biology of taste transduction. *BioEssays*, *15*(10), 645–650. doi:10.1002/bies.950151003

Martinez, K. K., Hart, J., & Ong, R. (2004). Sensor Network Applications. *Computer*, *8*, 50–56. doi:10.1109/MC.2004.91

Mascioli, F. M. F., & Martinelli, G. (1998). A constructive approach to neuro-fuzzy networks. *Signal Processing*, *64*, 347–358. doi:10.1016/S0165-1684(97)00200-4

Mascioli, F. M. F., Rizzi, A., Panella, M., & Martinelli, G. (2000). Scale-based approach to hierarchical fuzzy clustering. *Signal Processing*, *80*, 1001–1016. doi:10.1016/S0165-1684(00)00016-5

MathWorks. The. (2009). *Neural Network Toolbox User's Guide*. Retrieved from http://www.mathworks.es/access/helpdesk/help/pdf_doc/nnet/nnet.pdf.

Matlab, (2009), *The Mathworks website*. Retrieved August 15, 2009 from http://www.mathworks.com

McCulloch, W. S., & Pitts, W. (1943). A logical calculus of the ideas immanent in nervous activity. *The Bulletin of Mathematical Biophysics*, *5*, 115–133. doi:10.1007/BF02478259

McDonough, J. (2004). Least Mean Square Error (LMSE) Estimation. *Lecture Notes of Interactive Systems Laboratories Institut für Logik, Komplexitat, und Deduktionssysteme Universitat Karlsruhe.*

McIntosh, A. R., Rajah, M. N., & Lobaugh, N. J. (1999). Interactions of prefrontal cortex in relation to awareness in sensory learning. *Science*, *284*, 1531–1533. doi:10.1126/science.284.5419.1531

Mead, C. (1989). *Analog VLSI and Neural Systems*. Addison Wesley.

Medrano-Marqués, N. J., & Martín-del-Brío, B. (2001). Sensor linearization with neural networks. *IEEE Transactions on Industrial Electronics*, *48*, 1288–1290. doi:10.1109/41.969414

Medrano-Marques, N. J., & Martín-del-Brio, B. (2002). A Flexible Tool for Conditioning Sensor Signals based on Neural Networks. In *Proceedings IEEE Industrial Electronics Conference, IECON 2002*, (pp. 96-101). Sevilla: IEEE Press.

Mehring, C., Rickert, J., Vaadia, E., de Oliveira, S. C., Aertsen, A., & Rotter, S. (2003). Inference of hand movements from local field potentials in monkey motor cortex. *Nature Neuroscience*, *6*(12), 1253–1254. doi:10.1038/nn1158

Meijer, G. (Ed.). (2008). *Smart Sensor Systems*. Wiltshire, UK: Wiley. doi:10.1002/9780470866931

Messinger, A., Squire, L. R., Zola, S. M., & Albright, T. D. (2005). Neural correlates of knowledge: stable representation of stimulus associations across variations in behavioral performance. *Neuron*, *48*, 359–371. doi:10.1016/j.neuron.2005.08.035

Metta, G., Sandini, G., & Konczak, J. (1999). A developmental approach to visually-guided reaching in artificial systems. *Neural Networks*, *12*, 1413–1427. doi:10.1016/S0893-6080(99)00070-2

Miller, G. A. (1967). *The psychology of communication*. London: Penguin.

Minsky, M. L., & Pappert, S. A. (1969). *Perceptrons*. Cambridge, MA: MIT Press.

Mitchell, C. J., De Houwer, J., & Lovibond, P. F. (2009). The propositional nature of human associative learning. *The Behavioral and Brain Sciences*, *32*, 183–198. doi:10.1017/S0140525X09000855

Mitra, S., & Hayashi, Y. (2000). Neuro-fuzzy rule generation: Survey in soft computing framework. *IEEE Transactions on Neural Networks*, *11*, 748–768. doi:10.1109/72.846746

Mitri, S., Floreano, D., Magnenat, S., & Keller, L. (2007). Evolutionary Conditions for the Emergence of Communication in Robots. *Current Biology*, *17*(6), 514–519. doi:10.1016/j.cub.2007.01.058

Moerland, P., & Fiesler, E. (1996). Neural Network Adaptation to Hardware Implementations . In Fiesler, E., & Beale, R. (Eds.), *Handbook of Neural Computation*. New York: Oxford Press.

Mohseni, P., Najafi, K., Eliades, S. J., & Wang, X. (2005). Wireless Multichannel Biopotential Recording Using an Integrated FM Telemetry Circuit. *IEEE Transactions on Neural Systems and Rehabilitation Engineering*, *13*(3), 263–271. doi:10.1109/TNSRE.2005.853625

Montero, J., Lopez, V., & Gomez, D. (2007). The Role of Fuzziness in Decision Making . In Wang, D. P., Ruan, D., & Kerre, E. E. (Eds.), *Fuzzy Logic: A Spectrum of Theoretical & Practical Issues* (pp. 337–350). New York: Springer.

Moraga, C., Trillas, E., & Guadarrama, S. (2003). Multiple-valued Logic and Artificial Intelligence Fundamentals of Fuzzy Control Revisited. *Kluwer-Artificial Intelligence Review*, *20*(3-4), 169–197. doi:10.1023/B:AIRE.0000006610.94970.1d

Morgavi G., Morando M., Biorci G., & Caviglia D. (2005, June). Growing up: emerging complexity in living being. *Cybernetics and Systems: an International Journal.* Boca Raton, FL: Taylor and Francis ed.

Morgavi, G., & Marconi, L. (2008). Growing Up of Autonomous Agents: an Emergent Phenomenon. In *AIP Proceedings* 1051 (pp.187-194). Dubois Ed.

Moritz, C. T., Perlmutter, S. I., & Fetz, E. E. (2008). Direct control of paralysed muscles by cortical neurons. *Nature*, *456*, 639–642. doi:10.1038/nature07418

Musallam, S., Corneil, B. D., Greger, B., Scherberger, H., & Andersen, R. A. (2004). Cognitive Control Signals for Neural Prosthetics. *Science*, *305*, 258–262. doi:10.1126/science.1097938

Narasimhan, K. (2004). Scaling up neuroscience. *Nature Neuroscience*, *7*(5), 425. doi:10.1038/nn0504-425

Nauck, D., & Kruse, R. (1999). Neuro-fuzzy systems for function approximation. *Fuzzy Sets and Systems*, *101*, 261–271. doi:10.1016/S0165-0114(98)00169-9

Nauck, D. (1997). Neuro-fuzzy systems: Review and prospects. In *Proc. Fifth European Congress on Intelligent Techniques and Soft Computing*, 1044-1053.

Navabi, Z. (1998). *Analysis and Modeling of Digital Systems* (2nd ed.). New York: McGraw Hill.

Nedjah, N., & Mourelle, L. M. (2007). Reconfigurable Hardware for Neural Networks: Binary radix vs. Stochastic . *Journal of Neural Computing and Applications*, *16*(3), 249–155. doi:10.1007/s00521-007-0086-x

Newell, A. (1990). *Unified Theories of Cognition*. Cambridge, MA: Harvard University Press.

Nicolelis, M. A. L., Dimitrov, D., Carmena, J. M., Crist, R., Lehew, G., & Kralik, J. D. (2003). Chronic, multisite, multielectrode recordings in macaque monkeys. *Proceedings of the National Academy of Sciences of the United States of America*, *200*(19), 11041–11046. doi:10.1073/pnas.1934665100

Nicolelis, M. A. L., Chapin, J. K., & Wessberg, J. (2007). United States of America Patent No. Official Gazette of the United States Patent and Trademark Office Patents: U. S. P. a. T. Office.

Nilsson, N. J. (1965). *Learning Machines: Foundations of Trainable Pattern-Classifying Systems*. New York: McGraw-Hill.

Nolfi, S., & Parisi, D. (1997). Neural networks in an artificial life perspective., In W.Gerstner, A.Germond, M.Hasler, and J.D.Nicoud (Eds.) *Artificial Neural Networks (ICANN97)*. In *Proceedings of the 7th International Conference on Artificial Neural Networks*. Berlin, Germany: Springer Verlag, pp. 733-738

Nowrouzian, B. (1989). Minimal Multiplier Realization of Bilinear-LDI Digital All-Pass Networks. *IEE Proceedings on Devices and Systems*, *G-136*, 114–117. doi:10.1049/ip-g-2.1989.0018

Nowrouzian, B., Mercier, P., & Kilambi, S. M. (2007). Optimization of FRM FIR Digital Filters over CSD and CDBNS Multiplier Coefficient Spaces Employing a Novel Genetic Algorithm. *Journal of Computers*, *2*(7), 20–31.

Ogden, C. K., & Richards, I. A. (1960). *The Meaning of Meaning. A Study of the Influence of Language upon Thought and of the Science of Symbolism*. London: Routledge.

O'Halloran, M., & Sarpeshkar, R. (2004). A 10-nW 12-bit Accurate Analog Storage Cell with 10-aA Leakage. *IEEE Journal of Solid-state Circuits*, *39*(11), 557–560. doi:10.1109/JSSC.2004.835817

O'Halloran, M., & Sarpeshkar, R. (2006). An Analog Storage Cell with 5e-/sec Leakage. *Proceedings of the IEEE International Symposium on Circuits and Systems (ISCAS)*, 557-560.

Olsson, R. H. III, & Wise, K. D. (2005). A Three-Dimensional Neural Recording Microsystem With Implantable Data Compression Circuitry. *IEEE Journal of Solid-state Circuits*, *40*(12), 2796–2804. doi:10.1109/JSSC.2005.858479

Orna, M. V., & Stock, J. (1989). *Electrochemistry, Past and Present*. Columbus: American Chemical Society.

Osuna, R. G-., & Nagle, H. T. (1999). A Method for Evaluating Data-preprocessing Techniques for Odour Classification with an Array of Gas Sensors. *IEEE Transactions on Systems, Man, and Cybernetics . Part B*, *29*(5), 626–632.

Pandya, A. S., & Macy, R. B. (1995). *Pattern Recognition with Neural Networks in C*. CRC Press.

Pandya, A. S., & Venugopal, P. (1991). A Stochastic Parallel Algorithm for Supervised Learning in Neural Networks. *IEEE Transactions on Information Systems . E (Norwalk, Conn.)*, *77-D*(4), 376–384.

Panella, M. (2007). *Martinelly, Giuseppe*. Binary Neuro-Fuzzy Classifiers Trained by Nonlinear Quantum.

Pardo, M., & Sberveglieri, G. (2004). Feature Evaluation for an Electronic Node. *Proceedings of the IEEE*, *2*, 595–596. doi:10.1109/ICSENS.2004.1426235

Parker, A. E., & Skellern, D. J. (1997). A realistic large-signal MESFET model for SPICE. *IEEE Transactions on Microwave Theory and Techniques*, *45*(9), 1563–1571. doi:10.1109/22.622923

Passos, M. G., Silva, P. H. da F., & Fernandes, H. C. C. (2007). Applications of modular RBF/MLP neural networks in the modeling of microstrip photonic band gap structures. *Proceedings of Progress In Electromagnetics Research Symposium*, *2*(5), 695–700.

Patnaik, A., & Mishra, R. K. (2000). ANN techniques in microwave engineering. *IEEE Microwave Magazine*, *1*(1), 55–60. doi:10.1109/6668.823828

Pavlov, I. (1927). *Conditioned Reflexes: (1927)*. New York, NY, US: Oxford University Press.

Pearlmutter, B. A. (1995). Gradient calculations for dynamic recurrent neural networks: A survey . *IEEE Transactions on Neural Networks*, *6*, 1212–1228. doi:10.1109/72.410363

Pearson, M. J., Pipe, A. G., Mitchinson, B., Gurney, K., C. Melhuish, C., Gilhespy, I. & Nibouche, M. (2007). Implementing spiking neural networks for real-time signal-processing and control applications: a model-validation FPGA approach. *IEEE Transactions on Neural Networks, 18*(5), 1472-1487.

Perelman, Y., & Ginosar, R. (2008). *The Neuroprocessor: An Integrated Interface to Biological Neural Networks*. Springer-Verlag. Porto, A. B., & Pazos, A. (2006). Neuroglial Behaviour in Computer Science . In Rabuna, J. R., & Dorado, J. (Eds.), *Artificial Neural Networks in Real-life Applications* (pp. 1–21). London: Idea Group Publications.

Perfiliva, I. (2007). Analytical Theory of Fuzzy IF-THEN Rules with Compositional Rule of Inference . In Wang, D. P., Ruan, D., & Kerre, E. E. (Eds.), *Fuzzy Logic: A Spectrum of Theoretical & Practical Issues* (pp. 173–192). New York: Springer.

Pertijs, M., Bakker, A., & Huijsing, J. H. (2001). A high-accuracy temperature sensor with second-order curvature correction and digital bus interface. In *Proceedings IEEE International Symposium on Circuits and Systems (ISCAS)* (pp. 368-371). Sydney: IEEE Press.

Pesaran, B., Pezaris, J. S., Sahani, M., Mitra, P. P., & Andersen, R. A. (2002). Temporal structure in neuronal activity during working memory in macaque parietal cortex. *Nature Neuroscience*, *5*(8), 805–811. doi:10.1038/nn890

Peterson, W. D. (2002). *WISHBONE system-on-chip (SoC) interconnection architecture for portable IP cores, revision: B.3*. Retrieved from http://www.opencores.org/.

Pfurtscheller, G., Neuper, C., Schlogl, A., & Lugger, K. (1998). Separability of EEG signals recorded during right and left motor imagery using adaptive autoregressive parameters . *IEEE Transactions on Rehabilitation Engineering*, *6*(3), 316–324. doi:10.1109/86.712230

Pierce, D., & Kuipers, B. (1997). Map learning with uninterpreted sensors and effectors. *Artificial Intelligence Journal*, *92*, 169–229. doi:10.1016/S0004-3702(96)00051-3

Pinar, A., & Heath, M. T. (1999). Improving performance of sparse matrix-vector multiplication. *Proceedings of the 1999 ACM/IEEE conference on Supercomputing - Supercomputing '99*, 30-es. New York: ACM Press.

Pinker, S. (1994). *The Language Instinct*. London: Penguin.

Plate, T. A. (2003). *Holographic Reduced Representation*. Stanford, CA: CSLI Publications.

Popa, C. (2005). Current-mode Euclidean Distance Circuit Independent Technological Parameters. *Proceedings of IEEE Semiconductor Conference*, *2*, 459–462.

Potter, S.M (2007). What can AI Get from Neuroscience. *Lecture Notes in Artificial Intelligence*, 174-185.

Prasad, G., McGinnity, T. M., Leng, G., & Coyle, D. (2010). On-line identification of self-organizing fuzzy neural networks for modelling time-varying complex systems . In Plamen, (Eds.), *Evolving Intelligent Systems* (pp. 302–324). New York: John Wiley. doi:10.1002/9780470569962.ch9

Quiroga, R. Q., Reddy, L., Kreiman, G., Koch, C., & Fried, I. (2005). Invariant visual representation by single neurons in the human brain. *Nature*, *435*, 1102–1107. doi:10.1038/nature03687

Rabinowitch, I., & Segev, I. (2008). Two Opposing Plasticity Mechanisms Pulling a Single Synapse. *Trends in Neurosciences*, *31*(8), 377–383. doi:10.1016/j.tins.2008.05.005

Rabrenovic, D., & Lutovac, M. (1994). Elliptic Filters with Minimal Q-factors. *IEE Electronics Letters*, *30*(3), 206–207. doi:10.1049/el:19940180

Radisic, V., Qian, Y., Coccioli, R., & Itoh, T. (1998). Novel 2-D photonic band-gap structures for microstrip lines. *IEEE Microwave Guided Wave Letters*, *8*(2), 69–71. doi:10.1109/75.658644

Raghuram, R. (1989). *Computer simulation of electronic circuits*. New Delhi: Wiley Eastern Limited.

Rainer, G., Lee, H., & Logothetis, N. K. (2004). The effect of learning on the function of monkey extrastriate visual cortex. *PLoS Biology*, *2*, E44. doi:10.1371/journal.pbio.0020044

Rainer, G., & Miller, E. K. (2000). Effects of visual experience on the representation of objects in the prefrontal cortex. *Neuron*, *27*, 179–189. doi:10.1016/S0896-6273(00)00019-2

Rapoport, B. I. (2007). *Neural Prosthetics for Paralysis: Algorithms and Low-Power Analog Architectures for Decoding Neural Signals*. Cambridge, Massachusetts: Massachusetts Institute of Technology.

Rapoport, B. I., Wattanapanitch, W., Penagos, H. L., Musallam, S., Andersen, R. A., & Sarpeshkar, R. (2009). *A Biomimetic Adaptive Algorithm and Low-Power Architecture for Implantable Neural Decoders*. Paper presented at the 31st Annual International Conference of the IEEE Engineering in Medicine and Biology Society (EMBC 2009).

Rayas-Sanchez, J. E. (2001). *Neural space mapping methods for modeling and design of microwave circuits*. (Doctoral dissertation, McMaster University, 2001).

Reaz, M. B. I., Islam, S. Z., Ali, M. A. M., & Sulaiman, M. S. (2002). FPGA realization of backpropagation for stock market prediction. *9th International Conference on Neural Information Proceedings of ICONIP'02. 2*, 960-964.

Reed, D. R., Tanaka, T., & McDaniel, A. H. (2006). Diverse tastes: genetics of sweet and bitter perception. *Physiology & Behavior*, *88*(3), 215–226. doi:10.1016/j.physbeh.2006.05.033

Rescorla, R. A. (1973). Effect of US habituation following conditioning. *Journal of Comparative and Physiological Psychology*, *82*, 137–143. doi:10.1037/h0033815

Rescorla, R. A., & Wagner, A. R. (1972). A theory of Pavlovian conditioning: Variations in the effectiveness of reinforcement and non-reinforcement . In Black, A. H., & Prokasy, W. F. (Eds.), *Classical Conditioning II*. New York: Appleton-Century-Crofts.

Richardson-Burns, S. M., Hendricks, J. L., & Martin, D. C. (2007). Electrochemical polymerization of conducting polymers in living neural tissue. *Journal of Neural Engineering*, *4*, L6–L13. doi:10.1088/1741-2560/4/2/L02

Ridmiller, M., & Braun, H. (1993). *A direct adaptive method for faster backpropagation learning: The RPROP algorithm*. Paper presented at the IEEE International Conference on Neural Networks, San Francisco, EUA.

Riedel, G., Platt, B., & Micheau, J. (2003). Glutamate Receptor Function in Learning and Memory. *Behavioural Brain Research*, *140*, 1–47. doi:10.1016/S0166-4328(02)00272-3

Riul, A. Jr, de Sousa, H. C., Malmegrim, R. R., dos Santos, D. S. Jr, Carvalho, A. C. P. L. F., & Fonseca, F. J. (2004). Wine classification by taste sensors made from ultra-thin films and using neural networks. *Sensors and Actuators. B, Chemical*, *98*, 77–82. doi:10.1016/j.snb.2003.09.025

Riul, A. Jr, dos Santos, D. S. Jr, Wohnrath, K., Di Tommazo, R., Carvalho, A. C. P. L. F., & Fonseca, F. J. (2002). Artificial taste sensor: efficient combination of sensors made from Langmuir-Blodgett films of conducting polymers and a ruthenium complex and self-assembled films of an Azobenzene-containing polymer. *Langmuir*, *18*, 239–245. doi:10.1021/la011017d

Rizzi, A., Panella, M., & Maxioli, F. M. F. (2002). Adaptive resolution of min-max classifiers . *IEEE Transactions on Neural Networks*, *13*(2), 402–414. doi:10.1109/72.991426

Rokni, U., Richardson, A. G., Bizzi, E., & Seung, H. S. (2007). Motor Learning with Unstable Neural Representations. *Neuron*, *54*, 653–666. doi:10.1016/j.neuron.2007.04.030

Rosenblatt, F. (1958). The Perceptron: A Probabilistic Model for Information Storage and Organization in the Brain. *Psychological Review*, *65*, 386–408. doi:10.1037/h0042519

Rosenblatt, F. (1962). *Principles of Neurodynamics*. Washington, DC: Spartan Books.

Rosenblatt, F. (1958) The Perceptron: A probabilistic model for information storage and organization in the brain. *Psychological Review, 65*(6), p. 386-408. Retrieved February 06, 2010, from http://www.ling.upenn.edu/courses/Fall_2007/cogs501/Rosenblatt1958.pdf.

Rosenthal, O., Fusi, S., & Hochstein, S. (2001). Forming classes by stimulus frequency: behavior and theory. *Proceedings of the National Academy of Sciences of the United States of America*, *98*, 4265–4270. doi:10.1073/pnas.071525998

Ross, P., Hart, E., Lawson, A., Webb, A., Prem, E., Peolz, P., & Morgavi, G. (2003). *Requirements for getting a robot to grow up*. Lectures Notes in Artificial Intelligence.

Rothenberg, A. (1990). Creativity health and alcoholism. *Creativity Research Journal*, *3*, 179–202. doi:10.1080/10400419009534352

Rovithakis, G. A., & Christodoulou, M. A. (2000). *Adaptive Control with Recurrent High-order Neural Networks*. London: Springer-Verlag.

Roy, A., Steinmetz, P. N., Hsiao, S. S., Johnson, K. O., & Niebur, E. (2007). Synchrony: A Neural Correlate of Somatosensory Attention. *Journal of Neurophysiology*, *98*, 1645–1661. doi:10.1152/jn.00522.2006

Rumelhart, D. E., Hinton, G. E., & Williams, R. J. (1986). Learning Representations by Backpropagating Errors. *Nature*, *32*, 533–536. doi:10.1038/323533a0

Rumelhart, D. E., Hinton, G. E., & Williams, R. J. (1986). Learning internal representations by error propagation. In D. E. Rumelhart & J. L. McClelland (Ed.), *Parallel Distributed Processing: Explorations in the microstructure of cognition, Vol. 1: Foundations* (pp. 318-362). Cambridge, MA: MIT Press.

Rutkowski, L. (2004). *Flexible Neuro-fuzzy Systems: Structures, Learning and Performance Evaluation*. Boston: Kluwer.

Saint-Jones, P., & Gu, D. (2003). *Fractional Fixed Point Neural Network: an introduction*. Department of Computer Science, University of Essex.

Sakr, N., & Groza, V. (2005). Run-time Reconfigurable Hardware Blocks for Multimedia Applications. *Proceedings of Canadian Conference on Electrical and Computer Engineering*: *(1996-1999)*.

Salthouse, C., & Sarpeshkar, R. (2003). A Practical Micropower Programmable Bandpass Filter for use in Bionic Ears. *IEEE Journal of Solid-state Circuits*, *38*(1), 63–70. doi:10.1109/JSSC.2002.806286

Sanchez, E. N., & Perez, J. P. (2003). Input-to-state stabilization of dynamic neural networks. *IEEE Transactions on Systems, Man, and Cybernetics A*, *33*(4), 532–536. doi:10.1109/TSMCA.2003.811509

Sanchez, J. C., Erdogmus, D., Principe, J. C., Wessberg, J., & Nicolelis, M. A. L. (2005). Interpreting spatial and temporal neural activity through a recurrent neural network brain machine interface. *IEEE Transactions on Neural Systems and Rehabilitation Engineering*, *13*(2), 213–219. doi:10.1109/TNSRE.2005.847382

Santhanam, G., Ryu, S. I., Yu, B. M., Afshar, A., & Shenoy, K. V. (2006). A high-performance brain-computer interface. *Nature*, *442*, 195–198. doi:10.1038/nature04968

Santos, A. L., Romariz, A. R. S., & Carvalho, P. H. P. (1997). Neural model of electrical devices for circuit simulation. *Proceedings of the SBMO/IEEE MTT-S International Microwave and Optoelectronics Conference, Vol. 1,* 253-258.

Sarpeshkar, R. (1998). Analog Versus Digital: Extrapolating from Electronics to Neurobiology. *Neural Computation*, *10*, 1601–1638. doi:10.1162/089976698300017052

Sarpeshkar, R. (2006). Brain Power: Borrowing from Biology Makes for Low-Power Computing. *IEEE Spectrum*, *43*(5), 24–29. doi:10.1109/MSPEC.2006.1628504

Sarpeshkar, R., Lyon, R. F., & Mead, C. (1997). A low-power wide-linear-range transconductance amplifier. *Analog Integrated Circuits and Signal Processing*, *13*(1-2), 123–151. doi:10.1023/A:1008292213687

Sarpeshkar, R., Salthouse, C., Sit, J.-J., Baker, M., Zhak, S., & Lu, T. (2005). An Ultra-Low-Power Programmable Analog Bionic Ear Processor. *IEEE Transactions on Bio-Medical Engineering*, *52*(4), 711–727. doi:10.1109/TBME.2005.844043

Sarpeshkar, R., Wattanapanitch, W., Arfin, S. K., Rapoport, B. I., Mandal, S., & Baker, M. W. (2008). Low-Power Circuits for Brain-Machine Interfaces. *IEEE Transactions on Biomedical Circuits and Systems*, *2*(3), 173–183. doi:10.1109/TBCAS.2008.2003198

Sarpeshkar, R., Baker, M., Salthouse, C., Sit, J.-J., Turicchia, L., & Zhak, S. (2005). An Analog Bionic Ear Processor with Zero-Crossing Detection. *Proceedings of the IEEE International Solid State Circuits Conference (ISSCC)*, 78-79.

Sarpeshkar, R., Wattanapanitch, W., Rapoport, B., Arfin, S. K., Baker, M. W., Mandal, S., et al. (2007). Low-Power Circuits for Brain-Machine Interfaces. *Proceedings of the IEEE Symposium on Circuits and Systems*, 2068-2071.

Sasaki, M., Inoue, T., Shirai, Y., & Ueno, F. (1990). Fuzzy Multiple-input Maximum and Minimum Circuits in Current-mode and Their Analyses Using Bounded Difference Equations. *IEEE Transactions on Computers*, *39*(6), 768–774. doi:10.1109/12.53598

Sato, Y. D., Wolff, C., Wolfrum, P., & von der Malsburg, C. (2007). Dynamic Link Matching between Feature Columns for Different Scale and Orientation. *Lecture Notes In Computer Science*. Retrieved from http://portal.acm.org/citation.cfm?id=1423142.

Savov, S. V. (2002). An efficient solution of a class of integrals arising in antenna theory. *IEEE Antennas and Propagation Magazine*, *44*(5), 98–101. doi:10.1109/MAP.2002.1077781

Scassellati, B. M. (2002). Theory of mind for a humanoid robot. *Autonomous Robots*, *12*(1), 13–24. doi:10.1023/A:1013298507114

Schichman, H., & Hodges, D. A. (1968). Modeling and simulation of insulated-gate field-effect transistor switching circuits. *IEEE Journal of Solid-state Circuits*, *3*(3), 285–289. doi:10.1109/JSSC.1968.1049902

Schliebs, S., Defoin-Platel, M., & Kasabov, N. (2009). Integrated feature and parameter optimization for an evolving spiking neural network . In Köppen, M. (Ed.), *ICONIP 2008, Lecture Notes in Computer Science, Part I, 5506* (pp. 1229–1236). Berlin, Heidelberg: Springer-Verlag.

Schlogl, A., & Pfurtscheller, G. (2005). *Graz dataset IIIb description for the BCI 2005 data classification competition*. Retrieved October 14, 2005 from http://ida.first.fhg.de/projects/bci/competition_iii/desc_IIIb.pdf

Schrauwen, B., & Van Campenhout, J. (2006). Parallel hardware implementation of a broad class of spiking neurons using serial arithmetic. *European Symposium on Artificial Neural Networks ESANN'2006*, 623-628.

Scott, K. J. A. (1982). Concepts and issues in human motor behavior . In Scott Kelso, J. A. (Ed.), *Human Motor Behavior: An Introduction*. Hillsdale, NJ: Lawrence Erlbaum Associates.

Sepulchre, R., Jankovic, M., & Kokotovic, P. (1997). *Constructive Nonlinear Control*. New York: Springer-Verlag.

Serruya, M. D., Hatsopoulos, N. G., Fellows, M. R., Paninski, L., & Donoghue, J. P. (2003). Robustness of neuroprosthetic decoding algorithms. *Biological Cybernetics*, *88*(3), 219–228. doi:10.1007/s00422-002-0374-6

Seul, J., & Sung, S. K. (2007). Hardware Implementation of a Real-Time Neural Network Controller With a DSP and an FPGA for Nonlinear Systems . *IEEE Transactions on Industrial Electronics*, *54*(1), 265–271. doi:10.1109/TIE.2006.888791

Severinson-Eklund, K., Green, A., & Hüttenrauch, H. (2003). Social and collaborative aspects of interaction with a service robot . *Robotics and Autonomous Systems*, *42*, 223–234. doi:10.1016/S0921-8890(02)00377-9

Shain, W., Spataro, L., Dilgen, J., Haverstick, K., Retterer, S., & Isaacson, M. (2003). Controlling cellular reactive responses around neural prosthetic devices using peripheral and local intervention strategies. *IEEE Transactions on Neural Systems and Rehabilitation Engineering, 11*, 186–188. doi:10.1109/TNSRE.2003.814800

Shanks, D. R., & Darby, R. J. (1998). Feature- and rule-based generalization in human associative learning. *Journal of Experimental Psychology. Animal Behavior Processes, 24*, 405–415. doi:10.1037/0097-7403.24.4.405

Shenoy, K. V., Meeker, D., Cao, S. Y., Kureshi, S. A., Pesaran, B., & Buneo, C. A. (2003). Neural prosthetic control signals from plan activity. *Neuroreport, 14*(4), 591–596. doi:10.1097/00001756-200303240-00013

Sherrington, C. S. (1933). *The Brain and Its Mechanism. New London*. Cambridge University Press.

Shimodaira, H. (2001). A Diversity-Control-Oriented Genetic Algorithm (DCGA): Performance in Function Optimization. Proceedings of 2001 Congress on Evolutionary Computation, 1, *44-51.*

Shirai, Y., Ueno, F., & Inoue, T. (2007). Configuration of Fuzzy Membership Function Circuits Using Current-mode. *Wiley Interscience Electronics and Communications in Japan, 70*(8), 59–67.

Sigala, N., & Logothetis, N. K. (2002). Visual categorization shapes feature selectivity in the primate temporal cortex. *Nature, 415*, 318–320. doi:10.1038/415318a

Sigman, M., Pan, H., Yang, Y., Stern, E., Silbersweig, D., & Gilbert, C. D. (2005). Topdown reorganization of activity in the visual pathway after learning a shape identification task. *Neuron, 46*, 823–835. doi:10.1016/j.neuron.2005.05.014

Silva, P. H. da F., & Campos, A. L. P. S. (2008). Fast and accurate modeling of frequency selective surfaces using a new modular neural network configuration of multilayer perceptrons. *IET Microwaves . Antennas & Propagation, 2*(5), 503–511.

Silva, P. H. da F., Melo, M. A. B., & Neto, A. D. D. (2002). Using neural network models for efficient GaAs MESFET time-domain nonlinear circuit analysis . *Proceedings of the International Joint Conference on Neural Networks, 3*, 2282–2287.

Silva, P. H. da F., Passos, M. G., & D'Assunção, A. G. (2007). Fast and accurate analysis for the directivity of circular-shape antennas using optimal neural networks. *Microwave and Optical Technology Letters, 49*(11), 2721–2726. doi:10.1002/mop.22839

Silva, P. H. da F., Passos, M. G., & Fernandes, H. C. C. (2007). Novel neural network models of Q-type integrals and their use for circular-loop antenna analysis. *Proceedings of Progress In Electromagnetics Research Symposium, 1*, 2137–2141.

Silva, P. H. da F. (2002). *Modelos através de redes neurais artificiais sem realimentação para dispositivos e circuitos de RF/Microondas.* (Doctoral dissertation, Federal University of Campina Grande, 2002).

Silva, P. H. da F., Lacouth, P., Fontgalland, G., Campos, A. L. P. S., & D'Assunção, A. G. (2007), Design of frequency selective surfaces using a novel MoM-ANN-GA technique. *Proceedings of the SBMO/IEEE MTT-S International Microwave and Optoelectronics Conference, Vol. 1,* 275-279.

Silva, P. H. da F., Melo, M. A. B., & Neto, A. D. D. (2001). Fast and accurate neural network GaAs MESFET model for time-domain circuit simulation. *Proceedings of the SBMO/IEEE MTT-S International Microwave and Optoelectronics Conference, Vol. 1,* 53-56.

Simpson, P. K. (1992). Fuzzy min-max neural networks-Part 1: Classification. *IEEE Transactions on Neural Networks, 3*, 776–786. doi:10.1109/72.159066

Simpson, P. K. (1993). Fuzzy min-max neural networks-Part 1: Clustering. *IEEE Transactions on Fuzzy Systems, 1*, 32–45. doi:10.1109/TFUZZ.1993.390282

Sinclair-de-Zwart, H. (1973). Language acquisition and cognitive development . In Moore, T. (Ed.), *Cognitive development and the acquisition of language*. New York: Academic Press.

Smith, S. S., Ward, T. B., & Finke, R. A. (Eds.). (1995). *The creative cognition approach* (pp. 27–52). Cambridge, MA: MIT Press.

Snyder, L. H., Batista, A. P., & Andersen, R. A. (1997). Coding of intention in the posterior parietal cortex. *Nature*, *386*, 167–170. doi:10.1038/386167a0

Soltic, S., & Zuppicich, A. (2008). Comparison between software and FPGA implementation of ESNN in terms of processing speed. *15th Electronics New Zealand Conference ENZCon08*, 56-61.

Soltic, S., Wysoski, S. G., & Kasabov, N. (2008), Evolving spiking neural networks for taste recognition. *International Joint Conference on Neural Networks*, 2092-2098.

Song, Y.-K., Patterson, W. R., Bull, C. W., Borton, D. A., Li, Y., Nurmikko, A. V., et al. (2007). *A Brain Implantable Microsystem with Hybrid RF/IR Telemetry for Advanced Neuroengineering Applications*. Paper presented at the 29th Annual International Conference of the IEEE Engineering in Medicine and Biology Society.

Sontag, E. O. (1989). A universal construction of artstein's theorem on nonlinear stabilization. *Systems & Control Letters*, *13*, 117–123. doi:10.1016/0167-6911(89)90028-5

Sontag, D. E., & Qiao, Y. (1999). Further results on controllability of recurrent neural networks. *Systems & Control Letters*, *36*, 121–129. doi:10.1016/S0167-6911(98)00068-1

Sontag, D. E., & Sussmann, H. (1997). Complete controllability of continuous-time recurrent neural networks. *Systems & Control Letters*, *30*, 177–183. doi:10.1016/S0167-6911(97)00002-9

Soucek, B. (1992). *Fast Learning and Invariant Object Recognition*. New York: John Wiley & Sons.

Sovrano, V. A., Bisazza, A., & Vallortigara, G. (2002). Modularity and spatial reorientation in a simple mind: encoding of geometric and non-geometric properties of a spatial environment by fish. *Cognition*, *85*, B51–B59. doi:10.1016/S0010-0277(02)00110-5

Spaepen, L. (2003). *Goal oriented reaching*. Cambridge, MA: Harvard University Press.

Spelke, E. S., Breinlinger, K., Macomber, J., & Jacobson, K. (1992). Origins of knowledge. *Psychological Review*, *99*(4), 605–632. doi:10.1037/0033-295X.99.4.605

Srinivas, M., & Patnaik, L. M. (1994). Adaptive Probabilities of Crossover and Mutation in Genetic Algorithms . *IEEE Transactions on Systems, Man, and Cybernetics*, *24*, 656–667. doi:10.1109/21.286385

Srinivasan, L., Eden, U. T., Mitter, S. K., & Brown, E. N. (2007). General-purpose filter design for neural prosthetic devices. *Journal of Neurophysiology*, *98*, 2456–2475. doi:10.1152/jn.01118.2006

Srivastava, A. K., Srivastava, S. K., & Shukla, K. K. (1997). On the Design Issue of Intelligent Electronic Nose System. *Proceedings of the International Conference on Industrial Technology*, *1*, 243–248.

Stark, E., & Abeles, M. (2007). Predicting movement from multiunit activity. *The Journal of Neuroscience*, *27*(31), 8387–8394. doi:10.1523/JNEUROSCI.1321-07.2007

Steels, L. (1999). Discovering the Competitors. *Journal of Adaptive Systems*, *4*(2).

Stein, J. F., & Stoodley, C. J. (2006). *Neuroscience: an introduction*. John Wiley and sons.

Stitt, J. P., Gaumond, R. P., Frazier, J. L., & Hanson, F. E. (1997). A comparison of neural spike classification techniques. *The 19th International Conference IEEE/EMBS*, 1092-1094.

Stoica, A. (2000). Evolvable Hardware: From On-Chip Circuit Synthesis to Evolvable Space Systems. In *Proceedings of IEEE 30th International Symposium on Multiple-Valued Logic*, (ISMVL), 161.

Subramanian, C. S., Pinelli, J. P., Lapilli, C. D., & Buist, L. (2005). A Wireless Multipoint Pressure Sensing System: Design and Operation. *IEEE Sensors Journal*, *5*(5), 1066–1074. doi:10.1109/JSEN.2005.854135

Sugeno, M., & Kang, G. T. (1988). Structure identification of fuzzy model. *Fuzzy Sets and Systems*, *28*(15), 33.

Sugeno, M., & Yasukawa, T. (1993). A Fuzzy Logic Based Approach to Qualitative Modeling. *IEEE Transactions on Fuzzy Systems*, *1*(1), 7–31. doi:10.1109/TFUZZ.1993.390281

Suner, S., Fellows, M. R., Vargas-Irwin, C., Nakata, G. K., & Donoghue, J. P. (2005). Reliability of signals from a chronically implanted, silicon-based electrode array in non-human primate primary motor cortex. *IEEE Transactions on Neural Systems and Rehabilitation Engineering*, *13*(4), 524–541. doi:10.1109/TNSRE.2005.857687

Sussman-Fort, S. E., Narasimhan, S., & Mayaram, K. (1984). A complete GaAs MESFET computer model for SPICE. *IEEE Transactions on Microwave Theory and Techniques*, *32*(4), 471–473. doi:10.1109/TMTT.1984.1132707

Takagi, T., & Sugeno, M. (1985). Fuzzy identification of systems and its applications to modeling and control. *IEEE Transactions on Systems, Man, and Cybernetics*, *15*, 116–132.

Takagi, T., & Sugeno, M. (1985). Fuzzy Identification of Systems and Its Application to Modeling and Control. *IEEE Transactions on Systems, Man, and Cybernetics*, *20*(2), 116–132.

Takagi, T., & Sugeno, M. (1983). Derivation of fuzzy control rules from human operator's control action, *Proc. of the IFAC Symp. on Fuzzy Info., Knowledge Rep. and Decision Analysis*, (pp. 55-60).

Taube, J. S. (1995). Head Direction Cells Recorded in the Anterior Thalamic Nuclei of Freely Moving Rats. *The Journal of Neuroscience*, *15*(1), 70–86.

Taylor, D. M., Tillery, S. I. H., & Schwartz, A. B. (2002). Direct Cortical Control of 3D Neuroprosthetic Devices. *Science*, *296*, 1829–1832. doi:10.1126/science.1070291

Teel, A. (1999). Asymptotic convergence from L_p stability. *IEEE Transactions on Automatic Control*, *44*, 2169–2170. doi:10.1109/9.802938

Temam, O., & Jalby, W. (1992). Characterizing the behavior of sparse algorithms on caches. In *Proceedings of the 1992 ACM/IEEE conference on supercomputing* (pp. 578-587). Minneapolis: IEEE Computer Society Press.

Temel, T., & Karlik, B. (2007). An improved Odor Recognition System Using Learning Vector Quantization with a New Discriminant Analysis. *Neural Network World*, *4*(7), 287–294.

Temel, T. (2007). High-performance Current-mode CMOS Simultaneous Implementation of Window-literal Operations for Multi-valued Logic. *IET ElectronicsLetters*, *43*(15), 785–786. doi:10.1049/el:20070434

Temel, T., & Morgul, A. (2004). Implementation of Multi-Valued Logic Gates Using Full Current-mode CMOS Circuits. *Kluwer . Analog Integrated Circuits and Signal Processing*, *39*, 191–204. doi:10.1023/B:ALOG.0000024066.66847.89

Temel, T. (2009). Technical Report no: 4, Project no: 107E059 for Turkish Scientific and Technical Research, 2009.

Temel, T., (2008). Technical Report no: 3, Project no: 107E059 for Turkish Scientific and Technical Research, 2008.

Temel, T. (2008). A New, High-performance Current-mode Loser-take-all Minimum Circuit. *IET Electronics Letters*, *44*(12), 718–719. doi:10.1049/el:20081174

Thayse, A., & Deschamps, J. P. (1977). Logic Properties of Unate Discrete and Switching Functions. *IEEE Transactions on Computers*, *C-26*(12), 1020–1212. doi:10.1109/TC.1977.1674781

Thelen, E., & Smith, L. (1994). *A Dynamical Systems Approach to the Development of Cognition and Action.* Cambridge, MA: MIT Press.

Theogarajan, L., Wyatt, J., Rizzo, J., Drohan, B., Markova, M., Kelly, S., et al. (2004). *Low power neural stimulator for a retinal prosthesis*. Paper presented at the Annual Meeting of the Association for Research in Vision and Ophthalmology.

Thorndike, E. L. (1911). *Animal intelligence. New York: Macmillan. Watson, J. B. (1958). Behaviorism*. Chicago: University of Chicago Press.

Thorpe, S., Delorme, A., & Van Rullen, R. (2001). Spike-based strategies for rapid processing. *Neural Networks*, *14*, 715–725. doi:10.1016/S0893-6080(01)00083-1

TMS320C54x BGA Mechanical Data (Document MP-BG021C). (2002). Texas Instruments Incorporated.

TMS320C55x Technical Overview (Literature Number SPRU393). (2000). Texas Instruments Incorporated.

Tolman, E. C. (1948). Cognitive maps in rats and men. *Psychological Review, 55,* 189-208. Watson, J. B., & Rayner, R. (1920). Conditioned emotional reactions. *Journal of Experimental Psychology*, *3*, 1–14.

Toumazou, C., Ligey, F. J., & Haigh, D. G. (1990). *Analogue IC Design: The Current-mode Approach*. Herts, UK: Peregrinus Cop.

Toumazou, C., Lidgey, F. J., & Haigh, D. G. (1990). *Analogue IC Design: The Current-Mode Approach*. London: Peregrinus.

Tsai, S., Hong, P., & Chieu, B. (1992). Handwritten Digit Recognition via OCON Neural Network by Selective Pruning. *Proceedings of the IEEE 11th International Conference on Pattern Recognition,* 656–659.

Tsukamoto, Y. (1979). An approach to fuzzy reasoning method . In Gupta, M. M., Ragade, R. K., & Yager, R. R. (Eds.), *Advances in Fuzzy Set Theory and Applications* (pp. 137–149). Amsterdam: North-Holland.

Tuffy, F., McDaid, L. J., Kwan, V. W., Alderman, J., McGinnity, T. M., & Santos, J. A. (2007). Inter-Neuron Communications Strategies for Spiking Neural Networks . *Neurocomputing*, *71*(1–3), 30–44. doi:10.1016/j.neucom.2006.11.027

Valkenburg, V. (1965). *Introduction to Modern Network Synthesis*. New York: John Wiley and Sons.

Vallortigara G, Regolin L., Tommasi L., Zucca P., (2000). *Altro che cervello di gallina*, Le Scienze n.387

van der Horn, G., & Huijsing, J. L. (1998). *Integrated Smart Sensors, Design and Calibration*. Dordretch, The Netherlands: Kluwer Academic Publishers.

van der Velde, F., & de Kamps, M. (2008). The role of recurrent networks in neural architectures of grounded cognition: learning of control. In L. D. Raedt, B. Hammer, P. Hitzler, W. Maass (Eds.) *Recurrent Neural Networks-Models, Capacities, and Applications. Dagstuhl Seminar Proceedings 08041* (pp. 237-288). http://drops.dagstuhl.de/opus/ volltexte/2008/1421.

Varela, F. J., Thompson, E., & Rosch, E. (1991). *The Embodied Mind: Cognitive Science and Human Experience*. Cambridge, MA: MIT Press.

Varkevisser, B., Peterson, D., Ogura, T., & Kinnamon, S. C. (2001). Neural networks distinguish between taste qualities based on receptor cell population responses. *Chemical Senses*, *26*, 499–505. doi:10.1093/chemse/26.5.499

Vastenhouw, B., & Bisseling, R. H. (2005). A Two-Dimensional Data Distribution Method for Parallel Sparse Matrix-Vector Multiplication. *SIAM Review*, *47*(1), 67. .doi:10.1137/S0036144502409019

Vazquez, F., Garzon, E. M., Martinez, J. A., & Fernandez, J. J. (2009). The sparse matrix vector product on GPUs.

Velliste, M., Perel, S., Spalding, M. C., Whitford, A. S., & Schwartz, A. B. (2008). Cortical control of a prosthetic arm for self-feeding. *Nature*, *453*(7198), 1098–1101. doi:10.1038/nature06996

Verhagen, J. V., & Engelen, L. (2006). The neurocognitive bases of human multimodal food perception: sensory integration. *Neuroscience and Biobehavioral Reviews*, *30*(5), 613–650. doi:10.1016/j.neubiorev.2005.11.003

Verleysen, M. (1992). *Neural Networks and Content-Addressable Memories for Vision: From Theory to VLSI.* PhD Dissertation*:* UCL.

Verret, R. (2003). *TMS320VC5510 Power Consumption Summary (Application Report)*. Texas Instruments Incorporatedo. Document Number.

Vida, V. F. (1996). *Design of Mixed-Signal CMOS Neuro-Fuzzy Controllers*. (PhD Dissertation).

von Neumann, J. (1958). *The Computer and the Brain*. New Haven: Yale University Press.

Vuduc, R., Demmel, J. W., & Yelick, K. A. (2005). A library of automatically tuned sparse matrix kernels . In *Institute of Physics Publishing*. OSKI.

Vuduc, R., Demmel, J. W., Yelick, K. A., Kamil, S., Nishtala, R., Lee, B., et al. (2002). Performance optimizations and bounds for sparse matrix-vector multiply. In *Supercomputing '02: Proceedings of the 2002 ACM/IEEE conference on Supercomputing* (pp. 1--35). {Baltimore, Maryland: IEEE Computer Society Press. Retrieved from http://portal.acm.org/citation.cfm?doid=762761.762822#.

Wachowiak, M., Cohen, L. B., Zochowski, M., & Falk, C. X. (2000). The Spatial Representation of Odors by Olfactory Receptor Neuron Input to the Olfactory Bulb is Concentration Invariant. *The Biological Bulletin, 199*(2), 162–163. doi:10.2307/1542876

Waldemark, J., Millberg, M., Lindblad, T., Waldemark, K., & Becanovic, V. (2000). Implementation of a pulse coupled neural network in FPGA. International Journal of Neural Systems. *Special Issue on Hardware Implementations, 10*(3), 171–177.

Wang, H., Hu, Z., & Zhao, Y. (2007). An Efficient Algorithm for Generalized Discriminant Analysis Using Incomplete Cholesky Decomposition. *Pattern Recognition Letters, 28*, 254–259. doi:10.1016/j.patrec.2006.07.008

Wang, W. J. (1997). New similarity measures on fuzzy sets and on elements. *Fuzzy Sets and Systems, 85*, 305–309. doi:10.1016/0165-0114(95)00365-7

Wang, F., & Zhang, Q. J. (1997). Knowledge based neural models for microwave design. *IEEE Transactions on Microwave Theory and Techniques, 45*(12), 2333–2343. doi:10.1109/22.643839

Wang, J. S., & Lee, C. S. G. (2001). Efficient neuro-fuzzy control systems for autonomous underwater vehicle control. *Proc. of 2001 IEEE Int'l Conf. on Robotics and Automation*, 2986-2991.

Wang, L. X. (1992). Fuzzy systems are universal approximators. In *Proc. Int. Conf. Fuzzy Syst.*, 1163-1170, 1992.

Ward, T. B., Patterson, M. J., & Sifonis, C. M. (2004). The role of specificity and abstraction in creative idea generation. *Creativity Research Journal, 16*, 1–9. doi:10.1207/s15326934crj1601_1

Warland, D., Reinagel, P., & Meister, M. (1997). Decoding visual information from a population of retinal ganglion cells. *Journal of Neurophysiology, 78*(5), 2336–2350.

Watson, P. M., & Gupta, K. C. (1996). EM-ANN models for microstrip vias and interconnects in datasets circuits. *IEEE Transactions on Microwave Theory and Techniques, 44*(12), 2495–2503. doi:10.1109/22.554584

Watson, P. M., Gupta, K. C., & Mahajan, R. L. (1998). *Development of knowledge based artificial neural networks models for microwave components*. Paper presented at the IEEE MTT-S International Microwave Symposium, Baltimore.

Wattanapanitch, W., Fee, M., & Sarpeshkar, R. (2007). An Energy-Efficient Micropower Neural Recording Amplifier. *IEEE Transactions on Biomedical Circuits and Systems, 1*(2), 136–147. doi:10.1109/TBCAS.2007.907868

Wehr, M., & Laurent, G. (1996). Odour Encoding by Temporal Sequences of Firing in Oscillating Neural Assemblies. *Nature, 384*(6605), 162–166. doi:10.1038/384162a0

Weisberg, R. W. (1995). Prolegomena to theories of insight in problem solving: Definition of terms and a taxonomy of problems . In Sternberg, R. J., & Davidson, J. E. (Eds.), *The nature of insight* (pp. 157–196). Cambridge, MA: MIT Press.

Werbos, P. (2009). Intelligence in the brain: a theory of how it works and how to build it. *Neural Networks, 22*(3), 200–212. doi:10.1016/j.neunet.2009.03.012

Werbos, P. J. (1974). *Beyond Regression: New Tools for Prediction and Analysis in the Behavioral Sciences,* Unpublished Ph.D. dissertation: Harvard University.

Wertheimer, M. (1959). *Productive thinking*. New York: Harper and Row.

Wessberg, J., & Nicolelis, M. A. L. (2004). Optimizing a Linear Algorithm for Real-Time Robotic Control using Chronic Cortical Ensemble Recordings in Monkeys. *Journal of Cognitive Neuroscience*, *16*(6), 1022–1035. doi:10.1162/0898929041502652

Wessberg, J., Stambaugh, C. R., Kralik, J. D., Beck, P. D., Laubach, M., & Chapin, J. K. (2000). Real-time prediction of hand trajectory by ensembles of cortical neurons in primates. *Nature*, *408*, 361–365. doi:10.1038/35042582

Widrow, B. & Hoff, M. E. (1960). Adaptive Switching Circuits. *IRE WESCON Convention Record*. 96-104.

Wiener, N. (1948). *Cybernetics: Or, Control and Communication in the Animal and the Machine*. New York: John Wiley & Sons.

Wilamowski, B., Jaeger, R. C., & Kaynak, O. (1999). Neuro-fuzzy Architecture for CMOS Implementation. *IEEE Transactions on Industrial Electronics*, *46*(6), 1132–1136. doi:10.1109/41.808001

Williams, G. P. (1997). *Chaos Theory Tamed*. London: Taylor and Francis.

Williams, S., Oliker, L., Vuduc, R., Shalf, J., Yelick, K., & Demmel, J. (2009). Optimization of sparse matrix–vector multiplication on emerging multicore platforms. *Parallel Computing*, *35*(3), 178–194. doi:10.1016/j.parco.2008.12.006

Willson, A., & Orchard, H. (1995). Insights into Digital Filters Made as the Sum of Two All-Pass Functions. *IEEE Transactions on Circuits and Systems*, *42*, 129–137. doi:10.1109/81.376877

Wise, K. D., Anderson, D. J., Hetke, J. F., Kipke, D. R., & Najafi, K. (2004). Wireless implantable microsystems: High-density electronic interfaces to the nervous system. *Proceedings of the IEEE*, *92*(1), 76–97. doi:10.1109/JPROC.2003.820544

Wolfrum, P., Wolff, C., Lücke, J., & von der Malsburg, C. (2008). A recurrent dynamic model for correspondence-based face recognition. *Journal of vision*, *8*(7), 34.1-18.

Wu, S., & Er, M. J. (2000). Dynamic fuzzy neural networks-a novel approach to function approximation. *IEEE Transactions on Systems, Man, and Cybernetics. Part B, Cybernetics*, *30*(2), 358–364. doi:10.1109/3477.836384

Wu, S., Er, M. J., & Gao, Y. (2001). A fast approach for automatic generation of fuzzy rules by generalized dynamic fuzzy neural networks. *IEEE Transactions on Fuzzy Systems*, *9*, 578–594. doi:10.1109/91.940970

Wu, W., Black, M. J., Mumford, D., Gao, Y., Bienenstock, E., & Donoghue, J. P. (2004). Modeling and decoding motor cortical activity using a switching Kalman filter. *IEEE Transactions on Bio-Medical Engineering*, *51*(6), 933–942. doi:10.1109/TBME.2004.826666

Wu, W., Gao, Y., Bienenstock, E., Donoghue, J. P., & Black, M. J. (2006). Bayesian population decoding of motor cortical activity using a Kalman filter. *Neural Computation*, *18*(1), 80–118. doi:10.1162/089976606774841585

Wu, W., & Hatsopoulos, N. G. (2008). Real-Time Decoding of Nonstationary Neural Activity in Motor Cortex. *IEEE Transactions on Neural Systems and Rehabilitation Engineering*, *16*(3), 213–222. doi:10.1109/TNSRE.2008.922679

Wu, Q.-X., Bell, D., & Cai, J. (2006). Knowledge representation and learning mechanism based on network of spiking neurons, *IEEE International Conference on Systems, Man, and Cybernetics*, 2796-2801.

Wu, W., Shaikhouni, A., Donoghue, J. P., & Black, M. J. (2004). Closed-loop neural control of cursor motion using a Kalman filter. *Proceedings of the IEEE Engineering in Medicine and Biology Society*, 4126-4129.

Wu, Y., & Nowrouzian, B. (2008). A Novel Technique for the Design and DCGA Optimization of Bilinear-LDI Lattice-Based Digital IF Filters. Proceedings of IEEE International Symposium on Circuits and Systems, (ISCAS), 1184-1187.

Wysoski, S., Benuskova, L., & Kasabov, N. (2008). Adaptive spiking neural networks for audiovisual pattern recognition . In Ishikawa, M. (Eds.), *ICONIP2007, Lecture Notes in Computer Science, Part II, 4985* (pp. 406–415). Berlin, Heidelberg: Springer-Verlag.

Wysoski, S. G., Benuskova, L., & Kasabov, N. (2006). On-line learning with structural adaptation in a network of spiking neurons for visual pattern recognition . In Kollias, S. (Eds.), *ICANN 2006, Lecture Notes in Computer Science, Part I, 4131* (pp. 61–70). Berlin, Heidelberg: Springer-Verlag.

Xilinx Inc. (2007). *Spartan 3 Generation User Guide*. San Jose.

Xilinx Inc. (2008). *Virtex-4 FPGA User Guide*. San Jose.

Xilinx, Inc. (2009). *Foundation Series Software*. Retrieved from http://www.xilinx.com

Yamakawa, T. (1993). A Fuzzy Inference Engine in Nonlinear Analog Mode and Its Application to a Fuzzy Logic Control. *IEEE Transactions on Neural Networks, 4*(3), 496–522. doi:10.1109/72.217192

Yang, T., & Maunsell, J. H. (2004). The effect of perceptual learning on neuronal responses in monkey visual area V4. *The Journal of Neuroscience, 24*, 1617–1626. doi:10.1523/JNEUROSCI.4442-03.2004

Yang, H., & Sarpeshkar, R. (2006). A Bio-inspired Ultra-Energy-Efficient Analog-to-Digital Converter for Biomedical Applications. [Special Issue on Life Sciences and System Applications]. *IEEE Transactions on Circuits and Systems I, 53*(11), 2349–2356. doi:10.1109/TCSI.2006.884463

Yoshimura, H., Kato, N., Sugai, T., Honjo, M., Sato, J., Segami, N., & Onoda, N. (2004). To-and-fro optical voltage signal propagation between the insular gustatory and perietal oral somatosensory areas in rat cortex slices. *Brain Research, 1015*, 114–121. doi:10.1016/j.brainres.2004.04.056

Zadeh, L. A. (1965). Fuzzy sets. *Information and Control, 8*, 338–353. doi:10.1016/S0019-9958(65)90241-X

Zadeh, L. A. (1994). *Soft computing and fuzzy logic*. IEEE Soft.

Zadeh, L. (1973). Outline of a New Approach to the Analysis of Complex Systems and Decision Processes. *IEEE Transactions on Systems, Man, and Cybernetics, 3*(1), 28–44.

Zhak, S., Baker, M., & Sarpeshkar, R. (2003). A Low Power Wide Dynamic Range Envelope Detector. *IEEE Journal of Solid-state Circuits, 38*(10), 1750–1753. doi:10.1109/JSSC.2003.817599

Zhang, Q. J., & Gupta, C. (2000). *Neural networks for RF and microwaves design*. Norwood, MA: Artech House.

Zhao, F.-l., Shen, T., Kaya, N., Lu, S.-G., Cao, Y., & Herness, S. (2005). Expression, physiological action, and coexpression patterns of neuropeptide Y in rat taste-bud cells. *National Academy of Sciences of the United States of America, 102*(31), 11100–11105. doi:10.1073/pnas.0501988102

Zuppicich, A., & Soltic, S. (2008). FPGA implementation of an evolving spiking neural network . In Köppen, M. (Ed.), *ICONIP 2008, Lecture Notes in Computer Science, Part I, 5506* (pp. 1129–1136). Berlin, Heidelberg: Springer-Verlag.

About the Contributors

Turgay Temel, received his PhD in 2002 in the area of hybrid-mode circit design based on multi-valued logic and higher radices. In the field, he just completed a state-funded project which aims at using analog-wise information processing with digital concepts as a microarchitecture. The project was the first in this field in literature to his knowledge. His research interest diversifies, which spans to machine learning, neuroscience, biomedical engineering, sensor networks, biologically-inspired system and circuit design and high-performance circuit design. Recently, he has been focusing on reconfigurable analog systems with the hope that major units of intelligence can be emulated in an evolvable manner. The sensor development for biological information processing and bio-sensor systems have been at the core of his current scope. He has also developed unsupervised learning, i.e. clustering, techniques and currently working on single-step methods for high-performance pattern recognition.

* * *

Syed Bokhari received his BSc, and MSc degrees in electrical engineering from the University of Alberta, Edmonton, Alberta, Canada, in 2007 and 2010, respectively. His thesis topic was the design and discrete optimization of frequency response masking digital filters incorporating IIR interpolation subfilters through the use of diversity controlled genetic algorithms.

Jörg Bornschein studied physics at the Ruhr-University Bochum in Germany where he graduated with a diploma-degree under supervision of Prof. Christoph von der Malsburg. The topic of this thesis was "Efficient simulation of artificial neural networks using FPGAs". As of 2008, Jörg Bornschein is working at the Frankfurt Institute for Advanced Studies (FIAS)/ Goethe University in the context of the Bernstein Network Computational Neuroscience. His main research interest are generative models, large scale machine learning, efficient use of massive parallel computer systems and connectionist systems. He is currently working on his PhD thesis under supervision of Prof. Volker Lindenstruth, head of the Department of High Performance Computer Architecture.

Belén Calvo received the BSc degree in Physics in 1999 and the Ph. D. degree in Electronic Engineering in 2004, both from the University of Zaragoza, Spain. Currently she is Research Staff at the Group of Electronic Design, Aragon Institute for Engineering Research (GDE-I3A) of the University of Zaragoza. Her research interests include analogue and mixed-mode CMOS IC design, on-chip programmable circuits, integrated optical receivers, low-voltage low-power monolithic sensor interfaces and wireless sensors networks.

Santiago Celma was born in Zaragoza, Spain. He received the BSc, MSc, and PhD degrees in Physics from the University of Zaragoza, Zaragoza, Spain, in 1987, 1989, and 1993, respectively. Currently, he is a Full Professor of the Group of Electronic Design (GDE-I3A), Aragon Institute of Engineering Research, University of Zaragoza. He has coauthored more than 60 technical papers and 190 international conference contributions. His research interests include circuit theory, mixed-signal integrated circuits, high-frequency communication circuits, and wireless sensor networks.

Damien Coyle received a first class degree in computing and electronic engineering in 2002 and a doctorate in Intelligent Systems Engineering in 2006 from the University of Ulster where he is now a lecturer at the School of Computing and Intelligent Systems and a member of the Intelligent Systems Research Centre. He is involved in the computational neuroscience research team (CNRT) and brain computer interface (BCI) team. His research interests include biosignal processing, bio-inspired cognitive, adaptive systems and BCI technology. More recently he has been investigating computational models of neural systems and neurodegeneration related to Alzheimer's disease (AD). Dr. Coyle is the 2008 recipient of the IEEE Computational Intelligence Society Outstanding Doctoral Dissertation Award.

Rossana M. S. Cruz received the Technologist in Telecommunications degree from Federal Institute of Education, Science and Technology of Paraiba (IFPB), João Pessoa, in 2003. She received the M.S.E.E. degree from the Federal University of Rio Grande do Norte (UFRN), Natal, RN, Brazil, in 2005, and the doctoral degree from the same university, in 2009. She is currently teaching at the Federal Institute of Education, Science and Technology of Paraíba, João Pessoa, PB, Brazil. Her interest research areas are neural networks, frequency selective surfaces and propagation.

Adaildo Gomes d'Assunção received the B.S.E.E. degree (with honors) from the Federal University of Rio Grande do Norte, RN, Brazil, in 1974, and the M.S. and doctoral degree in electrical engineering from the State University of Campinas, SP, Brazil, in 1977 and 1981, respectively. From 1975-1976, he worked with radar and telemetry systems at the Launching Center of Barreira do Inferno, Natal, RN, Brazil. He has been with the Federal University of Rio Grande do Norte since 1976, where he is a Professor of Electrical and Electronics Engineering. From 1985-1987, he was a Postdoctoral Visiting Scientist in the Department of Electrical and Electronics Engineering at North Dakota State University, Fargo. He is currently teaching and conducting research on antennas, microwave integrated circuits, millimeter waves, and optical communications. Dr. d'Assunção is a member of the Brazilian Microwave and Optoelectronics Society (SBMO), the Microwave Theory and Techniques Society (MTT-S) and of the Antennas and Propagation Society (AP-S).

Rodrigo Martins da Silva received an engineering degree in Electronics. He also holds a MSc degree in Electronics engineering. His interests are architectures for embedded systems in particular and for intelligent systems in general.

Nikola Kasabov is the Director and Founder of the Knowledge Engineering and Discovery Research Institute (KEDRI) (www.kedri.info). He holds a Chair of Knowledge Engineering at the School of Computing and Mathematical Sciences at Auckland University of Technology. He is a Fellow of IEEE, Fellow of the Royal Society of New Zealand, Fellow of the New Zealand Computer Society. He is the current President of the International Neural Network Society (INNS) and a Past-President of the

Asia Pacific Neural Network Assembly (APNNA). Kasabov is Associate Editor of several international journals including Neural Networks, IEEE TrFS, Information Science. His main research is in intelligent information systems, neuroinforamics, bioinformatics, data mining, knowledge engineering. He has more than 400 publications and 28 patents. Kasabov is a Guest Professor at the Shanghai Jiao Tong University. Among the received awards are the RSNZ Science and Technology Medal, the Bayer Science Innovation Award, APNNA Excellent Service Award.

Ziqian Liu is currently an Assistant Professor of Electrical Engineering at State University of New York Maritime College, Throggs Neck, New York, USA. He received the BS and MS degrees from Hefei University of Technology, China, and the PhD degree from Southern Illinois University Carbondale, USA. Between 2005 and 2007, he worked for Ingersoll-Rand Co. Ltd, USA. From 1989 to 1999, he worked for the Department of Electrical Engineering at Hefei University of Technology, China. His research interests include recurrent neural networks, intelligent control systems, nonlinear optimal control, motor control systems, DSP or microprocessor based embedded systems, power electronics and drives, and computational modeling.

Martin McGinnity holds the post of Professor of Intelligent Systems Engineering within the Faculty of Computing and Engineering, University of Ulster. He has a first class honours degree in physics, and a doctorate from the University of Durham, is a Fellow of the IET, senior member of the IEEE, and a Chartered Engineer. He is currently Director of the Intelligent Systems Research Centre, which encompasses the research activities of over 85 researchers. He is also currently a Director of both the University's technology transfer company, UUTech and a spin out company Flex Language Services. He is the author or co-author of over 200 research papers, and has been awarded both a Senior Distinguished Research Fellowship and a Distinguished Learning Support Fellowship by the University in recognition of his contribution to teaching and research. His current research interests are focussed on the creation of bio-inspired intelligent computational systems which explore and model biological signal processing.

Nicolás Medrano received the BSc degree and PhD degree in Physics from the University of Zaragoza, Zaragoza, Spain, in 1989 and 1998, respectively. Currently, he is an Associate Professor of Electronics at the Faculty of Physics, University of Zaragoza, and a member of the Group of Electronic Design (GDE-I3A), Aragon Institute of Engineering Research, University of Zaragoza. His research interests include implementation of neural networks for signal processing, integrated sensor interfaces and smart sensors, wireless sensor networks, and intelligent instrumentation.

Giovanna Morgavi is doctor in Electronic Engineering and in Psychology. Since 1981 she has been working at the Institute of Electronic, Information and Telecommunication Engineer (IEIIT), within the Italian National Research Council (CNR), where she is senior researcher. Her research interests started from physical models of biological cells to arrive to chaotic behaviour analysis and to adaptive intelligent systems. Her today interest is focused on Adaptive Intelligence and Epigenetic Robotics. She is the coordinator of the research team on Cognitive Systems and Robotics at IEIIT. She has been author of more than 120 papers and conferences communications. She and her team have been involved in several European projects. She has been evaluator for many EC IST and Italian Ministery and Regional Scientific Project Proposal calls on cognitive, ICT, robotics and bio-inspired systems.

Luiza de Macedo Mourelle is an associate professor in the Department of System Engineering and Computation at the Faculty of Engineering, State University of Rio de Janeiro, Brazil. Her research interests include computer architecture, embedded systems design, hardware/software co-design and reconfigurable hardware. Mourelle received her Ph. D. in Computation from the University of Manchester - Institute of Science and Technology (UMIST), England, her M.Sc. in System Engineering and Computation from the Federal University of Rio de Janeiro (UFRJ), Brazil and her Engineering degree in Electronics also from UFRJ, Brazil.

Nadia Nedjah is an associate professor in the Department of Electronics Engineering and Telecommunications at the Faculty of Engineering, State University of Rio de Janeiro, Brazil. Her research interests include embedded systems and reconfigurable hardware design as well as cryptography. Nedjah received her PhD in Computation from the University of Manchester - Institute of Science and Technology (UMIST), England, her M.Sc. in System Engineering and Computation from University of Annaba, Algeria and her Engineering degree in Computer Science also from University of Annaba, Algeria.

Behrouz Nowrouzian received his BSc degree in electrical engineering from Arya-Mehr (Sharif) University of Technology, Tehran, Iran, in 1975. He received his M.Sc., D.I.C., and PhD degrees from the Imperial College of Science and Technology, University of London, London, U.K., in 1976, 1977, and 1983, respectively. Currently, he is a Professor at the Department of Electrical and Computer Engineering, University of Alberta, Edmonton, Alberta, Canada. His main research interests include VLSI digital signal processing and evolvable hardware, computer arithmetic and architecture, high-level synthesis, and application of optimization to circuits and systems.

Girijesh Prasad received the B.Tech. degree in electrical engineering from Regional Engineering College, India, in 1987, the M.Tech. degree in computer science and technology from the University of Roorkee, India, in 1992, and the PhD degree from the Queen's University, Belfast, UK in 1997. He has been a member of academic staff at the University of Ulster, Magee Campus, Londonderry, UK since 1999 and holds the post of Reader. He is an executive member of the Intelligent Systems Research Centre at the Magee Campus where he leads the Brain-Computer Interface and Assistive Technology team. His research interests are in self-organising hybrid intelligent systems, neural computation, type-1 and type-2 fuzzy logic, evolutionary algorithms, adaptive predictive modeling and control with applications in complex industrial and biological systems including brain-computer interface (BCI) and assistive robotic systems. He has published over 90 peer reviewed academic papers in international journals, books, and conference proceedings. Dr. Prasad is a Chartered Engineer, a Member of the IET and a Senior Member of IEEE.

Benjamin I. Rapoport received the BA degree in physics and mathematics and the MA degree in physics from Harvard University in 2003, the MSc degree in mathematics from Oxford University in 2004, and the MS degree in physics from the Massachusetts Institute of Technology (MIT) in 2007. He is currently a student in the MD–PhD Program at Harvard Medical School and is jointly pursuing the MD at Harvard Medical School and the PhD in electrical engineering at MIT. His research and professional interests include bioimplantable electronic interfaces with the brain and nervous system, biological and computational neuroscience, and clinical neurosurgery.

María Teresa Sanz received the PhD degree in Electronic Engineering from the University of Zaragoza, Zaragoza, Spain, in 2004 and was a member of the Group of Electronic Design, University of Zaragoza, until 2008. She is currently a Full Researcher at the Electronics Department, National Institute for Astrophysics, Optics and Electronics (INAOE), Mexico. Her research interests include analog and mixed IC design, integrated optical receivers and integrated sensor interfaces.

Rahul Sarpeshkar received the Bachelor's degrees in electrical engineering and physics from the Massachusetts Institute of Technology (MIT), and the Ph.D. degree from the California Institute of Technology (Caltech). After completing the Ph.D. degree at Caltech, he joined Bell Labs as a member of the technical staff. Since 1999, he has been on the faculty of MIT's Electrical Engineering and Computer Science Department where he heads a research group on Analog VLSI and biological Systems, and is currently an Associate Professor. His research interests include analog microelectronics, ultra-low power circuits and systems, biologically inspired circuits and systems, biomedical systems, feedback systems, neuroscience, and molecular biology. Dr. Sarpeshkar has received several awards, including the Packard Fellow award given to outstanding faculty, the ONR Young Investigator Award, the National Science Foundation Career Award, the Indus Technovator Award, and the junior Bose award for excellence in teaching. He holds more than 25 patents and has authored many publications, including one that was featured on the cover of *Nature*.

Paulo Henrique da Fonseca Silva received the B.S.E.E. and the M.S.E.E. degree from the Federal University of Rio Grande do Norte, RN, Brazil, in 1996 and 1998, respectively, and the doctoral degree in electrical engineering from the Federal University of Campina Grande, PB, Brazil, in 2000. He is currently teaching at the Federal Institute of Education, Science and Technology of Paraíba, João Pessoa, PB, Brazil. His interest research areas are artificial neural networks, natural optimization algorithms, RF/microwave devices and circuits, antennas, and propagation. Dr. Silva is a member of the Brazilian Microwave and Optoelectronics Society (SBMO).

Snjezana Soltic received the BE and MSc degrees in electrical engineering from University of Zagreb, Croatia, and the PhD degree in Computing and Mathematical Sciences from Auckland University of Technology, New Zealand. Currently, she is a senior lecturer in the School of Electrical Engineering at Manukau Institute of Technology, Auckland, New Zealand. Her research interests are in the areas of neuro-computing, data mining, knowledge discovery, colour management in imaging systems and optimization of light source spectra.

Frank van der Velde is a cognitive scientist at Leiden University (The Netherlands). His research concerns the understanding of the neural basis of higher levels of (human) cognition, in particular cognitive processes which are combinatorial and productive. The research topics include visual attention, working memory, language, reasoning and learning. The focus is to develop neural architectures of grounded cognition that produce and process complex cognitive structures in language, reasoning and vision. In 2006, he published a target paper in Behavioral and Brain Sciences (with Dr. M. De Kamps) on the way neural blackboard architectures, based on grounded neural assemblies, can code for complex cognitive structures in language and vision. The aim of his current research is to enlarge these neural blackboard architectures into an overall neural and grounded architecture of human-like) cognition, fit for fully parallel implementation.

Guillermo Zatorre received the BSc degree in Physics and the Ph. D. degree in Electronic Engineering from the University of Zaragoza, Zaragoza, Spain, in 2001 and 2010, respectively. Currently, he is working at the Microelectronic Design Department at INCIDE S.A. His research interests include auto-tuning techniques for integrated continuous time filters, basic blocks for neural network integration, and neural networks application for smart sensors.

Index

D

E

F

G

N

O

P

R

S

T

U

V

W

Z

Breinigsville, PA USA
07 December 2010
250864BV00006B/85-140/P

9 781609 600181